FIRST EDITION

DISCOVER RADIOLOGY:
CHEST X-RAY INTERPRETATION

Julian Dobranowski, MD, FRCPC
Director, Center for Radiological Anatomy (CORA)
Associate Professor, Faculty of Health Sciences
McMaster University, Hamilton, Ontario

Alexander J Dobranowski, MBBS

Anthony J Levinson, MD, FRCPC, MSc, MA
Director, Division of e-Learning Innovation and machealth.ca
John Evans Chair in Educational Research & Instructional Development
Associate Professor, Faculty of Health Sciences
McMaster University, Hamilton, Ontario

Foreword by:

Deborah Cook, MD, FRCPC, MSc(Epi), FRS
Professor of Medicine, Clinical Epidemiology & Biostatistics
McMaster University, Hamilton, Canada

J2D Publishing Inc.

DISCOVERY RADIOLOGY: CHEST X-RAY INTERPRETATION, First Edition

Julian Dobranowski, Alexander J Dobranowski and Anthony J Levinson

With 784 figures in 1581 separate illustrations, 147 in color, 41 tables, and 53 job aides.
© 2014, J2D Publishing Inc.

Library and Archives Canada Cataloguing in Publication

Dobranowski, Julian, 1955-, author
    Discover radiology : chest X-ray interpretation / Julian Dobranowski, Alexander J Dobranowski, Anthony J Levinson. -- First edition.

Includes bibliographical references and index.
ISBN 978-0-9918753-0-6 (pbk.)

    1. Chest--Radiography--Textbooks. I. Dobranowski, Alexander J. 1984-, author II. Levinson, Anthony J. 1969-, author III. Title.

RC941.D63 2013   617.5'407572   C2013-904441-8

ISBN 978-0-9918753-0-6
e-ISBN 978-0-9918753-1-3
First Edition
14 13 12 11 10 / 10 9 8 7 6 5 4 3 2 1

Printed in China

© 2014, J2D Publishing Inc.
J2D Publishing Inc.
Suite 196
1063 King St. West
Hamilton, Ontario CANADA L8S 4S3

To purchase additional copies of this book:
Visit J2D Publishing Inc. on the internet: at www.j2dpublishing.com

DISCOVERY RADIOLOGY: CHEST X-RAY INTERPRETATION, First Edition
Julian Dobranowski, Alexander J Dobranowski and Anthony J Levinson

© 2014, J2D Publishing Inc.

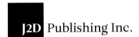 Publishing Inc.

J2D Publishing Inc.
Suite 196
1063 King St. West
Hamilton, Ontario CANADA L8S 4S3

Creative Director & Production Editor:
Shelley Jacobs, PhD
Biomedical Illuminations,
www.biomedicalilluminations.com

Cover design:	Shelley Jacobs
Cover illustration:	Edward Mallon, BSc
Inner folio illustration:	Edward Mallon
Layout:	Shelley Jacobs
Contributing designers:	Carla Pareja
	Hilary Rathbone
Lead illustrator:	Edward Mallon
Contributing illustrators:	Sama Anvari
	Shelley Jacobs
	Chandan Vatish

As this is a first edition and a novel approach we look forward to any feedback from our readers. We plan to develop additional instructional materials to accompany the book, including web-based e-learning modules and practice exercises, as well as digital versions of our performance support materials. You can learn more about these and subscribe to updates on our website:

www.j2dpublishing.com.

TABLE OF CONTENTS

Section I. Getting Started

Section II. Radiological Anatomy and Pathology

Section III. Putting it Together

LIST OF JOB AIDES

Checklists

How To's

Visual Search Aides

LIST OF ABBREVIATIONS

A – Anterior
ACR – American College of Radiologists
ALARA – As Low As Reasonably Achievable
ALARP – As Low As Reasonably Possible
AMSER – Alliance for Medical Student Educators in Radiology
AP* – Anterior Posterior
AP* – Aortopulmonary
ARDS – Acute Respiratory Distress Syndrome
AV – Aortic Valve
AV – Atrioventricular (pacemaker)
C5, C6 – Cervical vertebrae 5,6
CAD – Computer Assisted Diagnosis
CAR – Canadian Association of Radiologists
CHF – Congestive Heart Failure
cm – centimeters
COPD – Chronic Obstructive Pulmonary Disease
CR – Computed Radiology
CT – Computed Tomography
CTA – Computed Tomography Angiogram
CTPA – Computed Tomography Pulmonary Angiogram
CVC – Central Venous Catheter
CVP – Central Venous Pressure
CXR – Chest X-ray
DDx – Differential Diagnosis
DIP – Desquamative Interstitial Pneumonia
DR – Digital or Direct Radiology
ECG – Electrocardiogram
ED – Emergency Department
EHz – Exahertz
EKG – Electrocardiogram
ER – Emergency Room
ETT – Endotracheal Tube
EXP – Intentional Expiration
GI – Gastrointestinal
Gy – Gray
HRCT – High Resolution Computed Tomography
ICU – Intensive Care Unit
INS – Intentional Inspiration
IPF – Idiopathic Pulmonary Fibrosis
IVC – Inferior Vena Cava
km – kilometers
KUB – Kidney Ureter Bladder
kVp – peak kilovoltage
L – Left (patient's left side)
L1, L2, L3 – Lumbar vertebrae 1,2,3
LA – Left Atrium
LIP – Leukocytic Interstitial Pneumonia
LPA – Left Pulmonary Artery
LLL – Left Lower Lobe
LUL – Left Upper Lobe
LV – Left Ventricle
ml – milliliters
mm – millimeters
MPA – Main Pulmonary Artery
MRI – Magnetic Resonance Imaging
mSV – millisievert
MV – Mitral Valve

NG – Nasogastric (tube)
OSCE – Objective Structured Clinical Examination
P – Posterior
PA – Posterior Anterior
PACS – Picture Archiving and Communication System
PET – Positron Emission Tomography
PHz – Pica Hertz
PV – Pulmonary Valve
R* – Right (patient's right side)
R* – Roentgen
RA – Right Atrium
rad – Radiation Absorbed Dose
RAE – Radiation Absorption Event
RANZCR – Royal Australian and New Zealand College of Radiologists
RCR – Royal College of Radiologists
rem – Roentgen equivalent man
RPA – Right Pulmonary Artery
RML – Right Middle Lobe
RLL – Right Lower Lobe
RUL – Right Upper Lobe
RV – Right Ventricle
SPN – Solitary Pulmonary Nodule
STP – Standard Temperature & Pressure
Sv – Sievert
SVC – Superior Vena Cava
T4 – Thoracic vertebra (4th)
TV – Tricuspid Valve
US – Ultrasound
VQ – Ventilation-Perfusion
WR – radiation weighting factor
2D – two dimensional
3D – three dimensional

* both are used in clinical practice.

FORWARD

Learning how to interpret a radiograph is among the most important skills to master in caring for patients. The textbook, "DISCOVERY RADIOLOGY: CHEST X-RAY INTERPRETATION" is the newest and most inviting text available to ensure the realization of this goal. Written by a multidisciplinary group of authors, their collective skills and wisdom has created a special resource that will provide a solid foundation for the beginner, refine the skills of the seasoned clinician, and serve as a crucial resource for clinical teachers.

In a world characterized by information overload, this textbook acknowledges the importance of bite-size pieces of information to aid digestion. Each section on a page has clear messages, delivered by different vehicles. Words are presented using manageable text length, and key points are presented in bullet format or call-out boxes. Tables have adaptive lay-outs to aid the learner, such as compare and contrast functions, or relational messages to facilitate reasoned memory. Visual images are thoughtfully selected - either radiographs themselves, photographs or schematics. Classical arrows and sketched overlays are used to underscore key findings. Together, the variety of formats used is refreshing and inviting.

The examples are numerous, detailed, and enliven the book immensely. Many learning strategies and take-home points are underscored in this book, such as encouraging laser-sharp focus, the value of repetition, and the need to distinguish observation from inference. Consultancy skills are highlighted such as collaboration with radiologists in the care of patients, and thoughtful interpretation of radiographic reports.

"DISCOVERY RADIOLOGY: CHEST X-RAY INTERPRETATION" is patient-centered, problem-oriented, and vividly visual. This book will accelerate mastery of the chest radiograph, refine differential diagnoses, improve diagnostic accuracy, and hasten appropriate further tests or treatments. Thus, this text has the potential to improve patient care. It is 'a must-read', and with anticipation, I look forward to others in this series.

Deborah Cook, MD, FRCPC, MSc(Epi), FRS
Professor of Medicine, Clinical Epidemiology & Biostatistics
McMaster University, Hamilton, Canada

ACKNOWLEDGEMENTS

The authors would like to thank the many McMaster University medical students, residents and fellows who over the years questioned and sought answers. The idea for this book developed from this quest for knowledge, and our goals to enhance their education and training.

We would like to thank the many learners that spent time at the Center for Radiological Anatomy educational venue at St. Joseph's Healthcare, Hamilton. Many of the pedagogical approaches used in this book have been refined thanks to your feedback.

We thank the many visiting students from various countries for your insight.

The creation of a textbook of this magnitude is the result of the dedication of the authors, their families and the entire project team.

Special thanks to our project team especially our project coordinator Shelley Jacobs. The project would not have been possible without her excellent project management and editorial skills. We owe our gratitude to her artistic contribution in the form of her excellent detailed color illustrations and to her creativity in designing the striking book cover.

Also special thanks to our lead illustrator Edward Mallon. Edward used his science background to help shape the valuable pedagogic structure of this book through his excellent art work.

Last but not least we wish to thank our families for their support and patience during the past 4 long years.

"There is no more difficult art to acquire than the art of observation, and for some men it is quite as difficult to record the observation in brief and plain language."

Sir William Osler, Aphorisms From Bedside Teachings and Writings (1)

INTRODUCTION

Medical Imaging is an exciting, constantly evolving field. The tools of radiology are special because they represent an extension of our senses. Imaging extends the limits of our touch and sight, allowing us to look inside the body. No wonder medical imaging was chosen by the editors of the New England Journal of Medicine (NEJM) as one of the eleven most significant developments in medicine in the last 1000 years (2).

Radiology has evolved momentously over the last 100 years. From an early start with exciting but limited applications, radiology now plays an important role at almost every level of patient care from antenatal to end of life. As the costs of health care escalate, the understanding of radiology – particularly the appropriate ordering of radiological examinations – becomes increasingly more vital. The current focus in healthcare on patient safety has made radiation exposure awareness among healthcare providers an important quality priority.

Despite the increasing utilization of radiology, very little progress has been made in integrating radiology into the medical school curriculum. Medical students are expected to interpret radiological examinations without formal teaching and understanding of this technology (3). There may be little or no formal instruction in radiology in the pre-clerkship portion of medical school, as it seldom fits in with the traditional structure of curricula focused on organ systems or the more established clinical disciplines.

Radiological learning is usually dependent upon student radiology elective programs. Some radiology electives are well organized but many are informal, ad hoc experiences. We know that medical students do not fare well when it comes to chest x-ray interpretation (4). Anxiety, discomfort, apprehension or confusion may be some of the emotions felt by a learner when asked to interpret a chest x-ray for the very first time. Expectations are high and exceed reality. The reason for these emotions stems from a lack of basic information and confidence in understanding of the technology. Pressure is placed on the student to accurately interpret a chest x-ray without the underlying knowledge foundation.

> ! Learn not to look at a chest x-ray but to study the image and to unravel the secrets it contains.

The goals of undergraduate medical training need to shift from acquiring knowledge and cramming for examinations, to building procedural and strategic skills necessary for proper understanding and competency in x-ray interpretation.

The interpretive process need not stir up negative emotions. With the proper grounding in knowledge, procedures and principles, chest x-ray interpretation can be rewarding to the learner and more importantly can lead to extraction of accurate information leading to better patient care and improved patient outcomes. With the appropriate skills, training and tools, inappropriate examinations will be reduced leading to decreased patient radiation exposure and decreased overall healthcare costs.

Learning to interpret the chest x-ray can be compared to learning to drive a car. First the basics, then guided learning, then – on the road. The new roadmap for chest x-ray interpretation should include an understanding of the technology. It should include how the images are created and a thorough understanding of the issues related to radiation exposure and patient safety. The conceptual appreciation of the technologies is important because they are changing and evolving. The new roadmap should also guide the learner to an understanding of conventional anatomy and how this anatomy looks from a grayscale x-ray image perspective; and a consideration of how the x-ray grayscale changes in various pathological conditions. The roadmap should help familiarize the learner with the terms used to describe radiological findings, and the skills to summarize the radiological findings and how to formulate a differential diagnosis based on this summary.

The objective of this book is to provide this new roadmap. It is to focus on the needs of the learners and to address the aforementioned teaching issues - to provide the learner the building blocks necessary for successful chest x-ray interpretation.

Learning to interpret x-ray images is an intellectual journey.
A journey to understand the truths the x-ray is trying to show us and the truths the x-ray is hiding.

During the journey through the book you will review and understand:
- the radiological anatomy of the chest.
- the importance of the lateral chest x-ray.
- concepts of radiological pathology.
- the importance of the differential diagnosis.
- appropriate ordering of radiological examinations.

"DISCOVERY RADIOLOGY: CHEST X-RAY INTERPRETATION" is divided into 3 sections.

The first section provides a description of the technology, the patient journey, how the x-ray image is created, and the elements needed for interpretation.

The second section analyses how normal anatomical structures appear on an x-ray and how pathology modifies that appearance.

The third section then concentrates on the interpretive process and specific problems related to chest imaging.

Throughout the book, we incorporate evidence-based techniques to enhance learning and skill development. We use best practices in designing graphics for learning when creating the instructional images. The sections of the book are deliberately segmented and sequenced to facilitate transfer of concepts and skills. Each chapter has a structured introduction as an advanced cognitive organizer to help situate the material, as well as a case-based example to activate prior knowledge, provide authentic context, and reinforce the material. To improve application of the knowledge in the clinical setting, the book is filled with valuable checklists and job aides that provide performance support tools.

AMSER "DISCOVERY RADIOLOGY: CHEST X-RAY INTERPRETATION" brings together several hallmarks of modern medical education: problem-based, evidence-based, and conceptually-based; and now with the additional innovation of performance support to improve the transfer of competencies to the clinical setting.

The Alliance of Medical Student Educators in Radiology (AMSER) has published a comprehensive curriculum in radiology for medical students (5,6). This is the most comprehensive curriculum outline that we have identified. The key elements from this curriculum are identified and highlighted in this book (as indicated in the margin) allowing the student to fulfil the AMSER curriculum mandates while following the text.

"DISCOVERY RADIOLOGY: CHEST X-RAY INTERPRETATION" is the first in a series of radiology textbooks concentrating on the teaching of x-ray interpretation through a focus on anatomy, radiological anatomy, concepts of pathology, differential diagnosis and important concepts and competencies. Use this book to systematically develop foundational skills in chest x-ray interpretation, as well as a reference tool with job aides to continue to improve your knowledge and skills in the clinical setting. This book is your 'one-stop-shop' to learn, master, and achieve chest x-ray interpretative success.

WHAT MAKES THIS BOOK DIFFERENT?

Conceptual approach to x-ray and grayscale interpretation

Evidence-informed content and instructional design

Mapped to specific competencies

Performance support tools, including over 50 job aides

Learner-centered, written with student input

References

1. Bean, R.B. (1961). *Osler, (Sir) William. Aphorisms from his bedside teachings and writings.* (1874–1944), 2nd ed. Bean, W.B., (Ed.). Springfield, IL,: Charles C Thomas.

2. The Editors. (2000). Looking back on the millennium in medicine. *New. Engl. J. Med., 342*:42–49.

3. Collins, J., Dottl, S.L., & Albanese, M.A. (2002). Teaching radiology to medical students: An integrated approach. *Acad. Radiol., 9*(9) 1046–1053.

4. Jeffrey, D.R., Goddard, P.R., Callaway, M.P., & Greenwood, R. (2003). Chest radiograph interpretation by medical students. *Clin. Radiol., 58*(6):478–814.

5. Lewis, P.J., Shaffer, K., & Donovan, A. (Eds.). (2012). AMSER National Medical Student Curriculum in Radiology. http://aur.org/Secondary-Alliances.aspx?id=141.

6. Lewis, P.J., & Shaffer, K. (2005). Developing a national medical student curriculum in radiology. *Am. Coll. Radiol. 2*(1):8–11.

HOW TO USE THIS BOOK

This book is written to allow maximum flexibility during the learning experience. It is recommended that first time around the learner experiences the book systematically from beginning to end. This is because each chapter builds on the previous and each section enhances the next. The chapters form building blocks each playing an important role in the understanding of the interpretive process.

The breakdown of the Sections in the book is as follows:

SECTION I	What is a chest x-ray? What is the chest x-ray image? What is the interpretive process?

SECTION II	Radiological anatomy How does pathology show on an x-ray?

SECTION III	Applying the interpretive process

Following the initial review of the entire book you can:

- Review individual chapters as needed found through the regular table of contents.
- Review the job aides listed in the "job aides" special table of contents.

We highly recommend using the job aides and checklists for reviewing practice cases, on electives, and in the clinical setting. Eventually, the procedural knowledge and principles will become automatic with consistent, structured practice and feedback from your preceptors.

How to Make the Best Use of this Book

AMSER In addition to the AMSER icons mentioned previously, there are various coloured call-outs throughout the chapters that indicate specific types of information.

Normal **variants** and **author recommendations** are highlighted within the text.

How To

Step by step guides, with annotated x-rays, to illustrate key skills needed to confidently interpret chest x-rays.

Visual Search

Numbered visual guides to illustrate the sequential checks that should be performed in a visual search of a given anatomical structure or radiological zone on a chest x-ray.

Radiological Checklist

Illustrated lists of items that should be evaluated for a given anatomical structure or radiological zone, in the process of interpreting a chest x-ray.

Additional Information

Information that the authors deem relevant for a deeper understanding of the content, but that is not critical for your understanding of chest x-ray interpretation.

Frequency Of Visualization

Statistics of the frequency that important structures can be identified on x-rays.

Important Point

Information that the authors deem to be extremely important to note about chest x-ray interpretation.

Radiological Anatomy

Descriptions of various anatomical structures as they would appear on PA and lateral chest x-rays. This infomation is further highlighted by its presentation on black pages.

SECTION I

GETTING STARTED

Section I of this book provides an overview of how x-rays are used to produce an image of the chest.

The section is divided into 5 chapters that examine the building blocks necessary for chest x-ray interpretation. The chapters review x-ray image production and the general concepts related to image appearance. With this background information you will then be introduced to the key components of the interpretation process.

This section will provide you with the essentials needed to comprehend the radiological anatomy presented in section two and the more detailed aspects of the interpretive process reviewed in section three.

CHAPTER 1
The X-RAY EXAMINATION

importance

There are very few innovations in this past century that have developed at the immense pace as that of diagnostic imaging. From the first x-ray examination in 1895, by William Roentgen (Fig. 1a), the technology has significantly evolved to the digital format used today (Fig. 1b).

The x-ray examination creates a unique perspective of the human body. The 3D information is gone. All colour is gone. To be able to extract clinical information from this perspective requires a clear understanding of the technology and how the image is formed. In this chapter, you will learn about what an x-ray is, how it is formed, and how it is used to create an image for medical use.

You need to understand the x-ray examination before you can start thinking about the interpretation of chest x-ray images. In this chapter, you will gain an understanding of the different x-ray views that are used when imaging the chest, and their applications. You will learn about the technical factors of the examination that affect the x-ray image quality and what defines a good chest x-ray image.

Other radiological modalities, such as Computed Tomography (CT), Magnetic Resonance Imaging (MRI), and Ultrasound (US), are used to image the chest. This chapter includes a brief overview of all of these modalities. Additionally, the basics of radiation and radiation exposure from x-rays are included in this chapter.

objectives

Skills

You will identify

- the different types of chest x-ray examinations.
- the different types of radiological imaging modalities.

Knowledge

You will review and understand

- what an x-ray is, how it is formed, and how it is stored.
- how a chest x-ray examination is performed.
- how to distinguish between a good and a poor quality examination.
- the patient's experience through an x-ray examination.
- radiation units, doses, and the issues involved with a chest x-ray examination.

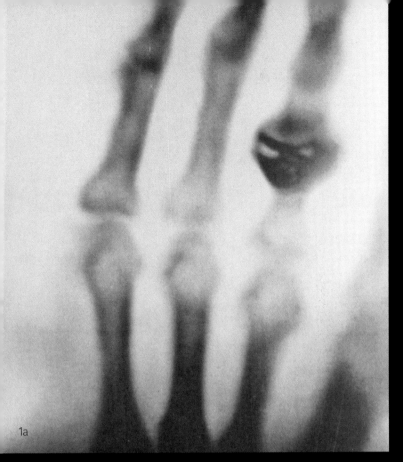

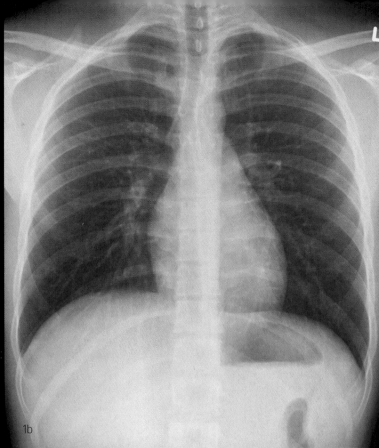

Figure 1. Evolution of the x-ray image. a, first x-ray taken by Roentgen in 1895 of his wife's hand, b, example of a modern digital chest x-ray. Courtesy of the National Library of Medicine.

associated resources

This chapter maps to the following AMSER curriculum content (1,2).

1) Techniques used to image this anatomical/physiological area.
Chest x-ray (CXR): Posterior-Anterior (PA), Anterior-Posterior (AP), lateral, decubitus, lordotic, expiratory, supine.

2) Limitations of modalities.
Patient cooperation
Language barriers

3) CXR equivalents of common examinations.
Chest CT

4) Radiation safety and risks.

5) Methods to reduce radiation exposure.
Reduction in unnecessary examinations (e.g., ICU x-rays)
Use of US and MRI

6) Imaging in pregnancy.

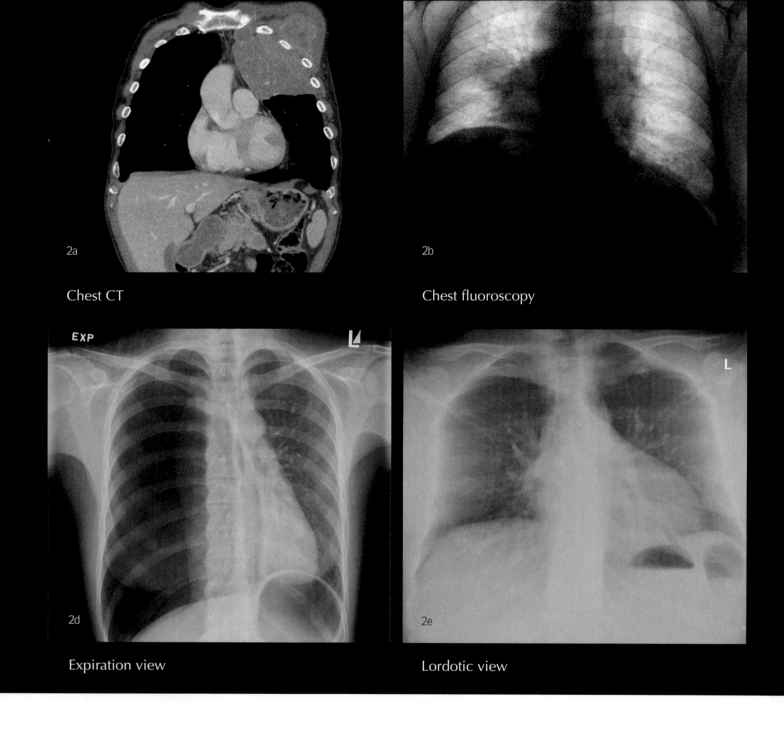

2a
Chest CT

2b
Chest fluoroscopy

2d
Expiration view

2e
Lordotic view

You are taking an OSCE examination and, at one station, you are asked to match the clinical situation with the appropriate imaging test (Fig. 2a,b,c,d,e,f).

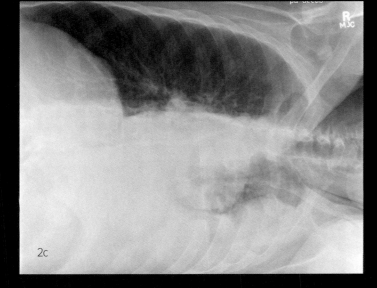

2c

Decubitus view

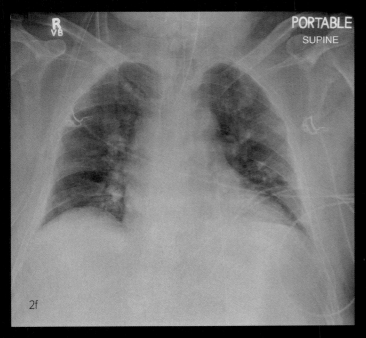

2f

Portable supine AP x-ray

The clinical scenarios are the following:

Differentiating pleural effusion
from pleural thickening

Suspected pneumothorax

Unconscious, unstable, intubated patient

Suspected paralysis of diaphragm

Staging of lung cancer

Apical lung disease

Can you match the clinical scenario above
with the appropriate imaging test?

WHAT ARE X-RAYS?

X-rays are a form of invisible, high-frequency, electromagnetic radiation, similar to light or radio waves. X-rays travel at the speed of light as discrete bundles of energy called photons. The wavelength of x-rays is between 10 and 0.01 nanometers, corresponding to a frequency of 30 petahertz (PHz) to 30 exahertz (EHz). The high frequency of x-rays makes them more energetic than light, giving x-rays the ability to penetrate the body.

HOW ARE X-RAYS FORMED?

Whenever electrons of high energy strike a heavy metal target, such as tungsten or copper, x-rays are produced by two distinct processes: characteristic and bremsstrahlung x-ray production (3).

When the high-energy electron beam strikes heavy metal, some of the electrons collide with electrons of the heavy metal atoms, causing the ejection of an electron from its native orbit (an inner valence shell). When this happens, a second electron will transition from a higher energy orbit (an outer shell) to fill the vacancy. The excess energy created in the movement from a state of higher energy to a lower one, will be released as photons (x-rays). This is called characteristic radiation (Fig. 3a,b), because the emitted x-ray photons will be of a specific energy that corresponds to (or is characteristic of) the amount of energy lost in the transition from an outer shell to an inner shell.

The second type of radiation, bremsstrahlung or braking radiation (Fig. 4), occurs when the incoming electrons do not interact directly with the electrons of the heavy metal, but are slowed or decelerated by the positively charged nucleus of the heavy metal atoms. The deceleration of these electrons results in a decrease in their energy and the release of this excess energy as photons (x-rays).

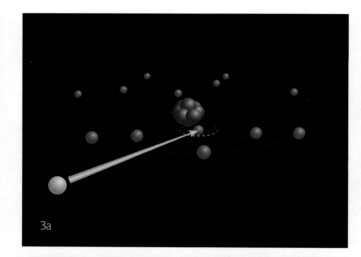

3a

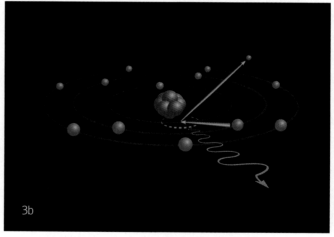

3b

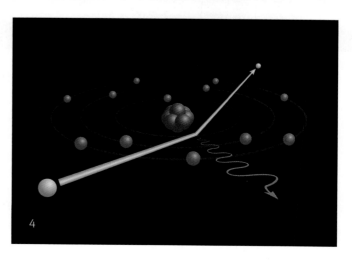

4

THE X-RAY DEVICE – WHAT IS IT?

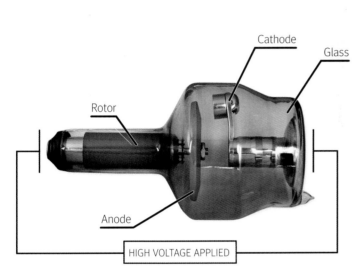

Cathode

Glass

Rotor

Anode

HIGH VOLTAGE APPLIED

5a

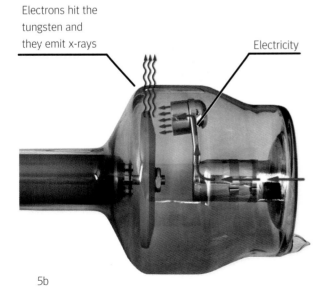

Electrons hit the tungsten and they emit x-rays

Electricity

5b

The heart of an x-ray machine is the x-ray tube, which consists of a cathode, an anode, a glass vacuum tube, and a high-voltage supply (Fig. 5a). An electrical current passing through the cathode causes the heating of the cathode, much like a light filament, and, as a result, electrons are emitted off of the surface. The anode, made of tungsten, draws the electrons across the tube and x-rays are produced (Fig. 5b).

The x-ray tube is surrounded by a thick lead shield. This keeps the newly-formed x-rays from escaping in all directions, and stops all low energy photons. A small window in the lead shield lets some of the x-ray photons escape in a narrow beam. This beam is aimed at the patient and is responsible for the creation of the x-ray image.

> Recently, researchers at the University of California, Los Angeles, have shown that peeling ordinary, transparent, sticky tape within a vacuum can generate x-rays (enough x-rays to take an image of one of the scientists' fingers). This kind of energy release is known as triboluminescence, and occurs whenever a solid (often a crystal) is crushed, rubbed or scratched (4).

Figure 3. Characteristic radiation. a, ejection of inner valence electron, b, transition of an outer valence electron into inner valence shell, and emission of a photon.

Figure 4. Bremsstrahlung (braking) radiation. Deceleration of an incoming electron causing emission of a photon.

Figure 5. The x-ray tube. a, inner structure of the x-ray tube, b, production of x-rays in the x-ray tube.

PRESERVING THE X-RAY IMAGE FOR VIEWING

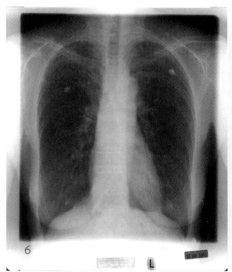 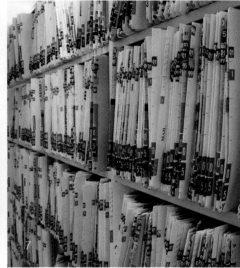 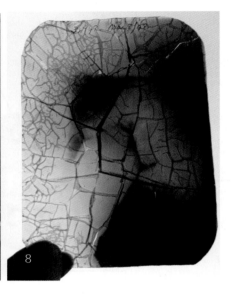

Historically, the capture and preservation (archiving) of the chest x-ray image has been a challenge. Initially, the images were captured and viewed on special photographic glass plates. This provided logistical problems related to handling and storage of these plates.

Glass plates were rapidly replaced by the use of light-sensitive photographic film. The light-sensitive film is placed inside a light-proof cassette. When an x-ray beam strikes the cassette, the radiation causes the crystals embedded in the internal surface of the cassette to emit light. This emitted light exposes the film, in a similar manner to film within a standard camera. The exposed film is chemically processed to produce a visible image (Fig. 6). The x-ray image, on the photographic film, can then be viewed on a light box.

Over the years, as the number of x-ray examinations continued to increase, problems arose relating to the storage and handling of the immense number of films (Fig. 7). Furthermore, if not properly processed, the x-ray films tended to degrade with time, limiting the possibilities for prior films to act as reference tools when imaging the same individual in future years (Fig. 8).

Another big limitation of x-ray images on film is the limited viewing. If the x-ray was taken in the emergency department, then the film was not simultaneously available for viewing in the intensive care unit (ICU), or in the radiology department – it had to be manually transported between departments, often with a delay in interpretation and in subsequent clinical interventions.

Currently, many institutions obtain x-ray examinations digitally. The x-ray source is the same as in previous x-ray imaging methods, but the detectors are modified. Modern detectors can either detect the x-rays directly (Direct or Digital Radiology – DR), or indirectly from information stored on a digital cassette (Computed Radiology – CR). The resulting images are transferred to, and stored in, a data handling and patient record system called the Picture Archiving and Communication System (PACS) (Fig. 9). This allows hospital- or clinic-wide viewing of images and reports. For example, with this technology, the same chest x-ray image can now be viewed simultaneously in the emergency department or the ICU, while being interpreted by the radiologist in the radiology department. In the future, images will be shared between cities and countries, allowing access to the best experts anywhere in the world.

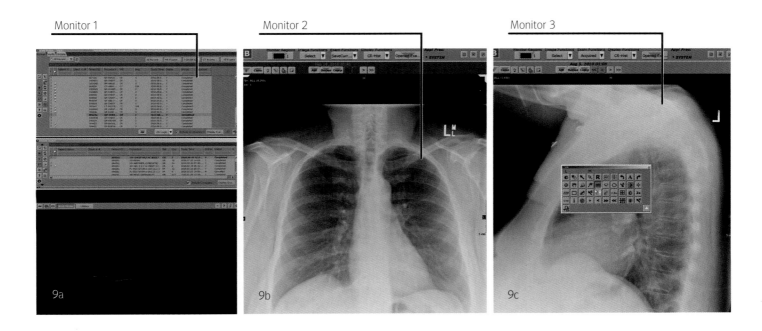

Monitor 1   Monitor 2   Monitor 3

9a   9b   9c

The storage of digital x-ray images is still a problem, even with PACS. A typical 12-bit medical x-ray may be 2048 pixels by 2560 pixels in dimension. This translates to a file size of 10,485,760 bytes (10 Megabytes). In a busy department, over time, Terabytes, and even PETABYTES (1 Petabyte = one quadrillion bytes, or 1000 Terabytes), of storage space may be required.

Figure 6. An x-ray film. X-ray image on photographic x-ray film.

Figure 7. X-ray film storage. X-ray film storage of conventional photographic x-ray films required a lot of space.

Figure 8. Deterioration of an old x-ray. Extreme deterioration of an x-ray film taken in 1947.

Figure 9. Picture archiving and communication system (PACS). Modern PACS workstation with a three monitor configuration, a, monitor 1, b, monitor 2, c, monitor 3.

X-RAY ABSORPTION

To create the final chest x-ray image, the thoracic tissues must absorb some of the x-rays, and yet, allow enough x-rays to pass through the thorax to expose the film. The final chest x-ray image will depend on what happens to the x-ray beam within the body – the x-rays can be absorbed, scattered, or travel through the body unaltered (Fig. 10).

How much of the x-ray beam is absorbed will depend (mostly) on tissue density: the higher the tissue density, the greater the absorption of the x-ray photons. Because fewer x-rays pass through denser tissue, denser tissue on an x-ray image will look whiter. Because more x-rays will pass through less dense tissue, less dense tissue on an x-ray image will look blacker. This is called differential x-ray absorption and forms the basis for x-ray image formation (Fig. 11).

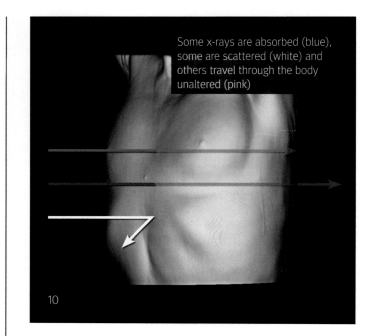

Some x-rays are absorbed (blue), some are scattered (white) and others travel through the body unaltered (pink)

10

Figure 10. X-ray beam disposition. Disposition of the x-ray beam in the human body. Blue arrow, absorbed, white arrow, scattered, pink arrow, travelled through unaltered.

Figure 11. X-ray beam disposition and the resulting grayscale. Disposition of the x-ray beam is related to absorption. The more the x-ray is absorbed (smaller arrows on right) the whiter the resulting grayscale, the less the x-ray is absorbed (larger arrows on the right) the blacker the resulting grayscale.

11

RADIATION DOSE

Exposure

Exposure is the amount of radiation delivered to a point, at a certain distance. The scientific (SI) unit of measurement is the roentgen, R; one roentgen equals the amount of radiation needed to produce one electrostatic unit of electricity (esu or statC), in one cubic centimeter of dry air, at standard temperature and pressure (STP) , or 1 R = 2.58 X 10-4 C/kg (1 esu ≈ 3.33564 X 10-10 C, standard air density of ~1.293 kg/m3).

Absorbed radiation dose

The absorbed radiation dose is the absorption of an amount of radiation energy per mass of absorbing material; the dose causing one joule of absorbed energy per one kilogram of matter.

Dose equivalent ('dose')

The dose equivalent is the weighted unit of radiation dose, to account for the fact that not all types of radiation are equally as harmful. The dose equivalent is equal to the "absorbed radiation dose" multiplied by a "radiation weighting factor" (WR for x-rays is 1). The SI unit of measurement for the 'dose', is the sievert (Sv), or millisievert (mSv); one seivert is approximately equal to the equivalent dose of absorbed radiation that has the same effect as one joule of gamma rays per one kilogram of tissue.

Effective dose

The effective dose is the computed average measure of the radiation absorbed by the whole body, that attempts to account for the relative sensitivities of each organ, or tissue, to different types of radiation. The effective dose is the sum of the weighted equivalent doses in all the organs and tissues of the body; effective dose is equal to the sum of the organ dose multiplied by the tissue-weighting factor, where the tissue-weighting factor represents the relative sensitivity of the organ. Like the dose equivalent, the SI unit of measurement for the effective dose is the Sv or mSv.

Discussing the radiation dose in terms of the effective dose allows for the quantification of risk and the comparison to more familiar sources of exposure, ranging from natural background radiation to radiographic medical procedures (5).

	NON-SI UNIT	SI UNIT	
Exposure	roentgen (R)	roentgen (R)	-
Absorbed radiation dose	rad (radiation absorbed dose)	gray (Gy)	1 Gy = 100 rad
Dose equivalent (effective dose)	rem (roentgen equivalent man)	sievert (Sv) or millisievert (mSv)	1 Sv = 100 rem

Table 1.1
Standard Radiation Units

How Much Radiation is in a Chest X-ray?

When compared to other radiological examinations, the radiation dose that patients receive during a chest x-ray examination is small. The effective dose of a chest x-ray is 0.1 mSv, which is the equivalent of 10 days of natural background radiation (6). This compares with 8 mSv, or two years of natural background radiation, from a Computed Tomography (CT) examination of the chest. Even though the radiation dose is small, the effects of radiation are cumulative and, therefore, any examination involving radiation should only be ordered by evidence-based rules (7).

EXAMINATION	EFFECTIVE RADIATION DOSE	RELATIVE AMOUNT OF NATURAL BACKGROUND RADIATION
Chest x-ray	0.1 mSv	10 days
CT - chest	7-8 mSv	2 years
Lung tomosynthesis	0.77 mSv	2-3 months
VQ scan	1.3 mSv	4-5 months
MRI	zero	zero
US	zero	zero

Table 1.2
Effective Radiation Doses of Standard Radiological Imaging Technologies. CT, computed tomography; VQ, ventilation-perfusion; MRI, magnetic resonance imaging; US, ultrasound.

What About the Pregnant Patient?

All x-ray examinations should be avoided in pregnancy, if possible. If an emergency situation arises that requires a chest x-ray, the examination should be limited to the posterior-anterior (PA) projection. The risks to the developing fetus from the chest x-ray examination are very small. The accepted cumulative radiation dose during pregnancy is 5 rad (0.05 Gy), which is far greater than the dose of the chest x-ray examination. In fact, approximately 70,000 chest x-rays would be needed to reach the 5 rad (0.05 Gy) limit (8).

Despite the low radiation dose, if the examination is deemed necessary, the fetus should be protected by additional lead screening placed over the maternal abdomen and pelvis (7,9,10).

!

RISK OF DEATH FROM....	
1 CHEST X-RAY (radiation-induced cancer)	1/770 000
Smoking 20 CIGARETTES A DAY (cancer)	1/1000
DRIVING 50 km PER DAY (accident)	1/160

Table 1.3
Putting the Risk of a Chest X-ray in Perspective
*adapted from Radiobiology for the Radiologist, Forth Edition; Eric Hall 1994, J.B. Lippincott Company (11)

Reducing Radiation Exposure

The most important means of reducing radiation exposure is by reducing unnecessary x-ray examinations. Developing an evidence-based approach to ordering x-rays is paramount. The appropriate ordering of chest x-rays is discussed in detail in Chapter 23.

If the examination is to be performed, it is the responsibility of the radiology department to make sure that the technical parameters are optimized for dose reduction, and that appropriate shielding is used during the examination. The ALARA *"As Low As Reasonably Achievable"*, and ALARP *"As Low As Reasonably Practicable"* principles should be applied to each patient (12).

HAVING A CHEST X-RAY – THE PATIENT EXPERIENCE

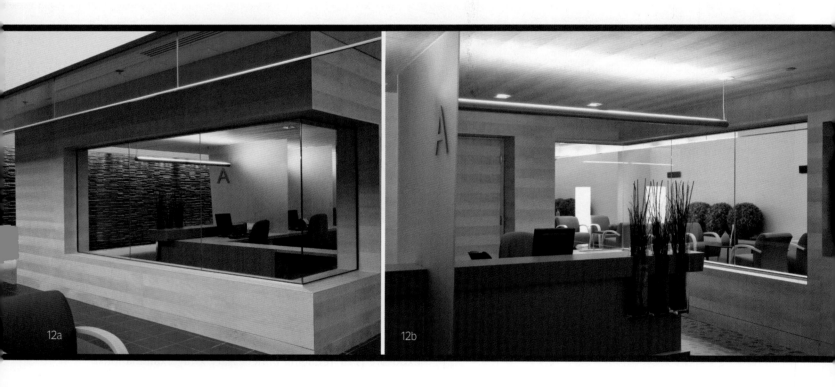

12a

12b

I am a 30-year-old female. Recently, my family doctor ordered a chest x-ray for me, after I complained of a productive cough and fever. I was given an x-ray requisition form, and told to go to the x-ray department.

After registering myself at the x-ray department reception, I was asked to sit in a waiting area. A few minutes later, a woman identifying herself as a medical radiation technologist introduced herself to me. She asked me how I was feeling and the reason for the examination. She also asked if I was pregnant and the date of my last menstrual period. When I asked why this last information was important, she explained that the chest x-ray examination involves radiation and that, although the radiation dose is small, all precautions are taken not to radiate pregnant females, especially during the early weeks of pregnancy.

I was then led to a dressing room and asked to remove all of my clothing from the waist up, and to put on a patient gown. When I was ready, the technologist led me into the x-ray room. The room was full of technical-looking equipment, as well as thick gowns on a wall hanger. (I later found out these are lead gowns that are worn by patients to protect parts of the body that are not being examined.)

I was asked to stand with my chest firmly against the front of a large square box. I had to lift my chin and place it on a supporting ledge. My hands were placed on my hips and my elbows were bent forward to touch the box in front of me. The technologist placed one of the lead gowns over my hips and upper legs. I was asked to take a deep breath. Almost immediately afterwards, I heard a beep and was told to breathe normally.

> Patients experience anxiety related to radiological examinations and procedures. Communication with the patient is important in controlling this anxiety. This responsibility lies with the radiology department, as well as with the referring physician (13).

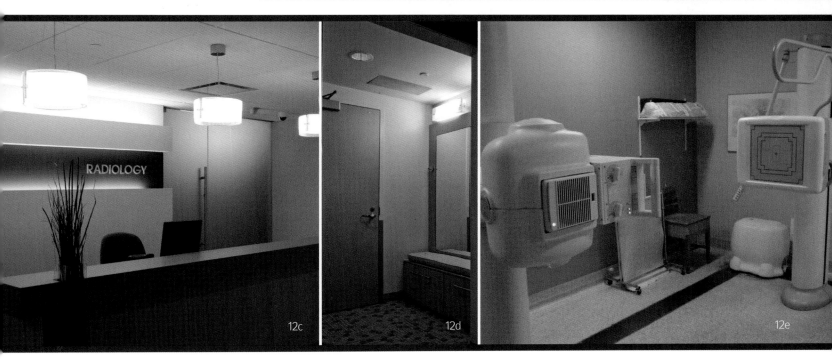

12c   12d   12e

The technologist then asked me to stand sideways, with the left side of my chest against the large square box – this time with my arms in the air, holding a support beam. I was again asked to take a deep breath and after the beep, I was told to breathe normally.

After about one minute, I was told that the examination was over; that I could change and go home. When I asked the technologist about the results of the test, she told me that the results would be sent to my family doctor after the examination was interpreted by a staff radiologist.

Figure 12. Modern x-ray department. a, entrance, b, reception area, c, waiting area, d, change rooms, e, x-ray room. Photos courtesy of A&D Architectural Design by architects Tillman, Ruth Robinson (aTRR, London, Ontario, Canada) in collaboration with Perkins & Will (P&W, Boston, Massachusetts, USA).

PATIENT PREREQUISITES FOR HAVING PA & LATERAL CHEST X-RAYS

- Able to stand or sit upright
- Able to take a deep breath
- Able to understand instructions ("take a deep breath")
- Is cooperative

Table 1.4
Patient Prerequisites for Having PA & Lateral Chest X-rays

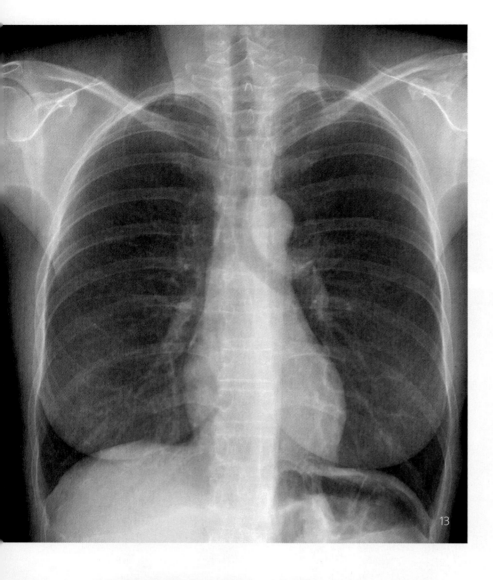

13

TYPES OF CHEST X-RAY EXAMINATIONS

The Posterior-Anterior (PA) X-Ray

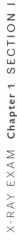

For non-critically ill patients, the frontal x-ray is usually performed in the x-ray department, with the patient standing with their anterior chest closest to the x-ray detector (as described in the patient experience). The x-ray beam courses through the chest from back to front – or from posterior to anterior (PA) (Fig. 13). This orientation minimizes the magnification of the heart. The exposure is taken at maximum inspiration, to ensure that the airspaces are filled to a maximum. This optimizes the contrast between pathology, which is usually white, and the blackness of the lungs. The more air in the lungs, the blacker they will appear on the x-ray, and any pathology within the lungs will be easier to identify.

For your reference, this example of a normal PA x-ray is also included inside the FRONT cover of this book.

Figure 13. Normal posterior-anterior (PA) chest x-ray.

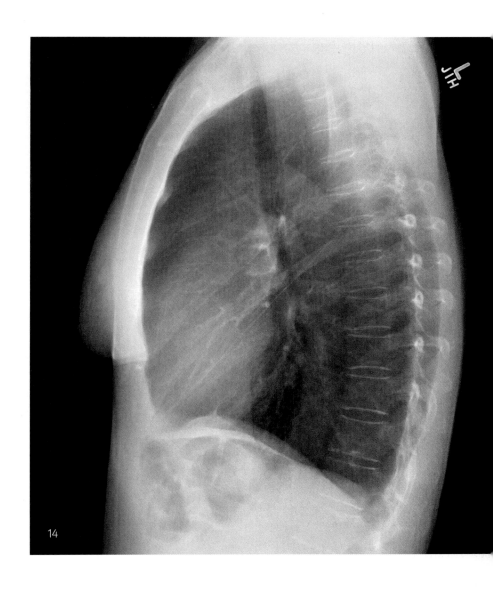

14

The Lateral Chest X-ray

The lateral chest x-ray is commonly ordered together with the PA view. The two examinations are complementary and, when combined, allow the viewer to create a mental 3D perspective of the chest (14). When a lateral x-ray is performed, the patient is positioned so that the left side of the chest lies adjacent to the x-ray detector. The x-ray beam courses through the chest from right to left (the lateral chest x-ray is sometimes called the left lateral chest x-ray) (Fig. 14). The exposure is taken at maximum inspiration. Although it is possible, it is technically very difficult to take a good lateral chest x-ray on the critically ill patient. Therefore, the lateral x-ray is usually only taken on fully cooperating, non-critically ill patients.

For your reference, this example of a normal LATERAL x-ray is also included inside the BACK cover of this book.

Figure 14. Normal lateral chest x-ray.

The AP Chest X-ray as Part of the Acute Abdomen Series

The chest x-ray can play an important role in the diagnosis of abdominal pathology. The acute abdomen x-ray examination series includes: an erect abdomen, a supine abdomen, a left lateral decubitus abdomen, and an erect AP view of the chest. The AP chest x-ray in this series plays an important role in the identification of free air, and in excluding thoracic causes of abdominal symptoms (i.e., lower lobe pneumonia causing abdominal pain).

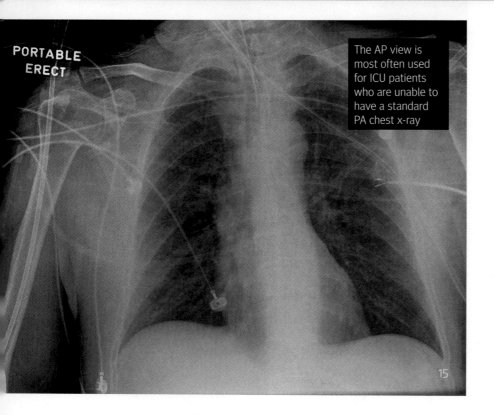

PORTABLE ERECT

The AP view is most often used for ICU patients who are unable to have a standard PA chest x-ray

15

The Anterior-Posterior (AP) X-ray

AMSER

Critically ill patients, who are bedridden, cannot have a standard PA x-ray and, therefore, will have a frontal x-ray taken in the sitting, or supine, position. This type of examination usually requires the use of mobile x-ray equipment, and the x-ray detector is positioned behind the patient's back. The x-ray beam courses through the chest from front to back – or from anterior to posterior (AP). The exposure is taken at maximum inspiration (for the same reasons mentioned previously) (Fig. 15).

Figure 15. Normal anterior-posterior (AP) chest x-ray, with patient erect

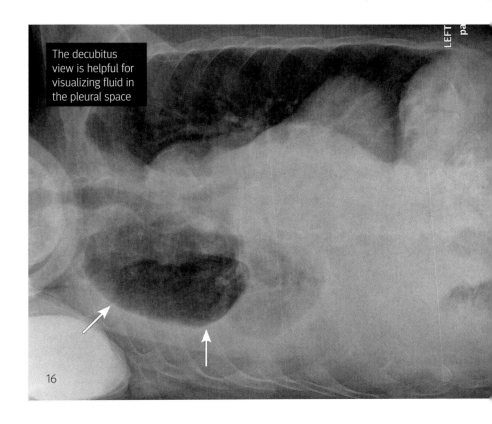

The decubitus view is helpful for visualizing fluid in the pleural space

The Decubitus View

On the PA, lateral or AP x-rays, it may be difficult to differentiate between pleural thickening, consolidation, and a pleural effusion. Ultrasound is the examination of choice in this scenario. If ultrasound is not available, a decubitus x-ray may be of value. For a decubitus x-ray, the patient is positioned horizontally, lying on the side of the questioned abnormality. The x-ray beam is directed through the patient, from front to back, covering the entire chest (Fig. 16). If pleural fluid is present, gravity will cause the fluid position to shift, and the fluid will layer in the most dependent part of the hemithorax. If there is no shift, the pleural opacity is caused by something other than fluid, such as scarring, or a tumor.

Figure 16. Decubitus chest x-ray with patient lying on the side – right side down. Pleural fluid (arrows) is layering within the most dependent part of the right hemithorax.

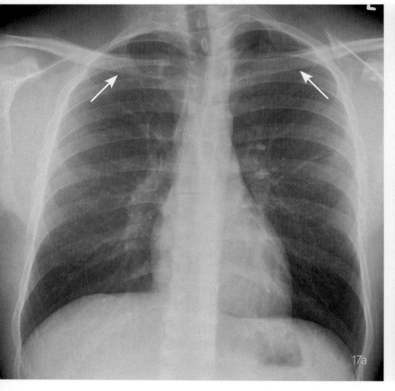

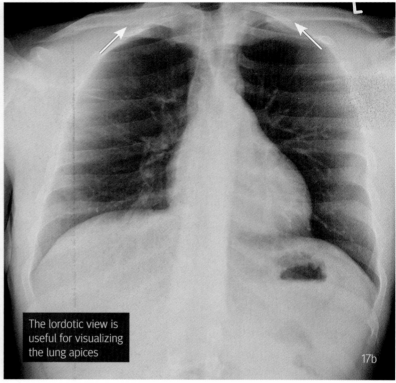

The lordotic view is useful for visualizing the lung apices

17a

17b

The Lordotic View

AMSER The lung apices can be a difficult region to evaluate due to the overlap of the ribs and the clavicles. In situations where a suspected apical pulmonary abnormality exists, the lordotic technique is used to confirm the finding (15). The lordotic technique is performed by orienting the x-ray beam cranially (i.e., upwards towards the head), thereby separating the anterior portion of the first ribs from the lung apices (Fig. 17a,b). The lordotic view has largely been replaced with CT imaging, but still has a role when access to CT is limited.

Figure 17. Normal PA x-ray versus lordotic view. a, normal PA chest x-ray; notice the clavicles (arrows) are positioned over the apex of the lungs, b, lordotic view of the same patient; notice the clavicles (arrows) now are positioned above the apex of the lungs.

X-RAY EXAM Chapter 1 SECTION I

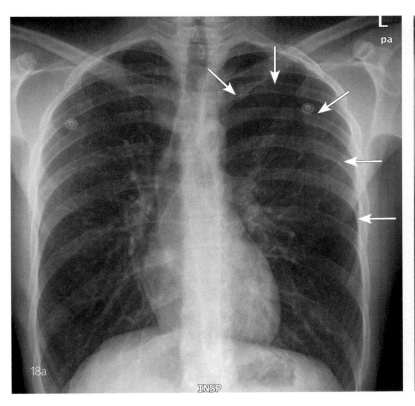

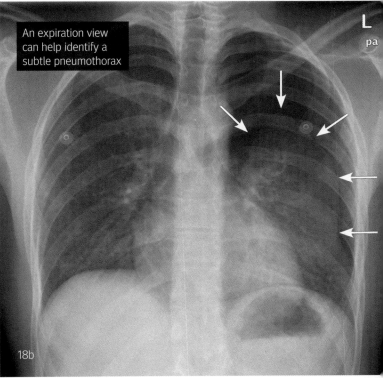

An expiration view can help identify a subtle pneumothorax

The Inspiration/Expiration Series

When the patient takes a limited inspiration, the opacity of the lungs will be greater than during a full inspiration, because there is less air within the lungs. Although in most scenarios this is not desirable, it is used to our advantage in patients with a pneumothorax. By making the lungs whiter by taking the x-ray during expiration (or limited inspiration), air outside the lungs in the pleural space will appear more obvious (Fig. 18a,b).

Figure 18. Inspiration/expiration series. a, inspiration chest x-ray with a subtle pneumothorax (arrows), b, expiration chest x-ray; this pneumothorax (arrows) is more conspicuous against the background of a whiter lung.

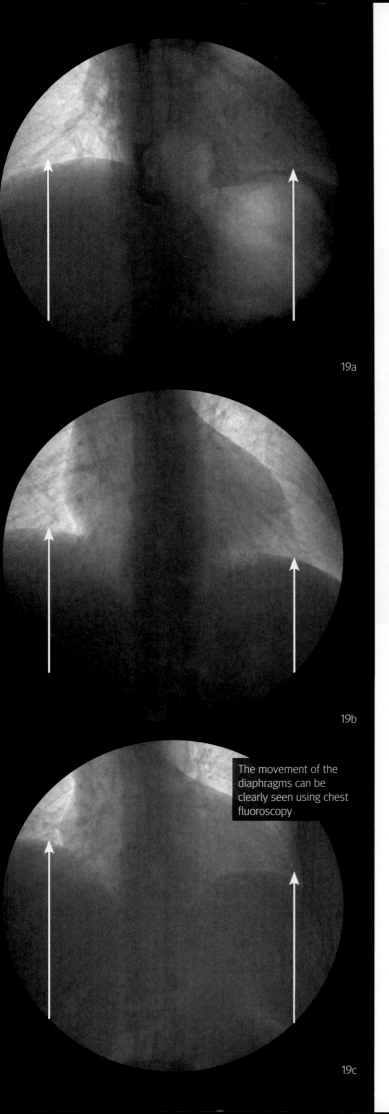

19a

19b

The movement of the diaphragms can be clearly seen using chest fluoroscopy

Chest Fluoroscopy

Fluoroscopy is an x-ray examination using a special x-ray camera that allows real-time, continuous, x-ray imaging. The patient stands in front of the fluoroscopic camera. When the exposure button is pressed by the radiologist, real-time images of the chest can be viewed and recorded (Fig. 19a,b,c).

This examination is useful when dynamic information, such as diaphragm movement, needs to be assessed. While the patient quickly exhales through the nose, the movement of the diaphragms is observed in real time. This is called the fluoroscopic sniff test. With phrenic nerve paralysis, there is paradoxical movement of the paralyzed diaphragm.

Figure 19. Chest fluoroscopy. Spot images captured during: a, normal breathing, b, maximum inspiration - diaphragms are lower, c, maximum expiration - diaphragms are higher. Arrows show the position of the diaphragms. The length of the arrows reflect the degree of movement of the diaphragms.

19c

Dual-Energy Chest X-ray

Dual-energy imaging enables the acquisition of two PA images of the chest, at different energy settings, separated by approximately 150 milliseconds.

These two acquisitions provide the radiologist with three images.

- The standard PA x-ray (Fig. 20a).

- A PA image of the chest with the bones removed (known as the soft-tissue image) (Fig. 20b).

- An image of the skeletal system of the chest (the bone image) (Fig. 20c).

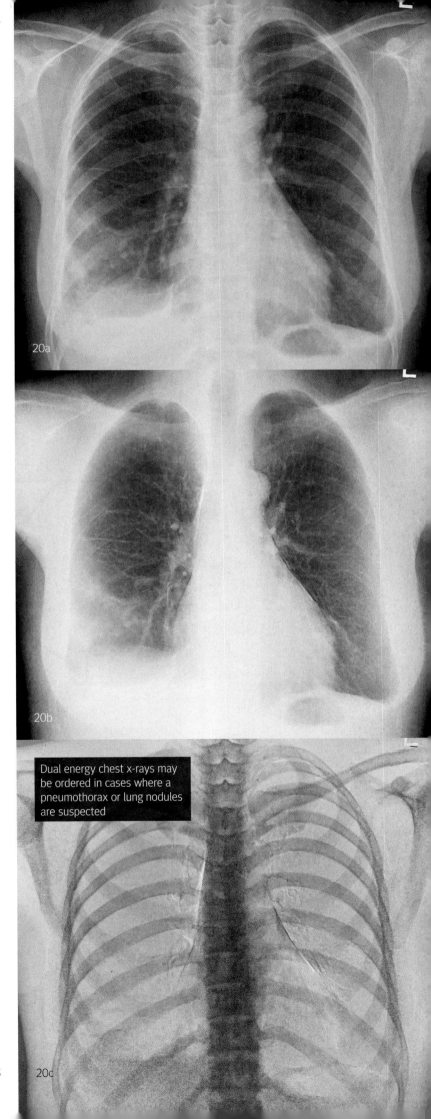

Dual energy chest x-rays may be ordered in cases where a pneumothorax or lung nodules are suspected

Figure 20. Dual energy chest x-ray series. a, full image, b, bones extracted, c, soft tissues extracted.

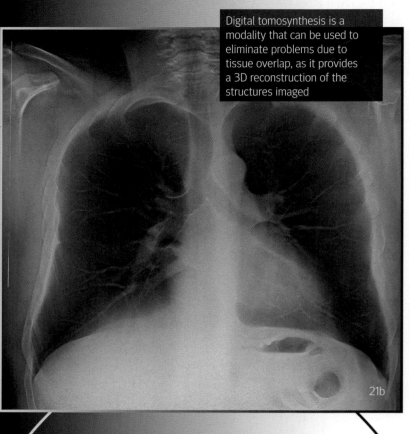

Digital tomosynthesis is a modality that can be used to eliminate problems due to tissue overlap, as it provides a 3D reconstruction of the structures imaged

21b

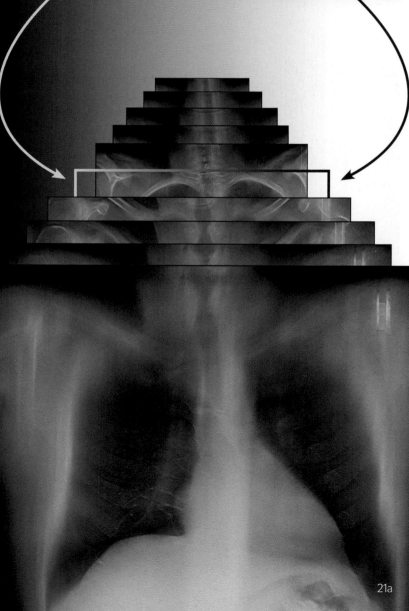

21a

Digital Tomography (Tomosynthesis)

Digital tomography, or tomosynthesis, is a method of producing sectional images using a digital detector, and a conventional x-ray system with a moving x-ray tube. Tomosynthesis allows the retrospective production of an arbitrary number of sectional images from a single pass of the x-ray tube. The acquired data is processed into slices that show anatomical structures at different depths and angles (16) (Fig. 21a,b).

Compared to a low-dose chest CT scan with a radiation dose of 2.5 mSv to 8 mSv, a 10-second lung tomosynthesis study has a radiation dose estimated at 0.77 mSv.

Figure 21. Chest tomography (tomosynthesis). a, series (stack) of digital x-ray slices through the thorax, b, selected image from the series at the level of the carina.

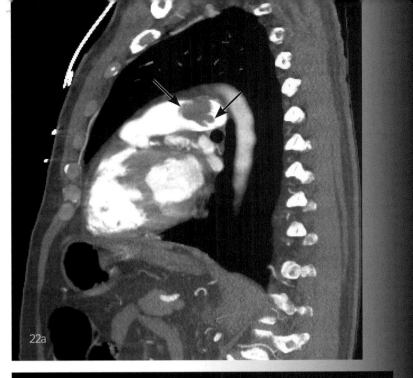

22a

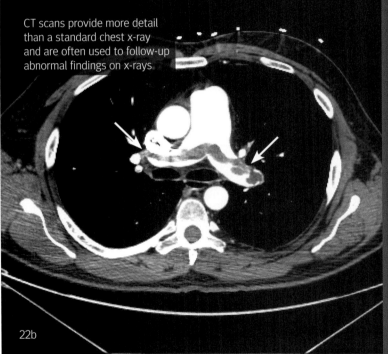

CT scans provide more detail than a standard chest x-ray and are often used to follow-up abnormal findings on x-rays

22b

Computed Tomography (CT)

Computed tomography (CT) is an x-ray technology that produces cross-sectional images of the body (Fig. 22a,b,c). The CT scanner consists of a doughnut-shaped scanning apparatus, and an x-ray table that moves into the hole of the x-ray scanner. A rotating x-ray tube is mounted around the edge of the hole, along with an array of x-ray detectors. The x-ray tube and the detectors revolve around the patient and, with each revolution, slices of the body are obtained. X-ray density information is recorded and used to produce 2D and 3D images.

To enhance the appearance of certain tissues or pathologies and to increase the diagnostic power of the scan, CT scans can be performed with contrast media.

Figure 22. Computed tomography (CT). a, sagittal CT of the thorax, b, transverse (horizontal) CT of the thorax, c, coronal CT of the thorax. Arrows highlight emboli within the pulmonary arteries, bilaterally.

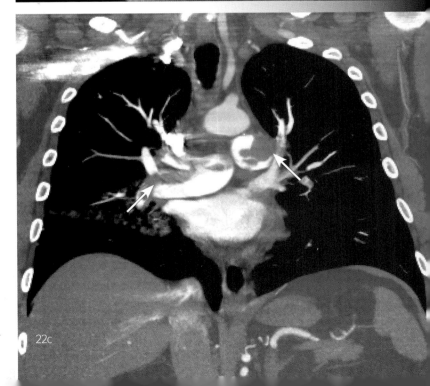

27

22c

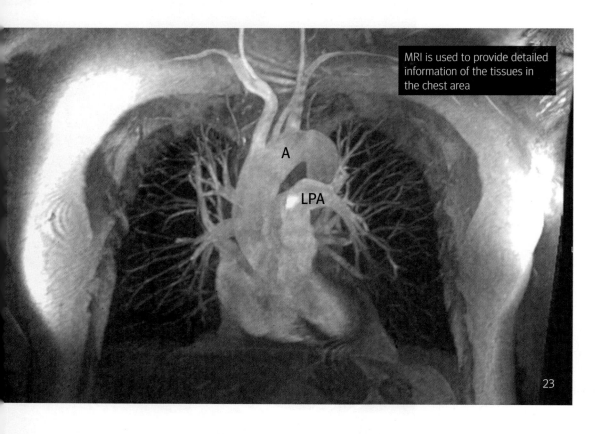

MRI is used to provide detailed information of the tissues in the chest area

A

LPA

23

Magnetic Resonance Imaging (MRI)

AMSER In an MRI examination, the patient is placed in a strong electromagnetic field, and positioned at the appropriate level so that an image of the desired organ(s)/structure(s) of interest can be obtained. Within the electromagnetic field, the hydrogen atoms in the body align themselves parallel with the magnetic field: either in the same direction as, or opposite to, the direction of the field.

A short, powerful radio signal (a form of electromagnetic energy) is then sent through the patient's body, perpendicular to the main magnetic field. The hydrogen atoms within the tissues, which have the same frequency as the radio signal, will become 'excited', or raised to a higher state of energy, and start to resonate with the exciting radio wave.

When the radio signal is turned off, the hydrogen atoms will (after a period of time) return to their original energy state, releasing energy in the form of radio waves. The MRI machine detects these signals, and uses the information to pinpoint their origin. The time it takes for the excited hydrogen atoms to return to their original energy level – which depends on the number of atoms and characteristic physical properties of the various tissue types – is also measured and analyzed by a computer. Then, on the basis of these measurements, combined with the information on the position of the signal, an image of the tissues within the body is constructed (Fig. 23).

To enhance the appearance of certain tissues or pathologies and to increase the diagnostic power of the scan, MRI can also be done with contrast media (17).

Figure 23. **Magnetic resonance imaging (MRI).** Coronal MRI of the thorax showing thoracic vessels; A, aorta; LPA, left pulmonary artery,

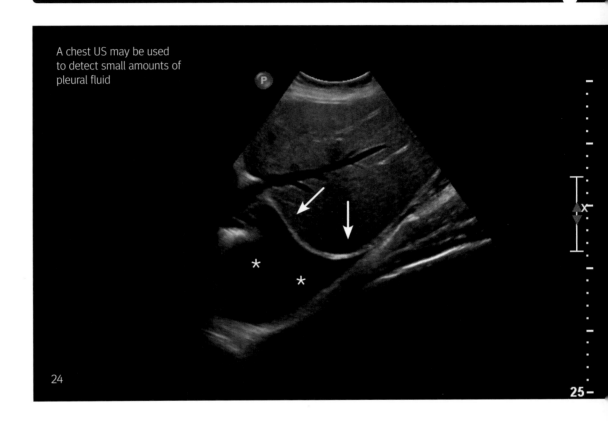

> Current literature shows that high-resolution ultrasound can play an important role in diagnosing a pneumothorax (18).

A chest US may be used to detect small amounts of pleural fluid

Ultrasound (US)

Ultrasound (US) is a non-radiation technology that uses the principles of sonar. During the ultrasound examination, a hand-held transducer is used to examine the target organ. The transducer emits sound and detects the returning echoes that are caused by a border between two tissues that conduct sound differently. The echoes are then analyzed by a computer in the ultrasound machine and transformed into real-time images.

Ultrasound waves pass easily through fluids and soft tissues, but are unable to penetrate bone or gas, so ultrasound is of limited use for examining regions surrounded by bone, or for areas that contain gas or air. Even so, ultrasound imaging is used to examine the thorax. The main indication for use of ultrasounds in thoracic imaging is for the localization of pleural fluid prior to thoracocentesis, and for confirming a pleural effusion (Fig. 24).

Other modalities used to image the thorax include Positron Emission Tomography (PET) scanners, PET/CT, and ventilation/perfusion nuclear lung scanning.

Figure 24. Ultrasound (US). Ultrasound of the thorax showing a pleural effusion; (asterisks) posterior to the diaphragm (arrows).

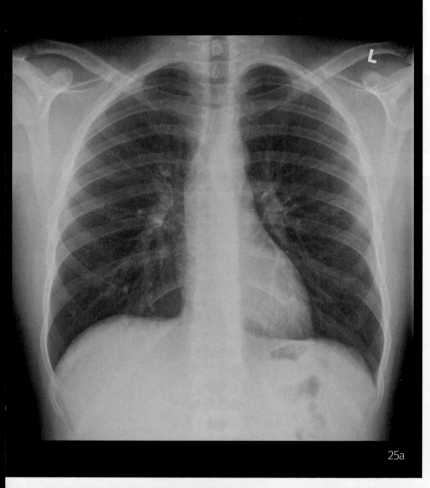

25a

WHAT IS A GOOD CHEST X-RAY IMAGE? IMAGE QUALITY

Your ability to spot a good or bad image will require knowledge of radiological anatomy, your interpretive skills, and your experience.

A good quality chest x-ray image is one that allows the interpreter to extract the maximum clinically important information from it. False positive and false negative interpretations will increase significantly with poor quality x-ray images. The quality of the chest x-ray image relates to the patient positioning on the image, the quality of inspiration, technical exposure factors (e.g., contrast and resolution), sharpness, and the presence (or lack) of artifacts (3).

Position:

Centering

The entire thorax should be visible and should be positioned in the center of the image (Fig. 25a). The image should include the apices of the lungs, the costophrenic angles, the spine and the sternum. The medial edge of the scapula should lie lateral to the chest wall. The patient's arms and chin should not overlap the upper lung fields.

Rotation

There should be no patient rotation. If the patient is rotated, the lung closest to the x-ray detector may look whiter, and the anatomy can appear distorted (Fig. 25b).

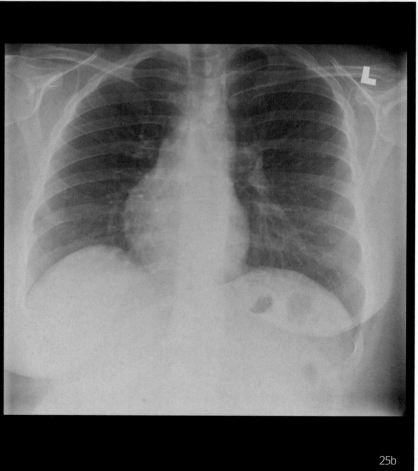

25b

Figure 25. Patient positioning on the x-ray is important. Example PA x-rays with, a, good positioning, b, poor positioning. The rotation of the patient is causing distortion of the cardiac shadow.

Quality of Inspiration:

The quality of the inspiration is difficult to assess without spirometry. However, assuming that the patient has taken a good inspiration and does not have restrictive lung disease, the outline of the tenth posterior rib should be seen above the right hemidiaphragm (Fig. 26a).

If a limited inspiration (or an expiration) image was taken, the blood vessels in the lungs will look crowded and larger than normal (Fig. 26b).

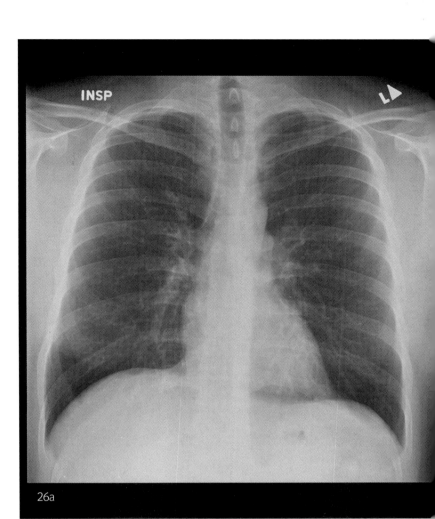

26a

26b

Figure 26. Inspiration quality. The proper degree of inspiration is important for a good chest x-ray. Example PA chest x-rays of the same patient with, a, adequate full inspiration, b, poor inspiration (in this case the patient purposely exhaled).

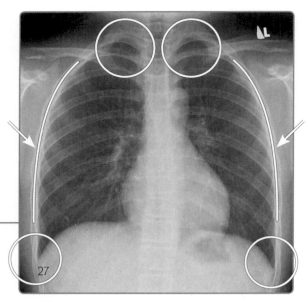

27

How to assess for proper positioning of the patient on the PA x-ray

Patient centering is evaluated by the visualization of all of the lung fields. All lung fields should be visible on the x-ray image, and the radiographic shadows of the scapula and chin should not be superimposed on the lungs.

Patient rotation is evaluated by defining the position of the medial aspect of the clavicles relative to the thoracic spinous processes.

STEP 1
Identify the lung apices, the costophrenic angles, and the lateral margins of both lungs (Fig. 27).

The patient is properly centered when the lung apices, the costophrenic angles, and the lateral lung margins are all included on the image.

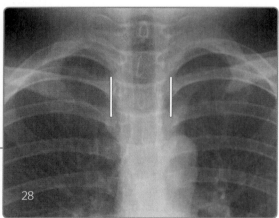

28

STEP 2
Identify the medial end of both clavicles (Fig. 28).

STEP 3
Identify the spinous processes of the thoracic spine, at the level of the clavicles (Fig. 29).

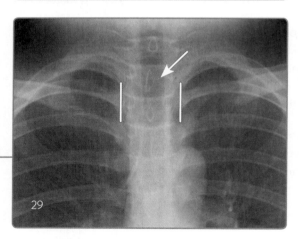

29

The patient is properly positioned when the distance between the medial end of one clavicle and the spinous process is the same as the distance between the medial end of the other clavicle and the spinous process (X) (Fig. 30).

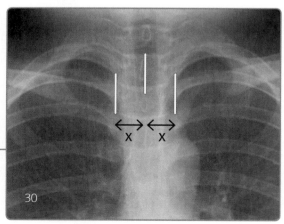

30

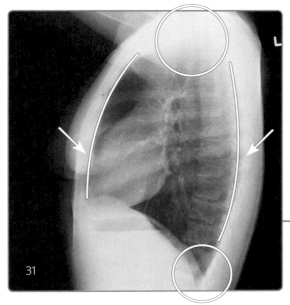

31

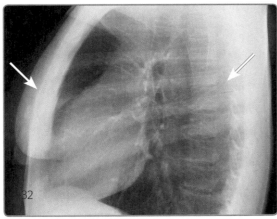

32

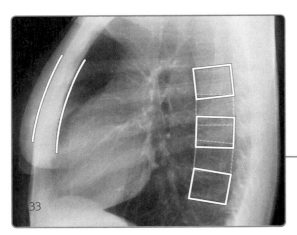

33

How to assess for proper positioning of the patient on the lateral x-ray

Patient centering is evaluated by the visualization of all of the lung fields. All lung fields should be visible on the x-ray image, and the radiographic shadows of the arms and shoulders should not be superimposed on the lungs.

Patient rotation is evaluated by identifying the sternum and the vertebral bodies in profile.

STEP 1
Identify the lung apices, the costovertebral angles, and the anterior and posterior margins of both lungs (Fig. 31).

The patient is properly centered when the lung apices, the costovertebral angles, and the anterior and posterior lung margins are all included on the image.

STEP 2
Identify the sternum and vertebral bodies (Fig. 32).

STEP 3
The patient is properly positioned when the anterior and posterior cortical outline of the sternum is clearly seen, or when the vertebral bodies and spinous processes are seen in profile as stacked rectangles (Fig. 33).

The effect of rotation on the image quality is discussed in Chapter 1 (Pg. 30).

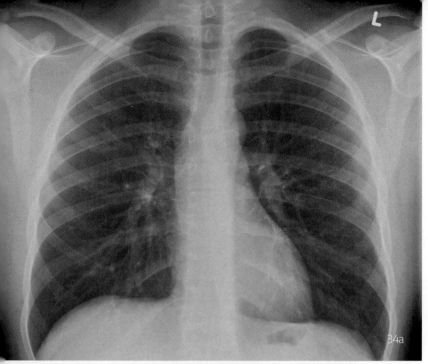

34a

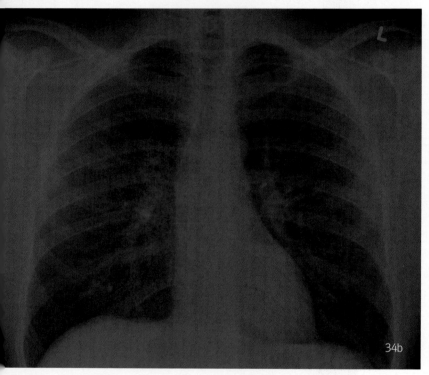

34b

Technical Exposure Factors (Contrast and Resolution):

Exposure

The exposure is optimum when the anatomy is clearly visible (Fig. 34a). On an adequately penetrated PA chest x-ray, the outlines of the thoracic vertebral bodies and the disc spaces should be visualized through the heart shadow and mediastinum. Vascular markings should be visible behind the heart.

When an x-ray is poorly exposed, it can either be over- or underexposed.

Overexposure causes a loss of anatomical detail because everything looks darker (Fig. 34b). If this occurs, some information can be extracted by increasing the brightness in the darkened areas of the image. When x-rays are on film, this is done by shining a bright light behind the part of the film being examined.

Underexposure also causes a loss of anatomical detail (Fig. 34c). The underexposed image will look too white everywhere. Unfortunately, no additional detail can be extracted by changing the image brightness. The underexposed x-ray causes a significant diagnostic problem because congestive heart failure can easily be over-diagnosed on underexposed chest x-rays.

Resolution and contrast

Exposure can be affected by contrast and resolution.

The degree of difference between the light and dark areas on the chest x-ray is called contrast. Resolution is a term used to describe the detail that is found on the x-ray

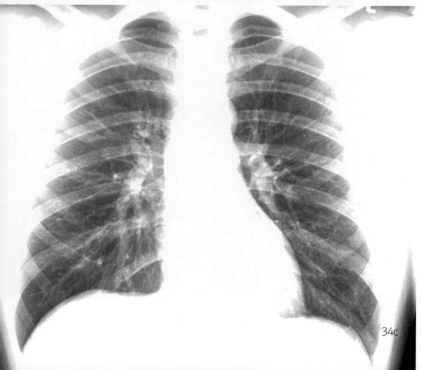

34c

image. Spatial resolution is the measure of how closely lines can be resolved on the x-ray. Contrast resolution is the ability to distinguish between differences in intensity on the x-ray.

Contrast and resolution are determined by the film-detector system, x-ray energy, and the amount of scatter radiation.

Film detector system

Equipment used should be of the highest quality standard to ensure optimum quality.

X-ray energy

X-ray images produced by using higher voltage (125 to 150 kVp) provide more information than images produced by lower voltage techniques.

Scatter radiation

When x-rays strike an object, secondary (scatter) radiation is produced in all directions. If this scatter radiation hits the detectors, the image detail will be degraded (Fig. 35). X-ray grids should be used to reduce this negative effect of scatter radiation.

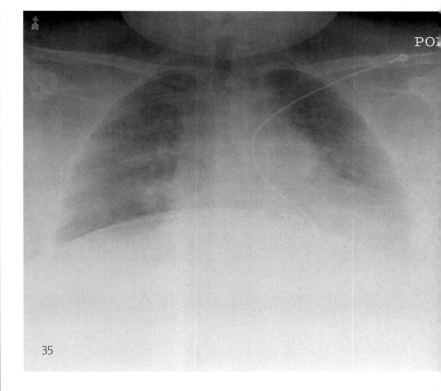

35

Figure 34. Effect of exposure on the appearance of the chest x-ray. Example PA chest x-rays that are, a, normal exposure, b, overexposed – too dark, c, underexposed – too white.

Figure 35. Morbidly obese patient. PA chest x-ray of a morbidly obese patient. The whiteness over the lungs is caused by scatter artifact.

How to assess for adequate exposure on a chest x-ray

To assess for an adequately penetrated chest x-ray, check the exposure in the following four areas (Fig. 36).

1

The lungs centrally – good, if not too black or too white. You should be able to see distinct vessel markings.

2

The lungs peripherally – good, if not too black or too white.

3

The central portion of the x-ray (the mediastinum over the spine) – good, if you can still perceive the cortical outline of the tenth thoracic vertebra.

4

The region of the heart (the cardiac zone) – good, if you can still distinguish the spine.

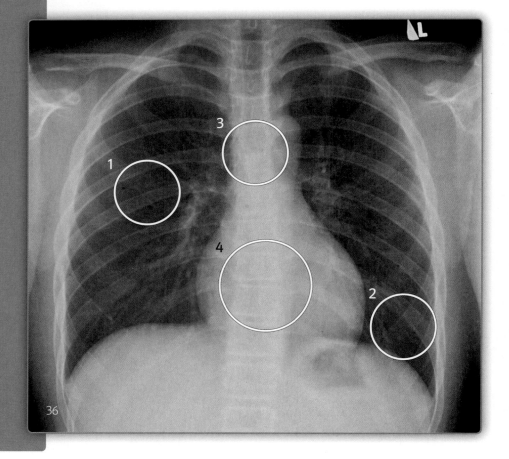

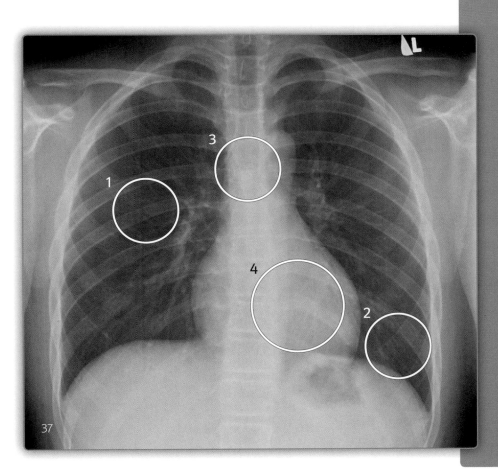

37

How to assess for adequate contrast on a chest x-ray

To assess for adequate contrast on a chest x-ray, check the contrast in the following four areas (Fig. 37).

1

The lungs centrally – good, if the blood vessels can be easily traced.

2

The lungs peripherally – good, if the peripheral blood vessels can be easily traced to the lung periphery and the vessels can be seen through the diaphragms on the PA x-ray.

3

The central portion of the x-ray (the mediastinum over the spine) – good, if the trachea and proximal bronchi are clearly visible.

4

The region of the heart (the cardiac zone) – good, if the pulmonary vessels can be easily seen behind the heart.

?

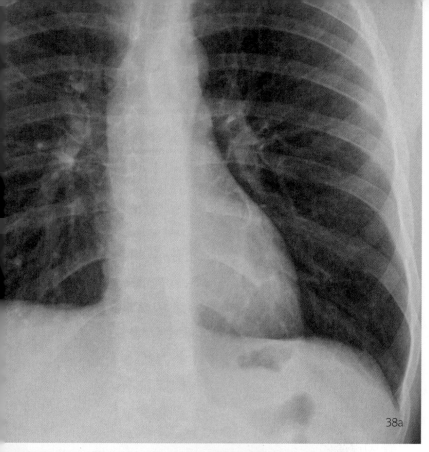

38a

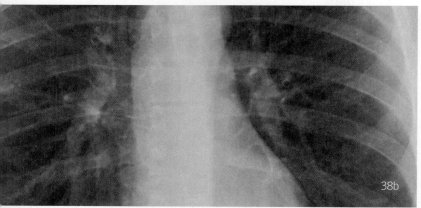

38b

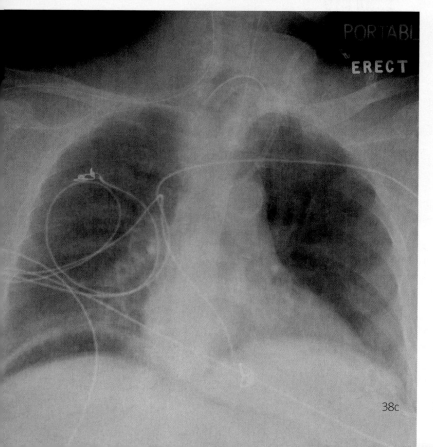

PORTABL

ERECT

Figure 38. Motion artifacts. Motion of the patient during a chest x-ray can cause the image to be blurry. Example chest x-rays with, a, a clear outline of heart and diaphragms, b, the pulmonary vessels clearly visible, c, blurred structures due to motion.

Figure 39. External artifacts. External objects can cause artifacts on chest x-rays. Example chest x-rays with, a, hair (arrows), b, clothing (shirt collar) (arrows), c, external lines (arrows).

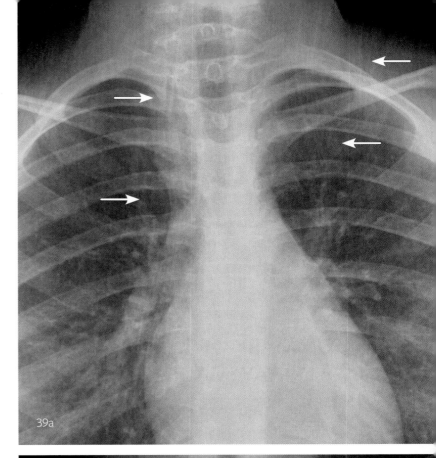

39a

Artifacts and Sharpness

Patient motion can decrease the quality of the x-ray because the image will be blurred. The outline of the heart and diaphragms should be sharp (Fig. 38a), with no distortion related to patient motion. The pulmonary vessels should be clearly visible in all of the lung fields, especially those around the heart (Fig. 38b).

If the x-ray is not sharp, the anatomical structures will look blurry and lack clarity (Fig. 38c). Subtle abnormalities may be completely obscured.

In addition, there should be no artifacts from external objects, such as hair, clothes, or lines (Fig. 39a,b,c).

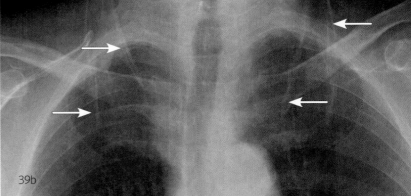

39b

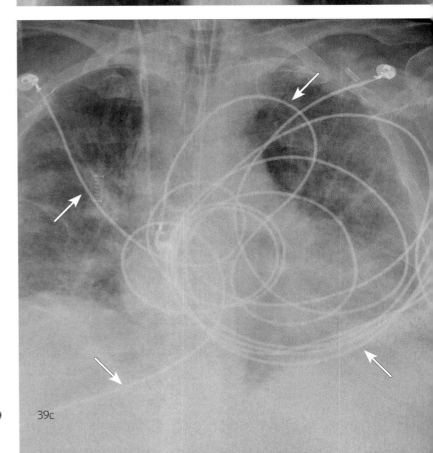

39c

SUMMARY OF THE EFFECTS OF POOR X-RAY QUALITY ON X-RAY IMAGE APPEARANCE & INTERPRETATION

	X-RAY IMAGE APPEARANCE	EFFECT ON INTERPRETATION
PATIENT POSITIONING:		
Rotation	Hila look distorted. One lung will look whiter, and the other will look blacker	Over-diagnose hilar pathology Increase false positives
Centering	Missed information	Under-diagnose pathology because information incomplete Increase false negatives
QUALITY of INSPIRATION:		
Poor inspiration	Vessels look engorged	Over-diagnose CHF Increase false positives
EXPOSURE:		
Underexposed	Lungs look congested	Over-diagnose CHF Increase false positives
Overexposed	Vessels less visible	Under-diagnose CHF Increase false negatives
ARTIFACTS & SHARPNESS:		
Movement	Blurry image	Miss small abnormalities Increase false negatives
Artifacts present	Structures obscured Pathology mimicked by artifacts	Increase false positives and false negatives

Table 1.5

Summary of the Effects of Poor X-ray Quality on X-ray Image Appearance and Interpretation. CHF, congestive heart failure.

Chest X-ray Quality Checklist

In order to make sure that the chest x-ray examination is of good quality, all parts of the checklist should indicate good quality.

rc

PATIENT POSITIONING

1 Is the patient position correct?
(rotation/centering)

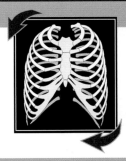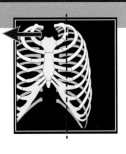

If **NO**, then describe.
Rotated right/left.
Shifted right/left.

QUALITY of INSPIRATION

2 Did the patient take a good inspiration?

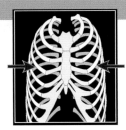

If **NO**, then describe.
Give number of posterior ribs visible.

EXPOSURE

3 Is the x-ray of adequate exposure?

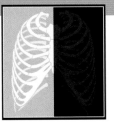

If **NO**, then describe.
Underexposed/overexposed.

ARTIFACTS & SHARPNESS

4 Is the x-ray free from external artifacts?
(Are artifacts obscuring part of the image?)

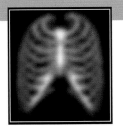

If **NO**, describe.
Hair/clothes/lines/jewellery.

5 Is the x-ray sharp?
(not blurry due to motion artifact)

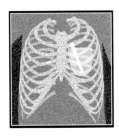

If **NO**, may need to
repeat chest x-ray.

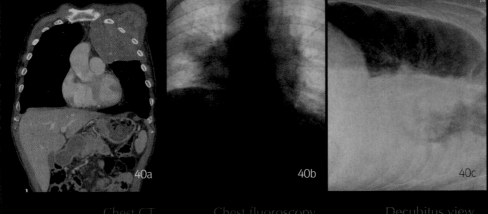

40a	40b	40c
Chest CT	Chest fluoroscopy	Decubitus view

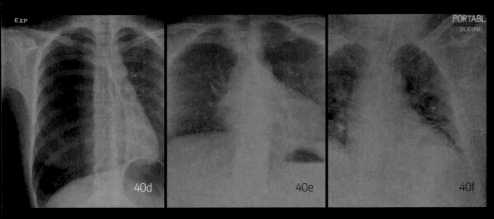

40d	40e	40f
Expiration view	Lordotic view	Portable supine AP x-ray

Can you match the clinical scenario with the appropriate imaging test?

CASE STUDY

You are taking an OSCE examination and, at one station, you are asked to match the clinical situation with the appropriate imaging test (Fig. 40a,b,c,d,e,f).

The clinical scenarios are the following:

Differentiating pleural effusion from pleural thickening; suspected pneumothorax; unconscious, unstable, intubated patient; suspected paralysis of diaphragm; staging of lung cancer; apical lung disease.

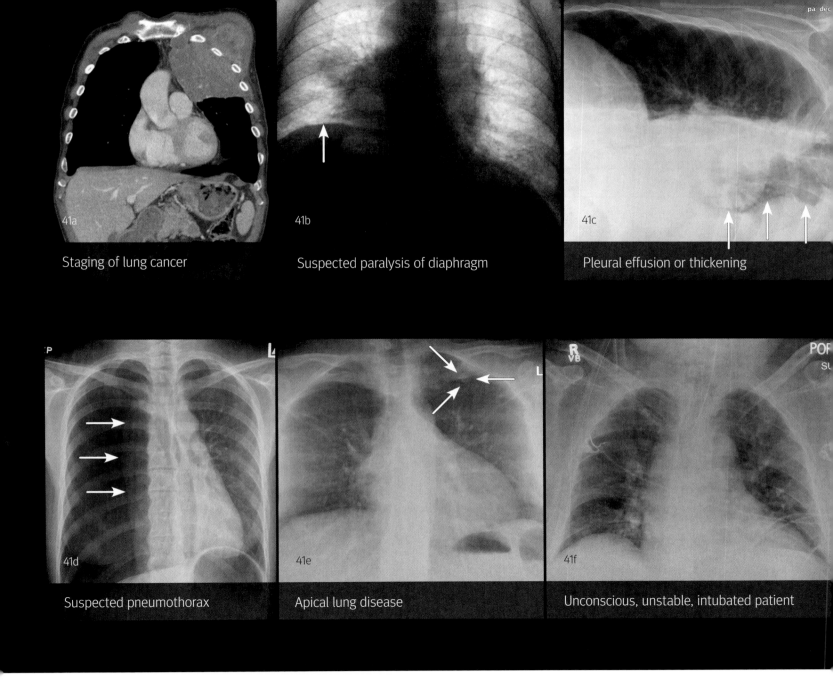

Staging of lung cancer

41a

Suspected paralysis of diaphragm

41b

Pleural effusion or thickening

41c

Suspected pneumothorax

41d

Apical lung disease

41e

Unconscious, unstable, intubated patient

41f

Figure 41. Appropriate imaging tests for clinical scenarios. a, chest CT showing lung cancer invading through the chest wall, b, suspected paralysis of diaphragm on chest fluoroscopy; paradoxical movement of left hemidiaphragm with the sniff test consistent with phrenic nerve paralysis (note high left diaphragm, arrow), c, pleural effusion or thickening seen on a decubitus x-ray; layering of a left pleural effusion is visible (arrows), d, suspected pneumothorax confirmed on an expiration x-ray; right tension pneumothorax is visible (arrows), e, apical lung disease on a lordotic x-ray; visible as nodules (arrows) in left apex, f, an AP (supine) x-ray of an unconscious, unstable, intubated patient.

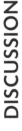

DISCUSSION

References

1. Lewis, P.J., Shaffer, K., & Donovan, A. (Eds.). (2012). AMSER National Medical Student Curriculum in Radiology. http://aur.org/Secondary-Alliances.aspx?id=141.

2. Lewis, P.J., & Shaffer, K. (2005). Developing a national medical student curriculum in radiology. *Am. Coll. Radiol. 2*(1):8–11.

3. Pavlinsky, G.V. (2008). *Fundamentals of X-ray Physics*. Cambridge, UK: Cambridge International Science Publishing.

4. Camara, C.G., Escobar, J.V., Hird, J.R., & Putterman, S.J. (2008). Correlation between nanosecond x-ray flashes and stick–slip friction in peeling tape. *Nature, 455*(7216):1089–1092.

5. Mettler, F.A. Jr., Huda, W., Yoshizumi, T.T., & Mahesh, M. (2008). Effective doses in radiology and diagnostic nuclear medicine: a catalog. *Radiology, 248*:254–263.

6. National Council on Radiation Protection and Measurements. (2009). Ionizing radiation exposure of the population of the United States: NCRP Report No 160. http://www.ncrponline.org/Publications/Press_Releases/160press.html.

7. Fazel, R., Krumholz, H.M., Wang, Y., et al. (2009). Exposure to low dose ionizing radiation from medical imaging procedures. *N. Engl. J. Med., 361*:849–857.

8. Toppenberg, K.S., Hill, A., & Miller, D.P. (1999). Safety of radiographic imaging during pregnancy. *Am. Fam. Physician, 59*(7):1813–1818.

9. Verdun, F.R., Bochud, F, Gundinchet, F., et al. (2008). Quality initiatives radiation risk: what you should know to tell your patient. *Radiographics, 28*:1807–1816.

10. International Commission on Radiological Protection (ICRP). (2001). Radiation and your patient: a guide for medical practitioners. *Ann. ICRP, 31*(4):5–31.

11. Hall, E. (2006). *Radiobiology for the Radiologist* (6th ed.). Philadelphia, PA: Lippincott Williams & Wilkins.

12. Willis, C.E., & Slovis, T.L. (2005). The ALARA concept in pediatric CR and DR: Dose reduction in pediatric radiographic exams - A white paper conference. *AJR Am. J. Roentgenol., 184*:373–374.

13. Flory, N., & Lang, E.V. (2011). Distress in the radiology waiting room. *Radiology, 260*:166–173.

14. Gaber, K.A., McGavin, C.R., & Wells, I.P. (2005). Lateral chest X-ray for physicians. *J. R. Soc. Med., 98*(7):310–322.

15. Chung, M.J., Goo, J.M., Im, J.G., et al. (1989). The influence of the lordotic projection on the interpretation of the chest radiograph. *Clin. Radiol., 40*:360–364.

16. Dobbins, J.T. (2009). Tomosynthesis imaging: At a translational crossroads. *Med. Physics., 36*(6):1956.

17. Bittner, R.C., & Felix, R. (1998). Magnetic resonance (MR) imaging of the chest: state-of-the-art. *Eur. Resp. J., 11*(6):1392–1404.

18. Chung, M.J., Goo, J.M., Im, J.G., et al. (2005). Value of high-resolution ultrasound in detecting a pneumothorax. *Eur. Radiol., 15*(5):930–935.

CHAPTER 2
The X-RAY IMAGE

importance

Looking at grayscale images is the cornerstone of radiology. This chapter explains the concept of grayscale and describes the five main densities seen on an x-ray. You will learn how the 3D structures in the body create a 2D x-ray image, and gain an understanding of the concept of radiation absorption events (RAEs). This chapter will help you to recognize anatomical structures on the x-ray image through the use of common shapes, such as rectangles, circles, and arches. Finally, you will learn all about interfaces and overlap – their uses for interpretation, and the problems associated with them.

objectives

Skills

You will identify

- the grayscale appearance of various anatomical structures on the PA and lateral chest x-rays.

- the interfaces created by anatomical structures on the PA and lateral chest x-rays.

Knowledge

You will review and understand

- the relationship between x-ray absorption and x-ray grayscale.

- the concept of radiation absorption events (RAEs) and how they impact on x-ray grayscale appearance.

- various grayscale shapes found on x-rays and how they are formed.

- where the 'problem spots' on chest x-rays are - those in which pathology can hide.

This chapter maps to the following AMSER curriculum content (1,2).

1) What produces density differences on radiographs?

2) The silhouette sign

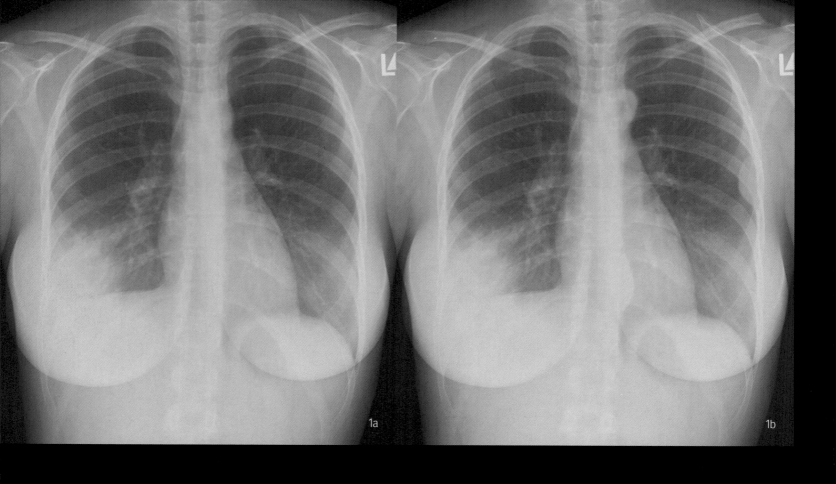

1a 1b

48

CASE STUDY

There are 5 differences between the two PA x-rays in the following two cases (Figs. 1a,b and 2a,b).

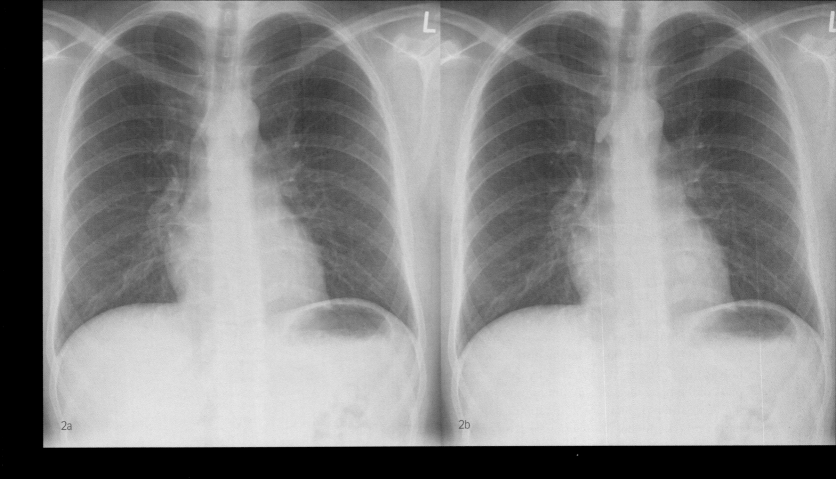

2a

2b

Can you find the differences?

THE CHEST X-RAY IMAGE

Y ou now understand how the x-ray examination is performed and you are looking at the chest x-ray images that you ordered. Before you can begin to interpret the images to provide your diagnosis, you need to understand the information found on the images. To start, you need to orient yourself to the chest x-ray images.

Patient Orientation on the X-ray Image - The Anatomical Position

The PA chest x-ray (Fig. 3a), is viewed as though the subject is standing upright and facing the observer. The right side of the patient is seen on the left-hand-side of the observer. The parts of the body closest to the observer are anterior. Parts of the body furthest from the observer are posterior (this is true for both PA and AP x-ray examinations). The parts of the body that are superior, or positioned towards the head of the patient, are at the top of the image. The parts of the body that are inferior, or positioned towards the feet of the patient, are at the bottom of the image.

On the lateral x-ray (Fig. 3b), the sternum is seen on the left, and the spine on the right, of the x-ray image. The structures positioned closer to the sternum are anterior (ventral) and the structures positioned closer to the spine are posterior (dorsal). Superior and inferior are the same as for the PA x-ray.

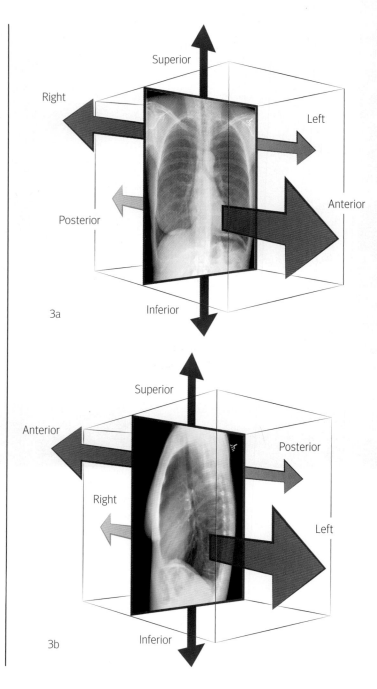

3a

3b

Figure 3. Patient anatomical orientation on chest x-rays. Illustrations of the anatomical orientation of, a, PA chest x-ray, b, lateral chest x-ray.

Patient Orientation on the CT Image - The Anatomical Position

Although CT scanning is beyond the scope of this book, throughout the book, CT images will be used to highlight important anatomical points related to the chest x-ray. For this reason, it is important to understand the patient orientation on a CT image.

In the CT scanner, the patient is almost always lying supine (Fig. 4a). The orientation of the body on the CT image corresponds to viewing the patient from the bottom of their feet (Fig. 4b). In this case, the right side of the patient is on the left side of the monitor – just like on the chest x-ray. Anterior anatomical structures lie more ventral, towards the sternum, and are seen on the top of the CT image. Posterior anatomical structures lie more dorsal, towards the spine, and are seen on the bottom of the CT image. Superior anatomical structures will be found in slices that are closer to the head, and inferior anatomical structures will be found on slices that are closer to the patient's feet.

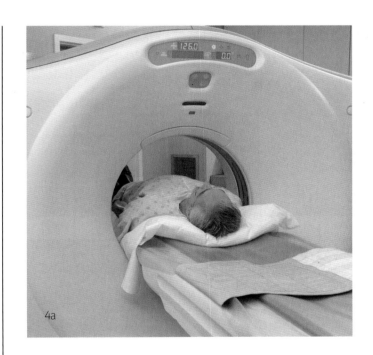
4a

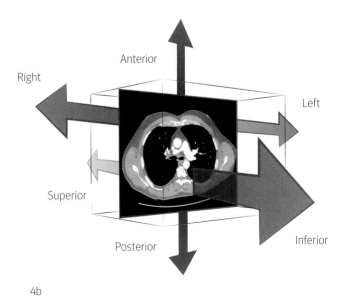
4b

Figure 4. Patient anatomical orientation on CT. Illustrations of a, patient positioned in scanner, b, patient anatomical orientation on the CT image. Photo courtesy: Craig Peters.

Anatomical markers are placed on x-ray and CT images to help understand the position of the patient and to indicate how the examination was performed (Fig. 5a,b). These markers can be either physical, made of lead, or digital.

Commonly used markers are:

R for patient's right side   **Exp** for intentional expiration x-ray   **Supine**   **Semi-erect**
L for patient's left side   **Ins** for intentional inspiration x-ray   **Erect**

Frequently, the initials of the technologist performing the examination are also visible.

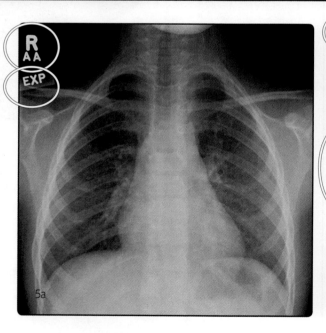

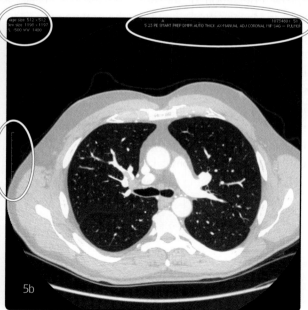

Figure 5. Markers are commonly found on x-rays and CT scans. a, PA chest x-ray with x-ray markers circled, R, right, EXP, expiration, AA, technologist initials, b, chest CT scan with CT markers circled.

THE X-RAY AS A GRAYSCALE IMAGE

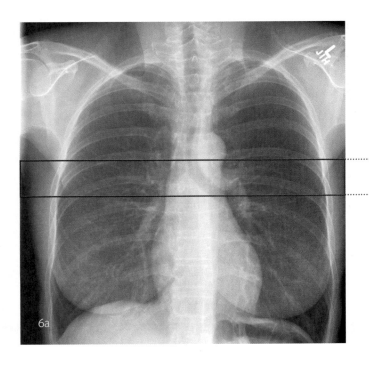

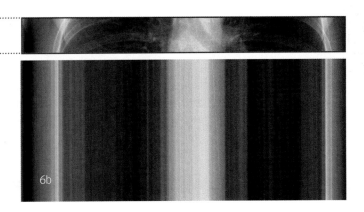

Whether on film or in digital format, the chest x-ray image is a 2D grayscale composite of radiological densities that represent the anatomical structures within the thorax. Understanding the grayscale of a chest x-ray will help you to extract the information necessary for accurate interpretation. The concept of 'the x-ray as a grayscale image' can be clarified through a discussion of the following concepts: grayscale, interfaces, geometrical shapes and familiarity.

By reading this book, you will learn the grayscale appearance of the normal anatomical structures (Fig. 6a,b).

Figure 6. Chest x-rays are 2D grayscale composites. a, normal PA chest x-ray, b, highlighted section from the same x-ray revealing the multiple changes in grayscale along the highlighted strip.

UNDERSTANDING GRAYSCALE

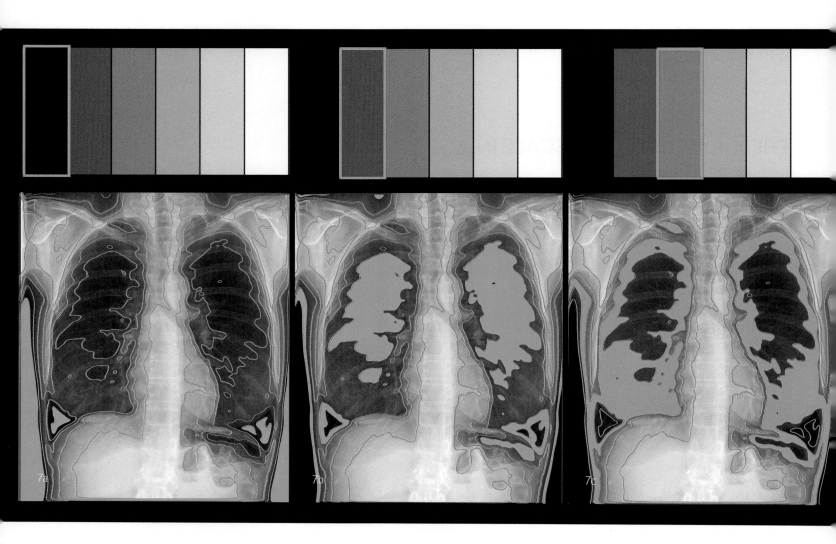

A grayscale image is an image in which each pixel carries only information about intensity.

Images of this sort are also known as black-and-white, and are composed exclusively of shades of gray, varying from black at the weakest intensity, to white at the strongest (4).

AMSER The normal chest x-ray image is a mosaic of various grayscale shapes that are a reflection of the underlying anatomy (Fig. 7a-f). As mentioned in the previous chapter, the anatomical structures within the thorax have varying propensities to absorb x-rays – they have different radiodensities. Black is the darkest possible shade and occurs when there is total absence of x-ray absorption. White is the lightest possible shade and occurs when there is total absorption of the x-rays.

Figure 7. A chest x-ray can be divided into regions of different grayscales. Series of images illustrating the division of a chest x-ray into six shades of gray from, a, completely black, to f, completely white. In each x-ray image the highlighted (orange) region of the x-ray corresponds to the (orange) region on the grayscale bar above it. Correlate with the normal PA chest x-ray found inside the front cover of this book.

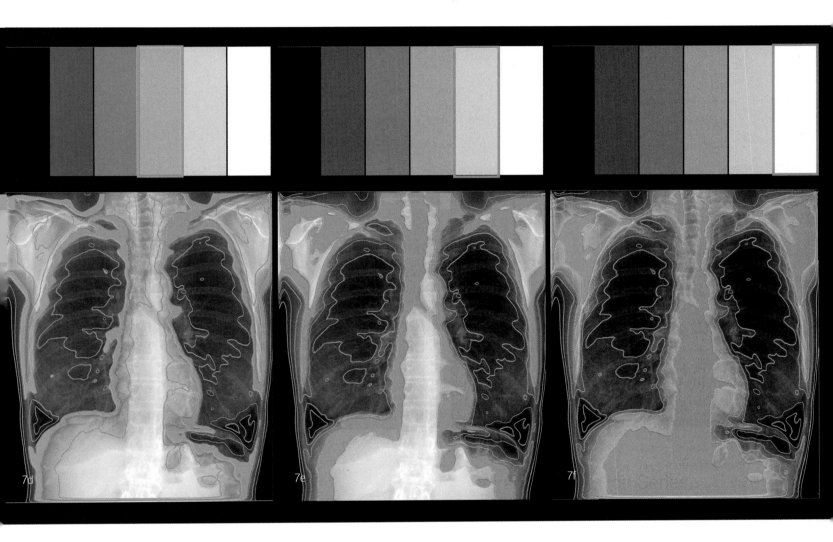

7d 7e 7f

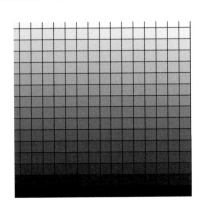

8

An 8-bit digital imaging system supports 256 shades of gray. A 10-bit system supports 1,024, and a 16-bit system supports 65,536. Most humans need a 1% change in brightness to discriminate between two shades of gray, so most humans should be able to discriminate about 100 different shades of gray in an 8-bit system (3) (Fig. 8).

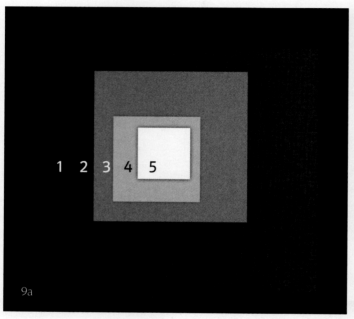

9a

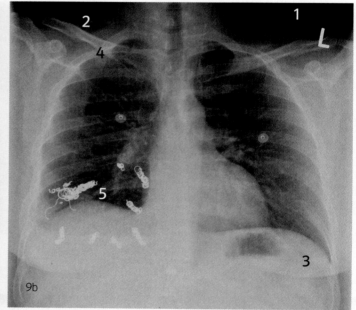

9b

AMSER Structures on the chest x-ray can be divided into four main grayscale densities: air, fat, soft tissue/fluid and bone/calcium (Fig. 9a,b). Air is the most radiolucent, has the weakest image intensity, and is black. Fat, soft tissues and fluids are gray, with fat lying in the blacker end of the spectrum. Bone has the strongest intensity for a normal anatomical structure, lying on the whiter end of the spectrum.

A fifth density is also frequently seen on chest x-rays – this density is not intrinsic to the human body, and represents metal or contrast material (Fig. 9b,c). Metal (or contrast material) has the strongest intensity and is very white.

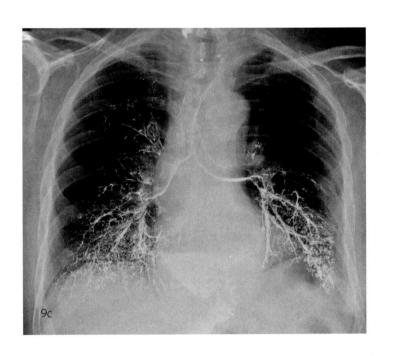

9c

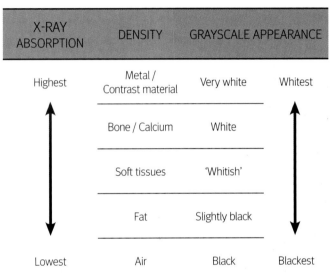

X-RAY ABSORPTION	DENSITY	GRAYSCALE APPEARANCE	
Highest	Metal / Contrast material	Very white	Whitest
	Bone / Calcium	White	
	Soft tissues	'Whitish'	
	Fat	Slightly black	
Lowest	Air	Black	Blackest

Table 2.1
The Relationship Between X-ray Absorption and Grayscale Appearance

Figure 9. Five main grayscale densities. a, illustration of the five main densities that can be seen on an x-ray, b, PA chest x-ray with the five main grayscale densities, (1) air, (2) fat, (3) soft tissues, (4) bone, and (5) metal/ contrast, metallic coils used to embolize A-V malformation in the right lung, c, PA chest x-ray showing an example of the fifth main grayscale density, contrast material; barium in lungs.

WHAT ARE RAEs ?
(RADIATION ABSORPTION EVENTS)

As the x-ray beam travels from the x-ray tube to the detector plate it passes through the entire thorax. The human body is complex, and therefore when the x-ray travels through the body, it will pass through a number of structures. As an x-ray beam travels through each structure, some of the energy of the x-ray photons is absorbed. This absorption of energy is called a radiation absorption event (RAE).

The number of RAEs will depend on the number of atoms with which the x-ray photons collide. Each time an x-ray photon collides with an atom, a single RAE occurs (Fig. 10a). Therefore, the amount of energy remaining in the photon upon exiting the material depends on the total of the individual RAEs along the path of the x-ray. The grand total of all RAEs an x-ray photon experiences along its path is the sum of all of the RAEs occurring through each structure it passes (Fig. 10b). In fact, a similar number of RAEs can be encountered in a larger, less dense, structure and in many smaller dense structures.

The differential absorption of the x-ray photons - or, in other words, the different number of RAEs experienced by photons - as they pass through the body produces the varied grayscale appearance on the resulting x-ray image. The more RAEs that cause absorption, the whiter the resulting x-ray image. For example, if we follow the paths of narrow portions of the x-ray beam, (illustrated on this CT image (Fig. 11a)), the corresponding point on the resulting 2D standard x-ray will have information regarding the anterior chest wall, ribs, lung, heart, etc., (Fig. 11b). The paths encountering more RAEs produce regions that are more white on the resulting x-ray.

Figure 10. What are radiation absorption events (RAEs)? Artistic representation of RAEs, a, a photon loses energy in an RAE as it strikes a series of atoms in a material; the more atoms it strikes, the more energy absorbed, and the less energy exiting, b, the total of all RAEs along the path of an x-ray is determined by the sum of the number of atoms encountered in each structure (due to its density or size) and the number of structures crossed. Notice how the same exiting energy can be produced by an x-ray encountering 3 RAEs in each of 2 structures, 2 RAEs in each of 3 structures, or 6 RAEs in 1 structure.

Figure 11. How a chest x-ray is formed from RAEs? a, the path of the x-ray through thoracic structures shown on a CT scan; the white structures are the most dense (the x-ray would encounter the highest number of RAEs), b, the resulting chest x-ray features (asterisks). Notice how the two regions, A and B, have a similar grayscale appearance on the x-ray, and yet are caused by vary different pattern of RAEs: A passes through many smaller more dense structures and B passes through a larger less dense structure, and yet must have a similar total number of RAEs. to generate a similar grayscale appearance on the resulting chest x-ray.

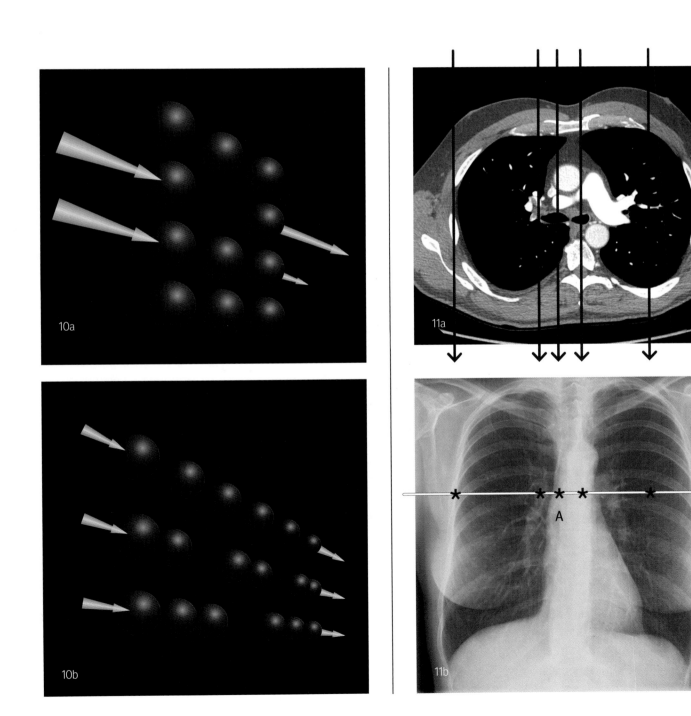

10a

10b

11a

11b

A

B

59

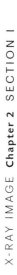
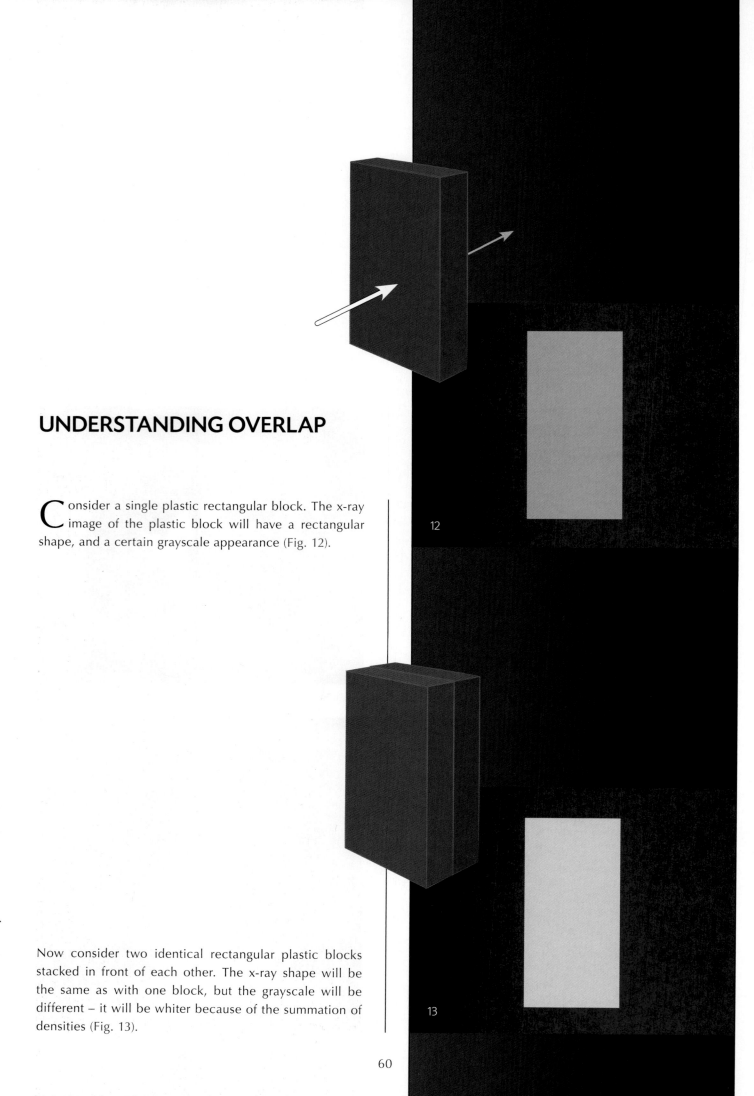

UNDERSTANDING OVERLAP

Consider a single plastic rectangular block. The x-ray image of the plastic block will have a rectangular shape, and a certain grayscale appearance (Fig. 12).

12

Now consider two identical rectangular plastic blocks stacked in front of each other. The x-ray shape will be the same as with one block, but the grayscale will be different – it will be whiter because of the summation of densities (Fig. 13).

13

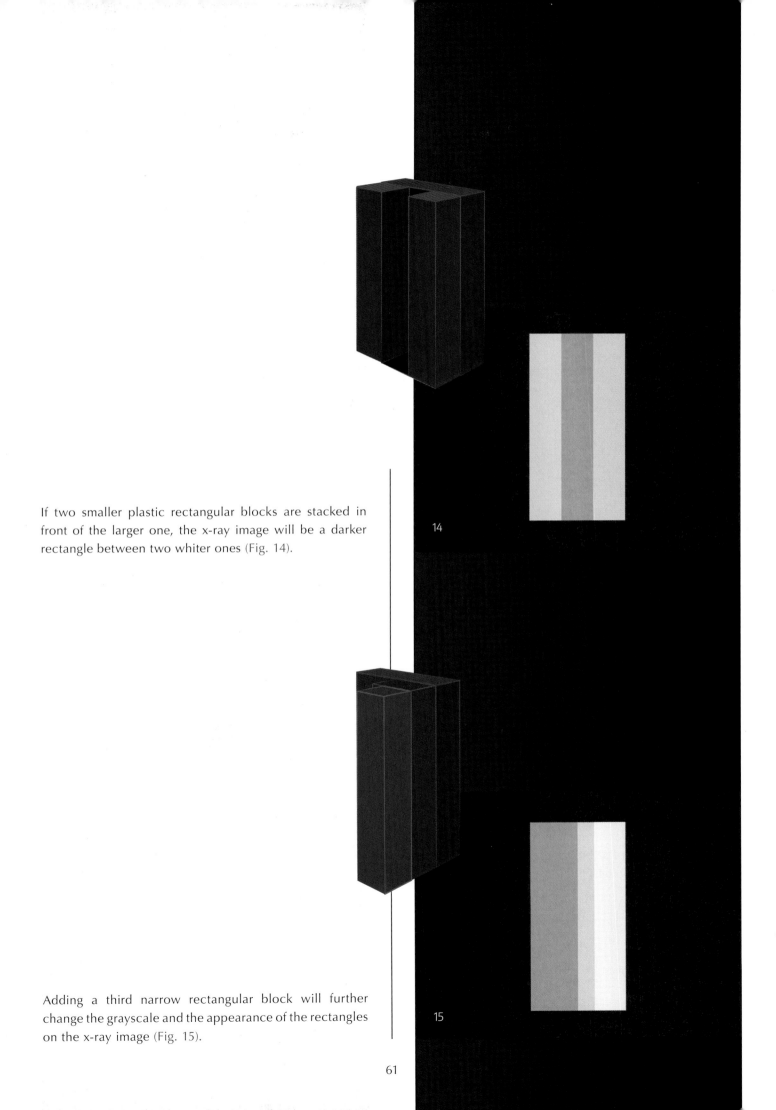

If two smaller plastic rectangular blocks are stacked in front of the larger one, the x-ray image will be a darker rectangle between two whiter ones (Fig. 14).

14

Adding a third narrow rectangular block will further change the grayscale and the appearance of the rectangles on the x-ray image (Fig. 15).

15

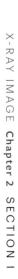

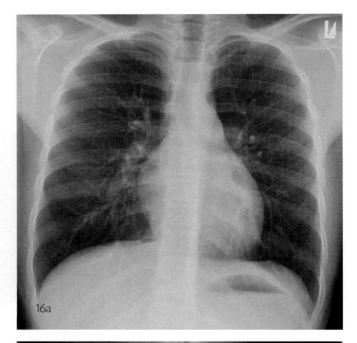

The Problem with Overlap

In a corresponding manner, the grayscale of an anatomical structure on a chest x-ray will be influenced by the overlap of other anatomical structures. For example, the grayscale of the heart will be influenced by the opacity of the lungs. Therefore, if, when examining an x-ray, the heart appears too white, this resulting abnormal grayscale could be a result of a pathology of the heart itself (e.g., chamber enlargement), or as a result of pathology in one of the structures that overlap the cardiac zone (e.g., pneumonia in the lungs). Similarly, the grayscale of the lungs will be influenced by the size and density (or percentage of adipose tissue) of the breasts (Fig. 16a,b,c).

Areas on a chest x-ray where the overlap of anatomical structures can obscure pathology are summarized in **Table 2.2** and **Table 2.3** (Pg. 64-65).

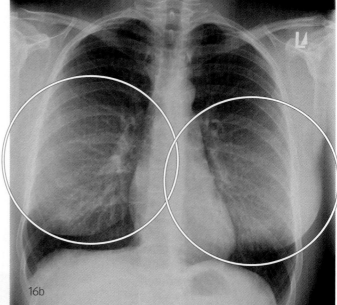

Figure 16. The grayscale of the lungs is altered by the overlap (or absence of) structures. a, normal PA chest x-ray; notice the grayscale of the lungs, b, PA chest x-ray where the lungs are too white because of overlapping breast tissue (highlighted), c, PA chest x-ray where the lungs are too white because of overlapping breast implants (highlighted).

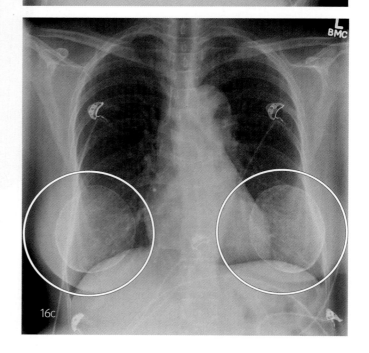

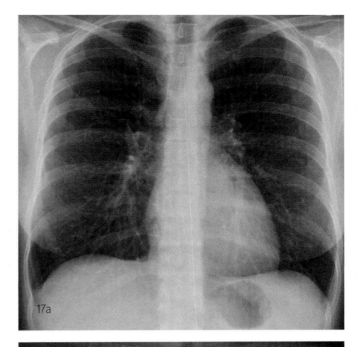

17a

The Specific Problem with Adipose Tissue

An excess of adipose tissue will cause an overall increase in whiteness of the x-ray. This is caused by the overlap effect of the increased tissues, and because of increased scatter radiation.

When the x-ray beam penetrates the body, some of the photons are deflected by tissue in the body, but still reach the x-ray detector. This is called scatter radiation.

Scatter radiation contains no useful clinical information as it arrives from random directions. It does, however, produce a uniform graying, or fogging, of the x-ray image, and can obscure useful information. The amount of scatter increases with an increase in adipose tissue (Fig. 17a,b,c).

17b

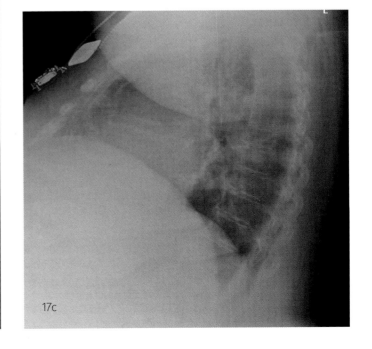

17c

Figure 17. Scatter radiation is increased with adipose tissue. a, normal PA chest x-ray, b, PA chest x-ray of an obese patient, c, lateral chest x-ray of an obese patient.

SUMMARY OF PARTICULARLY PROBLEMATIC AREAS DUE TO OVERLAP

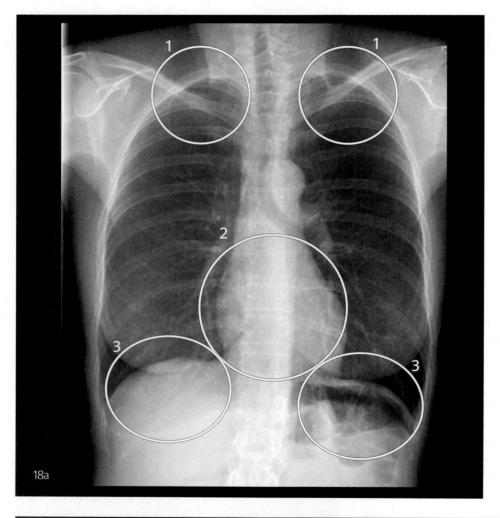

18a

PA X-RAY		
PROBLEMATIC AREA	REASON	RESULT
1. Apices of lungs	Overlapping ribs and clavicles	Undercall apical pathology
2. Retrocardiac region	Overlapping heart and spine	Undercall LLL, mediastinal and paraspinal pathology
3. Below dome of diaphragm(s)	Overlapping liver on the right, and the stomach and bowel gas on the left	Undercall LLL pathology and small effusions

Table 2.2
Summary of Particularly Problematic Areas Due to Overlap on the PA X-ray. LLL, left lower lobe.

> Not all difficult areas on the PA chest x-ray are the same on the lateral chest x-ray. Use of both the PA and lateral images can help identify most pathology – even in the difficult areas.

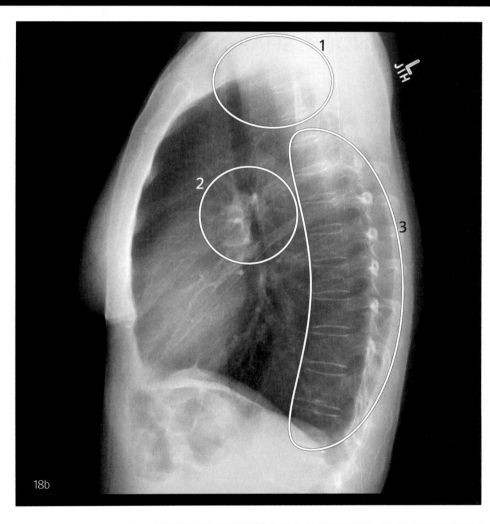

18b

LATERAL X-RAY		
PROBLEMATIC AREA	REASON	RESULT
1. Apices of lungs	Overlap of humerus and upper arm soft tissues	Undercall apical pathology
2. Hilar region	Overlap of the pulmonary arteries and the superior pulmonary veins	Overcall or undercall hilar pathology
3. Posterior lungs	Overlapping spine	Undercall mediastinal and lower lobe pathology

Table 2.3
Summary of Particularly Problematic Areas Due to Overlap on the Lateral X-ray

UNDERSTANDING SHAPES

We now know that the chest x-ray image is comprised of a pattern of varying grayscales. Similarly, the chest x-ray is comprised of a pattern of various geometric shapes. The shape of an object in space refers to the part of space occupied by the object, as determined by its external borders. Potential shapes that can be identified on chest x-rays include circles, arches and rectangles (Fig. 19a-f).

Anatomical Shapes and Familiarity

In the real world, identification of common geometrical shapes is easy, because of our familiarity with these shapes from an early age. In fact, if we superimpose common shapes onto a chest x-ray, these are easy to identify, even for someone with no medical experience. For example, a fork superimposed on a chest x-ray (Fig. 21) is easily and confidently identified. However, we have no intrinsic familiarity with the shape of the aorta or of the pulmonary arteries. Understanding the radiological shape of the various anatomical structures, such as the aorta (Fig. 21a,b), on an x-ray will allow you to then look for these structures in a way analogous to finding Waldo in the Where's Waldo books (4). This requires patience on the part of the learner, and practice.

The radiological shape of each of the anatomical structures of the thorax will be described individually in Section II.

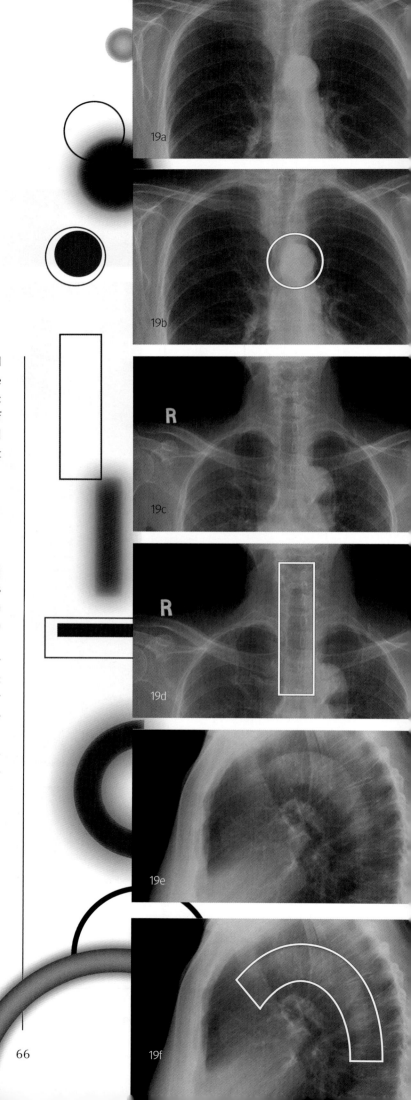

19a

19b

19c

19d

19e

19f

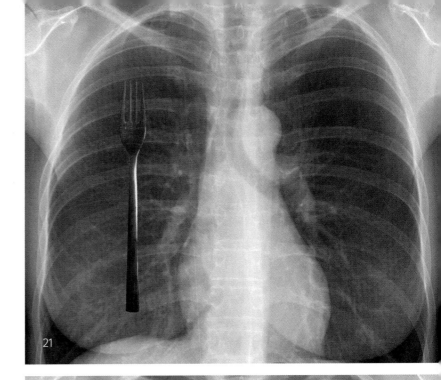

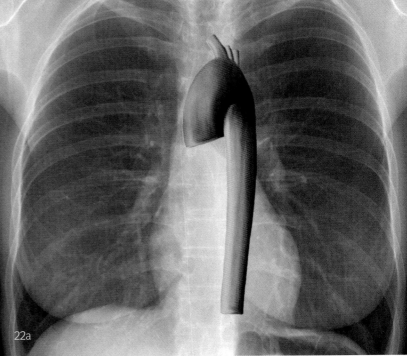

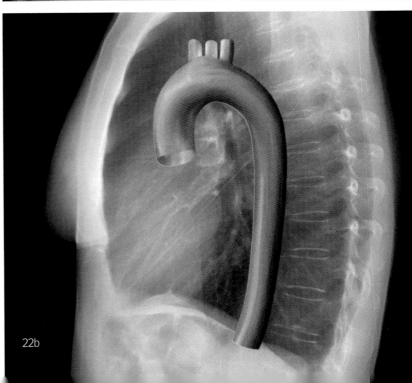

Figure 19. An x-ray is made of many geometrical shapes. Examples of shapes on an x-ray. a, white circle, b, white circle highlighted, c, black rectangle, d, black rectangle highlighted, e, white arch, f, white arch highlighted.

Figure 20. Familiar objects are easy to identify on an x-ray. For example, the fork superimposed on this chest x-ray.

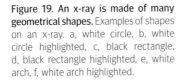

Figure 21. Anatomical structures can be thought of as familiar shapes on a chest x-ray. Once we know the aorta has a familiar shape of a 3D arch, it can then be easily identified on the a, PA and, b, lateral chest x-rays.

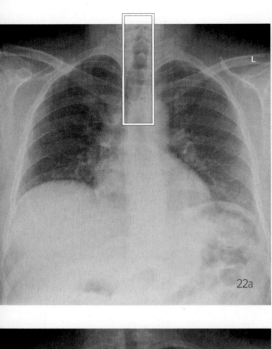

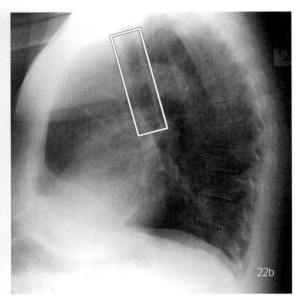

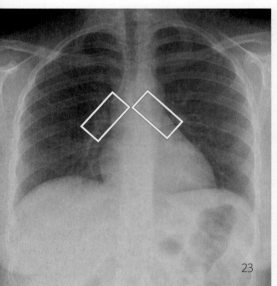

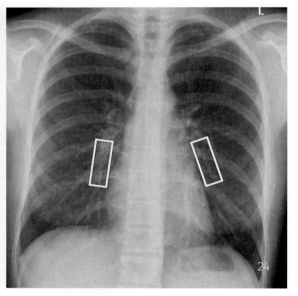

Rectangles

The radiological shadow of the trachea on the PA and lateral chest x-rays is a black rectangle that is vertically oriented, extending from the neck region, inferiorly to the carina in the mid-thorax (Fig. 22a,b).

Two smaller black rectangles extend from the trachea. These course obliquely and are created by the main stem bronchi (Fig. 23).

Examples of white rectangles are the blood vessels that are orientated perpendicular to the x-ray beam (Fig. 24t).

Figure 22. Geometric shapes on chest x-rays - large rectangles. The trachea forms a large black rectangle on both the a, PA and, b, lateral x-rays.

Figure 23. Geometric shapes on chest x-rays - small rectangles. Smaller black rectangles are formed by the airways when they lie perpendicular to the x-ray beam.

Figure 24. Geometric shapes on chest x-rays - small rectangles. Smaller white rectangles are formed by the blood vessels when they lie perpendicular to the x-ray beam.

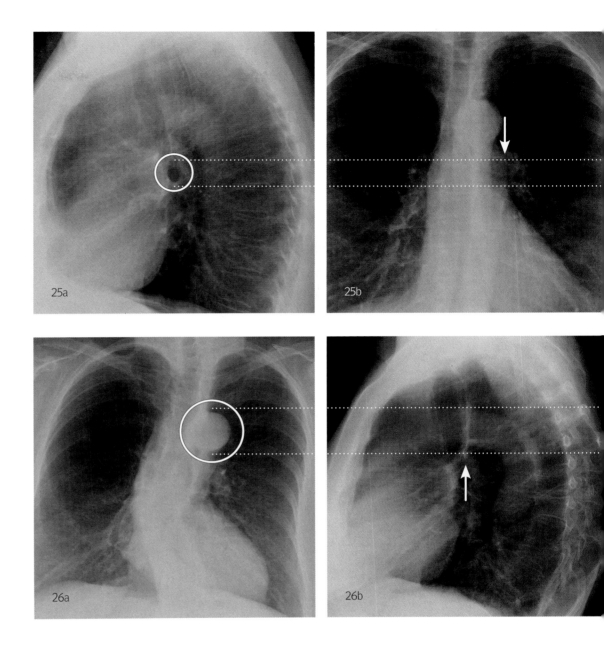

Circles

The radiological shadow of any round or spherical structure will be a circle. Normally there are no round structures in the thorax. However, black or white circles are seen on x-rays when elongated cylindrical structures, such as blood vessels or airways, are viewed end-on. In this case, the circle will only be seen in one plane; so it will be visible either on the PA, or the lateral x-rays (Figs. 25a,b and 26a,b).

Figure 25. Geometric shapes on chest x-rays - black circles. Black circles on x-rays can be formed by the airways. a, if a bronchus lies parallel to the x-ray beam it will appear as a black circle as on this lateral chest x-ray, b, a corresponding circle will not be seen on the PA chest x-ray.

Figure 26. Geometric shapes on chest x-rays - white circles I. White circles on x-rays can be formed by the blood vessels. a, if a vessel lies parallel to the x-ray beam it will appear as a white circle as on this PA chest x-ray, b, a corresponding circle will not be seen on the lateral chest x-ray.

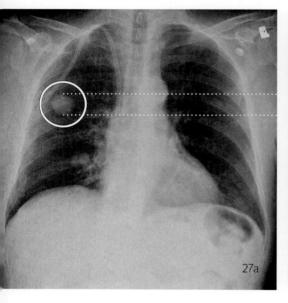

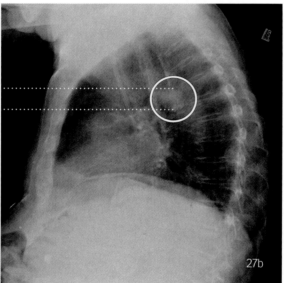

27a

27b

On the other hand, tumors in the lung will often exhibit a spherical form and will, therefore, be visible as a circle on an x-ray. Importantly, since tumors have a spherical form, the circle will be present on both the PA and lateral x-rays (Fig. 27a,b).

Figure 27. Geometric shapes on chest x-rays - white circles II. White circles on an x-ray can also be formed by a tumor; unlike the blood vessels, the white circle will be seen on both the a, PA and, b, lateral x-rays.

Figure 28. Geometric shapes on chest x-rays - white arches. White arches are also found on x-rays: a, the left pulmonary artery (LPA) forms a white arch on the PA x-ray, b, the aorta forms a large white arch on the lateral x-ray.

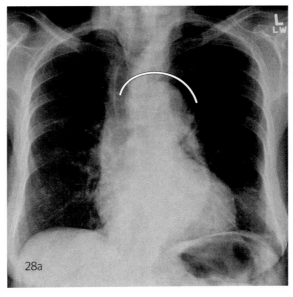

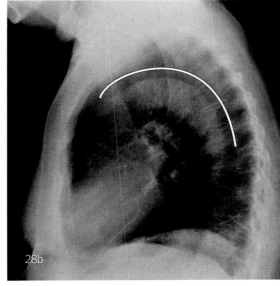

28a

28b

Arches

We have already described rectangles and how rectangular radiological shadows form. Arches can be thought of as curved rectangles. Arching occurs with the blood vessels when the vessels are either changing direction (e.g., from cranial to caudal, like the aorta), or if the vessel is passing over another anatomical structure. Since, most often, the arches identified on x-rays are blood vessels, they will be seen as white arches (Fig. 28a,b).

RECTANGLES	Black	Trachea, bronchi
	White	Blood vessels
CIRCLES	Black	Bronchi
	White	Blood vessels
ARCHES	White	Aortic arch Left pulmonary artery (LPA)

Table 2.4
Geometrical Shapes on the Chest X-ray

How X-ray Shapes Are Formed

The resulting 2D x-ray shapes 'cast' by the 3D structures in the body can be explained using the analogy of light shining on objects and their cast shadows.

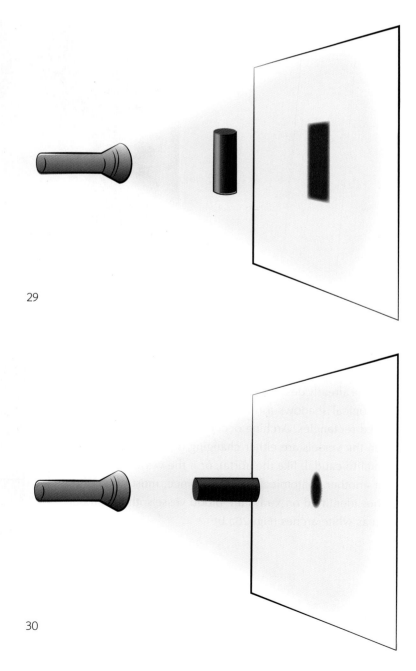

If you shine a light on a solid cylinder that lies perpendicular to the axis of the light beam, the shadow will look like a rectangle (Fig. 29).

29

If you now angle the cylinder so that the long axis of the cylinder is parallel to the axis of the light beam, the shadow will now look like a circle (Fig. 30).

30

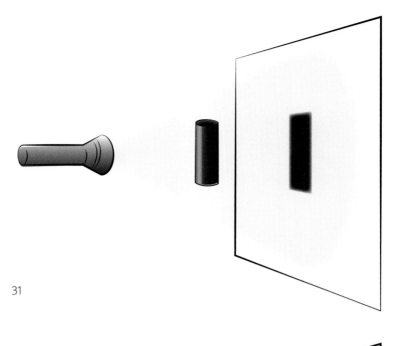

If the cylinder is hollow and perpendicular to the light beam, it will remain a rectangle (Fig. 31).

31

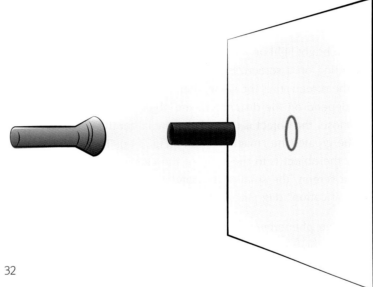

If the hollow cylinder is parallel to the light beam, it will look like a ring (Fig. 32).

32

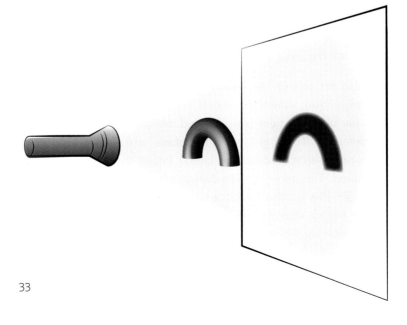

Curve the cylinder, and it will look like an arch (Fig. 33).

33

The Magnification Phenomenon
On Chest X-rays

Shine a bright light on an object and you will get a shadow projecting on a screen. If the distance between the light and the screen stays the same, then the size of the shadow will depend on the distance of the object from the light. The closer the object is to the light, the larger the shadow, or, the greater the "magnification" (Fig. 34a). The farther away the object is to the light, or the closer the object is to the screen, the smaller the shadow, or, the lesser the "magnification" (Fig. 34b).

The same phenomenon occurs on chest x-rays. Objects closer to the x-ray source will become magnified relative to objects farther away from the x-ray source. A good example of this phenomenon is the difference in the size of the heart on PA and AP chest x-rays. Since the heart is an anterior structure in the thorax, in the AP projection, the heart will be closer to the x-ray source than on the PA projection. The heart size will be magnified on the AP projection (Fig. 35a,b).

We also see this on the lateral chest x-ray with the ribs. By convention, when the lateral exposure is taken, the left side of the patient is positioned against the cassette or detector. The right ribs, therefore, are closer to the x-ray source, and on the lateral image they will be magnified. This allows you to distinguish between the left and right ribs on the lateral x-ray, and is also the basis for the big rib sign (the ribs appear big because they are magnified) (Fig. 36).

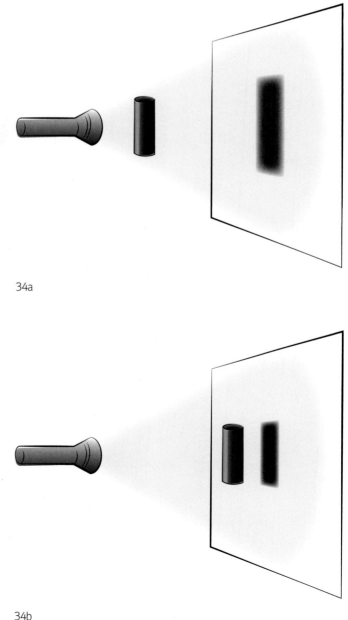

34a

34b

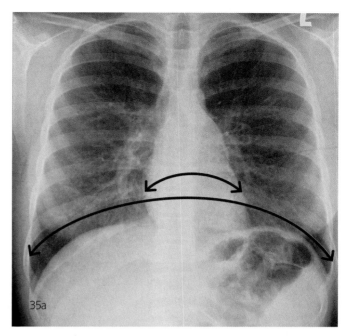

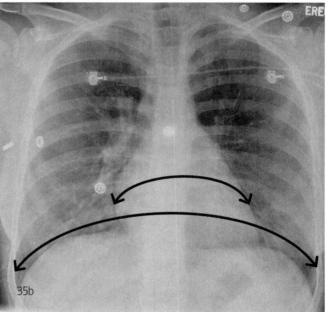

Figure 34. Illustration of the magnification phenomenon. Illustration of the resulting shadow created by an object when it is, a, close to the light source and magnified, b, far from the light source (closer to the screen) and smaller.

Figure 35. The magnification phenomenon. Example chest x-rays showing the magnification phenomenon as it relates to heart size. a, normal heart size on a PA x-ray, b, the normal heart size is magnified on an AP chest x-ray because it is closer to the x-ray source in the AP orientation.

Figure 36. Magnification phenomenon — big rib sign. Example chest x-rays showing the magnification phenomenon as it relates to the big rib sign. The right ribs (white arrows) will appear larger than the left ribs (purple arrows), or magnified, because they are closer to the x-ray source.

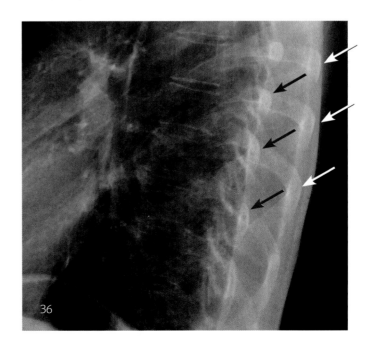

!

The concept of shape is directly linked with the concept of interface.
Without interfaces, there are no shapes.

UNDERSTANDING INTERFACES

An interface is a surface forming a common boundary between two things.

If the thorax were filled with a homogeneous soft tissue density, the chest x-ray grayscale appearance would be simple – a homogeneous gray. If the thorax were filled with a homogeneous air density, the chest x-ray grayscale appearance would be simple – a homogeneous black. Since the contents of the thorax are comprised of multiple anatomical structures of varying size, density and location, the chest x-ray becomes a composite of structures with varying grayscales. The structures can be separated from each other only if an interface exists between them.

In the normal chest, five different types of interfaces can be identified:

1. Interfaces between the lungs and the mediastinal structures.

2. Interfaces between mediastinal structures and the air in the airways.

3. Interfaces between mediastinal structures and bone.

4. Interfaces between the lungs.

5. Interfaces between the skin and the air surrounding the patient.

From a cross-section of the thorax (Fig. 37a,b), the number of interfaces that will occur on a chest x-ray can be easily established (Fig. 37c). On this example, there are three clear reasons for interfaces to occur between the mediastinal structures and other structures.

The concept of interfaces as they pertain to the chest x-ray will be thoroughly discussed in **Chapter 9**, The Mediastinum.

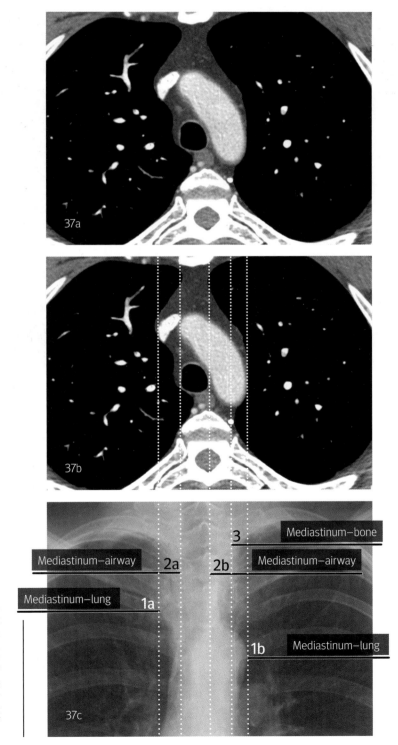

Figure 37. Predicting interfaces on a chest x-ray. Interfaces on a chest x-ray form when there is a common boundary between two structures. a, a CT scan of the thorax, b, predicted interfaces (dotted lines) on a CT scan of the thorax, c, corresponding interfaces (arrows) on a chest x-ray; 1a, superior vena cava, 1b, edge of aorta, 2a, right border of trachea, 2b, left border of trachea, 4, left paraspinal edge.

Mediastinum–bone

Mediastinum–airway

Mediastinum–airway

Mediastinum–lung

Mediastinum–lung

A spherical structure will have an infinite number of possible interfaces on an x-ray (Fig. 38).

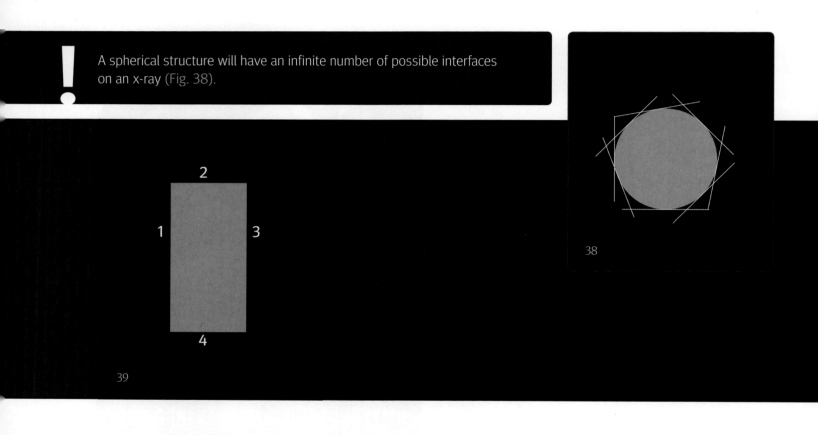

38

39

How Do Interfaces Work?

An x-ray interface will only exist if there is enough density difference between the adjacent structures, so that on the x-ray, the structures will be seen as distinct elements.

An x-ray of a rectangle made of plastic (Fig. 39) appears as a rectangle on an x-ray because the rectangle is surrounded by room air. Four interfaces will be identified, related to the four visible edges; left, right, upper and lower.

If we have two separate rectangles, but one is smaller than the other (Fig. 40a), the x-ray will show both rectangles as separate structures (and there will be eight interfaces). If we move the smaller rectangle so that it stands in front of the larger rectangle (Fig. 40b), the x-ray will show a structure with five interfaces.

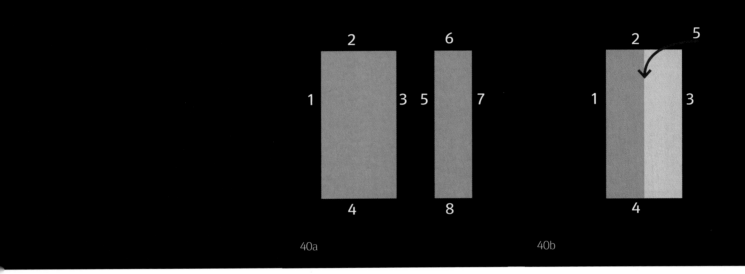

40a

40b

Figure 38. The interfaces of a sphere.
A sphere forms an infinite number of
interfaces on an x-ray.

Figure 39. The interfaces of a
rectangle. A plastic rectangle will form
four interfaces on an x-ray.

Figure 40. How do interfaces work?
PART I a, two plastic rectangles will
each create four interfaces on an x-ray,
for a total of eight interfaces, b, if one
rectangle is brought in front of the other,
they will form five interfaces.

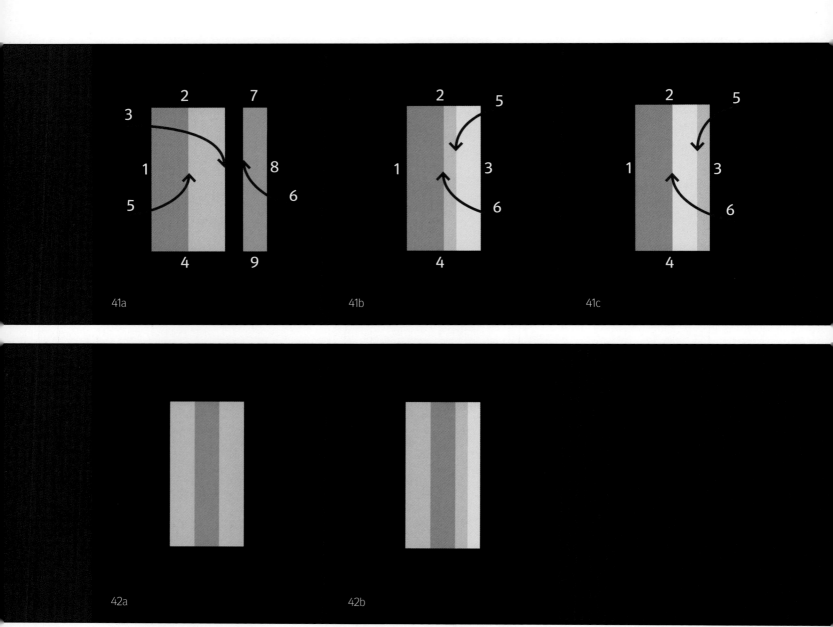

41a   41b   41c

42a   42b

If we now add a third, even narrower rectangle, the x-ray will show nine interfaces (Fig. 41a). If we position this third rectangle in front of the other two, as in Figure 41b, the x-ray will now show three rectangles and a total of six interfaces. By changing the position of the third rectangle so it lies more medially (Fig. 41c), the three rectangles remain visible and again there are six interfaces present. Only the position of the rectangles has changed.

By changing the location of the rectangles and adding additional rectangles (Fig. 42a,b), the appearance of the objects on the x-ray, and their grayscale, will change in a very predictable manner.

AMSER   Alternatively, if two structures are of a similar radiological density and abut one another, the interface between the two is lost and the two structures will be seen as one (Fig. 43a,b). This is called the silhouette sign (**Ch. 17, Pg. 654**) – an important indicator of pathology.

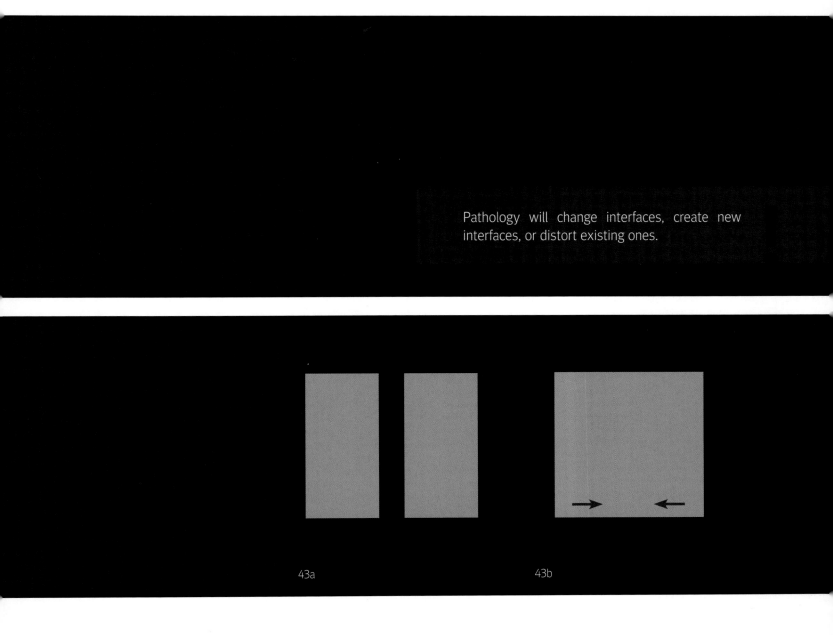

Pathology will change interfaces, create new interfaces, or distort existing ones.

43a 43b

In the normal individual, a number of interfaces are present in the cardiac and mediastinal regions between the lungs and surrounding soft tissues. When pathology exists that alters the appearance of aeration in the normal air-filled lung, one or more of these interfaces may be lost. For example, consolidation of the right lower lobe may make it difficult to see a part, or all, of the right diaphragm.

Figure 41. How do interfaces work? PART II. a, if a third rectangle is added there will be nine interfaces on the x-ray, b, if that rectangle is brought in front of the other two, there will be six interfaces on the x-ray.

Figure 42. How do interfaces work? PART III. When the a, shape, b, position or number of rectangles is changed, the number of interfaces on the x-ray will change in a predictable manner.

Figure 43. Interfaces and the silhouette sign. The silhouette sign is created when two objects of a similar density are brought next to each other and there is no interface formed between the two on the x-ray. a, two rectangles of similar density appear distinctly, b, when brought together the same two rectangles are now seen as one due to the lack of an interface formed between them.

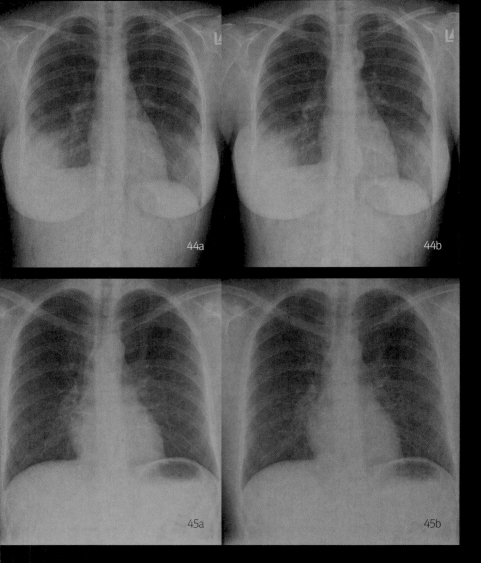

44a 44b

45a 45b

Can you find them?

Find five differences between the two PA x-rays in the following two cases (Figs. 44a,b and 45a,b).

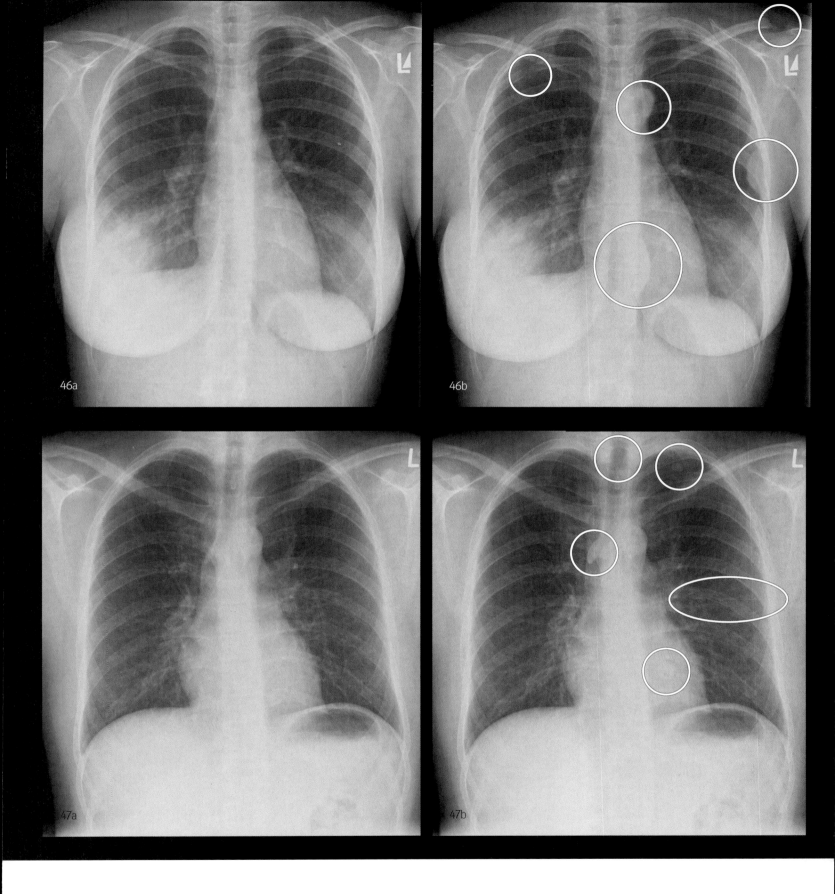

46a

46b

47a

47b

83

References

1. Lewis, P.J., Shaffer, K., & Donovan, A. (Eds.). (2012). AMSER National Medical Student Curriculum in Radiology. http://aur.org/Secondary-Alliances.aspx?id=141.

2. Lewis, P.J., & Shaffer, K. (2005). Developing a national medical student curriculum in radiology. *Am. Coll. Radiol. 2*(1):8–11.

3. Kimpe, T., & Tuytschaever, T. (2007). Increasing the number of gray shades in medical display systems-- how much is enough? *J. Digital Imag., 20*(4):422–32.

4. Handford, M. (1997). *Where's Waldo?* Somerville, MA: Candlewick Press.

CHAPTER 3
WHAT SHOWS UP on a CHEST X-RAY?

importance

To order x-rays appropriately, you will require an understanding of the value, and the limitations, of the technology.

This chapter gives an overview of various thorax pathologies and how they alter the grayscale of the chest x-ray image. You will learn how to correctly identify radiological patterns formed by pathology on a chest x-ray. These patterns form the basis for the radiological differential diagnosis.

objectives

Skills

You will identify

- the different kinds of pathology found within the thorax.
- the pathologies on PA and lateral chest x-rays that affect: the airspaces, the interstitium, the pleura, the pleural space, the mediastinum, the hilum, and the chest wall.

Knowledge

You will review and understand

- the classification of pathology, based on appearance, on a chest x-ray.
- the process of determining if the grayscale of the x-ray is abnormal.
- the pathological conditions within the thorax, and how they affect the grayscale of the x-ray.
- the basics of radiological signs and patterns.

associated resources

This chapter maps to the following AMSER curriculum content (1,2).

1) Terminology used in radiology (reports).
   Plain films/fluoroscopy
      Lucency, opacity
   Computed Tomography (CT)
      Attenuation, Hounsfield units
   Ultrasound
      Hyper- and hypo-echoic
   MRI
      Increased and decreased signal intensity

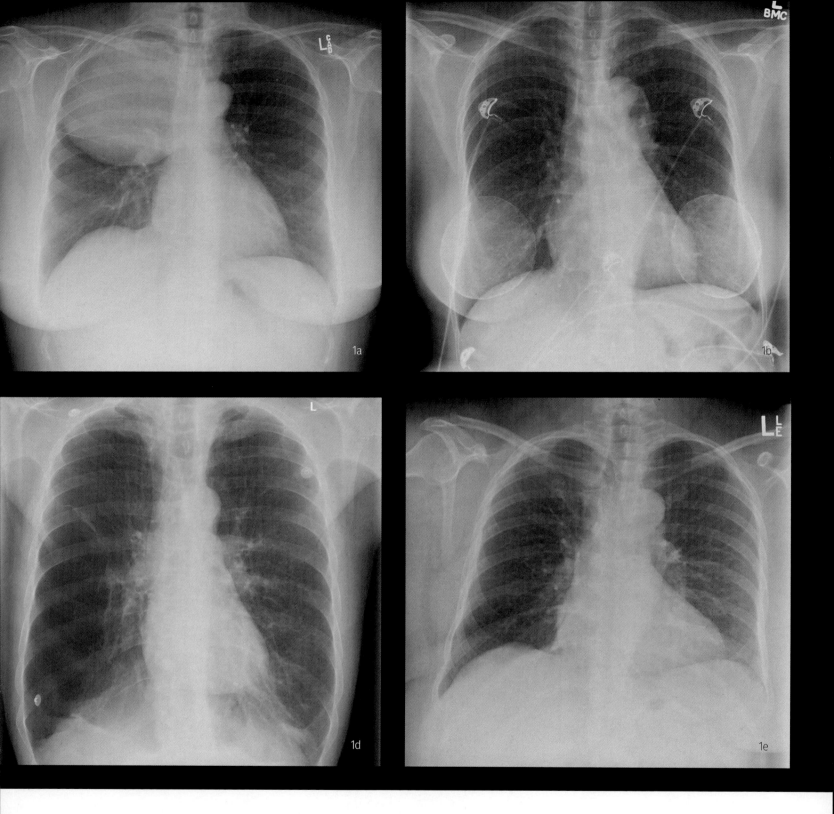

Pathology on chest x-rays will usually shift the grayscale of part, or all, of the x-ray to too white or too black. In each of the following six images there is an obvious abnormality (Fig. 1a,b,c,d,e,f).

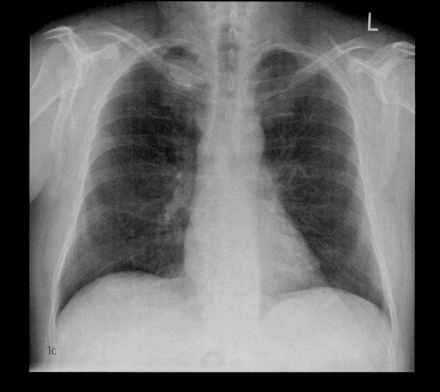

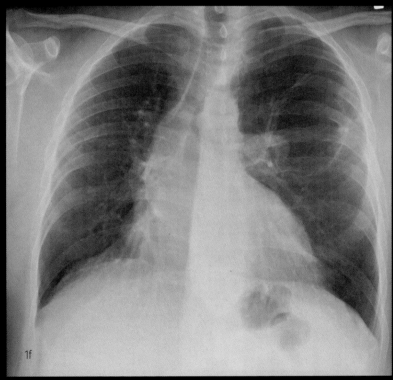

Describe the shift of the grayscale (too white or too black) caused by the abnormality as compared to the normal image found on the inside front cover.

THE CLASSIFICATION OF CHEST X-RAY PATHOLOGY BASED ON GRAYSCALE APPEARANCE

The concept of what is considered the normal grayscale appearance of individual anatomical structures on a chest x-ray is discussed in further detail in the chapters on radiological anatomy in Section II. In addition to the normal anatomical structures that will be described in **Chapters 7-14**, various pathological conditions will also manifest themselves on a chest x-ray, and can be classified in terms of how they alter the normal grayscale appearance.

AMSER   A pathological condition on a chest x-ray can be described as one that:

1) causes a change in the GRAYSCALE – "too white" or "too black" (Fig. 2a):

a) too white: pathological changes that will absorb more of the x-ray beam compared to normal and, therefore, will cause the grayscale of an anatomical structure, or region, to look 'too white' (shift of grayscale to white);

b) too black: pathological changes that will absorb less of the x-ray beam compared to normal and, therefore, will cause the grayscale of an anatomical structure, or region, to look 'too black' (shift of grayscale to black);

	NORMAL	"TOO WHITE"	"TOO BLACK"
X-ray	Normal density	Increased density Increased opacity Decreased lucency	Decreased density Decreased opacity Increased lucency
CT	Isoattenuation	Hyperattenuation Increase in Hounsfield units	Hypoattenuation Decrease in Hounsfield units
MRI	Isosignal intensity	Increased signal intensity	Decreased signal intensity
US	Isoechoic	Hyperechoic	Hypoechoic (anechoic)

Table 3.1
Terminology Used to Describe the Changes Caused by Pathology on X-ray, CT, MRI and US. CT, computed tomography, MRI, magnetic resonance imaging, US, ultrasound.

Figure 2. Changes to grayscale shadows due to pathology. a, pathology can cause the grayscale shift to "too white" or "too black".

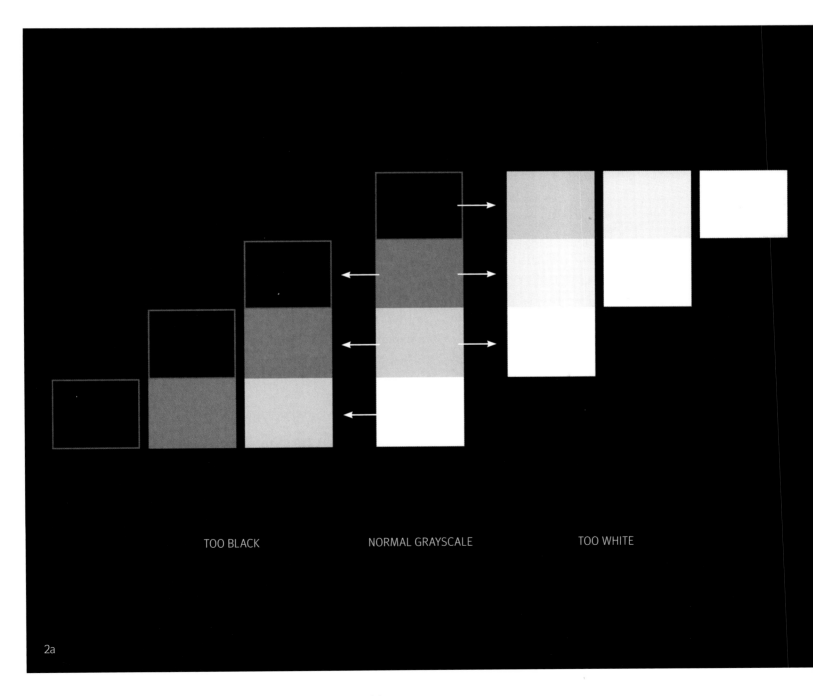

TOO BLACK   NORMAL GRAYSCALE   TOO WHITE

2a

2) does not change the shade of the grayscale, but alters the normal SIZE of the grayscale shadow cast by an anatomical structure or region - "too much white/black" or "too little white/black" (Fig. 2b):

a) too much white or black: pathology that causes an increase in the size, or extent, of the anatomical structure/region (e.g., too big, too long, or enlarged);

b) too little: those that cause a decrease in the size of the anatomical structure/region (e.g., too small, or shortened);

3) does not change the grayscale, but SHIFTS/DISPLACES the POSITION of the anatomical structure, or region, so that its shadow occupies a different position on the grayscale image (alters the configuration of the grayscale regions on the x-ray image) (Fig. 2c):

a) shifted vertically (i.e., more superior, inferior);

b) shifted horizontally (i.e, more lateral, medial, left of midline, right of midline);

4) does not change the grayscale, but alters or DISTORTS the SHAPE of the grayscale shadow cast by an anatomical structure or region (Fig. 2d):

a) widened or distended;

b) narrowed or pinched.

Figure 2. Changes to grayscale shadows due to pathology. Pathology can cause the grayscale shadow of a structure to, b, change in size, c, change in position, d, change in shape.

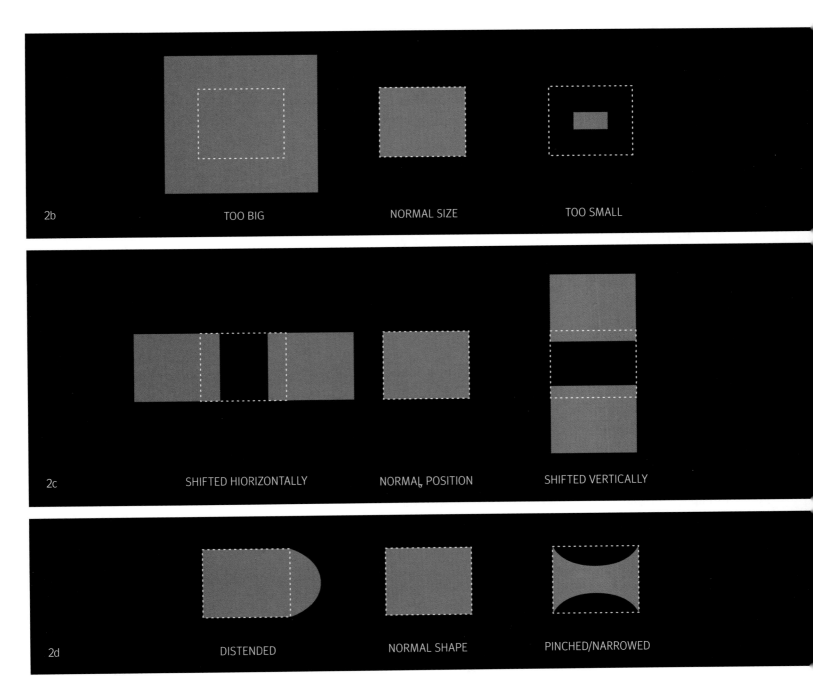

2b   TOO BIG   NORMAL SIZE   TOO SMALL

2c   SHIFTED HIORIZONTALLY   NORMAL POSITION   SHIFTED VERTICALLY

2d   DISTENDED   NORMAL SHAPE   PINCHED/NARROWED

HOW WILL YOU KNOW IF THE GRAYSCALE IS ABNORMAL?

To determine if the chest x-ray is abnormal requires a strong understanding of what the normal grayscale looks like. The grayscale pattern of a normal chest x-ray provides the comparative background or template. Pathology will represent what is remaining on a chest x-ray after the normal background has been removed or subtracted. The process is akin to the "spot the difference" puzzles in which you are required to identify the differences between two very similar pictures (Figs. 3a,b and 4a,b).

With experience, this becomes an automatic process. As a learner, it is important for you to have an example of a normal x-ray handy to be used for comparison (e.g., the normal x-rays on the inside covers of this book).

With practice, you will eventually establish a mental template based on this normal grayscale. Until then, one of the most important tools for determining whether the grayscale of an x-ray is normal or abnormal, is the patient's previous x-ray(s). The previous images give a template that can be used directly in the analysis.

If you suspect an abnormality that is too white, and no previous x-rays are available, you can confirm the suspicion by comparing the grayscale of the suspected area with the grayscale of other parts of the same structure (or when the structure is bilateral, with the contralateral structure). For example if a region of the right lung looks too white, you can compare that region with other regions of the right lung, and/or with similar regions of the left lung.

The following lists are given as an introduction to the concept of grayscale changes with pathology. More detailed descriptions of pathology on chest x-rays, specific to anatomical structures, will be given in the radiological anatomy section (**Section II**) of this book.

Figure 3. Spot the difference I. Spot the difference in grayscale between, a, pre-treatment, and b, post-treatment, on the x-rays. (Left effusion - cleared.)

Figure 4. Spot the difference II. Spot the difference in grayscale between, a, pre-treatment, and b, post-treatment, on the x-rays. (Left airspace consolidation - cleared.)

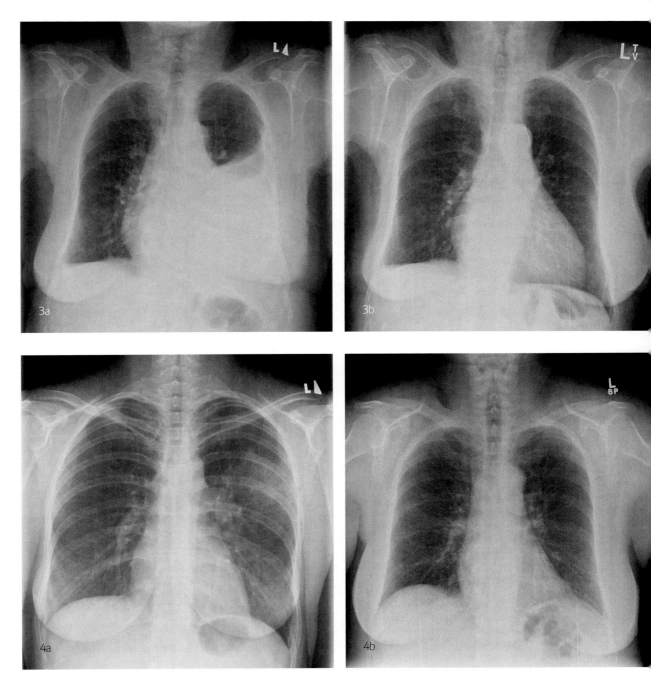

3a

3b

4a

4b

SUMMARY OF
PATHOLOGICAL CONDITIONS
WITHIN THE THORAX

AIRSPACES

Pneumonia (Fig. 5)
Hemorrhage
Fluid
Tumor

5

THAT CHANGE
THE GRAYSCALE
TO "TOO WHITE"

Inflammation (Fig. 6)
Infiltration
Tumor

Fluid (either exudate or transudate)(Fig. 7)
Calcification
Tumor

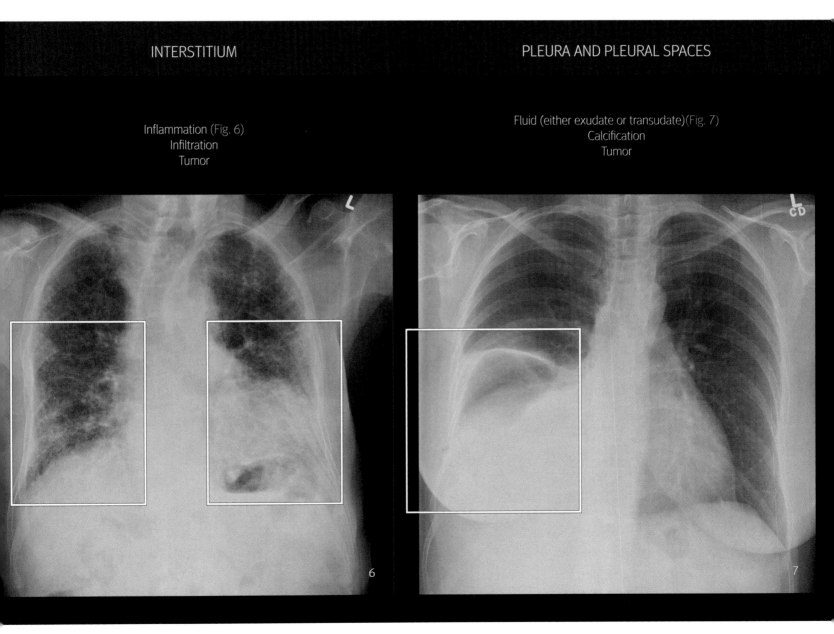

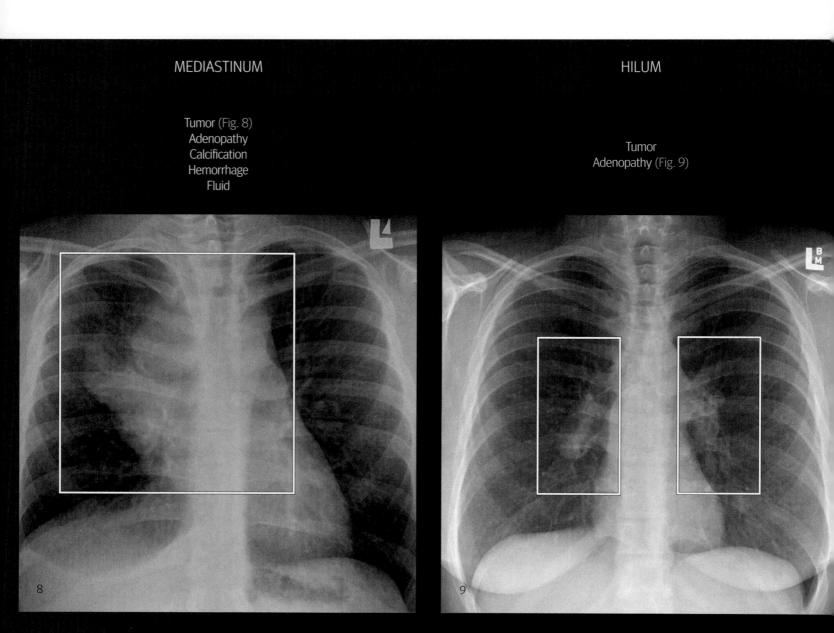

MEDIASTINUM

Tumor (Fig. 8)
Adenopathy
Calcification
Hemorrhage
Fluid

HILUM

Tumor
Adenopathy (Fig. 9)

8

9

CHEST WALL

Tumor (Fig. 10)
Infection
Chest wall hematoma

HEART AND PERICARDIUM

Calcification (Fig. 11)

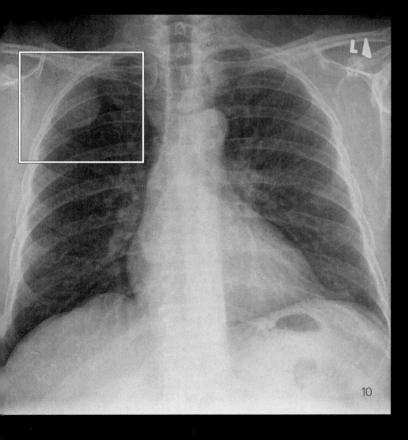

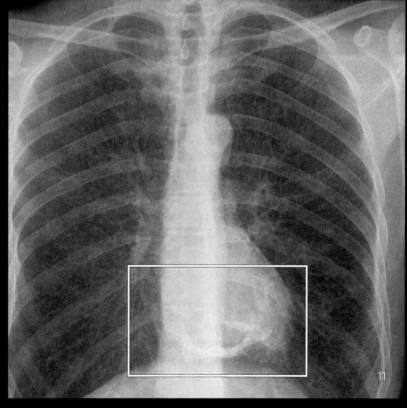

AIRSPACES

Bullae (Fig. 12)
Cysts
Cavity
Air trapping / Hyperinflation

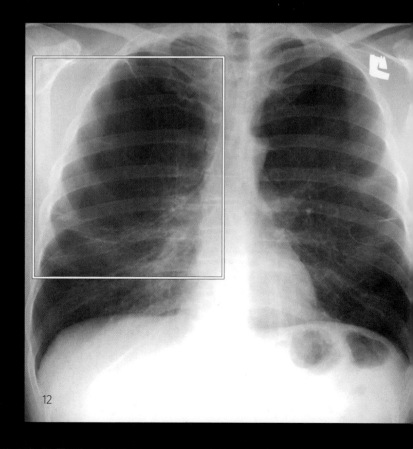

12

**THAT CHANGE
THE GRAYSCALE
TO "TOO BLACK"**

PLEURA AND PLEURAL SPACES

Pneumothorax (Fig. 13)
Air within a hydropneumothorax

MEDIASTINUM

Pneumomediastinum
Hiatus hernia (Fig. 14)
Air within an obstructed esophagus

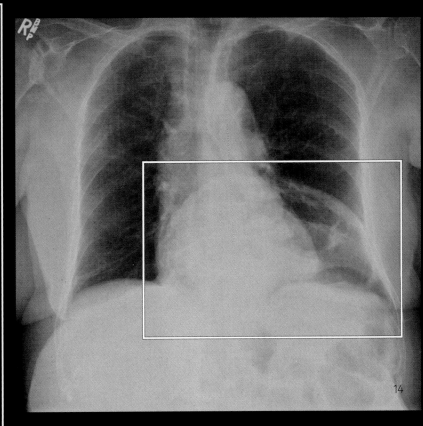

CHEST WALL

Surgical emphysema (Fig. 15)
Previous surgery

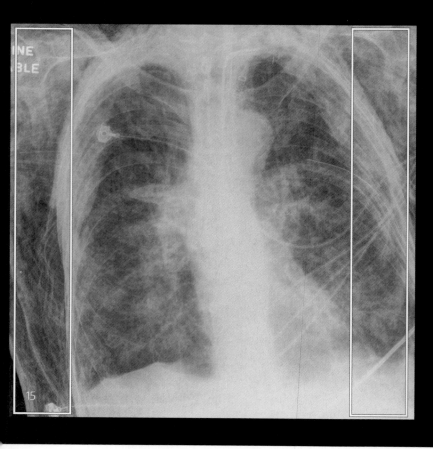

HEART AND PERICARDIUM

Pneumopericardium (Fig. 16)

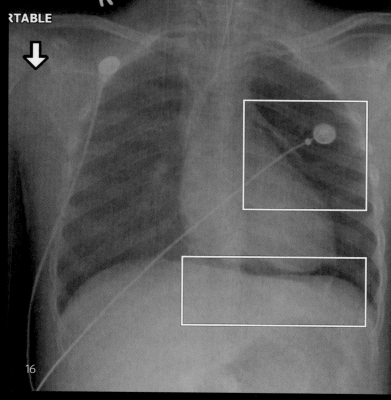

Hydropneumothorax (Fig. 17)

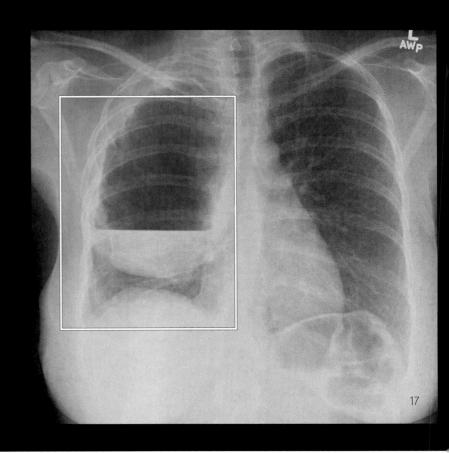

17

**THAT CHANGE
THE GRAYSCALE TO
"TOO BLACK & TOO WHITE"**

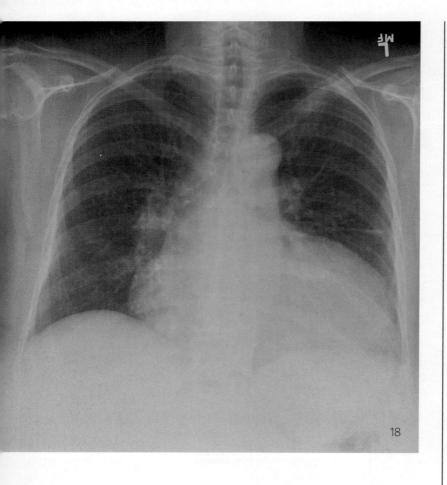

Pathological Conditions That Do Not Change the Grayscale, But Alter the Normal Size: "too much white" or "too much black"

In most clinical situations, the abnormality will present on an x-ray as a shift in the grayscale such that the previously normal grayscale is now too white or too black. However, in some scenarios, the grayscale stays the same, but there is too much of it (the anatomical structure is altered). For example, if the x-ray reveals that the patient has an enlarged heart, the grayscale region of the heart would not be too white or too black compared to normal, but would be larger than expected–too much white (Fig. 18).

Figure 18. Pathology can cause the grayscale shadow of a structure to change size - too much white. Too much white on this PA chest x-ray is caused by a massive heart.

104

Pathological Conditions
That Do Not Change the Grayscale,
But Alter the Normal Position or Shape
of the Grayscale Shadow

In some situations, the pathology is not seen directly, but, instead, is inferred because of its effect on other anatomical structures (e.g., this occurs frequently for pathology within the mediastinum). In these cases the pathological condition (the culprit) can cause other normal structures (the victims) to look abnormal from their displacement, rotation or compression. For example, a thyroid goiter (the culprit) will show up as a mediastinal mass (Fig. 19), but will obscure the outline of normal vessels in the thoracic inlet, and will narrow and displace the normal trachea (the victims). In fact, in some cases, these secondary effects may completely obscure the primary problem (e.g., a lung collapse may completely hide the underlying tumor that is causing the collapse (Fig. 20)).

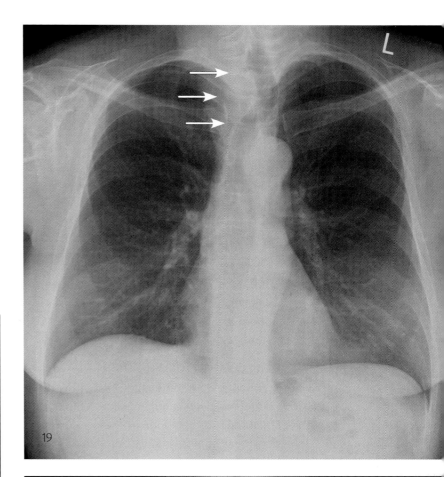

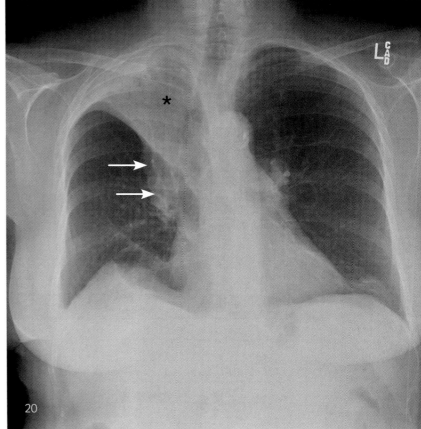

Figure 19. Pathology can cause the grayscale shadow of a structure to shift position. The position of the tracheal grayscale shadow is shifted to the left on this PA chest x-ray due to an enlarged thyroid (arrows).

Figure 20. Pathology can cause the grayscale shadow of a structure to change shape. The shape of the grayscale shadow of the right lung is altered on this PA chest x-ray due to collapse (asterisk); this change in grayscale is masking a tumor (arrows) obstructing the airways.

105

RADIOLOGICAL PATTERNS

A radiological pattern refers to a radiological appearance, or several radiological findings, that can be caused by one, or several, predictable pathological processes.

The identification of a radiological pattern leads to a radiological differential diagnosis. However, a clinically relevant differential diagnosis can only be established when the radiological pattern is linked with appropriate clinical information. The importance of the clinical context in a diagnosis is illustrated in Table 3.3.

The radiological pattern of certain disease processes can evolve over time. Additionally, a secondary pathology may show patterns that overlap those of the primary pathological process; for example, alveolar edema may completely obscure the interstitial changes related to cardiac failure. For both of these reasons, patterns are best identified in the earlier stages of disease before changes or overlap make pattern recognition difficult (4).

Patterns are usually discussed based on location and imaging characteristics.

Types of Chest X-ray Patterns

Chest x-ray patterns can be classified based on different characteristics (Table 3.2). Patterns related to various anatomical structures and zones of the thorax will be discussed in each of the specific chapters in **Section II.**

CHARACTERISTIC OF PATTERN	EXAMPLE
Anatomical location	Mediastinal mass
Distribution	Upper versus lower lung zone
Radiological grayscale appearance	Too white or too black
Change over time	Acute versus chronic
Simple	One finding
Complex	Multiple findings

Table 3.2
Types of Chest X-ray Patterns

THE IMPORTANCE OF CLINICAL CONTEXT

The chest x-ray of your patient reveals the presence of airspace disease (Fig. 21). However, an airspace (air-bronchogram) pattern can be caused by the presence of blood, pus, water, or tumor within the lungs. Therefore, clinically relevant information must be used in order to form a CLINICALLY RELEVANT diagnosis (Table 3.3).

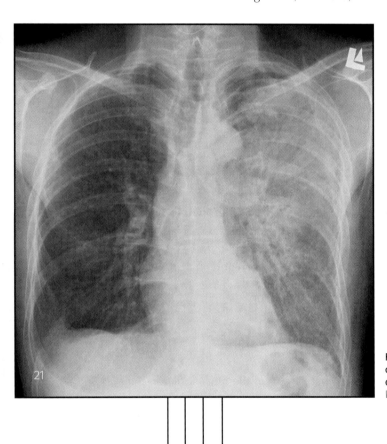

Figure 21. The importance of clinical context in airspace disease. Airspace disease in the left lung (note the air bronchograms).

CLINICAL CONTEXT	The patient has a productive cough.	The patient has hemoptysis and recent chest trauma.	The patient has been recently treated for cardiac failure.	The patient has been treated for infection that is still unresolved, or worse.
PREFERRED DIAGNOSIS	PNEUMONIA	PULMONARY HEMORRHAGE	UNRESOLVED PULMONARY EDEMA	SUSPECT TUMOR

Table 3.3
Applying Clinical Context to Narrow a Differential Diagnosis

RADIOLOGICAL SIGNS

A radiological sign (Fig. 22a,b,c,d,e,f) is an objective indication of some medical fact or quality that is detected by a physician during the examination of a radiograph (i.e., standard x-ray, CT scan, MRI) (5). It refers to a specific radiological appearance that narrows the differential diagnosis to a specific pathological process; in fact, the differential diagnosis for a sign will be narrowed significantly (6).

For example, the air-bronchogram sign is one such sign that helps narrow a differential diagnosis.

The list of possible disease processes that can make the lungs look too white is long, and includes: tumor, fibrosis, consolidation, and atelectasis. If the area of the lungs that is too white contains patent black airways – the air bronchogram sign – the differential diagnosis is narrowed to consolidation.

However, the concept of a pattern or a sign is not so clearly distinguished. When a pattern is found to be characteristic of a pathological process, it may be called a sign. In either case, the presence of a sign or pattern is an important diagnostic indicator that should trigger a specific differential diagnosis.

Figure 22. Radiological Signs. Examples of radiological signs on chest x-rays. a, luftsichel sign, arrows outline the crescent of lucency adjacent to the the aortic arch, b, silhouette sign, notice the loss of the left heart border due to the presence of pathology (arrows), c, pseudotumor sign, notice the opacity (arrow) in the right lung which resembles a mass, and yet is due to the presence of fluid within the horizontal fissure, d, 1,2,3 sign, characteristic pattern of adenopathy in sarcoidosis, 1, right paratracheal, 2, right hilar, 3, left hilar node enlargement, e, double contour sign, lateral border of the enlarged left atrium (arrows) seen distinctly, and separate, from the lateral contour of the right atrium (arrow heads), f, incomplete border sign., There is a distinct inferior border (arrows). The superior border (?) is not clearly defined.

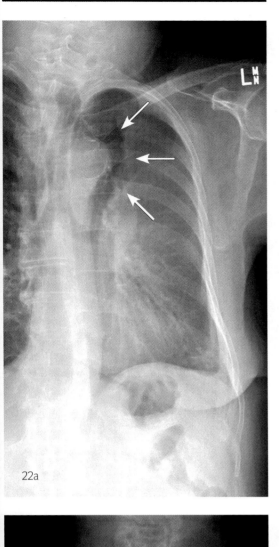

22a

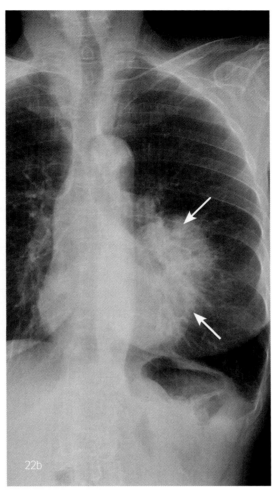

22b

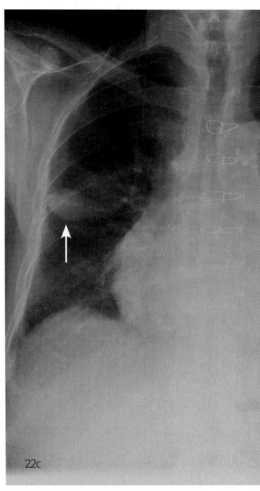

22c

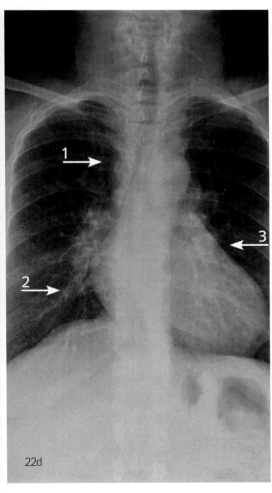

22d

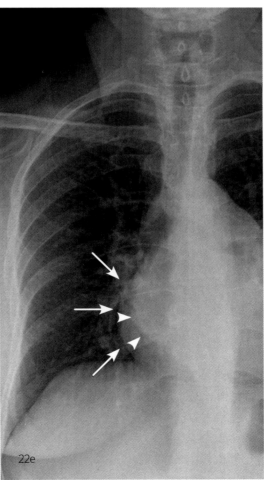

22e

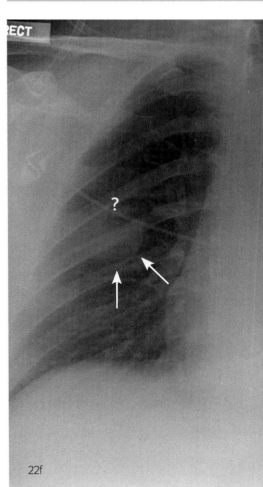

22f

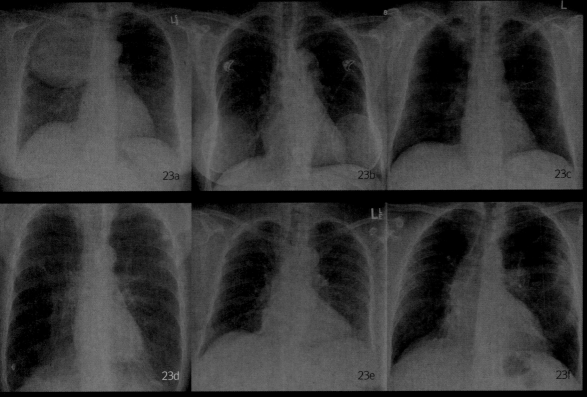

Describe the shift of the grayscale (too white or too black) caused by the abnormality as compared to the normal image found on the inside front cover.

Pathology on chest x-rays will usually shift the grayscale of part, or all, of the x-ray to too white or too black. In each of the following six images there is an obvious abnormality (Fig. 23 a,b,c,d,e).

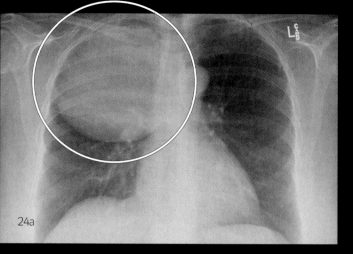

24a

The abnormality is too white. Homogeneous white region within the upper aspect of the right hemithorax (large mass) (Fig. 24a).

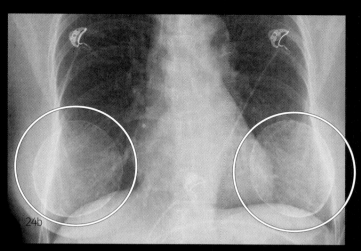

24b

The abnormality is too white. Rounded areas on both sides of the lower thorax and extending past the lateral borders of the rib cage (bilateral calcified breast implants) (Fig. 24b).

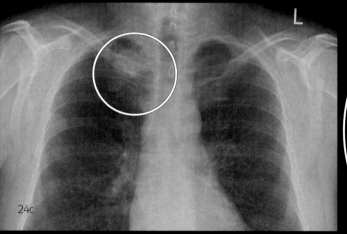

24c

The abnormality is too white. Small white area in the apex of the right hemithorax partially obscured by the medial aspect of the right clavicle (right apical lung cancer) (Fig. 24c).

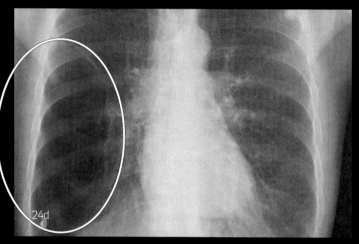

24d

The abnormality is too black. Oval area of too black within the inferior lateral aspect of the right hemithorax (large bulla) (Fig. 24d).

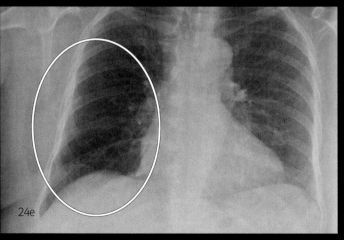

24e

The abnormality is too black. The inferior aspect of the right hemithorax is too black, as compared to the left (previous right mastectomy) (Fig. 24e).

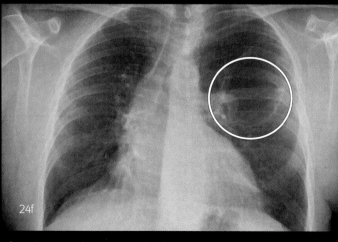

24f

The abnormality is too black. The black area is delineated by a thin white outline (lung cyst, bulla) (Fig. 24f).

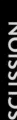

References

1. Lewis, P.J., Shaffer, K., & Donovan, A. (Eds.). (2012). AMSER National Medical Student Curriculum in Radiology. http://aur.org/Secondary-Alliances.aspx?id=141.

2. Lewis, P.J., & Shaffer, K. (2005). Developing a national medical student curriculum in radiology. *Am. Coll. Radiol., 2*(1):8–11.

3. The British Thoracic Society Standards of Care Committee, Pulmonary Embolism Guideline Development Group (2003). BTS guidelines for the management of suspected acute pulmonary embolism, 2003. *Thorax, 58*:470–484.

4. Felson, B. (1979). A new look at pattern recognition of diffuse pulmonary disease. *AJR Am. J. Roentgenol., 133*:183–189.

5. Algin, O., Gokalp, G., & Topal, U. (2011). Signs in chest imaging. *Diagn. Interv. Radiol., 17*:18–29.

6. Parker, M.S., Chasen, M.H., & Paul, N., (2009). Radiologic signs in thoracic imaging: case-based review and self-assessment module. *AJR Am. J. Roentenol., 192*:S34–S48.

CHAPTER 4
VISUAL PERCEPTION
and the CHEST X-RAY

importance

Our visual perception shapes how and what we see and is, therefore, a key part of the interpretive process. By reviewing this chapter you will learn about how the human visual system works and how humans perceive the data on x-ray images. Together with the interpretive process presented (in Chapters 5 and 16), a deeper understanding of visual perception will help you to minimize missing pathology on chest x-rays, and help you to avoid making common interpretive errors.

objectives

Knowledge

You will review and understand

- the technical and intellectual aspects of chest x-ray interpretation.

- why consultant doctors make x-ray interpretation mistakes.

associated resources

This chapter maps to the following AMSER curriculum content (1,2).

1) False positive and negative studies

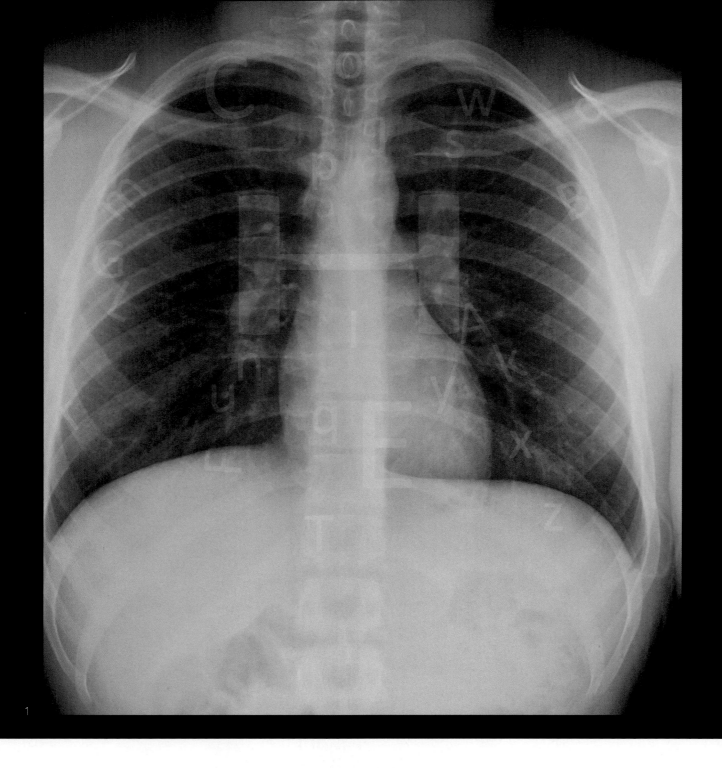

1

CASE STUDY

Hidden within Figure 1 is the entire alphabet.

Can you identify all of the letters of the alphabet starting from A?

VISUAL PERCEPTION AND THE CHEST X-RAY

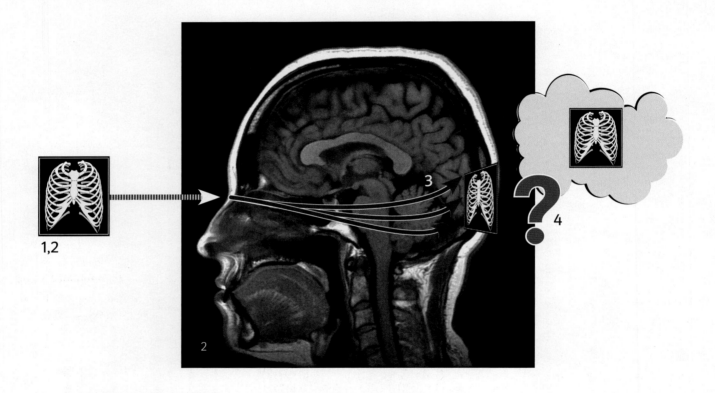

1,2

2

3

4

Visual perception is defined as the ability to interpret information from the visible light reaching the retina. This is also known as vision, or eyesight. However, what we see is not simply the translation of the retinal stimuli – the process of visual perception is very complex (3), and consequently, is a cause of interpretive errors.

There are four main elements of visual perception that are related to chest x-ray interpretation (Fig. 2):
- the viewing environment,
- the x-ray image,
- the visual pathway,
- the brain's cognitive processing of the image.

Figure 2. Visual perception and the chest x-ray. The interpretation of an x-ray image is affected by four areas of visual perception: the viewing environment (1), the x-ray image (2), the visual pathway (3), and the brain's cognitive processing of the image (4).

When you first put the ear tips of your stethoscope in your ears, you do not hear any clinically useful sounds, only noise related to the ear tip movement. Only after you shut out all external noise and distractions, do you start being able to discern the heart sounds. When looking at a chest x-ray, it is necessary to achieve this same level of concentration and diminish extrinsic cognitive load. To see what you are looking at requires concentration and focus. Get ready for this visual process by optimizing external lighting and by shutting out noise and other distractions.

The Viewing Environment

The viewing environment is important because of the potential for auditory distractions or excessive lighting to interfere with the perception of the x-ray. Conventional x-ray images, preserved on film, are viewed on an illuminated film viewer. The viewers come in a variety of sizes and shapes to accommodate from one to multiple x-rays simultaneously. The room in which the viewing takes place should have subdued background lighting. There should be enough space for the x-rays to be viewed from the distance of 1.5 to 3 feet, and from 6 to 8 feet. Pathology is generally easier to see at a distance closer to the film; the further distance allows for a more holistic view of the examination.

In the digital environment, the x-ray images are viewed on computer monitors from PACS. The top of the x-ray image should be positioned close to the top of the horizontal line of sight, with the rest of the screen positioned at an angle below this. The grayscale of the images can be affected by the quality of the monitors on which the images are viewed (4,5) Therefore, interpretation of x-ray images should, ideally, be performed using monitors specifically suited for PACS environments, because the resolution of the monitors needs to be optimum for x-ray viewing (6). There are no concrete rules for selecting the viewing distance within the PACS environment. However, since longer distances relax the eyes, it is best to view the x-ray from the furthest position at which the x-ray images are still clearly visible. PACS is further discussed in **Chapter 16**.

The X-ray Image

The x-ray image is a complex image for a learner to perceive. The learner is unfamiliar with the grayscale appearance of normal and abnormal structures. Additionally, technical factors such as over-exposure or under-exposure have a tremendous effect on the x-ray image and what is perceived (4,5).

The Visual Pathway

Visual perception is affected by visual acuity. Errors in interpretation can occur in situations where the individual reading the x-ray has less than ideal visual acuity. This can be related to uncorrected myopic or mydriatic vision.

Cognitive Processing of the Image

The human brain can be trained to make quick and accurate observations (4,7). During the visual interpretive process, objects are compared to memories of that object. If you do not know what an object looks like, it is difficult to perceive it. This process underlies the difference in the interpretive capacity between experienced and novice chest x-ray observers. It also explains the need for practice looking at chest x-rays to build up familiarity with normal and abnormal radiological appearances.

VISUAL PERCEPTION
AND PATTERN RECOGNITION

In radiology, pattern recognition is important because pattern identification is necessary for the formulation of a differential diagnosis.

Three steps to pattern recognition have been described (8):

First, features from the visual field are extracted by neurons in the eye and sent to the visual cortex. This step is usually rapid and without conscious thought. The extracted features relate to the location, size, shape, orientation and texture of the objects being perceived.

Then, this initial perception of the visual field is grouped into regions and simple patterns.

Finally, we process the visual information obtained, in order to make sense of what we see. We pay attention to certain patterns and if we are curious about something, we try and find an explanation for it.

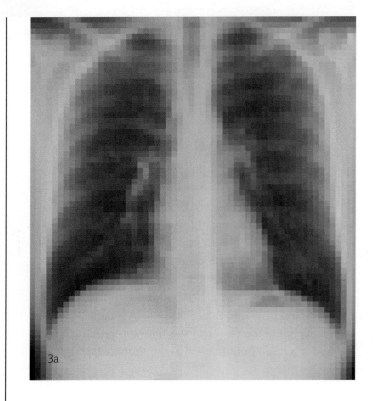

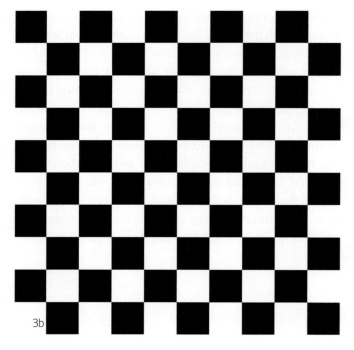

Figure 3. Pattern recognition and chest x-ray interpretation. a, PA chest x-ray that has been distorted, however, due to pattern recognition the PA chest x-ray can still be identified, b, example of an easily recognized checkerboard pattern.

GESTALT THEORY AND IMAGE PERCEPTION

The Gestalt theory in modern psychology is based on the concepts that people intuitively prefer the simplest and most stable of possibilities, that holistic approaches are necessary to understand the mind, and that the mental process is greater than the simple "summing of the component parts". According to Gestalt, our perception of the things around us (e.g., our experiences, sensory perceptions, etc.) is taken from 'the whole' in context, rather than combining information about the individual perceptual elements. In terms of visual perception, the contextualization of the visual information we obtain, is thought to shape how we interpret that which we see.

This is seen in daily practice, as experienced radiologists will perform a rapid assessment of the x-ray to determine if the examination is normal and to detect abnormal lesions. This has been called the global perspective, global impression or snapshot impression (9).

There are various principles associated with the Gestalt theory that are important for visual perception (9) – specifically relating to the perception of the chest x-ray image.

Principle of Proximities

The closer together objects are, the more likely we will mentally group them together (e.g., the anatomical structures of the mediastinum) (Fig. 4a,b). Even though the mediastinum is composed of various individual elements, it is perceived as one white structure in the mid-portion of the thorax. Pathology can easily be missed within the mediastinum if the observer cannot distinguish the individual elements.

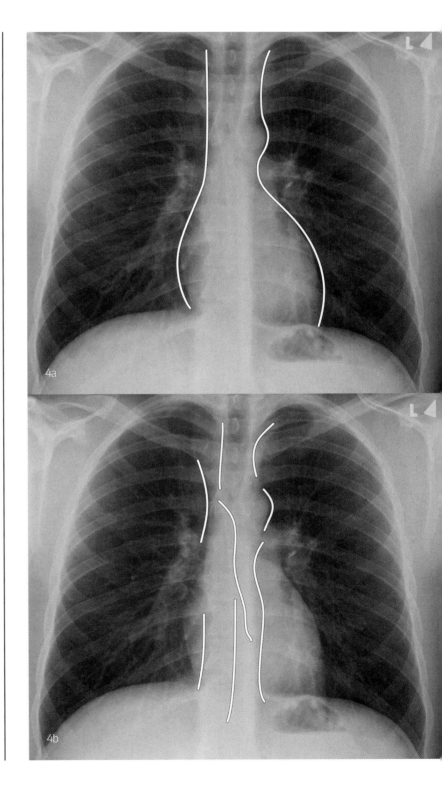

Figure 4. Principle of proximities. The mediastinum is perceived as one structure due to the principle of proximities. a, PA chest x-ray, with the margins of the mediastinum highlighted, b, the same PA chest x-ray with the components of the mediastinum highlighted.

121

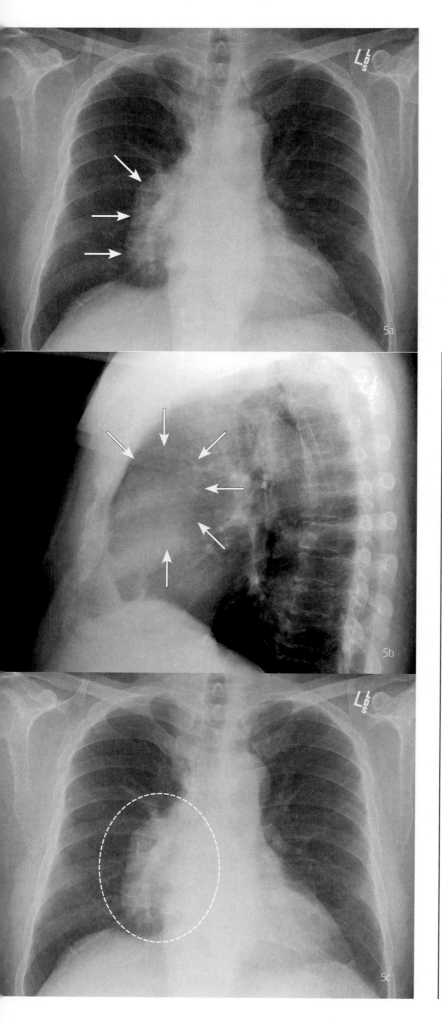

Principle of Similarities

We tend to link together parts of an image that are similar in color, grayscale, texture, and/or shape. For example, at first glance, the heart and an anterior mediastinal mass overlying the heart will be seen as one structure (Fig. 5a). The use of both the lateral (Fig. 5b), and PA (Fig. 5c), chest x-rays may be necessary to help perceive the two as being separate (8).

Principle of Continuity

We prefer figures that are continuous. We tend to perceive that a line continues in a particular, anticipated direction, even when the line has stopped. In the example in Figure 6, due to the principle of continuity, our perception of the first rib gives the illusion of a cyst in the upper lung lobes (Fig. 6a,b,c).

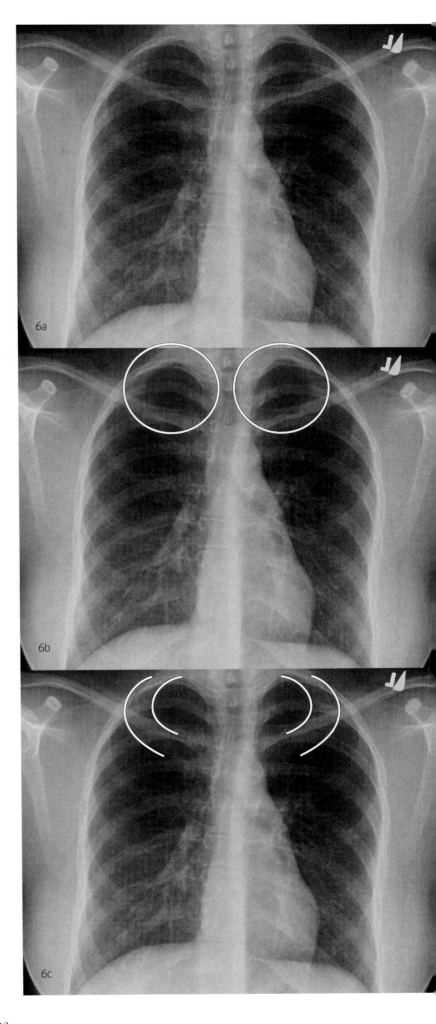

Figure 5. Principle of similarities. Due to the principle of similarities a mass in the mediastinum may be overlooked. a, a PA chest x-ray with the perceived border of the mediastinum highlighted (arrows), b, the corresponding lateral chest x-ray reveals the presence of a mass (arrows), c, the PA chest x-ray with the mass in the mediastinum highlighted.

Figure 6. Principle of continuity. Due to the principle of continuity we perceive the contour of the first ribs to represent abnormalities (oval cysts) in the apices of the lungs. a. a PA chest x-ray, b, the same PA chest x-ray with the perceived cysts highlighted, c, the same PA chest x-ray with the border of the first ribs highlighted.

Principle of Closure

Cognitively, our brains prefer to perceive a complete form; if parts of a line are missing, we fill in the missing parts to make the line complete. We normally see the lines of the cortex of a rib. With rib destruction, portions of these cortical lines disappear. Due to the principle of closure we may perceive that the cortical lines are complete (Fig. 7a,b, c). When examining a chest x-ray pay close attention to the integrity of the complete cortical outline of all bones to make sure rib fractures or rib destruction is not overlooked, due to the principle of closure.

Principle of Figure and Ground

When viewing an object or scene, the focus of visual attention becomes the figure and all other visual input becomes the ground. The perception of the object will, therefore, change, depending on what is taken to be the figure and what is taken to be the ground. Objects that are smaller, brighter, and more centrally located on the image usually become the figure and, therefore, the focus of our attention (Fig. 8) (9).

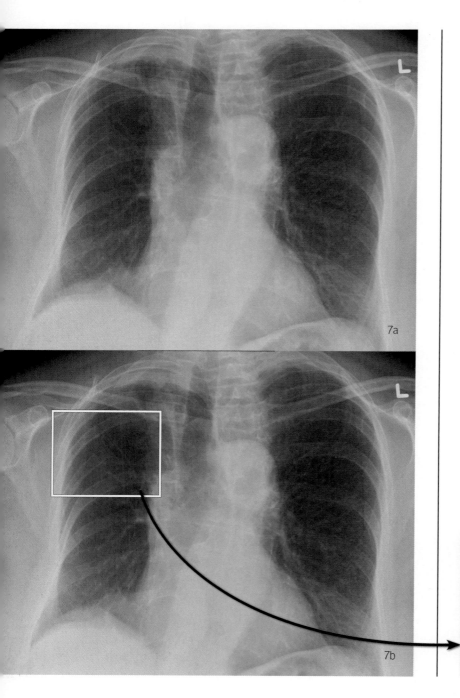

7a

7b

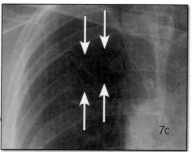

7c

124

When viewing a chest x-ray, be aware of the "tricks" that your eye can play, and do not be quick to call pathology. With experience, catching yourself before the illusion fools you will become easier (4,9).

Figure 7. Principle of closure. Due to the principle of closure we perceive lines as continuous. a, PA chest x-ray with destruction in one rib that is easily overlooked, b, same PA chest x-ray with region containing rib destruction highlighted, c, magnified region of the same PA chest x-ray, highlighting the obvious rib destruction (no cortex visible, arrows).

Figure 8. Principle of figure and ground. Due to the principle of figure and ground, the eyes will automatically go to whitest area on a chest x-ray. a, PA chest x-ray with an aortic stent (arrows). When such an object is present, caution should be used to ensure that no other abnormality is overlooked.

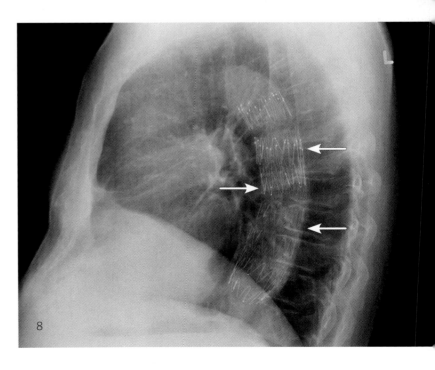

125

OPTICAL ILLUSIONS
AND THE CHEST X-RAY

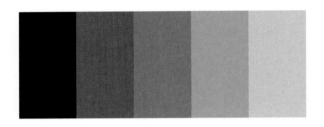

9a

Various optical illusions have been described, related to chest x-rays. One of the most frequently encountered optical illusions is called the Mach band effect. This illusion relates to the perception of a lighter (or darker) line/area between two regions that have a significant difference in grayscale (Fig. 9a). For example, each of the regions in Figure 9a have a uniform intensity; however, most people will perceive them to be lighter on the left and darker on the right. The Mach band effect is seen at the immediate border between two areas of differing lightness gradients (Fig. 9a,b,c) (9,10).

Another illusion similar to the Mach band is the cornsweet illusion. In this illusion (and contrary to the Mach band effect), a very small area (the central "edge") affects the perception of entire large areas, including portions that are distant from the "edge" (Fig. 10a,b,c) (9,10).

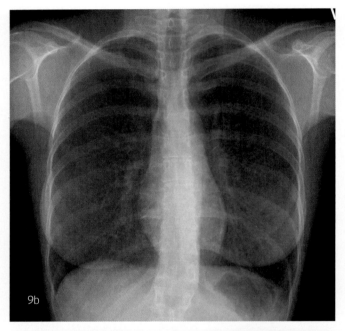

9b

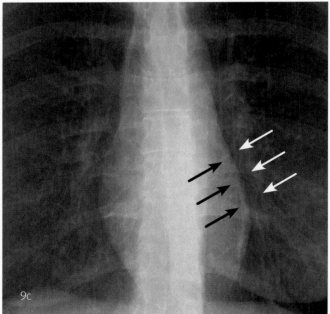

9c

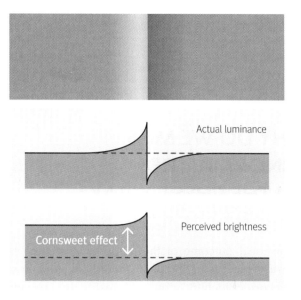

Actual luminance

Perceived brightness

Cornsweet effect

10a

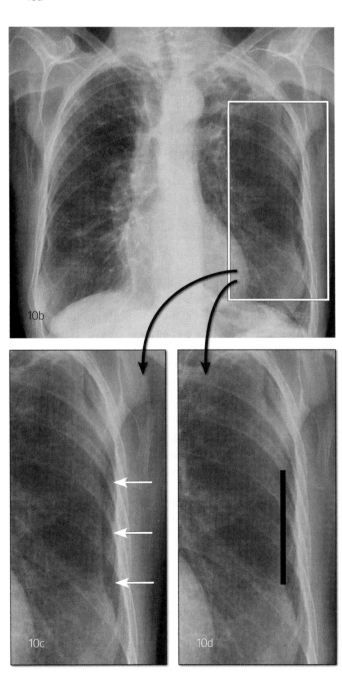

10b

10c

10d

Figure 9. The Mach band effect. The Mach band effect can cause erroneous perceptions of shifts in grayscale. a, an illustration of the Mach band effect, a vertical band of blackness is perceived between the grayscale changes, b, PA chest x-ray with an example of the Mach band effect occurring at the border of the heart shadow, c, a magnified region of the PA chest x-ray. The right edge of the heart shadow (purple arrows) is perceived as too white, and the left edge of the abutting lungs (white arrows) is perceived as too black.

Figure 10. The cornsweet illusion. The cornsweet illusion can result in the erroneous perception of shifts in grayscale. a, an illustration of the cornsweet illusion, b, a PA chest x-ray with an example of the cornsweet illusion occurring at the lateral border of the left lung due to a skin fold, c, a magnified region of the PA chest x-ray highlighting the cornsweet illusion. The outer portion of the lung (lateral to the skin fold, arrows) appears too black, d, the same magnified region with a black bar. When the edge is removed (hidden by the black bar) the edge effect is lost, and the lungs are seen as having a uniform appearance.

127

WHY DO WE MISS ABNORMALITIES ON THE CHEST X-RAY?

The ideal outcome of the interpretive process is the correct identification of an abnormality (true positive) or the correct identification of normality (true negative).

Two other outcomes can occur. An abnormality is called that does not exist (false positive), or an abnormality that does exist is not recognized (false negative).

Achieving interpretive perfection (only true positives and true negatives) is impossible. We can, however, decrease the number of false positives and false negatives with education and practice (11,12).

Errors of Interpretation

Error in the interpretation of the x-ray may arise from various issues. There are several systems for the classification of errors. Robinson (13) succinctly describes errors arising from 1) poor technique; 2) failures of perception; 3) lack of knowledge; and 4) misjudgments. Often, errors are produced by a combination of these factors, and exacerbated by problems in communication (11,14,15).

A second classification of errors in x-ray interpretation divides them into errors of perception and errors of cognition (15). Perception errors occur when the abnormality is featured on the image, but is not appreciated by the observer (false negative). Cognitive errors occur when the observer identifies the abnormality, but formulates the wrong conclusions about the findings (false positive).

Another classification system in x-ray interpretation divides the errors into the following categories (11).

Complacency

Errors of complacency are errors of overreading and misinterpretation. The interpreter appreciates the finding, but attributes it to the wrong cause (false positive).

Faulty reasoning

Errors of faulty reasoning are also errors of overreading and misinterpretation. The finding is appreciated and interpreted as abnormal, but attributed to the wrong cause. Misleading information and a limited differential diagnosis are included in this category (true positive, but misclassification).

Lack of knowledge

The finding is seen, but attributed to the wrong cause because of lack of knowledge by the viewer (true positive, but misclassification).

Underreading

Errors of underreading are errors in which the finding is missed. This may result from failure to isolate important material, or from satisfaction of search (false negative).

Satisfaction of search

Satisfaction of search is a phenomenon in which the detection of one radiographic finding interferes with that of others (16). Once you identify one finding, you stop looking for other abnormalities. A finding is identified (true positive) but other – sometimes more clinically relevant – findings are missed (false negative) (Fig. 11a,b).

Poor communication

Errors of poor communication are errors resulting from the lack of communication of identified findings to the clinician.

Miscellaneous (technical limitations)

Miscellaneous errors are the result of technical factors obscuring the findings (false negative).

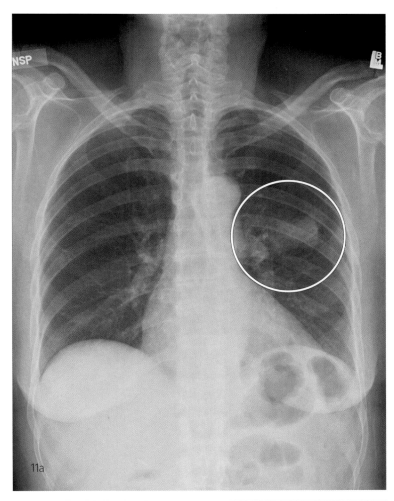

11a

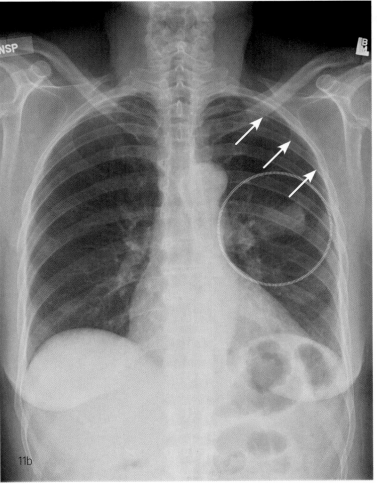

11b

Figure 11. Satisfaction of search. Due to the phenomenon of satisfaction of search, errors of underreading can occur. Once a single finding is noted, we are 'satisfied' and stop looking for other abnormalities. a, PA chest x-ray with an obvious mass is the left lung (highlighted), b, the same PA chest x-ray also contains a second abnormality, a pneumothorax (arrows), which could be missed due to satisfaction of search if the interpretation process stopped after the first finding was noted.

TRAINING PERCEPTION AND REDUCING ERRORS

Several authors have shown that formal art observation training can improve the visual diagnostic skills of learners (20,21). Medical students who took courses in Art Observation significantly improved their ability to make accurate visual observations.

There is no single method for learning observational skills in radiology. However, there are certain key factors that will lead to improved recognition of normal structures and pathology on chest x-rays.

The first is having a good understanding of the radiological appearance of normal anatomical structures. The second is the reinforcement of this understanding by repetition – by looking at normal examinations and systematically identifying specific anatomical structures. Normal examinations can be found in PACS, in teaching files on line, and on the inside covers of this textbook.

It is also necessary to fully understand how pathology can appear on x-ray examinations. If you identify an abnormality, the search does not stop there. Continue examining the x-ray until all the structures have been scrutinized.

Finally, avoid inferences. An inference is a hypothesis based on an observation. "The white area looks like a pneumonia", is an inference. "The opacity contains air bronchograms", is an observation.

METHODS TO DECREASE FALSE NEGATIVES
• Increasing education
• Increasing awareness of the problem
• Increasing research
• Improving technical standards
• Using computer-assisted diagnosis (CAD)

Table 4.1
Methods to Decrease False Negatives

VISUAL SEARCH AND THE CHEST X-RAY

Visual search is a visual task that involves an active scan of the chest x-ray for an abnormality among the expected normal anatomical structures. It has been hypothesized that this occurs in two distinct phases (22).

The first is the single glance, or flash viewing, phase. This involves the entire retina, as information from the entire field of view is compared to mental templates of similar images. In this phase, the context is established and gross deviations are identified. This phase can answer the question: is the x-ray normal or abnormal?

The second phase requires the use of the fovea to assess more minute details. This occurs through a series of checking fixations, and requires eye movement. In this phase, any missing detail is determined and any ambiguity is resolved.

These phases are somewhat analogous to Norman's descriptions of non-analytic/System 1 and analytic/System 2 models of clinical reasoning. Both approaches are complementary, and the combination of both may help to reduce diagnostic errors (4,23).

Visual search is a critical component of chest x-ray interpretation. A recommended systematic visual search (Fig. 12) of specific anatomical structures will be presented in each radiological anatomy chapter.

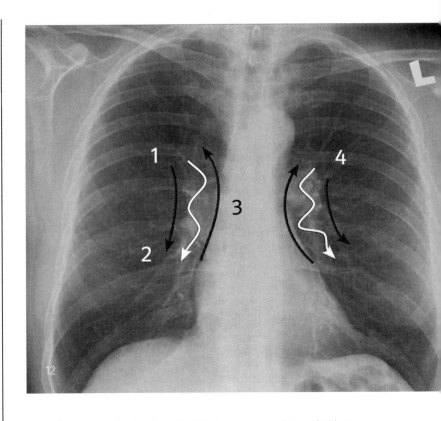

Figure 12. A systematic visual search. A PA chest x-ray superimposed with an example of a series of visual checks one would follow to perform a systematic visual search of the hila. 1, Start at the top of the right hilum, 2, Follow the lateral outline of the hilum inferiorly to the lower heart level, 3, Follow the medial outline of the right hilum superiorly, 4, Follow the same instructions on the left. White wavy line indicates the completion of the visual search by checking for any density changes across the hila from top to bottom.

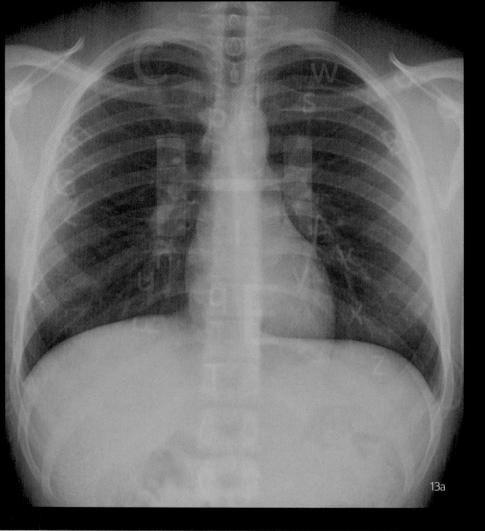

13a

Can you identify all of the letters of the alphabet starting from A?

Hidden within Fig 13a is the entire alphabet.

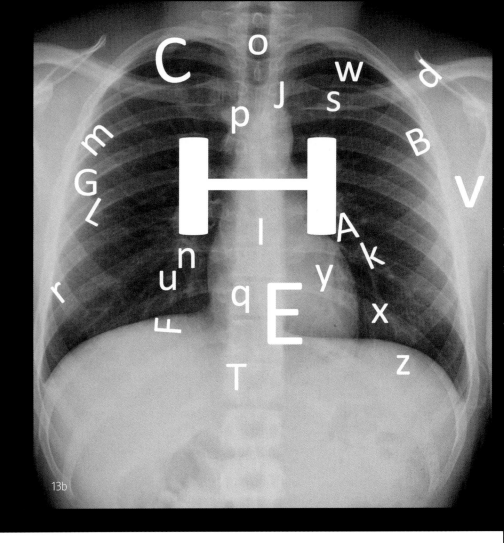

The alphabet highlighted (Fig. 13b).

References

1. Lewis, P., Shaffer, K., & Donovan, A. (Eds.). (2012). AMSER National Medical Student Curriculum in Radiology. http://aur.org/Secondary-Alliances.aspx?id=141.

2. Lewis, P.J., & Shaffer, K. (2005). Developing a national medical student curriculum in radiology. *Am. Coll. Radiol., 2*(1):8–11.

3. Berbaum, K., Franken, E., Caldwell, R., & Schwartz, K. (2009). Satisfaction of search in traditional radiographic imaging. In Samei, E. and E. Krupinski, (Eds.), *The Handbook of Medical Image Perception and Techniques.* New York, NY: Cambridge University Press.

4. Norman, G., Young, M., & Brooks, L. (2007). Non-analytical models of clinical reasoning: the role of experience. *Med. Educ., 41*:1140–1145.

5. Carrino, J.A. (2002). Chapter 3: Digital Image Quality: A Clinical Perspective. In Siegel, E.L., Reiner, B.I. & Carrino, J.A. (Eds.) *Quality Assurance – Meeting the Challenge in the Digital Medical Enterprise.* Great Falls, VA: The Society for Computer Applications in Radiology.

6. Bacher, K., Smeets, P., De Hauwere, A., et al. (2006). Image quality performance of liquid crystal display systems: Influence of display resolution, magnification and window settings on contrast-detail detection. *Eur. J. Radiol., 58* (3):471–479.

7. Pusic, M.,V., Andrews, J.S., Kessler, D.O., et al. (2012). Prevalence of abnormal cases in an image bank affects the learning of radiograph interpretation. *Med. Educ., 46*:289–298.

8. Ware, C. (2008). *Visual thinking for design* (Morgan Kaufmann Series in Interactive Technologies). Burlington, MA: Morgan Kaufmann.

9. Koontz, N.A., & Gunderman, R.B. (2008). Gestalt theory: implications for radiology education. *AJR Am. J. Roentgenol., 190*(5):1156–1160.

10. Chasen, M.H.(2001). Practical applications of Mach band theory in thoracic analysis. *Radiology, 219*(3):596–610.

11. Renfrew, D.L., Franken, E.A. Jr., Berbaum, K.S., et al. (1992). Error in radiology: classification and lessons in 182 cases presented at a problem case conference. *Radiology, 183*(1):145–150.

12. Brook, O.R., O'Connell, A.M., Thornton, E., et al., (2010). Quality initiatives: anatomy and pathophysiology of errors occurring in clinical radiology practice. *Radiographics, 30*(5):1401–1410.

13. Robinson, P.J.A. (1997). Radiology's Achilles heel: error and variation in the interpretation of the Röntgen image. *Br. J. Radiol., 70*:1085–1098.

14. Fitzgerald, R. (2001). Error in Radiology. *Clin. Radiology, 56*(12):938–946.

15. Kundel, H.L., (1989). Perception errors in chest radiography. *Semin. Respir. Crit. Care Med., 10*(3):203–210.

16. Ashman, C.J., Yu, J.S., & Wolfman, D. (2000). Satisfaction of search in osteoradiology. *AJR Am. J. Roentgenol., 175*(2):541–544.

17. Brogdon, B.G., Kelsey, C.A., & Moseley, R.D. Jr. (1983). Factors affecting perception of pulmonary lesions. *Radiol. Clin. North Am., 21*(4):633–654.

18. Samuel, S., Kundel, H.L., Nodine, C.F., & Toto, L.C. (1995). Mechanism of satisfaction of search: eye position recordings in the reading of chest radiographs. *Radiology, 194*(3): 895–902.

19. Manning, D.J., Ethell, S.C., & Donovan, T. (2004). Detection or decision errors? Missed lung cancer from the posteroanterior chest radiograph. *Br. J. Radiol., 77*(915):231–235.

20. Shapiro, J., Rucker, L., & Beck, J. (2006). Training the clinical eye and mind: using the arts to develop medical students' observational and pattern recognition skills. *Med. Educ., 40*(3): 263–268.

21. Bardes, C.L., Gillers, D., & Herman, A.E. (2001). Learning to look: developing clinical observational skills at an art museum. *Med. Educ., 35*(12):1157–1161.

22. Kundel, H.L., & Nodine, C.F. (1975). Interpreting chest radiographs without visual search. *Radiology, 116*(3):527–532.

23. Norman, G. (2009). Dual Processing and diagnostic errors. *Adv. Health Sci. Edu. 14*:37–49.

CHAPTER 5
An Introduction to CHEST X-RAY INTERPRETATION

importance

How do you interpret an x-ray? The interpretive process is not commonly taught in medical school. Students tend to jump directly to making an x-ray diagnosis. Without an approach to x-ray interpretation, you cannot perform a comprehensive assessment of the chest x-ray.

This chapter reviews the basic elements of the interpretive process. You will learn about the phases of x-ray interpretation: how to start, progress through, and finish a chest x-ray interpretation – complete with guidance for how to provide a proper description of the findings and a differential diagnosis.

objectives

Skills

You will identify

- important structures that are used as landmarks for the x-ray interpretive process.

- common pathology encountered during x-ray interpretation (including incidental findings).

Knowledge

You will review and understand

- the basic approach to chest x-ray interpretation.

- the steps of the interpretive process (including the six phases).

- the systematic approach to identifying pathology on the chest x-ray, based on structure and location.

APPROACH TO
CHEST X-RAY INTERPRETATION

Chest x-rays are ordered to identify, or to exclude, pathology. The identification of disease on a chest x-ray is done through the interpretive process. Correctly interpreting an x-ray requires an understanding of the interpretive process, and the mastering of all of the key interpretation elements.

This interpretive process can be divided into the following distinct phases:

1.   Preparatory phase

2.   Visual identification phase

3.   Descriptive phase

4.   Summary phase

5.   Differential diagnosis phase

6.   Communication phase (action phase)

1. The Preparatory Phase

The preparatory phase is necessary for verification that the chest x-ray you are viewing is correctly matched to the patient. In this phase, you will determine what type of chest x-ray examination was performed. The clinical questions, and any relevant clinical information, are reviewed. This includes a search for, review of, and comparison of previous relevant radiological examinations and reports.

The patient name, age (date of birth), date of examination and any markers on the radiograph should be evaluated (e.g., 'PA', 'Supine', and 'Expiration') (Fig. 1). In the era of film and patient film bags, it was not unusual for films to be misfiled. With PACS and digital imaging, mistakes are rare, but can still occur.

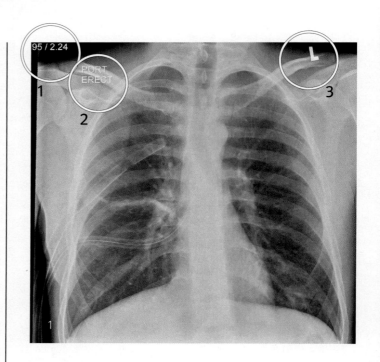

Figure 1. The preparatory phase. In the preparatory phase, you need to check the information on the chest x-rays. This is an example of a chest x-ray with identifiers (highlighted); 1, date of examination, 2, type of examination and patient positioning, 3, patient's left side.

Figure 2. The visual identification phase. During the visual identification phase, previous x-rays should be viewed. a. current chest x-ray shows obvious mass lesions in the lung, b, the corresponding previous, normal, chest x-ray.

After verification, the quality of the x-ray is assessed. This involves an evaluation of exposure, patient position, and degree of inspiration. A chest x-ray quality checklist is provided on page 41 (Chapter 1).

2. The Visual Identification Phase

In this phase, through a variety of cognitive processes that are dependent on knowledge and experience, the viewer will determine if the examination is normal or abnormal. An experienced radiologist makes this determination in a matter of seconds (1). Such a quick determination is possible only through a mental comparison of the viewed x-ray with a mental template of what a normal x-ray looks like, and the Gestalt processes described earlier (e.g., snapshot impression, global impression, and non-analytic processing).

A mental template is developed through the understanding of the grayscale representation of normal thoracic structures, and through experience. While you are developing experience, you should have printed, or digital images, of normal PA and lateral chest x-rays close at hand for comparison (or use the inside covers of this book).

A second visual process occurs when the current x-ray is compared with previous x-rays (Fig. 2a,b). Here, the comparison with the mental template is replaced with the direct visual information provided by the previous x-rays and radiological reports.

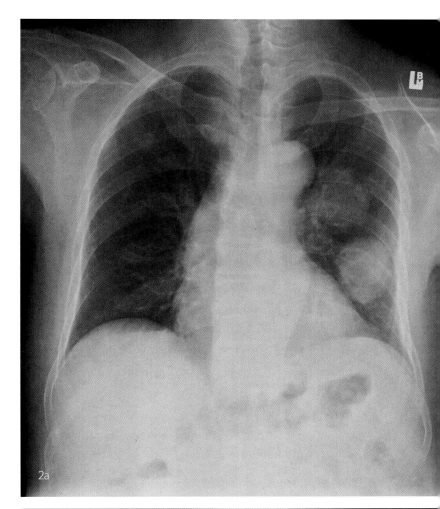

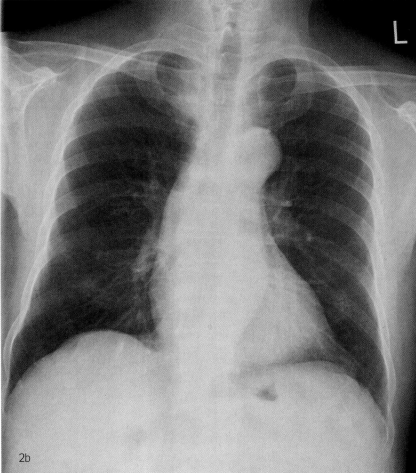

Using a Systematic Approach to Interpret Chest X-ray Images

The need for a systematic approach in chest x-ray interpretation has been a strong message throughout the history of radiology.

In 1940, Heusinkfeld said "to get the most out of the chest x-ray, an orderly approach is necessary" (2).

Lange reiterated this sentiment in 1990, when he stated that, "in assessing a chest radiograph, one should always proceed systematically" (3).

A systematic approach will help you identify any additional abnormalities after you have made the initial major observations. Also, if you do not identify an abnormality on the first glance, the systematic approach will help you work through the examination.

As a guide to the systematic approach, an x-ray interpretation checklist can be found at the end of each anatomical chapter (Chapters 7-14). A review of all checklists will be presented in Chapter 16.

Various systematic approaches have been proposed, many of which are variations of the ABC approach suggested by Talley and O'Connor (4,5).

1) The ABC approach by structures:

A » Airways
B » Bones
C » Cardiac
D » Diaphragms
E » Extras
F » Fields

2) Systematic approach based on location:

(i) Starting from center and moving out:
Trachea & Bronchi
Heart
Mediastinum
Hila
Lungs
Pleura
Chest wall

(ii) Starting from outside and moving in:
Chest wall
Pleura
Lungs
Hila
Mediastinum
Heart
Trachea & Bronchi

For you, as a learner, this approach may seem to have limited value. What does it mean to look at the mediastinum? The mediastinum, is composed of various anatomical structures and each of the structures contributes to the radiological appearance. To look at the mediastinum really means to look at each of the anatomical structures within the mediastinum individually, and to determine if each of these is normal or abnormal.

Each word used in the approach should trigger a response. The word "trachea" should trigger a search for the trachea as an object, and secondarily, a systematic detailed search for pathology involving the trachea. In this sense, the approach directs the chronology of the visual search. This guarantees that important components of the x-ray are not overlooked.

If, during rounds, and after using the approach, you still have not made the observations, changing the visual presentation of the x-ray may be helpful. In PACS, this can be done by magnifying the image, video inverting, or by changing the orientation of the images (i.e., looking at the images upside down). Image contrast and brightness can also be adjusted for further image enhancement.

The viewing, and interpreting, of x-rays should also be adjusted to the clinical context of each case. This will happen automatically, based on clinical information. For example, a patient presenting with a cough and sputum production will automatically trigger a search for pneumonia on their chest x-ray. Similarly, record of recent trauma to the chest will trigger a search for a pneumothorax, rib fractures, the accumulation of pleural fluid, and mediastinal widening.

Solitary pulmonary nodules are usually noticed by chance on a chest x-ray that was ordered for another reason. This is what is referred to as an incidental finding.

AUTHOR RECOMMENDATION:
Start from the center and work outward.
1, trachea and bronchi, 2, heart, 3, mediastinum, 4, hila, 5, lungs, 6, pleura, 7, chest wall.

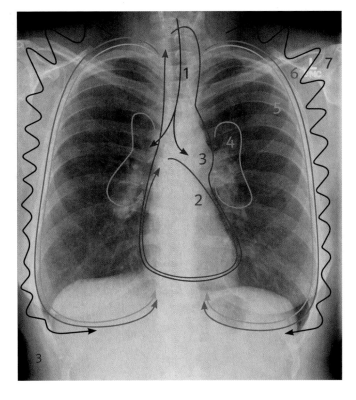

Figure 3. Systematic approach to x-ray interpretation. An example of a PA chest x-ray with the recommended "start from center and work out" systematic approach illustrated. 1, trachea and bronchi, 2, heart, 3, mediastinum, 4, hila, 5, lungs, 6, pleura, 7, chest wall.

In clinical practice, the terms "too white" and "too black" are not used. However, we encourage you to use these terms until you can use other appropriate radiological terms, such as an "opacity" or "lucency".

3. The Descriptive Phase

The chest x-ray is a composite of grayscale interfaces, and pathology will cause the grayscale to change and appear as an area that is too white or too black (when compared to the normal).

After determining that the x-ray examination is abnormal, the first step in the descriptive process is to determine if the abnormality is too white or too black. This is usually not too difficult if the abnormality is focal, but can be difficult if the abnormality is more diffuse.

The descriptive phase for a focal abnormality includes information related to:

- the shape,
- the size,
- the borders,
- the homogeneity of grayscale change,
- the localization to an anatomical structure, and to subdivisions of the structure (e.g., a lobe of the lung),
- any secondary effects (e.g., mass effect).

The descriptive phase for a diffuse abnormality includes information related to:

- the localization to an anatomical structure,
- the distribution,
- any secondary effects (e.g., decreased lung volume).

Figure 4. The descriptive phase. In the descriptive phase the pathology is described for the report. a, PA chest x-ray with an example of a well-defined mass, b. PA chest x-ray with an example of a heterogeneous mass with a central black area (a cavity).

CASE 1

Example description of a well-defined mass (Fig. 4a):

Abnormal. Abnormality in left lung. The abnormality is too white as compared to the grayscale of the normal right lung. The abnormality is homogeneously white with lobulated borders. There are no black areas within the abnormality.

CASE 2

Example description of a heterogeneous mass (Fig. 4b):

Abnormal. Abnormality in left lung. The abnormality is inhomogeneous. The abnormality is oval in shape with a lobulated border. The outside border is too white as compared to the grayscale of the normal right lung. The central portion, however, is too black.

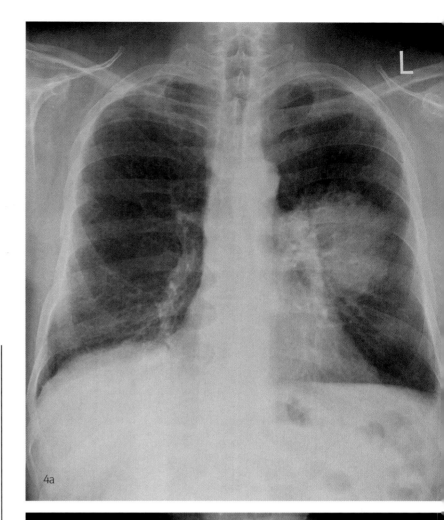

4a

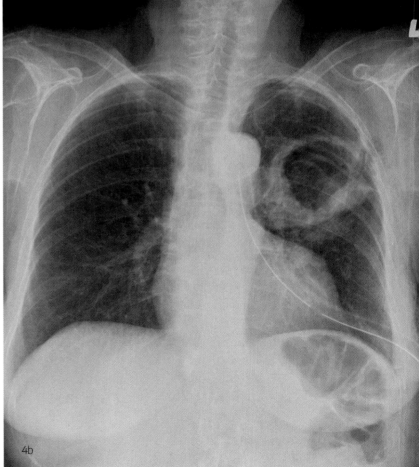

4b

4. The Summary Phase

A radiological summary is a group of words, or a statement, that best describes the findings. The summary is based on the key elements of the radiological description of the abnormality. The summary is not a pathological description and is not a guess at the pathology.

The summary is important because it is the trigger for the differential diagnosis.

In the case of multiple findings on the x-ray, the summary may have several components. Each component, in turn, will trigger a differential diagnosis. The findings should be listed in order of importance.

CASE 1

An example of a one-component summary is "anterior mediastinal mass". The words 'anterior mediastinal mass' are enough to trigger a differential diagnosis.

CASE 2

An example of a multi-component summary is "focal airspace disease with pleural effusion, and anterior mediastinal mass". Each of the three components can trigger a differential diagnosis, and before drawing conclusions that all three are related, the differential diagnosis from each component should be analyzed.

"A vague density in the right hemithorax" is an example of a poor summary. The description of the density is incomplete. There is no localization. A differential diagnosis is impossible.

5. The Differential Diagnosis Phase

The differential diagnosis is a list of the most common causes of a radiological finding. The differential diagnosis list should start with the cause that is most critical to the patient outcome – what in the list of possible causes can potentially kill the patient? For example, consider the case of a patient presenting in the emergency department with chest pain. The differential diagnosis for chest pain is long – however, in the first instance, you need to exclude critical diseases such as myocardial infarction, aortic dissection, or pulmonary embolism. Once these are excluded, you can consider possibilities that may be statistically more common than myocardial infarction, but are not medically considered to be life-threatening.

One additional essential element to the differential diagnosis phase is the review of the formulated differential diagnosis list with the clinical information at hand. For example, an x-ray finding in an immunocompromised patient can have a significantly different differential diagnosis to the same finding in a non-immunocompromised patient. An x-ray finding in a post-operative patient can also have completely different significance compared to the same finding in a patient without surgery. It is vital to carefully consider all of these factors prior to providing a differential diagnosis.

Textbooks have been written giving complete lists of differential diagnoses (6,7,8). In each book, all of the differential diagnoses listed are triggered by a specific finding or pattern: a radiological summary.

6. The Communication Phase (or Action Phase)

The communication phase involves giving further clinical guidance based upon the radiological findings.

In many cases, no urgent action is necessary, however, communication of the radiological findings is necessary to initiate appropriate patient management. For example, consider the finding of airspace consolidation in a

If the diagnosis is clear from the clinical presentation, a full differential diagnosis may not be necessary. For example, if the patient has suffered a thoracic injury from a motor vehicle accident, and the chest x-rays reveal air in the pleural space, the air in the pleural space is a pneumothorax. Further differential diagnosis is unnecessary.

patient with a cough and fever. Communication of the radiological findings enables the clinician to begin the appropriate treatment. (In this case, no further imaging is required unless the patient shows no improvement following appropriate treatment.)

However, if a pneumothorax is identified, then the finding needs to be communicated immediately to enable appropriate intervention to be initiated.

The radiological findings can also trigger further radiological investigation. For example, a CT scan may be required in a patient with chest x-ray findings of a mass. In some cases, a series of additional radiological investigations may be necessary (Fig. 5) – in all cases, radiation doses should be considered.

If the radiological findings do not correlate with the clinical symptoms, then further clinical correlation needs to be made. In these cases, you may need to re-evaluate the patient, considering the radiological findings and the differential diagnosis.

Figure 5. The communication or action phase. During the communication, or action, phase further clinical guidance is provided based on the radiological findings. An example of a clinical pathway for the management of a case.

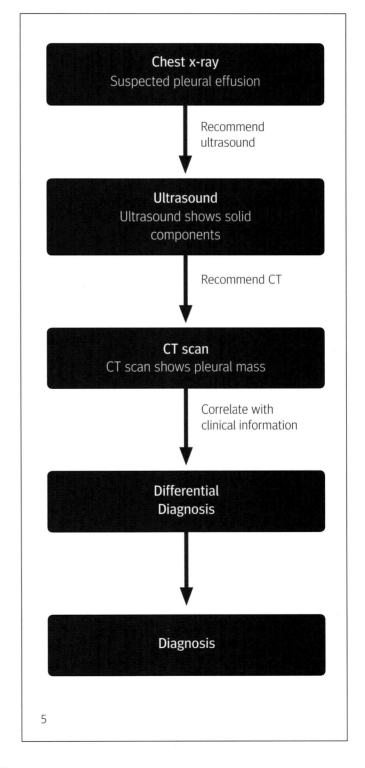

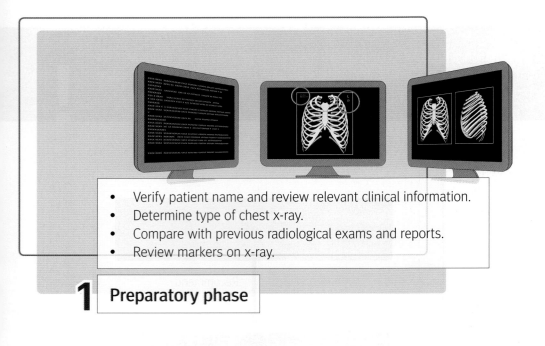

- Verify patient name and review relevant clinical information.
- Determine type of chest x-ray.
- Compare with previous radiological exams and reports.
- Review markers on x-ray.

1 Preparatory phase

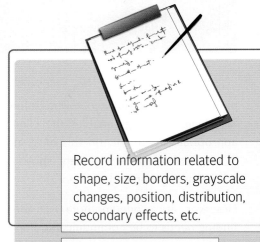

Record information related to shape, size, borders, grayscale changes, position, distribution, secondary effects, etc.

3 Descriptive phase

2 Visual identification phase

- Compare to normal.
- Scan x-ray using systematic approach.

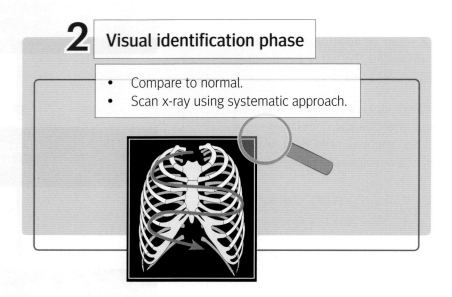

Summary

From your perspective as a learner, phase 1 of the interpretive process should be self-explanatory. Phases 2 and 3 may be more difficult to understand due to a lack of knowledge about basic anatomy and radiological anatomy. Phase 4 can also be challenging because you need to filter through what is relevant and what is not, in order to establish the summary. Moreover the differential diagnosis (phase 5) can only be given if a proper summary is established.

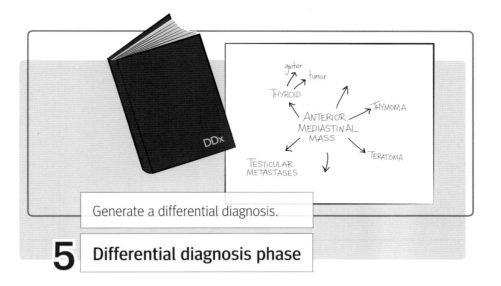

Generate a differential diagnosis.

5 **Differential diagnosis phase**

4 **Summary phase**

Generate a summary statement based on key findings.

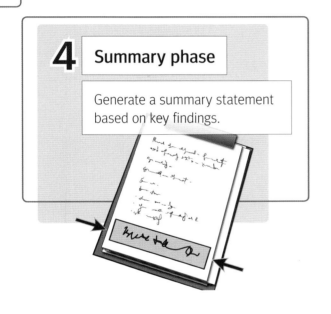

6 **Communication (action) phase**

Communicate the next steps (eg., treatment plan, further tests, etc.).

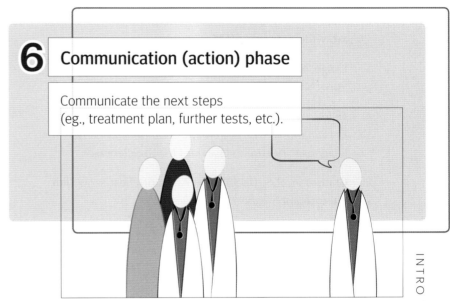

To complete the interpretive process successfully requires knowledge of anatomy, knowledge of how this anatomy appears on an x-ray, and knowledge of the radiological appearance of pathology. Just remember, chest x-ray interpretation is a combination of systematic analysis and finding patterns – and all of the phases take practice!

The following chapters will review the key elements to the interpretive process that are specific to each anatomical structure (**Chapters 7-14**). In addition, the interpretive process will be reviewed in the last section of this book, after you have developed confidence with the essential learning blocks.

References

1. Kundel, H.L., & Nodine, C.F. (1975). Interpreting chest radiographs without visual search. *Radiology, 116*(3):527–532.

2. Heusinkveld, D.W. (1940). Interpretation of chest x-ray films. *Chest, 6*(12): 373–376.

3. Lange, S. (1990). *Radiology of Chest Diseases*. New York, NY: Thieme Medical Publishers.

4. Talley, N.J., & O'Connor, S. (2009). *Clinical Examination: A Systematic Guide to Physical Diagnosis*. Australia: Elsevier Health Sciences.

5. Crausman, R.S. (1998). The ABCs of chest x-ray film interpretation. *Chest, 113*(1):256–257.

6. Reeder, M.M. & Felson, B. (2003). *Reeder and Felson's Gamuts in Radiology: Comprehensive Lists of Roentgen Differential Diagnosis*. New York, NY: Springer.

7. Reed, J.C. (2003). *Chest Radiology: Plain Film Patterns and Differential Diagnoses* (5th ed). Mosby, PA: Elsevier Health Sciences.

8. Davies, S.G., & Nakielny, R. (Eds.). (2009). *Aids to Radiological Differential Diagnosis*. Philadelphia, PA: W.B. Saunders.

RADIOLOGIC
ANATOMY and
PATHOLOGY

In Section I you learned about radiation and how the x-ray image is formed. You also reviewed the key elements to the visual interpretation process.

Section II is divided into 10 chapters. This section starts with a description of the radiological zones. The concept of radiological zones is introduced to give you a starting point in the understanding of the radiological anatomy of the chest. The next 8 chapters review in detail the radiological anatomy of specific anatomical structures and regions found within the thorax. The chapters also provide examples of how the x-ray image can change due to pathology. The final chapter explains how the individual structures come together to form the radiological image.

The focus of this section is on the anatomy of the normal PA and lateral chest x-ray - the radiological anatomy - and the basics of how pathology can alter this normal radiological appearance. Understanding this is the foundation for interpreting the more complex x-rays presented in Section III.

CHAPTER 6

The RADIOLOGICAL ZONES
of the THORAX
and KEY LANDMARKS

importance

The concept of radiological zones is introduced to facilitate discussion
about anatomy in general terms, while you are learning how to accurately
localize pathology to specific anatomical structures. The radiological
zones are used to describe anatomical areas. As you develop a better
understanding of the radiological anatomy of the chest, you will gradually
move away from the description of radiological zones to descriptions of
the specific anatomy.

In this chapter, you will learn how to define and locate the six radiological
zones on PA and lateral chest x-rays, and about some key landmarks
useful for localization.

objectives

Skills

You will identify

- the radiological zones on the PA and lateral chest x-rays;.the areas
  where the various radiological zones overlap on the PA and lateral
  chest x-rays.

Knowledge

You will review and understand

- how to accurately describe and localize each of the six radiological
  zones on the PA and lateral x-rays.
- the concept of using key landmarks to localize other structures within
  the thorax.

associated resources

This chapter maps to the following AMSER curriculum content (1,2).

1) Lungs
   Trachea and carina
   Right and left main bronchi

2) Heart
   Aorta

3) Mediastinum
   Right and left main pulmonary arteries

4) Bone and soft tissues
   Diaphragms

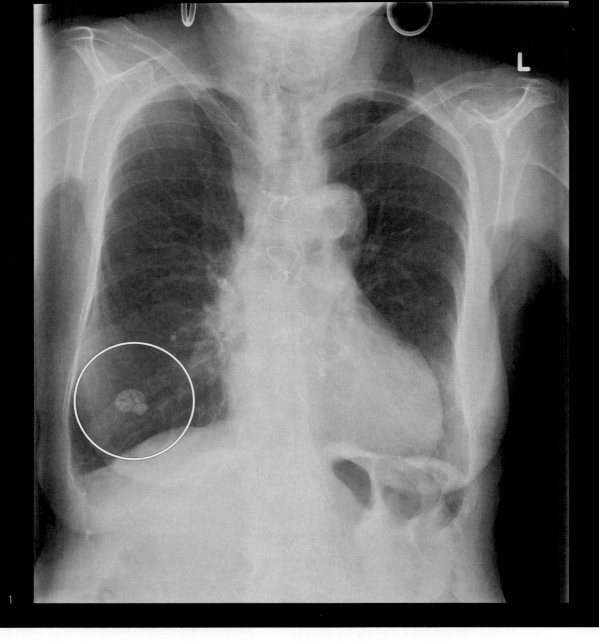

1

A 72-year-old female presents with mild exertional dyspnea. The patient has had a previous sternotomy and aortic valve replacement. The family doctor ordered a chest x-ray. You are on a radiology elective and are asked to comment on the PA chest x-ray (Fig. 1). You correctly identify a white oval lesion on the right, inferiorly.

Anterior pleura
Lung
Mediastinum
Posterior pleura
Posterior ribs
Soft tissues of the chest wall posteriorly

Without the aid of a lateral x-ray
and using the PA x-ray only,
select which of the above locations
are possible for the lesion in Figure 1.

THE RADIOLOGICAL ZONES

A photograph of the thorax gives a 2D image of the exterior surface of the 3D human body, whereas an x-ray of the thorax gives a 2D representation of the entire depth of the 3D human body – all external and internal structures. All organs and tissues of the chest from front to back (or side to side on a lateral x-ray) are collectively included. Because the process is all-inclusive (i.e., the x-rays go right through the body), there is considerable overlap of the anatomical structures on the image produced. The issue of overlap was discussed in greater detail in Chapter 2.

AMSER The overlap of anatomical structures sometimes makes it impossible to identify individual structures separately; for example, the lateral border of the descending thoracic aorta is clearly visible (Fig. 2a), whereas the medial border is not (Fig. 2b). It is present; we just do not see it as a separate structure.

To simplify the radiological anatomy for the purposes of interpretation and to lessen any ambiguity due to overlap, it is useful for you to divide the anatomical structures of the thorax into radiological zones. As you gain confidence in understanding radiological anatomy, the need to use the radiological zones will decrease and will be replaced with the use of names of the specific anatomical structures. Even so, the use of radiological zones will never be completely replaced because even with years of experience, in some circumstances it is impossible to accurately localize pathology based on standard x-rays alone. In these cases, accurate anatomical localization requires cross-sectional imaging.

Six zones are described on PA and lateral chest x-rays

Zone 1	Hilar Zone
Zone 2	Mediastinal Zone
Zone 3	Cardiac Zone
Zone 4	Pleural Zone
Zone 5	Lung Zone
Zone 6	Peripheral Zone

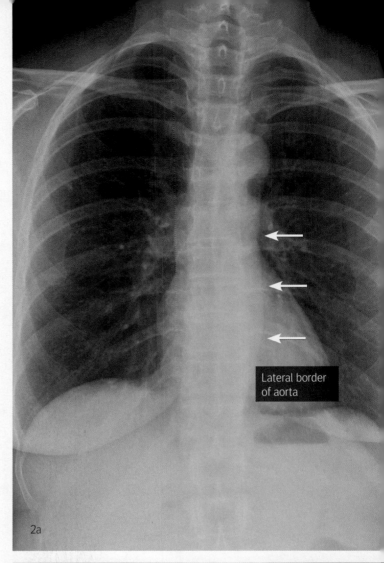

Lateral border of aorta

2a

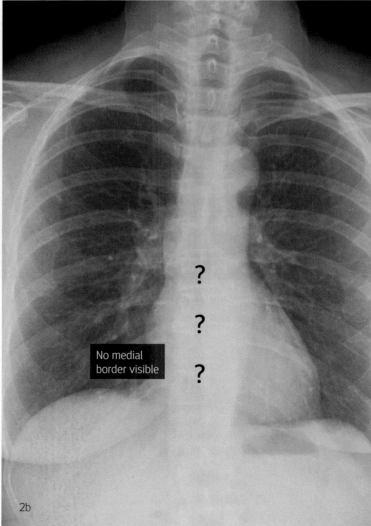

No medial border visible

?

?

?

2b

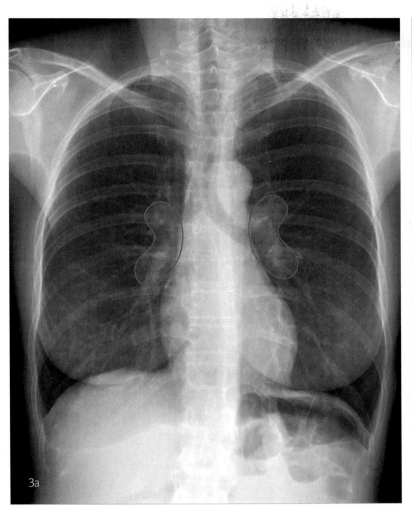

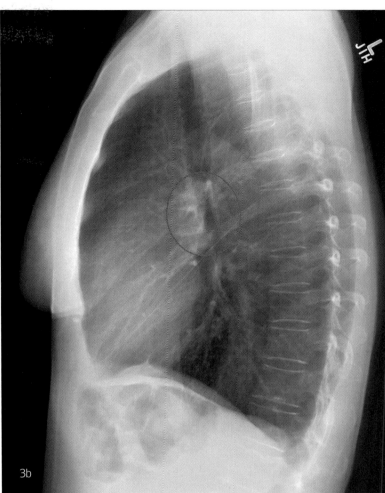

3a

3b

The zones are presented in an order to correspond with the chapter order in this Section.

Zone 1 - The Hilar Zones

The hilar zones are two medial areas in the thorax that correspond to the location of the proximal pulmonary arteries. On the PA x-ray (Fig. 3a), they appear as white extensions from the central part of the mediastinal zone. The shape of the hilar zone roughly resembles the letter H. On the lateral x-ray (Fig. 3b), the hilar zone lies centrally in the thorax. The details of the hilar zone will be presented in **Chapter 8**.

Figure 2. Overlap of anatomical structures. Overlap of structures can make it difficult to identify borders. a, PA chest x-ray in which the lateral border of the descending aorta is visible (arrows), b, the same PA chest x-ray in which the medial border of the descending aorta is hidden by adjacent structures within the mediastinum (?s).

Figure 3. The hilar zones. a, PA chest x-ray with the hilar zones outlined, b, lateral chest x-ray with the hilar zones outlined.

ZONES & LANDMARKS **Chapter 6** SECTION II

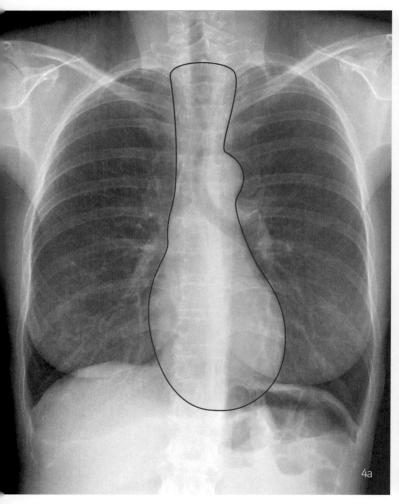

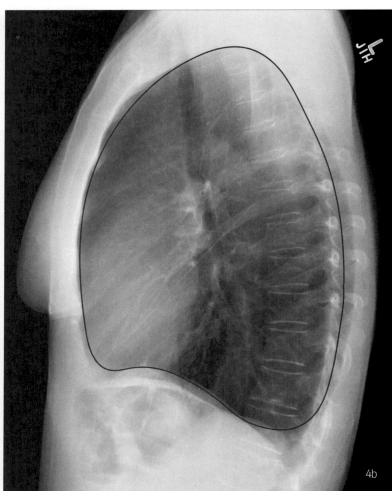

Zone 2 - The Mediastinal Zone

The mediastinal zone on the PA x-ray (Fig. 4a) is the area within the thorax lying between the medial edges of the lungs. The margins of this zone are clearly seen on the PA x-ray because a significant part of the mediastinum abuts the adjacent lungs. On the lateral x-ray (Fig. 4b), the mediastinal zone covers the same area as the pleural and lung zones from the front of the thorax to the back. The mediastinal zone will be discussed in more detail in Chapter 9.

Figure 4. The mediastinal zone. a, PA chest x-ray with the mediastinal zone outlined, b, lateral chest x-ray with the mediastinal zone outlined.

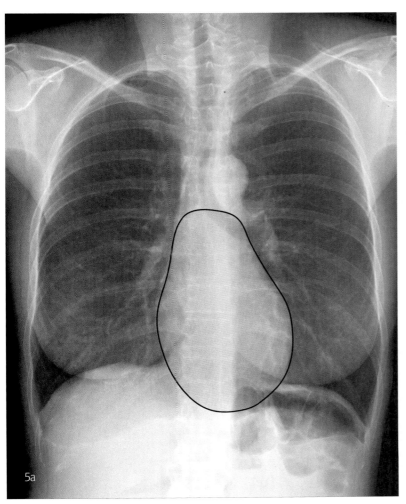

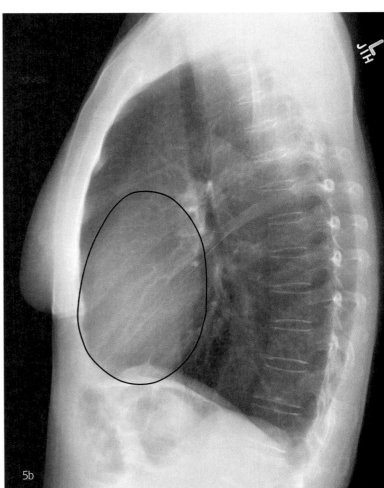

Zone 3 - The Cardiac Zone

The cardiac zone lies in the anterior and inferior part of the mediastinal zone. On both the PA (Fig. 5a) and lateral (Fig. 5b) x-rays, the outer edges of this zone are formed by the heart, pericardium and mediastinal fat. The specific heart chambers that contribute to the visible edges will be discussed in **Chapter 10**.

Figure 5. The cardiac zone. a, PA chest x-ray with the cardiac zone outlined, b, lateral chest x-ray with the cardiac zone outlined.

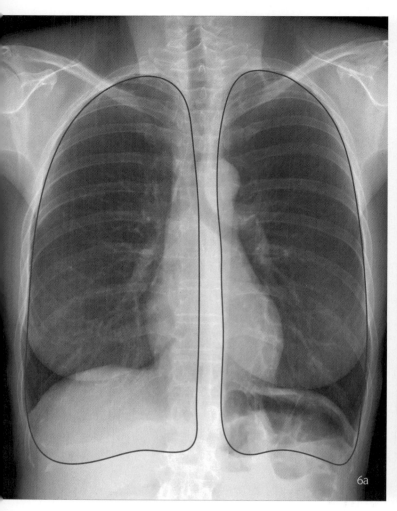

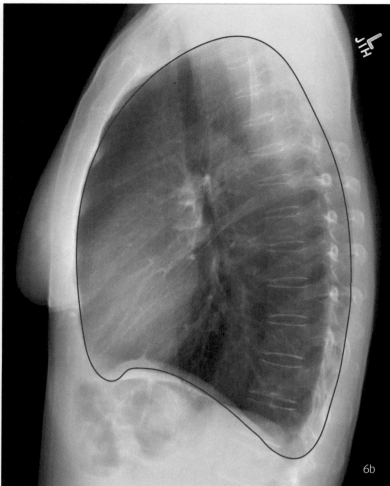

Zone 4 - The Pleural Zone

Because of the close relationship of the pleura to the lungs (the pleura surround the lungs), the pleural zone roughly corresponds to the lung zone on the PA (Fig. 6a) and lateral (Fig. 6b) x-rays. In Chapter 11, you will learn that the pleural zone is, in fact, larger than the lung zone - especially posteriorly and inferiorly.

Figure 6. The pleural zone. a, PA chest x-ray with the pleural zone outlined, b, lateral chest x-ray with the pleural zone outlined.

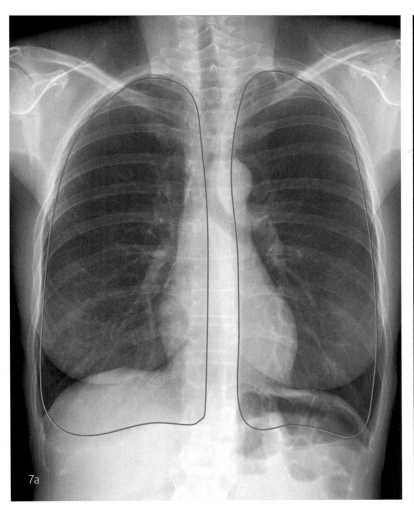

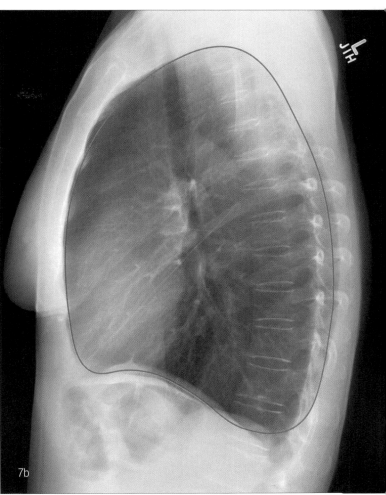

Figure 7. The lung zone. a, PA chest x-ray with the lung zone outlined, b, lateral chest x-ray with the lung zone outlined.

Zone 5 - The Lung Zone

The lung zone is the area in the thorax that contains the lungs and corresponds to the air-filled region between the ribs and the mediastinum medially. On the PA x-ray (Fig. 7a), the lung zone will have lateral, medial, superior and inferior borders. On the lateral x-ray (Fig. 7b), the lung zone has anterior, posterior, superior and inferior borders. The lung zone occupies a large percentage of the thorax. A common mistake made by learners is that they think the lungs only exist within the limits of the visible black areas on the chest x-ray. However, these are only the directly-visualized lung fields. Significant portions of the lungs are partially obscured because they overlap the mediastinum, heart and diaphragms. These portions of the lungs are visualized indirectly, through other structures. More information on the lung zone can be found in Chapter 12.

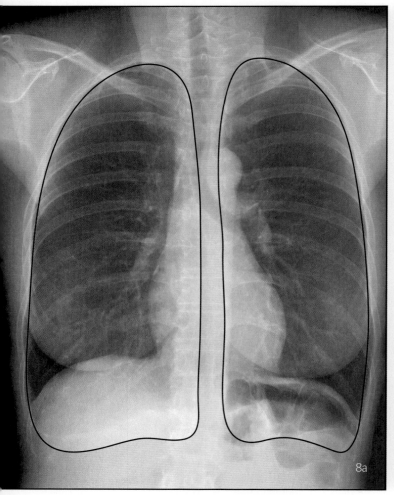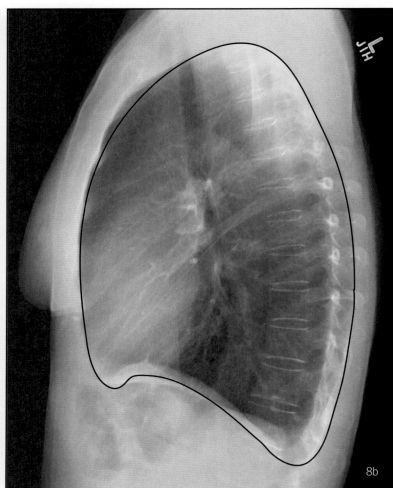

Zone 6 - The Peripheral Zone

The peripheral zone contains all of the remaining structures of the thorax not found in the other five zones. This zone extends from the pleural zone outward to cover the chest wall, lower neck and upper abdomen (Fig. 8a,b). The peripheral zone will be discussed in more detail in Chapter 14.

Figure 8. The peripheral zone. a, PA chest x-ray with the peripheral zone outlined, b, lateral chest x-ray with the peripheral zone outlined.

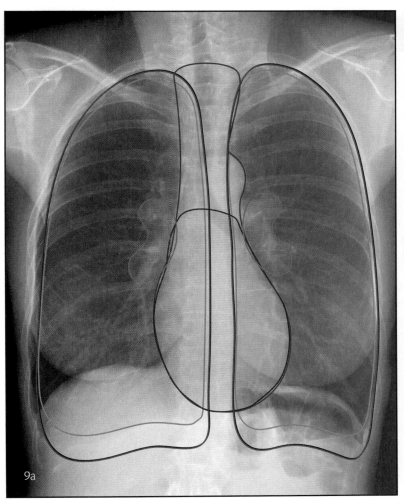

9a

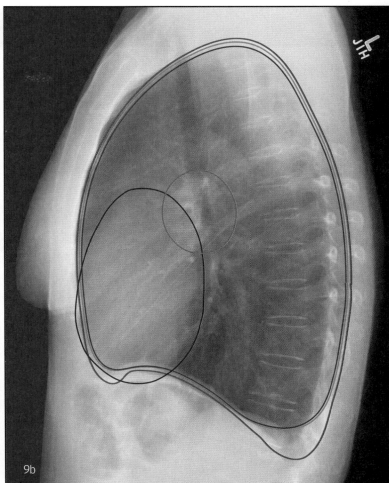

9b

On the lateral chest x-ray, the pleural, lung and mediastinal zones all completely overlap.

Overlap of the Zones

The overlap of the zones on the PA x-ray is highlighted in Figure 9a. The more central on the x-ray, the more overlap that occurs. The overlap is even more complex on the lateral x-ray (Fig. 9b) because the right and left-sided structures also overlap.

Figure 9. All zones overlap. a, PA chest x-ray with all of the overlapping zones outlined. b, lateral chest x-ray with all of the overlapping zones outlined.

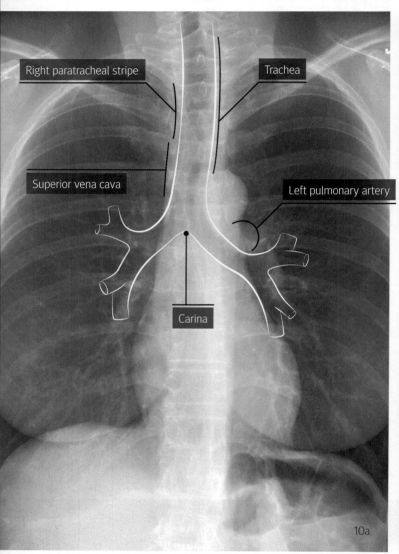

Right paratracheal stripe

Trachea

Superior vena cava

Left pulmonary artery

Carina

10a

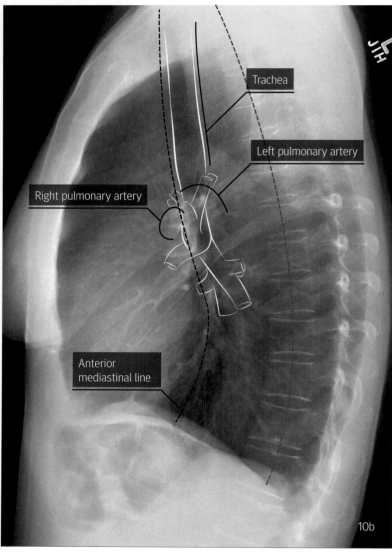

Trachea

Left pulmonary artery

Right pulmonary artery

Anterior mediastinal line

10b

AMSER **THE IMPORTANCE OF LANDMARKS**

One of the keys to identification of specific anatomical structures in the chest is through the recognition of important landmarks. A landmark should be easy to distinguish on a grayscale image. It should be present on most x-rays so that it can be used as a reliable starting point. A landmark should have unique and consistent features that make it a useful guide to locate and identify other anatomical structures – especially for those structures that may be difficult to identify on their own.

One of the most important landmarks is the trachea. The trachea is an easily recognizable, black, rectangular structure on both the PA and lateral

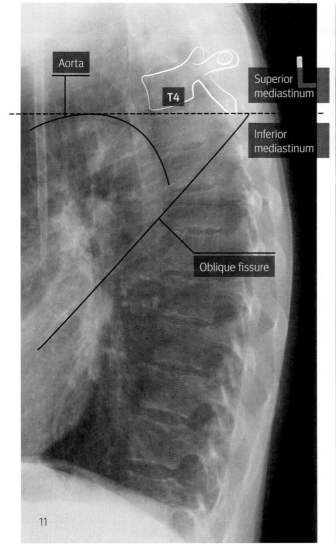

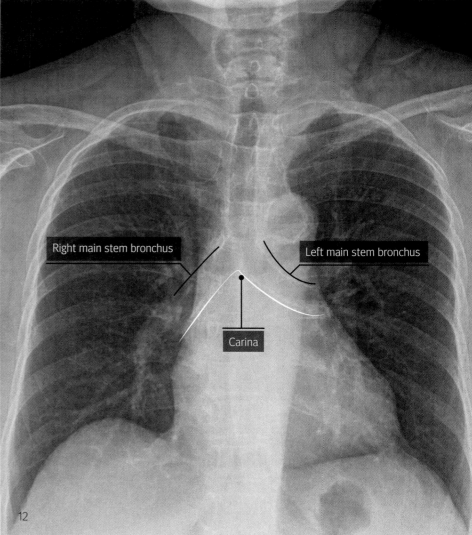

11

12

A second key landmark is the fourth thoracic vertebral body (T4). The bodies of the thoracic vertebrae are easy to identify, but can be difficult to number, especially on the lateral x-ray. A method for counting the thoracic vertebrae is discussed in Chapter 14 (Pg. 354). On the lateral x-ray, T4 is useful in identifying the aorta and the upper posterior margin of the oblique fissures, and is used to delineate the superior and the inferior mediastinum (Fig. 11).

Other important landmarks are the carina, the diaphragms and the aortic arch. The carina is used to identify the level of the main bronchi, and as a reference point for central line and endotracheal tube placement (Fig. 12)(Ch. 20, Pgs. 740, 750).

Figure 10. The trachea as a landmark. a, PA chest x-ray highlighting the trachea as a landmark for the left pulmonary artery, the aortic arch, superior vena cava (SVC) and right paratracheal stripe, b, lateral chest x-ray highlighting the trachea as a landmark for the left and right pulmonary arteries and the anterior mediastinal line (the border of the anterior and middle mediastinum).

Figure 11. T4 as a landmark. Lateral chest x-ray highlighting T4 as a landmark for the aorta, superior posterior limit of the oblique fissures, and the border of the superior and inferior mediastinum.

Figure 12. The carina as a landmark. PA chest x-ray highlighting the carina as a landmark. The carina defines the level where the main stem bronchi merge together.

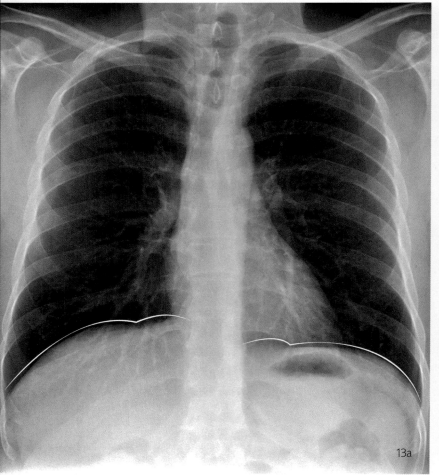

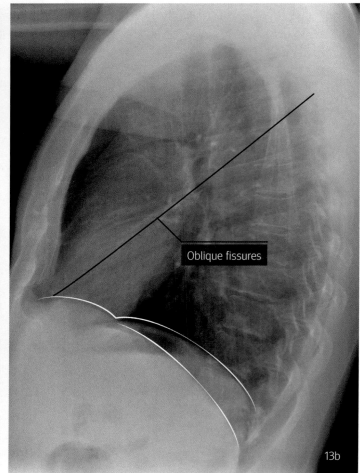

Oblique fissures

13a

13b

AMSER

LANDMARK	USEFUL TO LOCALIZE	
	On the PA x-ray	On the lateral x-ray
Trachea	• Left pulmonary artery • Aortic arch • Right paratracheal stripe • Superior vena cava	• Left pulmonary artery • Mediastinal divisions • Posterior paratracheal stripe • Right pulmonary artery
T4	———	• Upper posterior part of oblique fissures • Superior/inferior mediastinum • Angle of Louis • Top of aortic arch
Carina	• End of trachea • Origin of the main bronchi	———
Domes of the diaphragms	• Anterior inferior level of major fissures • Inferior border of the lungs laterally	• Anterior inferior level of major fissures • Inferior border of lungs anteriorly and posteriorly
Top of the aortic arch	• Posterior superior level of major fissures	• Posterior superior level of major fissures

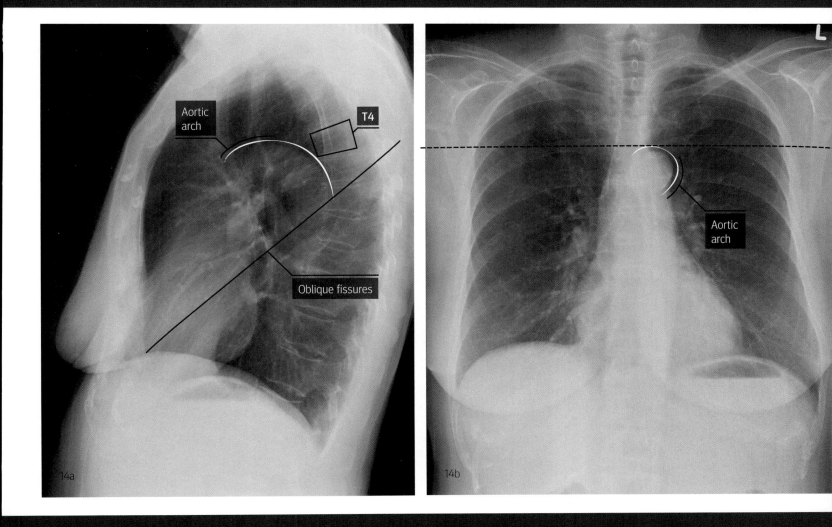

The domes of the diaphragms identify the anterior, inferior level of the major fissures (Fig. 13a,b)(Ch. 11, Pg. 398). The top of the aortic arch defines the superior level of the major fissures (Fig. 14a,b) (Ch. 11, Pg. 398).

Figure 13. The domes of the diaphragms as landmarks. The domes of the diaphragms can be used to define the position of the oblique fissures. a, PA chest x-ray highlighting the diaphragms as landmarks, b, lateral chest x-ray highlighting the diaphragms as landmarks.

AMSER

Figure 14. The top of the aortic arch as a landmark. The top of the aortic arch is used to define the position of the oblique fissure. a, lateral chest x-ray highlighting the aortic arch as a landmark, b, PA chest x-ray highlighting the aortic arch as a landmark. The line defines the superior limit of the oblique fissure.

The important message is that on a single x-ray view, the spatial positioning of an abnormality may be difficult to determine; having the second view allows for the correct localization.

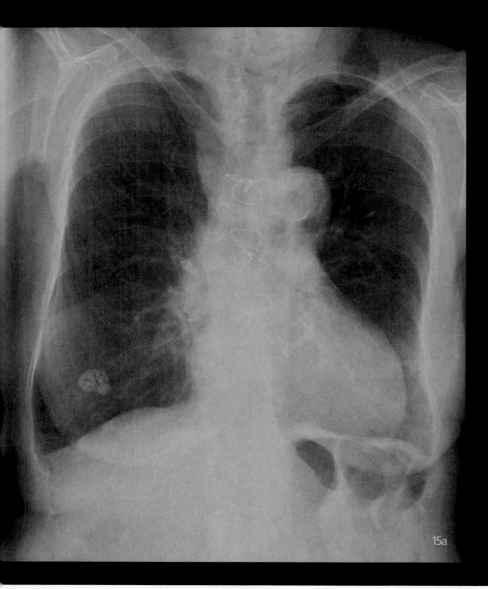

15a

Without the aid of a lateral x-ray and using the PA x-ray only, select which of the following locations are possible for the lesion in Figure 15a.

Soft tissues of the chest wall anteriorly
Anterior ribs
Anterior pleura
Lung
Mediastinum
Posterior pleura
Posterior ribs
Soft tissues of the chest wall posteriorly

CASE STUDY

A 72-year-old female presents with mild exertional dyspnea. The patient has had a previous sternotomy and aortic valve replacement. The family doctor ordered a chest x-ray. You are on a radiology elective and are asked to comment on the PA chest x-ray (Fig. 15a). You correctly identify a white oval lesion on the right, inferiorly.

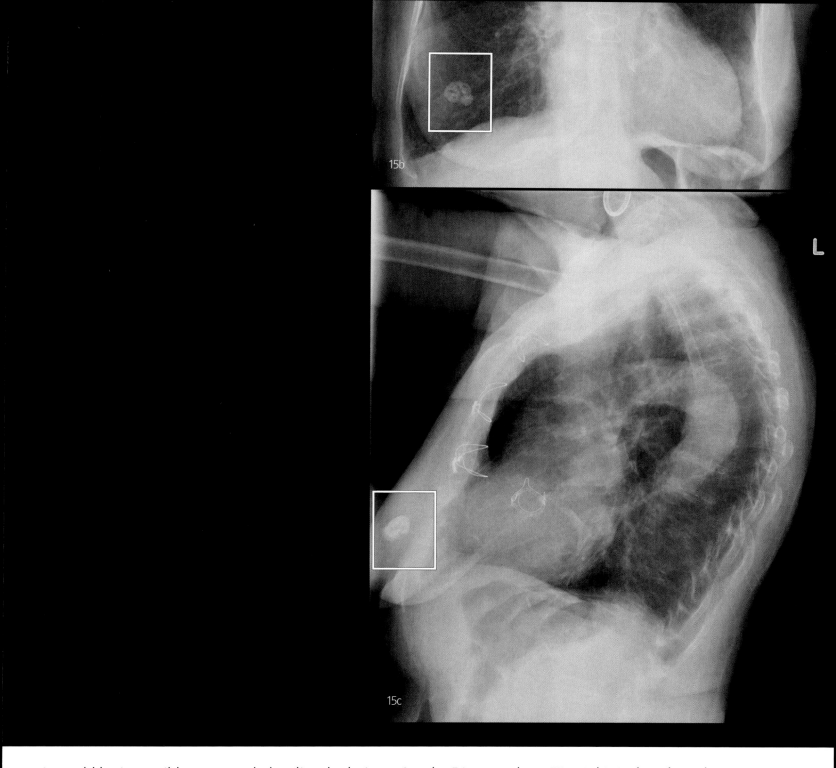

It would be impossible to correctly localize the lesion using the PA x-ray alone (Fig. 15b). In fact, from the PA x-ray alone, the lesion could lie in any one of the positions listed, except 5, the mediastinum. The lateral x-ray is essential to localize the lesion (Fig. 15c).

The lesion is found on the lateral x-ray anteriorly, outside of the chest cavity, within the right breast. In this case, even without knowledge of the radiological anatomy of the thoracic structure, a student can correctly localize the lesion.

The opacity of the lesion is very white, consistent with benign calcification. This represents an incidental finding and has no relationship to the patient's symptoms.

DISCUSSION

References

1. Lewis, P.J., Shaffer, K., & Donovan, A. (Eds.). (2012). AMSER National Medical Student Curriculum in Radiology. http://aur.org/Secondary-Alliances.aspx?id=141.

2. Lewis, P.J., & Shaffer, K. (2005). Developing a national medical student curriculum in radiology. *Am. Coll. Radiol., 2*(1):8–11.

3. Konen, E., Greenberg, I., & Rozenman, J. (2005). Visibility of normal thoracic anatomic landmarks on storage phosphor digital radiography versus conventional radiography. *Isr. Med. Assoc. J., 7*(8):495–497.

Knowledge

You will review and understand

- the anatomy of the trachea and main stem bronchi.

- the radiological appearance of the trachea and main stem bronchi.

- the relationship of the trachea and main stem bronchi to other anatomical structures.

- the role of the trachea in creating mediastinal interfaces.

- how pathology, intrinsic and extrinsic, can change the radiological appearance of the trachea and main stem bronchi.

- the common causes of tracheal narrowing and enlargement.

- the important radiological signs related to the major airways.

associated resources

This chapter maps to the following AMSER curriculum content (1,2).

1) Normal radiological anatomy
   Trachea and bronchi
   Right and left main bronchi

2) Pathological conditions affecting the trachea and bronchi
   Goitre

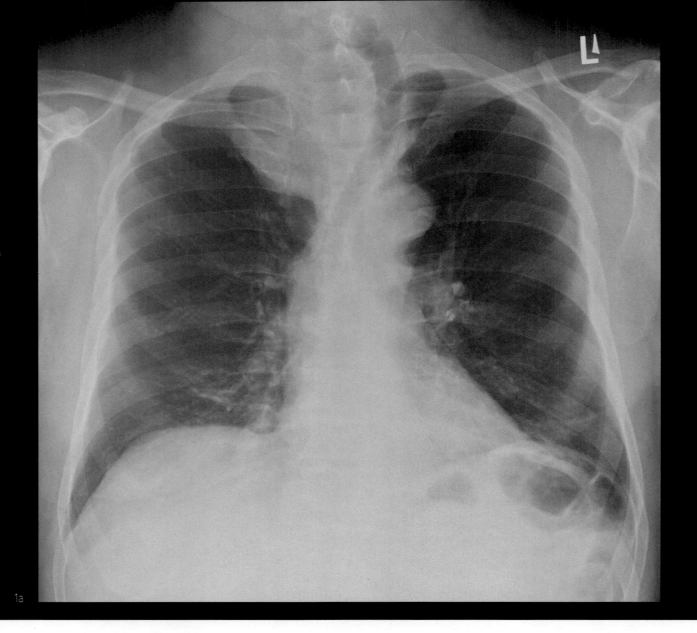

1a

You are the intern on call in the emergency department and you are called in to see a 70-year-old male patient who presents with stridor. You try to take a history from the patient, but he is very distressed and cannot communicate properly. On physical examination, you feel a large, firm mass in the lower neck region. Many differential diagnoses run through your mind and you decide that you need a chest x-ray to help eliminate some of them from your list. You order PA and lateral chest x-rays (Fig. 1a,b).

174

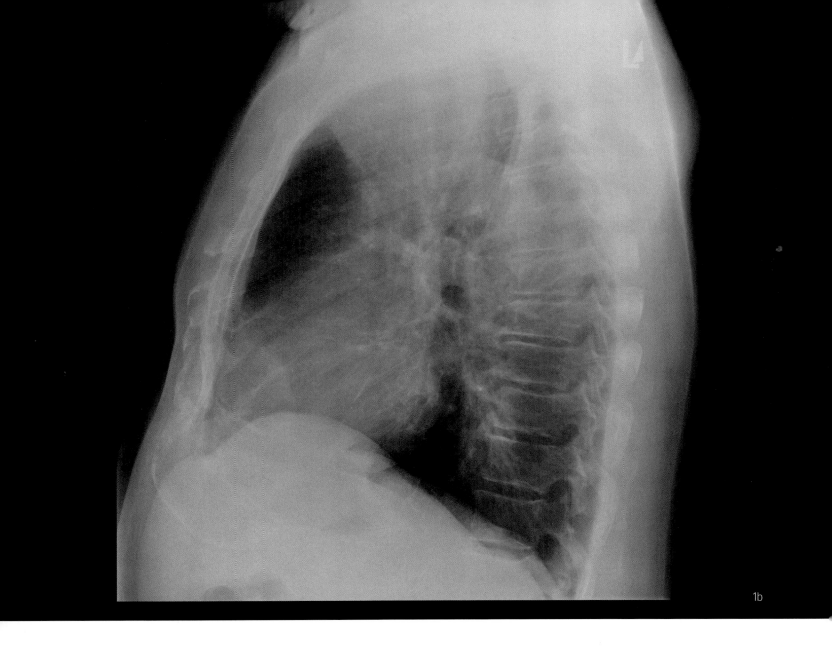

1b

What are
your findings?

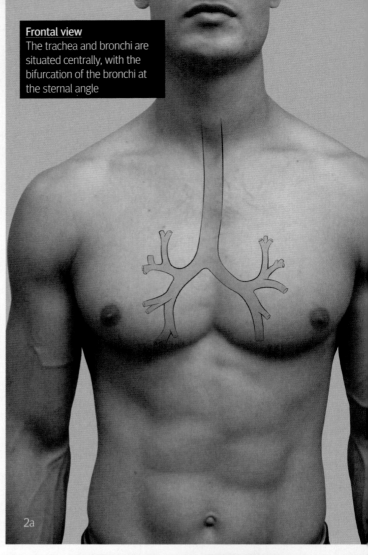

Frontal view
The trachea and bronchi are situated centrally, with the bifurcation of the bronchi at the sternal angle

2a

THE MAJOR AIRWAYS – THE TRACHEA & PROXIMAL BRONCHI

Snuggled within the mediastinum, but meriting their own discussion, are the lifelines that allow air to get into our lungs: the trachea and bronchi (Fig. 2a,b). The trachea starts at the larynx and terminates at the carina, where the right and left main stem bronchi begin. This tracheal bifurcation lies at the fourth or fifth thoracic vertebra (T4-T5), or at the level of the sternal angle.

From a functional perspective, the airways are divided into three zones (Fig. 3).

Zone 1: The conductive zone, which includes the trachea and bronchi to the level of the nonalveolated bronchioles.

Zone 2: The transitory zone, which includes the respiratory bronchioles, alveolar ducts and alveolar sacs.

Zone 3: The respiratory zone, which contains the alveoli.

In this chapter, the discussion will be limited to Zone 1 – the conductive zone: the trachea and bronchi.

Figure 2. Surface anatomy localization of the trachea and bronchi. a, frontal perspective, b, lateral perspective.

Figure 3. Functional respiratory zones. Illustration of the functional zones of the airways.

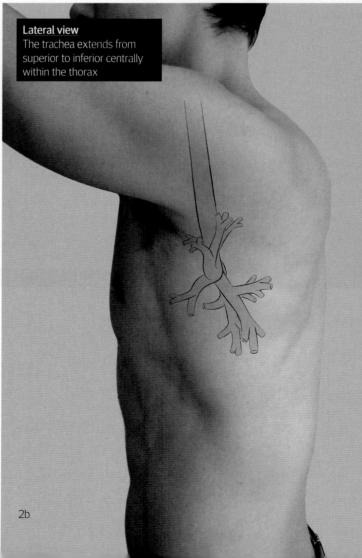

Lateral view
The trachea extends from superior to inferior centrally within the thorax

2b

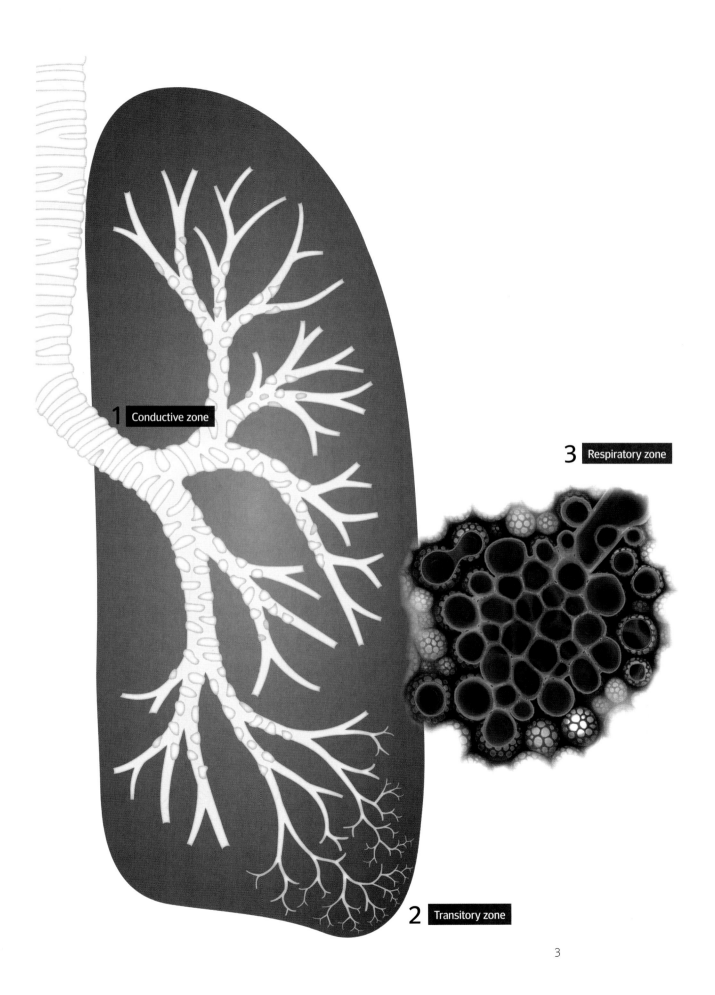

1 Conductive zone

3 Respiratory zone

2 Transitory zone

3

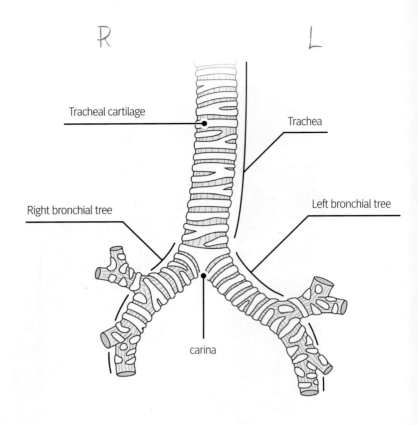

R   L

Tracheal cartilage

Trachea

Right bronchial tree

Left bronchial tree

carina

4a

The Trachea

The trachea, also referred to as the windpipe, is the major airway carrying air to the lungs. The word trachea originates from the Greek *arteria tracheia*, meaning rough artery, so called because of its bumpy appearance due to the rings of cartilage that encircle the airway.

As a geometrical structure, the trachea represents a hollow cylinder, approximately 8-13 cm in length (Fig. 4a,b,c). The trachea courses in a downward and posterior direction. Most of the trachea (6-9 cm) lies within the thorax – the intrathoracic portion. A shorter (2-4 cm) extrathoracic portion lies within the neck.

In adults, the trachea measures approximately 21 mm in its widest coronal diameter and 23 mm in its widest sagittal diameter in women; and approximately 25 mm in its widest coronal diameter and 27 mm in its widest sagittal diameter in men (3). This is about the diameter of your thumb.

The trachea contains 18-22 cartilaginous rings, giving the lumen of the trachea an irregular, wavy contour. The tracheal cartilage rings are incomplete posteriorly. Cartilaginous rings are also present in the walls of the proximal bronchi.

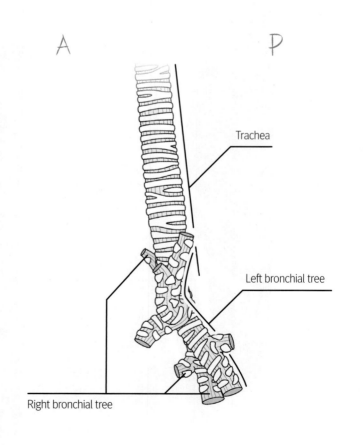

A   P

Trachea

Left bronchial tree

Right bronchial tree

4b

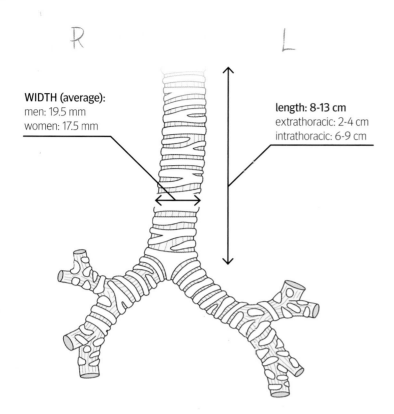

WIDTH (average):
men: 19.5 mm
women: 17.5 mm

length: 8-13 cm
extrathoracic: 2-4 cm
intrathoracic: 6-9 cm

4c

In the pediatric population, these measurements are smaller and vary considerably. **!**

LENGTH	TOTAL: 8-13 cm Extrathoracic: 2-4 cm Intrathoracic: 6-9 cm
DIAMETER (AVERAGE)	Adult Men: 19.5 mm 13-25 mm coronal 13-27 mm sagittal Adult Women: 17.5 mm 10-21 mm coronal 10-23 mm sagittal

Table 7.1
Normal Tracheal Measurements

The trachea is a key radiological structure because it represents an important landmark (Ch. 6, Pg. 164) used to identify other key anatomical structures that include:

- The right pulmonary artery.
- The left pulmonary artery.
- The compartments of the mediastinum.
- The paratracheal stripe.

Figure 4. Anatomy of the trachea and bronchi. Illustrations of the trachea and bronchi, a, frontal perspective, b, lateral perspective, c, with dimensions.

Radiological Shape and Grayscale of the Trachea

Because the trachea has a cylindrical shape, contains air, and is surrounded by the soft tissues of the mediastinum, it will appear as a vertical black rectangle on both the PA and lateral x-rays. The rectangle on the PA x-ray (Fig. 5a,b,c,d) will be directed from superior to inferior, and on the lateral x-ray (Fig. 6a,b,c,d) from superior anterior to inferior posterior. The borders of the rectangle may appear irregular because of the tracheal cartilage, which gives the appearance of corrugations. In the elderly population, tracheal cartilage can calcify. This calcified cartilage can help delineate the borders of the trachea.

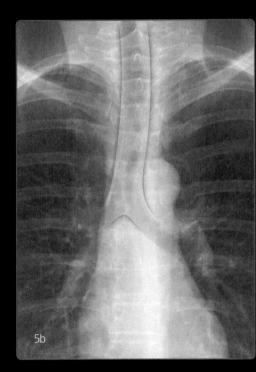

Figure 5. Radiological anatomy of the trachea from the frontal perspective. a, PA chest x-ray with the trachea outlined, b, PA chest x-ray with grayscale illustration of trachea overlay, c, PA chest x-ray cropped to highlight the trachea, d, magnification of PA chest x-ray highlighting calcification.

5a

5b

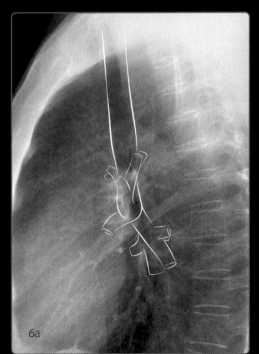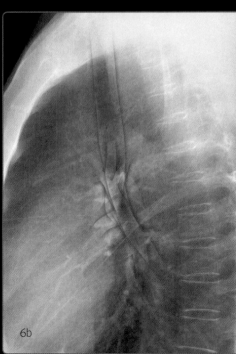

Figure 6. Radiological anatomy of the trachea from the lateral perspective. a, lateral chest x-ray with the trachea outlined, b, PA chest x-ray with grayscale illustration of the trachea overlay, c, lateral chest x-ray cropped to highlight the trachea, d, magnification of lateral chest x-ray highlighting corrugations.

6a

6b

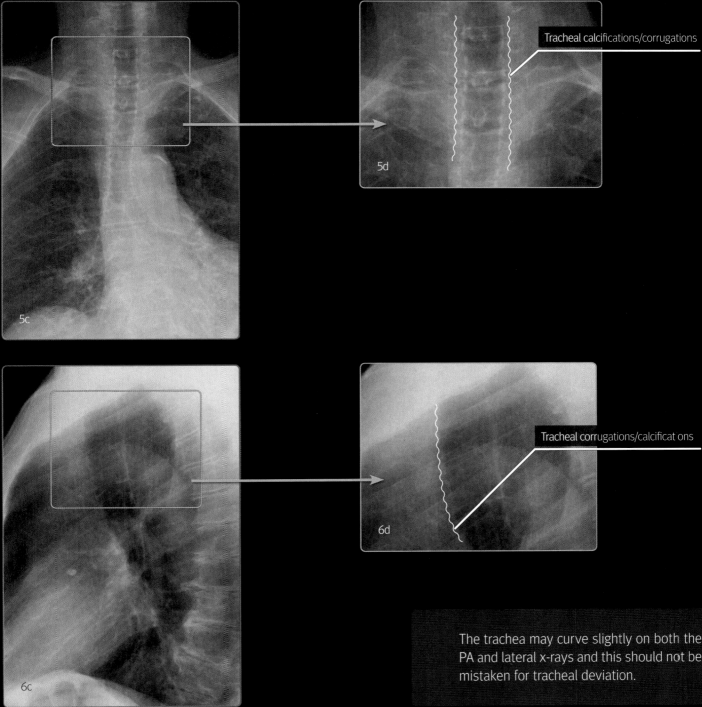

Tracheal calcifications/corrugations

5c

5d

Tracheal corrugations/calcificat ons

6c

6d

The trachea may curve slightly on both the PA and lateral x-rays and this should not be mistaken for tracheal deviation.

How to identify the trachea on the PA x-ray

STEP 1
Confirm that the patient is midline, and not rotated (Ch. 1, Pg. 32).

STEP 2
Focus your vision on the midline of the patient at the level of the lower neck/upper thorax (Fig. 7).

STEP 3
Identify a black rectangle that is oriented vertically. This rectangle measures approximately 2 cm from side to side (Fig. 8).

STEP 4
Confirm that this is the trachea by

A Identifying corrugations in the wall of the black rectangle caused by tracheal cartilage, or identifying tracheal cartilage calcification (Fig. 9).

B Identifying the main stem bronchi as continuations of the trachea inferiorly (Fig. 10).

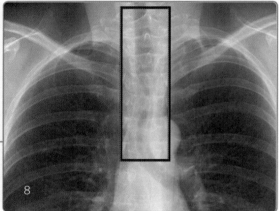

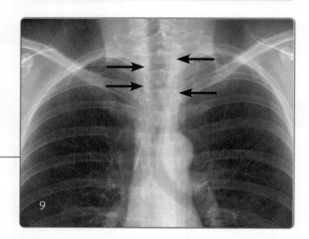

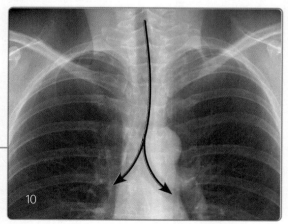

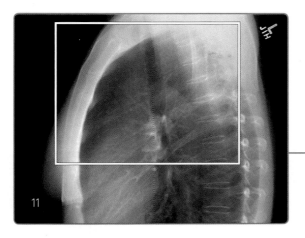

11

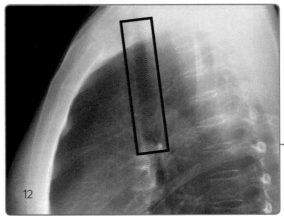

12

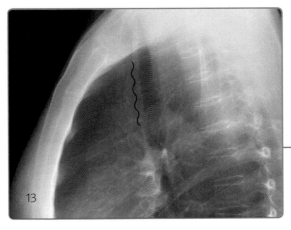

13

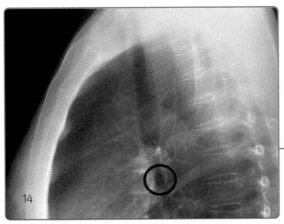

14

How to identify the trachea on the lateral x-ray

STEP 1
Focus your vision on the lower neck/ upper thorax (Fig. 11).

STEP 2
Identify a black rectangle oriented vertically, angled from superior anterior to inferior posterior (Fig. 12).

STEP 3
Confirm that this is the trachea by:

A   Identifying corrugations in the wall of the black rectangle caused by tracheal cartilage, or identifying tracheal cartilage calcification (Fig. 13).

B   Identifying the main stem bronchi as black circles within the black rectangle (Fig. 14).

?

The orientation of the scapulae wings can be up and down, framing air in the lungs as a vertical black rectangle on a lateral chest x-ray, and can, therefore, mimic a tracheal airway column (Fig. 15a,b,c). This can be distinguished from the trachea by a lack of corrugations or cartilage calcification.

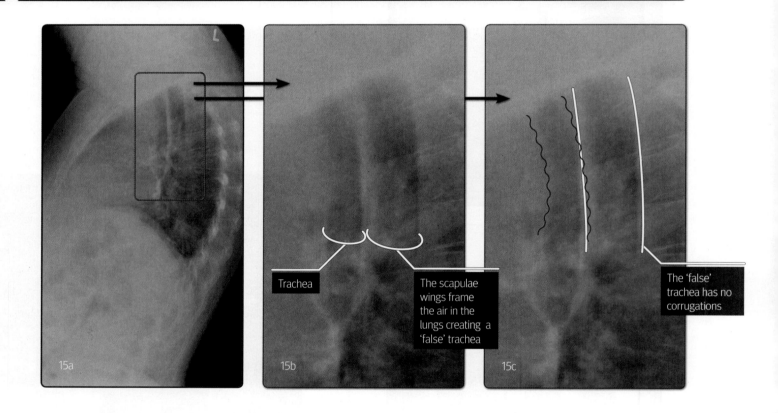

Trachea

The scapulae wings frame the air in the lungs creating a 'false' trachea

The 'false' trachea has no corrugations

15a

15b

15c

Figure 15. Scapulae wings can mimic the appearance of the trachea. On the lateral chest x-ray, the vertical white bands of the scapulae follow the course of the anterior and posterior walls of the trachea, and can be mistaken for the trachea. a, lateral chest x-ray, b, magnified region of the same lateral chest x-ray highlighting the trachea and 'false' trachea created by the scapulae, c, the same region of the lateral x-ray highlighting the lack of corrugations on the 'false' trachea (white).

ANATOMICAL RELATIONSHIPS OF THE TRACHEA

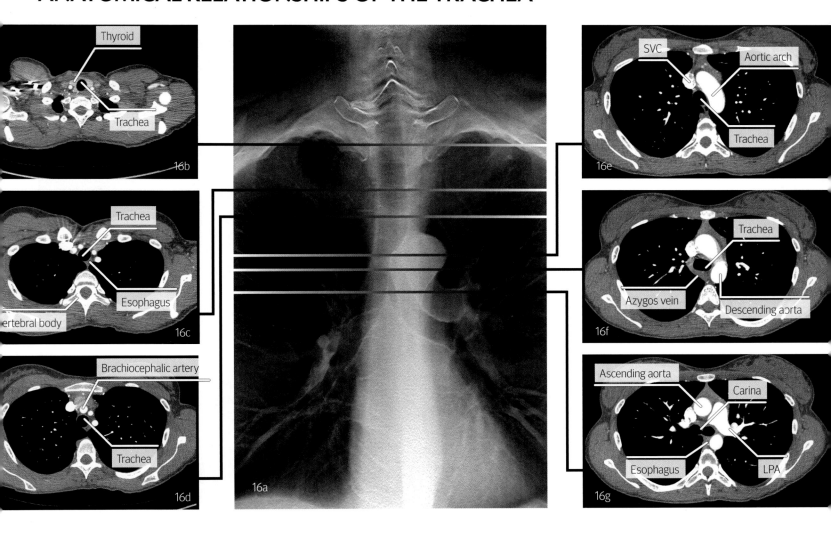

Figure 16. Spatial relationship of the trachea with other anatomical thoracic structures. a, Tomographical image of chest showing levels of cross sectional slices, b, slice 1 at the level of the thoracic inlet highlighting the thyroid gland, c, slice 2 through the superior trachea highlighting the esophagus and vertebral column, d, slice 3 midway down the trachea highlighting the brachiocephalic artery, e, slice 4 at the level of the aortic arch highlighting the aorta and superior vena cava (SVC), f, slice 5 just above the carina highlighting the azygos vein and descending aorta, g, slice 6 at the level of carina highlighting the ascending aorta, esophagus and left pulmonary artery (LPA).

Lying centrally in the thorax, the trachea forms many relationships with surrounding anatomical structures (3). Superiorly, in the lower neck, the thyroid gland lies anterior and lateral to the trachea. The proximal esophagus is found at the left posterior and superior border of the trachea. The vertebral bodies are at the right posterior border of the trachea. Midway down the trachea, the brachiocephalic artery lies anteriorly. At the level of the aortic arch, the aorta is found to the left, and the superior vena cava (SVC) to the right of the trachea. Below this, the descending aorta and the azygos vein can be found on the right and left of the trachea, respectively. At the level of the carina, anterior to the trachea the left pulmonary artery (LPA) can be seen to the left and the ascending aorta anteriorly on the right. Here, the esophagus can still be seen posteriorly.

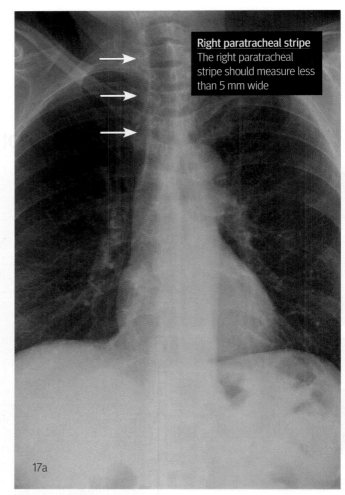

17a

INTERFACES RELATED TO THE TRACHEA

The lumen of the trachea is visible because of the air that lies within it. If the trachea touches the lung, then the wall of the trachea will be visible as the white line between the air in the lumen of the trachea and the air in the lung. An important interface on the PA chest x-ray is the right paratracheal stripe. This stripe represents the soft tissues lying adjacent to the right lateral border of the trachea and should measure less than 5 mm in thickness (Fig. 17a)(4). The right paratracheal stripe is also discussed on page 312 (Ch 9).

On the lateral chest x-ray, a white stripe is occasionally seen just posterior to the posterior aspect of the tracheal air column. This represents the soft tissues that lie between the posterior border of the trachea air column and the air within the esophagus, and is called the tracheoesophageal stripe. This stripe should measure no more than 5.5 mm in thickness (Fig. 17b)(5). Occasionally, an anterior tracheal stripe can also be visualized.

Figure 17. Right paratracheal stripe and tracheoesophageal stripe. a, PA chest x-ray with the right paratracheal stripe (white vertical stripe adjacent to the right border of the trachea) highlighted, b, lateral chest x-ray with the tracheoesophageal stripe (white vertical stripe posterior to the posterior border of the trachea) highlighted.

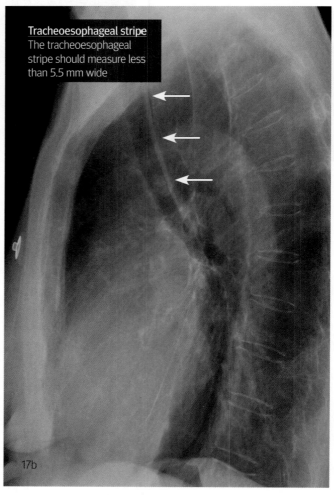

17b

The widening of the right paratracheal stripe is one of the most useful indicators of adenopathy in the mediastinum (Fig. 18a,b,c).

!

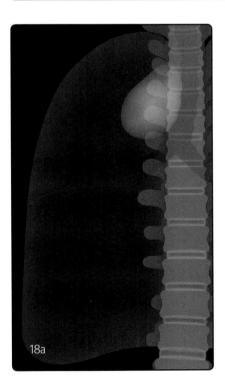
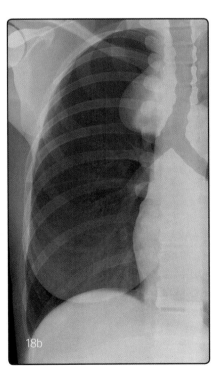
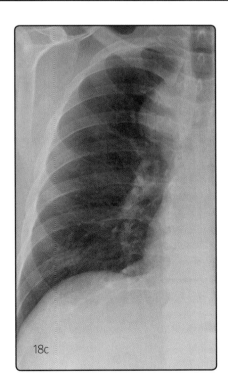

Figure 18. Widened paratracheal stripe. The paratracheal stripe can widen with pathology (adenopathy). a, artistic representation of a mediastinal mass causing widening of the right paratracheal stripe, b, artistic representation of the widened paratracheal stripe with all thoracic structures, c, PA chest x-ray with a widened paratracheal stripe

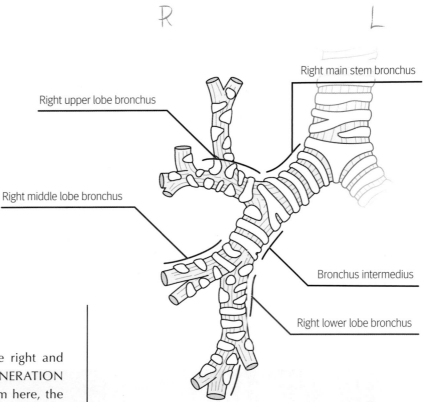

R   L

Right main stem bronchus

Right upper lobe bronchus

Right middle lobe bronchus

Bronchus intermedius

Right lower lobe bronchus

19a

The Bronchi

At the carina, the trachea bifurcates into the right and left main stem bronchi – the FIRST GENERATION BRANCHES of the tracheobronchial tree. From here, the bronchi branch a total of 22 times, with each generation of branches becoming increasingly smaller in diameter, before ending at the alveoli.

The Right Main Stem, Lobar and Segmental Bronchi

The right main stem bronchus measures approximately 2.5 cm in length (6).

The right lung has three lobes and each lobe is supplied by a lobar bronchus. The lobar bronchi are referred to as SECOND GENERATION BRANCHES of the tracheobronchial tree.

The right main stem bronchus gives rise to the right upper lobe (RUL) bronchus and then continues inferiorly as the bronchus intermedius (Fig. 19a,b). The bronchus intermedius gives rise to the right middle lobe (RML) bronchus, as well as the right lower lobe (RLL) bronchus.

The RUL bronchus lies above the right pulmonary artery (RPA) – epiarterial (above the artery). This is the only branch of the bronchi that originates above the artery. All the other branches originate below the pulmonary artery and are called hypoarterial (below the artery).

The THIRD GENERATION BRANCHES are called the segmental bronchi. The segmental bronchi of the RUL are the apical, anterior and posterior divisions. The RML bronchus divides into medial and lateral segmental

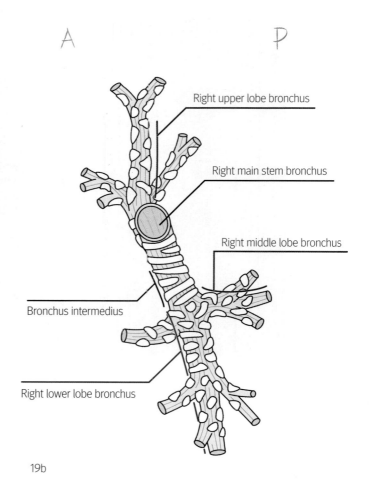

A   P

Right upper lobe bronchus

Right main stem bronchus

Right middle lobe bronchus

Bronchus intermedius

Right lower lobe bronchus

19b

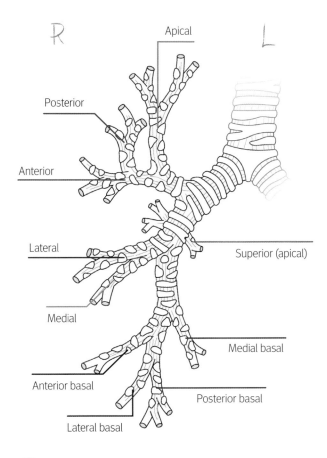

19c

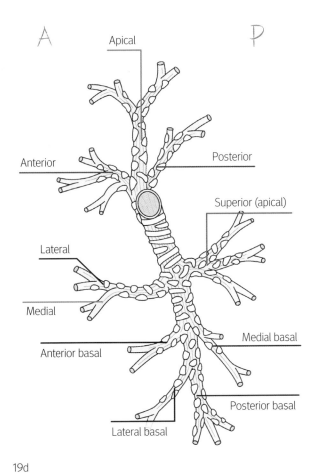

19d

branches. The RLL segmental bronchi are: superior, anterior basal, medial basal, lateral basal and posterior basal (Fig. 19c,d).

	SEGMENT	SEGMENT NUMBERING
RIGHT UPPER LOBE (RUL)	Apical	S1
	Anterior	S2
	Posterior	S3
RIGHT MIDDLE LOBE (RML)	Lateral	S4
	Medial	S5
RIGHT LOWER LOBE (RLL)	Superior (Apical)	S6
	Medial Basal	S7
	Anterior Basal	S8
	Lateral Basal	S9
	Posterior Basal	S10

Table 7.2
List of Segmental Bronchi in the Right Lung (7)

Figure 19. Anatomy of the right bronchi. a, illustration of the right main stem bronchus and main branches from the frontal perspective, b, illustration of the right main stem bronchus and main branches from the lateral perspective, c, illustration of the right segmental bronchi from the frontal perspective, d, illustration of the right segmental bronchi from the lateral perspective.

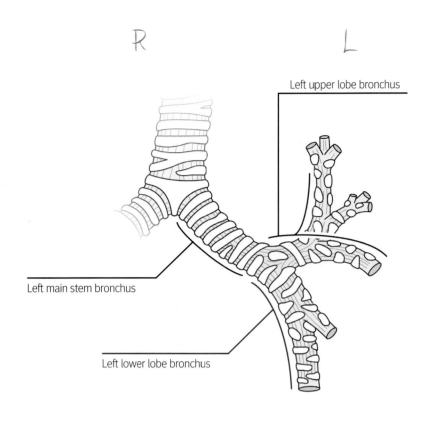

R L

Left upper lobe bronchus

Left main stem bronchus

Left lower lobe bronchus

20a

The Left Main Stem, Lobar and Segmental Bronchi

The left main stem bronchus is longer than the right - measuring approximately 5 cm in length (6).

The left lung has two lobes, with each supplied by a lobar (second generation) bronchus. These are called the left upper lobe (LUL) and left lower lobe (LLL) bronchi (Fig. 20a,b).

As on the right, the left lobar bronchi divide into the segmental (third generation) bronchi (Fig. 20c,d). The LUL bronchus divides into the apicoposterior, the anterior, as well as the superior and inferior lingual segmental bronchi. The LLL segmental bronchi are: the superior, the anteromedial basal, the lateral basal and the posterior basal segmental bronchi.

The more proximal bronchi, but not the peripheral bronchi, are visible on the chest x-ray because they form an interface with the mediastinal soft tissues. This is normal and does not constitute the pathological air bronchogram sign. The air bronchogram is described later in this chapter, on page 212.

The third generation bronchi continue to divide into smaller and smaller (sub-segmental) bronchi from generation four through nine, decreasing in size from 4 to 1 mm in diameter.

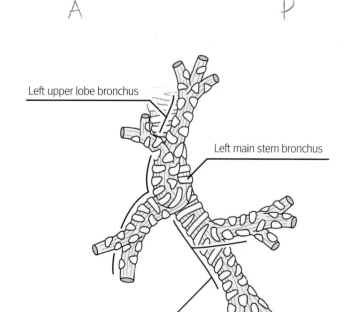

A P

Left upper lobe bronchus

Left main stem bronchus

Left lower lobe bronchus

20b

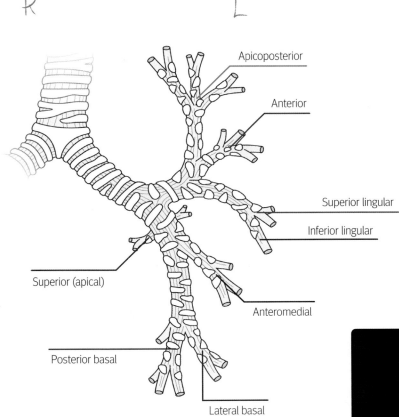

R   L

Apicoposterior

Anterior

Superior lingular

Inferior lingular

Superior (apical)

Anteromedial

Posterior basal

Lateral basal

20c

Remember, in contrast to the left lung, the right lung has separate apical and posterior upper lobe segments, and separate lower lobe anterior and media. segments.

!

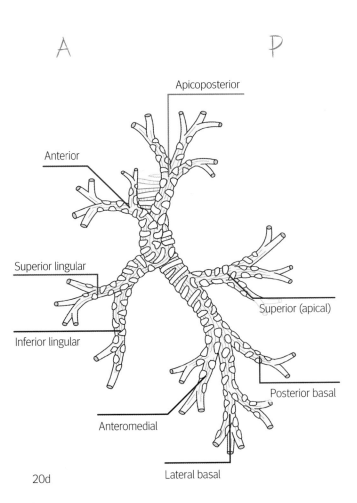

A   P

Apicoposterior

Anterior

Superior lingular

Inferior lingular

Superior (apical)

Posterior basal

Anteromedial

Lateral basal

20d

	SEGMENT	SEGMENT NUMBERING
LEFT UPPER LOBE - UPPER DIVISION	Apicoposterior	S1 + 3
	Anterior	S2
LEFT UPPER LOBE - LINGULAR DIVISION	Superior lingular	S4
	Inferior lingular	S5
LEFT LOWER LOBE	Superior (Apical)	S6
	Anteromedial	S7 + 8
	Lateral Basal	S9
	Posterior Basal	S10

Table 7.3
List of Segmental Bronchi in the Left Lung (7)

Figure 20. Anatomy of the left bronchi. a, illustration of the left main stem bronchus and main branches from the frontal perspective, b, illustration of the left main stem bronchus and main branches from the lateral perspective, c, illustration of the left segmental bronchi from the frontal perspective, d, illustration of the left segmental bronchi from the lateral perspective.

Radiological Shape and Grayscale of the Main Stem Bronchi

Because the main stem bronchi have a cylindrical shape, contain air and are surrounded by mediastinal soft tissue, they will appear as black rectangles on both the PA and lateral chest x-rays, similar to the trachea.

On the PA chest x-ray (Fig. 21a,b,c), the rectangles formed by the main stem bronchi will be directed from superior medial to inferior lateral. The borders of the rectangles may be irregular because of incomplete cartilage rings.

On the lateral chest x-ray (Fig. 22a,b,c), the main stem bronchi will look like inferior extensions of the trachea.

Figure 21. Radiological anatomy of the main stem bronchi from the frontal perspective. a, PA chest x-ray with the bronchi outlined, b, PA chest x-ray with grayscale illustration of the main bronchi overlay, c, PA chest x-ray cropped to highlight the main bronchi.

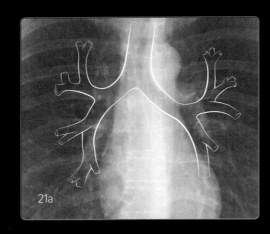

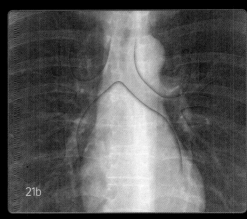

21a

21b

Figure 22. Radiological anatomy of the main stem bronchi from the lateral perspective. a, lateral chest x-ray with the bronchi outlined, b, lateral chest x-ray with grayscale illustration of the trachea overlay, c, lateral chest x-ray cropped to highlight the main bronchi.

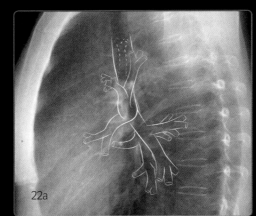

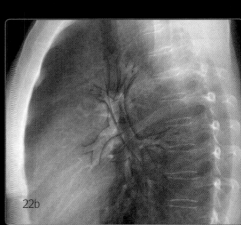

22a

22b

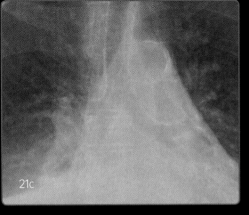

21c

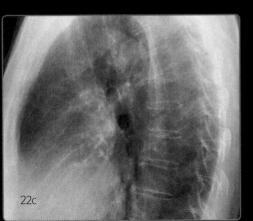

22c

Under normal circumstances only the proximal bronchi are visible on the PA and lateral chest x-rays.

Because of its more horizontal course, the left main stem bronchus can frequently be identified as a black circle within the airway column on the lateral chest x-ray (Fig. 23a,b). The right upper lobe bronchus is also horizontally oriented, and can sometimes be seen as a black circle within the airway column on the lateral chest x-ray (Fig. 23a,b). Some of the larger second-generation bronchi, if seen end-on, will also be visible (as black circles) on the PA and lateral chest x-rays.

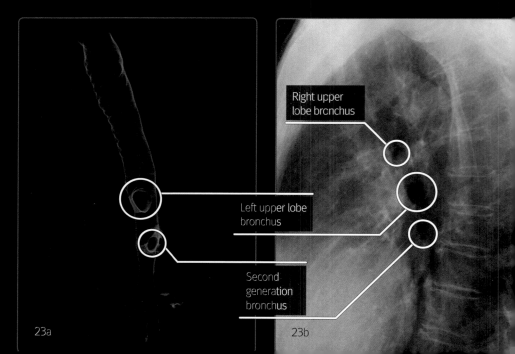

Figure 23. Relationship of the main stem bronchi on the lateral chest x-ray. The main stem bronchi can be seen as black circles on the lateral chest x-ray due to their horizontal orientation, a, 3D reconstruction of the trachea and main stem bronchi from the lateral perspective, b, lateral chest x-ray with the main stem bronchi highlighted.

Right upper lobe bronchus

Left upper lobe bronchus

Second generation bronchus

23a

23b

Variations on the Development of the Trachea & Bronchi

The most common developmental variants of the trachea and bronchi relate to the branching pattern of the lobar and segmental bronchi (8). These are usually of no clinical significance, but are important to recognize during bronchoscopy, or lung surgery. In rare cases, abnormal bronchi originating from the trachea or proximal bronchi can occur. These include the tracheal bronchus and the cardiac bronchus.

The cardiac bronchus is defined as an accessory bronchus that originates from the inner wall of the right main stembronchus (Fig. 24a,b). The cardiac bronchus can also originate from the bronchus intermedius, opposite to the origin of the right upper lobe bronchus (9).

The tracheal bronchus refers to a variety of accessory bronchi originating from the trachea or main bronchi, and directed to the upper lobes (Fig. 25)(10).

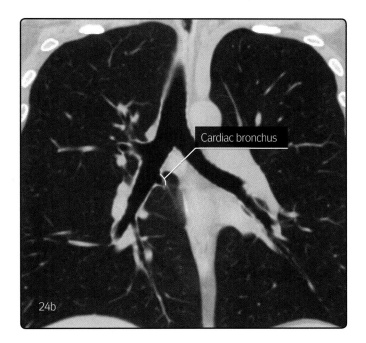

24a

Cardiac bronchus

Cardiac bronchus

24b

Figure 24. Cardiac bronchus. a, illustration of the cardiac bronchus, b, coronal CT image from a patient with a cardiac bronchus.

Figure 25. Tracheal bronchus. Illustration of the tracheal bronchus.

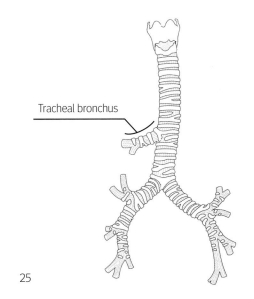

Tracheal bronchus

25

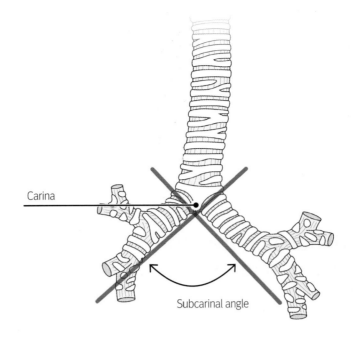

Carina

Subcarinal angle

THE SUBCARINAL AND INTERBRONCHIAL ANGLES

26a

The subcarinal angle is defined as the angle of divergence of the main stem bronchi, measured along their inferior border (Fig. 26a)(11). Normally, this angle is less than 90 degrees (Fig. 26b). The tip of this angle is called the carina. Carina in Latin means a keel-like part or shape.

The interbronchial angle is the angle between the vertical tracheal axis and the long axis of each of the main stem bronchi (Fig. 27a)(12). In the normal individual, the interbronchial angle is steeper on the right (Fig. 27b).

These angles are important because they will change when the bronchi are displaced by pathological processes – they are, therefore, important indicators of pathology. This is described on page 204.

Figure 26. Subcarinal angle. a, illustration of the trachea and bronchi depicting the subcarinal angle, b, PA chest x-ray with the subcarinal angle highlighted.

Figure 27. Interbronchial angle. a, illustration of the trachea and bronchi depicting the interbronchial angle, b, PA chest x-ray with the interbronchial angle highlighted.

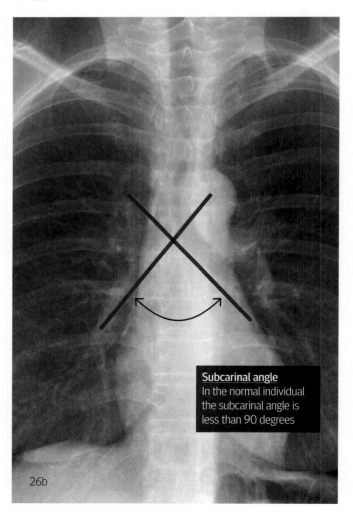

Subcarinal angle
In the normal individual the subcarinal angle is less than 90 degrees

26b

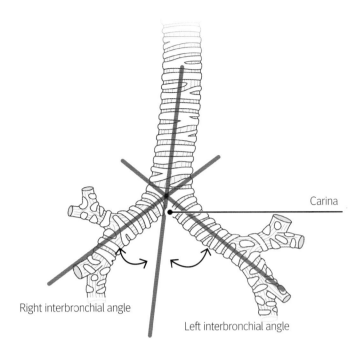

Carina

Right interbronchial angle

Left interbronchial angle

27a

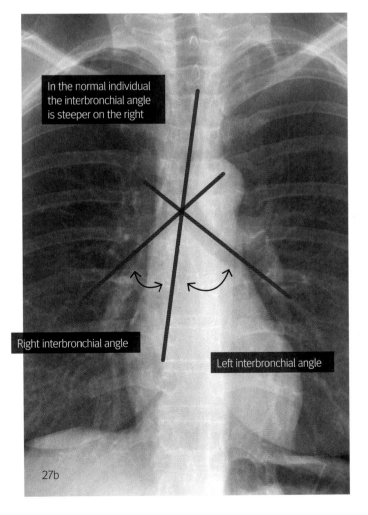

In the normal individual the interbronchial angle is steeper on the right

Right interbronchial angle

Left interbronchial angle

27b

Frequency of Visualization on the PA X-ray (13)

Trachea 100%
Carina 98%

Frequency of Visualization on the Lateral X-ray (13)

Trachea 100%
Orifice of RUL bronchus 50%
Orifice of LUL bronchus 77%
Posterior wall of bronchus intermedius 95%
Anterior wall of bronchus intermedius 56%

The left pulmonary artery lies on top of the left main stem bronchus. Finding the pulmonary artery can then help locate the left main stem bronchus and, therefore, the carina.

!

How to identify the carina on the PA x-ray

STEP 1
Confirm that the patient is midline and not rotated (Ch. 1, Pg. 32).

STEP 2
Identify the trachea (Pg. 182) (Fig.28).

STEP 3
Follow the right lateral border of the trachea inferiorly to the bifurcation of the bronchi and identify the superior border of the right main stem bronchus (Fig. 29). Do the same on the left.

STEP 4
Identify the lower inferior border of the right and left main stem bronchi (Fig. 30).

STEP 5
Now follow the inferior borders of the main stem bronchi medially until they join together. This point is the carina (Fig. 31).

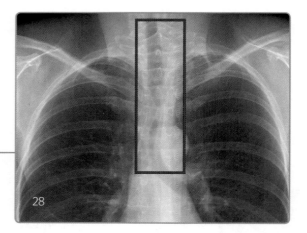
28

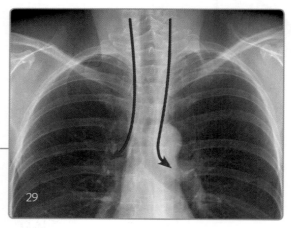
29

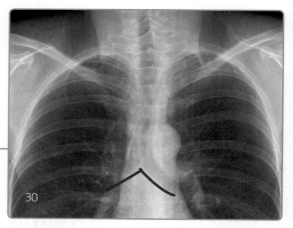
30

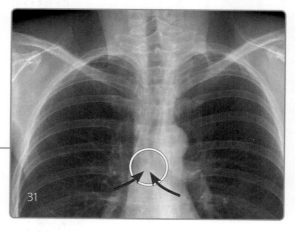
31

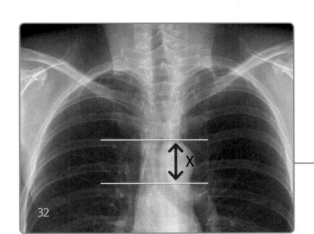

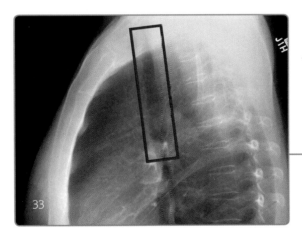

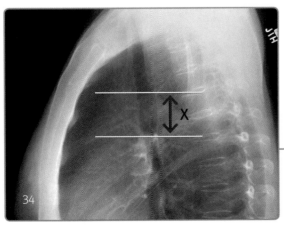

How to identify the carina on the lateral x-ray

STEP 1
On the PA x-ray, measure the distance (X) from the most superior edge of the aortic arch to the carina (Fig. 32).

STEP 2
On the lateral x-ray identify the trachea (Fig. 33).

STEP 3
Identify the most superior edge of the aortic arch and measure from this point inferiorly using the measurement (X) obtained in Step 1 (Fig. 34). This is the level of the carina.

?

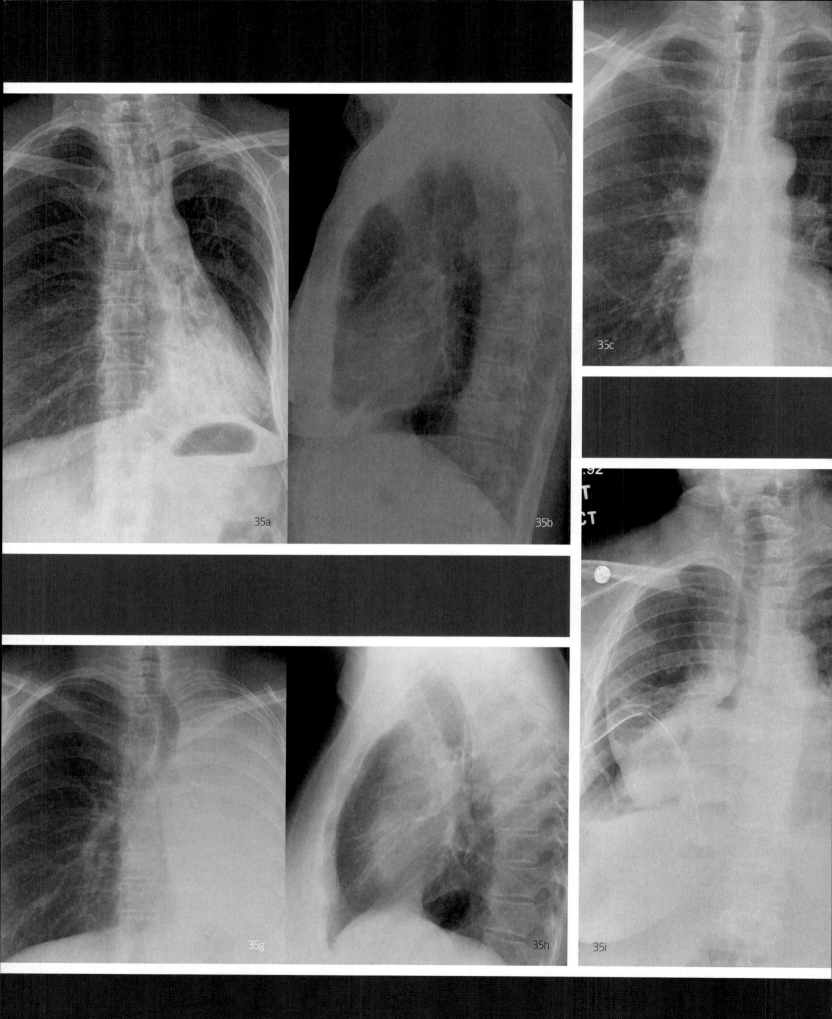

PATHOLOGY OF THE TRACHEA & PROXIMAL BRONCHI

Example images of diseases and conditions that affect the trachea and proximal bronchi.

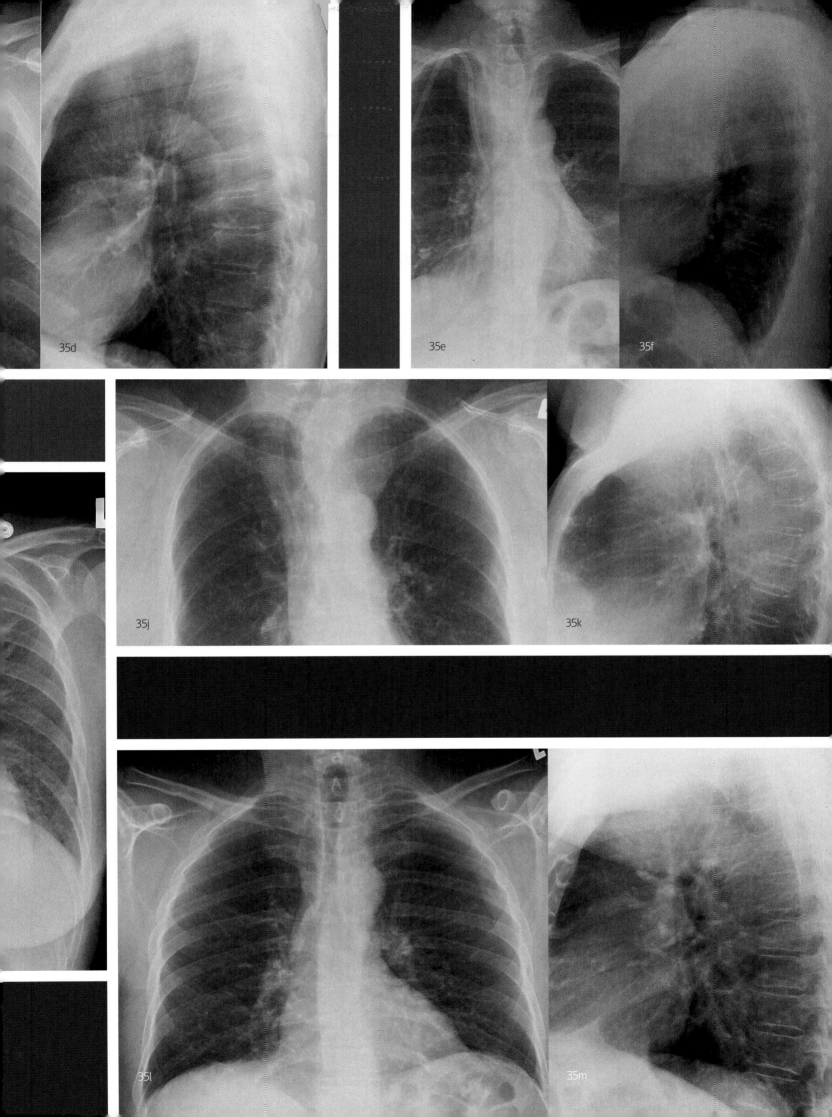

35d

35e

35f

35j

35k

35l

35m

THE ABNORMAL
TRACHEA & PROXIMAL BRONCHI

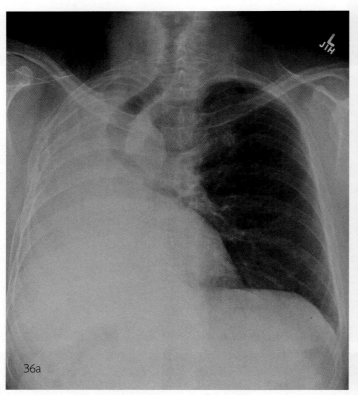

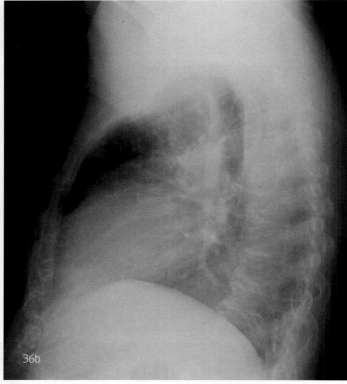

The Radiological Trachea & Proximal Bronchi Will Be Abnormal When

1) The position of the trachea, proximal bronchi, or both, is shifted.

2) The shape of the trachea, proximal bronchi, or both, is altered.

3) Special case: foreign bodies are present in the proximal bronchi.

Figure 36. Tracheal deviation following right pneumonectomy. Pathology can shift the position of the trachea, a, PA chest x-ray of a patient with a pneumonectomy showing the trachea deviated to the right, b, lateral chest x-ray of the same patient revealing the trachea skewed posteriorly.

Figure 37. Tracheal deviation due to anterior mediastinal mass. a, PA chest x-ray with an anterior mediastinal mass deviating the trachea to the left, b, the lateral x-ray also shows deviation of the trachea, posteriorly.

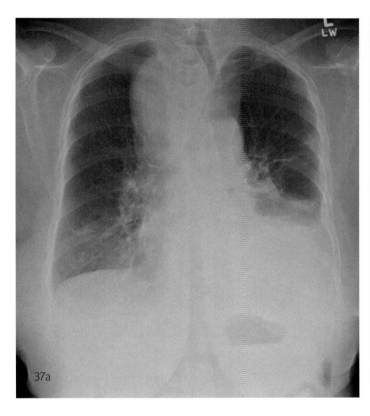

37a

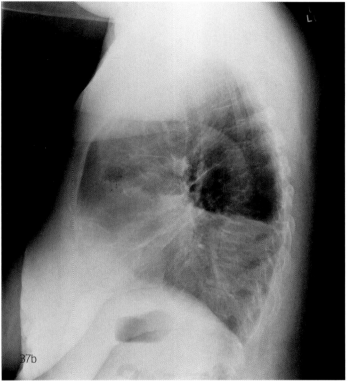

37b

1. Pathology that affects the position of the trachea or proximal bronchi

Tracheal displacement

Tracheal displacement is commonly seen following lung surgery, such as pneumonectomy (Fig. 36a,b); as the remaining lung hyperinflates, it pushes the trachea to the side of the surgery.

The trachea can also be displaced by pathology involving the mediastinum and hila. An example is an anterior mediastinal mass that will displace the trachea posteriorly and will narrow the caliber of the trachea (Fig. 37a,b). This posterior displacement is best seen on the lateral chest x-ray.

Conversely, middle and posterior mediastinal tumors, if large enough, will displace the trachea anteriorly.

Did you catch the examples on pages 200–201?
Figs. 35e,f and 35j,k – Deviated trachea due to mass
Fig. 35g,h – Deviated trachea post-operatively

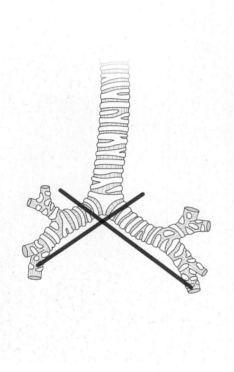

38a

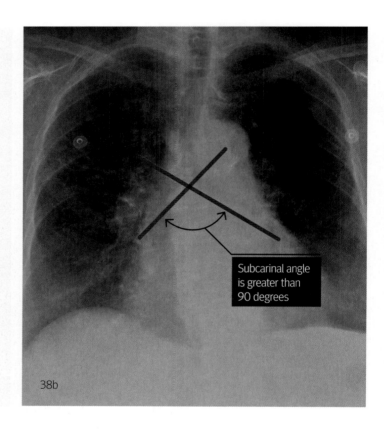

Subcarinal angle is greater than 90 degrees

38b

Bronchial displacement – the abnormal carina

Disease processes involving the trachea and bronchi, whether focal or diffuse, may affect the carina (14). The subcarinal angle will increase from extrinsic influences that cause lifting of the proximal bronchi (Fig. 38a,b). This includes the enlargement of the left atrium (especially in mitral valvular disease), generalized cardiomegaly, pericardial effusion, subcarinal masses and adenopathy. The subcarinal angle will also increase with fibrotic diseases involving the upper lobes that are causing superior retraction of the proximal bronchi, and in cases of lobar collapse.

Figure 38. Abnormal carina. Pathology can shift the position of the bronchi such that the carina angle is widened. a, illustration of a widened carina angle, b, PA chest x-ray of a patient with a mass resulting in a widened carina angle.

Figure 39. Saber sheath trachea. Pathology can alter the shape of the trachea. a, PA chest x-ray showing how the trachea is narrowed, b, lateral chest x-ray showing how the trachea is widened.

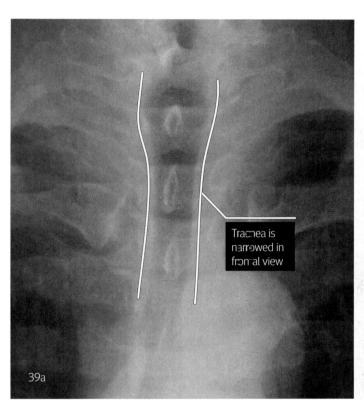

Trachea is narrowed in frontal view

39a

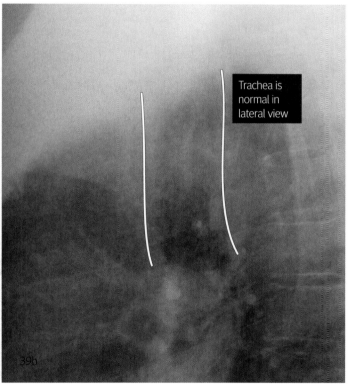

Trachea is normal in lateral view

39b

2. Pathology that alters the shape of the trachea and proximal bronchi

Tracheal widening AND narrowing

Often, with aging or with chronic obstructive pulmonary disease (COPD), the lateral (coronal) diameter of the trachea may decrease, with an increase in the anteroposterior (sagittal) diameter. Picture the shape you would expect if you pinched the trachea between your thumb and index finger. This abnormal appearance of the trachea is called saber sheath trachea (Fig. 39a,b)(15).

Did you catch the example on pages 200–201?
Fig. 35c,d – Saber sheath trachea

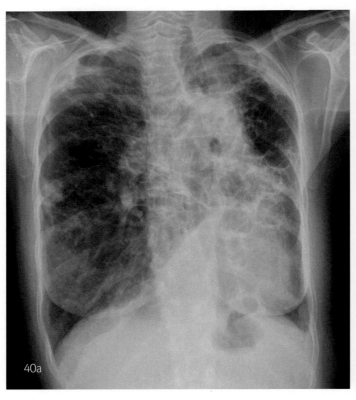

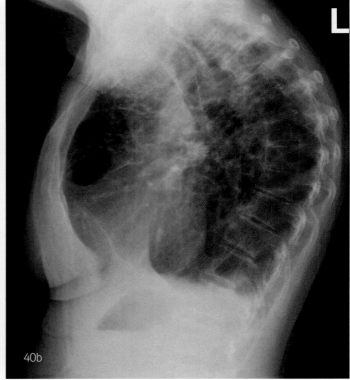

40a

40b

L

Tracheal or bronchial widening

Tracheal widening, or enlargement, can occur as the result of chronic disease processes that cause upper lobe lung fibrosis such as: cystic fibrosis, tuberculosis, histoplasmosis and sarcoidosis (16). Widening can also be seen in the congenital abnormality called tracheobronchomegaly (Mounier-Kuhn) (17).

Chronic infections can also lead to diffuse enlargement of the proximal bronchi. More commonly, chronic infections can lead to enlargement of more peripheral bronchi, a condition called bronchiectasis (Fig. 40a,b,c,d). Depending on the shape of the enlarged bronchi, they are described as cylindrical or cystic. Cylindrical are elongated and cystic are more spherical.

Figure 40. Bronchiectasis. a, FA chest x-ray from a patient with bronchiectasis, b, lateral chest x-ray from the same patient, c, CT scan from the same patient, d, coronal CT scan from a different patient showing elongated and dilated bronchi (arrows) in the lower lobes.

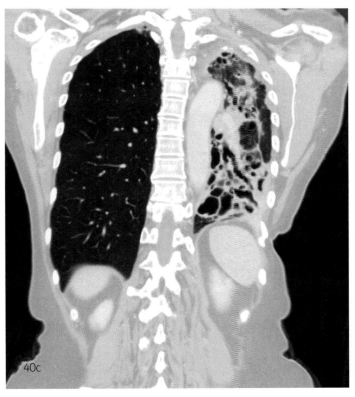

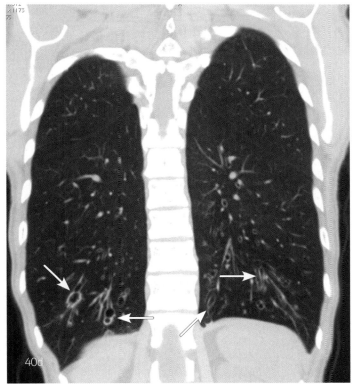

TRACHEAL WIDENING / ENLARGEMENT		
Adult men	Coronal diameter	›25 mm
	Sagittal diameter	› 27 mm
Adult women	Coronal diameter	› 21 mm
	Sagittal diameter	› 23 mm

Table 7.4
Pathological Tracheal Measurements (15)

BRONCHIAL WIDENING / ENLARGEMENT		
Adult Men	Left main stem bronchus diameter:	› 18 mm
	Right main stem bronchus diameter	› 21 mm
Adult Women	Left main stem bronchus diameter:	› 17.4 mm
	Right main stem bronchus diameter	› 19.8 mm

Table 7.5
Pathological Bronchial Measurements (15)

Did you catch the example on pages 200–201?

Fig. 35a,b – Bronchiectasis

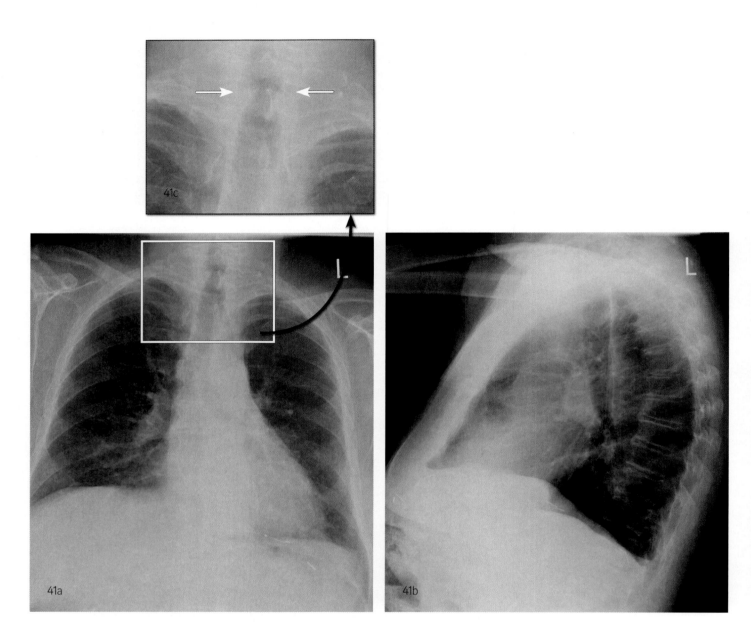

Tracheal narrowing

Tracheal or bronchial narrowing, or stenosis, can be focal or diffuse (18,19). Focal causes can be intrinsic, and include malignant tumors, benign tumors, foreign bodies and tracheal scarring (Fig. 41a,b,c). Extrinsic causes of focal narrowing are usually related to compression from an adjacent tumor (Fig. 42a,b,c) or adenopathy. The narrowing can lead to complete obstruction of the affected bronchus. When this occurs, the air within the bronchus will be completely lost (cut off).

Diffuse tracheal narrowing can be related to diffuse extrinsic compression from an adjacent tumor, or adenopathy. Rare causes of diffuse tracheal narrowing include tracheomalacia, relapsing polychondritis, or amyloidosis.

Figure 41. Tracheal stenosis - intrinsic. Pathology can alter the shape of the trachea. a, PA chest x-ray from a patient with tracheal scarring due to previous tracheal trauma causing narrowing of the trachea, b, lateral chest x-ray from the same patient is normal, c, magnification of the PA chest x-ray highlighting the narrowing of the trachea (arrows).

Figure 42. Tracheal stenosis - extrinsic. Pathology can alter the shape of the trachea. a, PA chest x-ray from a patient with a mass to the right of the trachea causing compression of the trachea, b, lateral chest x-ray from the same patient is normal, c, magnification of the PA chest x-ray highlighting the compression of the trachea (arrows).

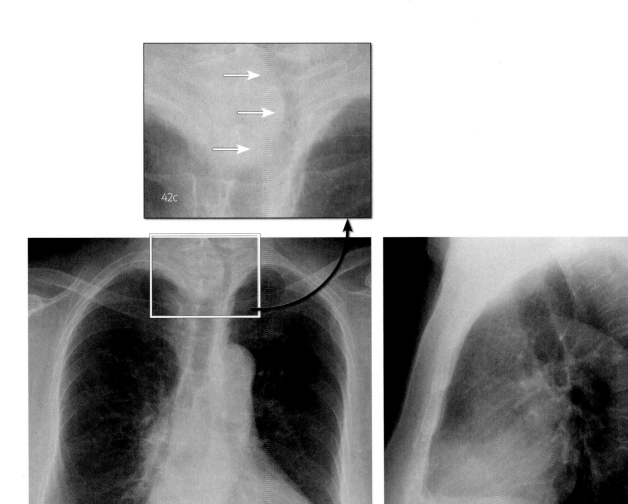

42c

42a

42b

What Are the Types of Stenosis (Tracheal Narrowing) ? (15)

Tracheobronchial stenosis can be classified as either structural or functional. Four types of structural stenosis have been identified.

Type 1:   Caused by exophytic intraluminal lesions, such as tumors or granulation tissue.

Type 2:   Caused by extrinsic compression.

Type 3:   Caused by distortion related to previous surgery, or extrinsic pathological processes causing traction on the trachea or bronchi.

Type 4:   Caused by scarring.

Two types of functional stenosis are described.

Type 1:   Caused by damaged cartilage.

Type 2:   Caused by a floppy posterior membrane.

Did you catch the examples on pages 200–201?

Fig. 35i – Cut-off bronchus

Fig. 35l,m – Tracheal stenosis

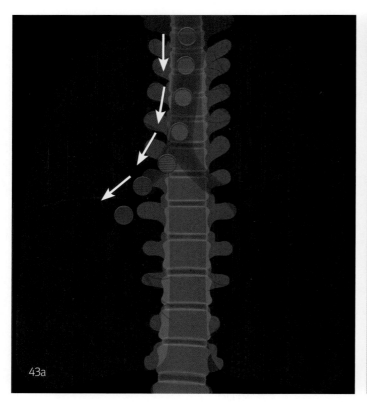

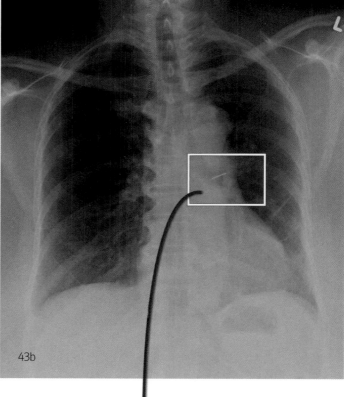

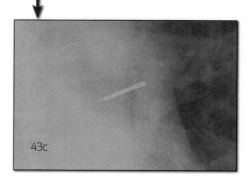

3. Special case: Foreign bodies

Foreign bodies in the airways are a common problem in children. The majority of aspirated foreign bodies will find their way into the right lung because of the more vertical orientation and wider orifice of the right main bronchus (Fig. 43a,b,c)(6). For the same reason, the right middle and lower lung lobes are the most common sites of infiltrate formation, due to aspiration in elderly and high-risk patients.

Figure 43. Foreign bodies. Foreign bodies will often find themselves in the airways. a, illustration of the typical path of a foreign body into the right main stem bronchus, b, PA chest x-ray from a patient with a foreign body (pin) in left main stem bronchus (highlighted), c, magnification of the PA chest x-ray highlighting the pin in the left main stem bronchus.

SUMMARY OF RADIOLOGICAL CHANGES
TO THE TRACHEA & PROXIMAL BRONCHI

RADIOLOGICAL CHANGES		ASSOCIATED FINDINGS, DISEASES AND CONDITIONS
1. Position shifted	Trachea	• Pneumonectomy • Tumors (e.g., thymoma) • Goitre
	Bronchi (abnormal carina)	• Enlargement of the left atrium (e.g., mitral valvular disease) • Cardiomegaly • Pericardial effusion • Subcarinal tumor • Adenopathy • Fibrotic diseases • Lobar collapse • Lobectomy
2. Shape altered	Narrowing (stenosis)	• Foreign bodies • Tracheal scarring • Tumor • Adenopathy • Tracheomalacia (rare) • Relapsing polychondritis (rare) • Amyloidosis (rare) • Cut-off bronchus
	Widening (enlargement)	• Cystic fibrosis • Tuberculosis • Histoplasmosis • Sarcoidosis • Congenital abnormality: tracheobronchomegaly (Mounier-Kuhn) • Bronchiectasis
	Widening & Narrowing	• Saber sheath trachea
3. Special case: Foreign bodies		• Aspiration in elderly and high-risk patients • Often in right main bronchus

Table 7.6
Summary of Radiological Changes to the Trachea & Proximal Bronchi

RADIOLOGICAL SIGNS
RELATED TO THE
TRACHEA & PROXIMAL BRONCHI

Air Bronchogram Sign (18)

Normally, the peripheral bronchi are not visible on the chest x-ray because the walls of these bronchi are not thick enough to create an interface. The blackness of the air within the bronchi blends with the blackness of the air in the alveoli. However, if the alveoli are opacified, and the bronchi remain patent and full of air, the bronchi will become visible on the x-ray. The visualization of black branching bronchi within an opacified lung is called an air bronchogram (Fig. 44a,b,c). An air bronchogram is indicative of airspace disease. Air bronchograms can be seen with pneumonia, pulmonary contusion and bleeding, pulmonary edema, and bronchoalveolar cell carcinoma and lymphoma. The presence of an air bronchogram helps localize pathology to the respiratory zone of the lungs.

If the bronchi also become filled with fluid, cells or blood, the opacity will still be visible, but the black rectangles will disappear. In this case, there is no air bronchogram sign, and the differential diagnosis will include a broader range of pathologies, including lung tumor.

Tram Line Sign

When there is thickening of the bronchial walls, along with diameter enlargement, the bronchi will become visible as parallel line shadows. These are similar to train tracks, and when present, are called the tram line or the tram track sign (Fig. 45a,b,c). Although this can occasionally be seen in normal patients, it is usually associated with cylindrical bronchiectasis.

Figure 44. Air bronchogram sign. a, artistic representation of the air bronchogram sign in the lung, b, artistic representation of the air bronchogram sign with all thoracic structures, c, PA chest x-ray with air bronchogram sign evident.

Figure 45. Tram line sign. a, artistic representation of the tram line sign in the lung, b, artistic representation of the tram line sign with all thoracic structures, c, PA chest x-ray with tram line sign present.

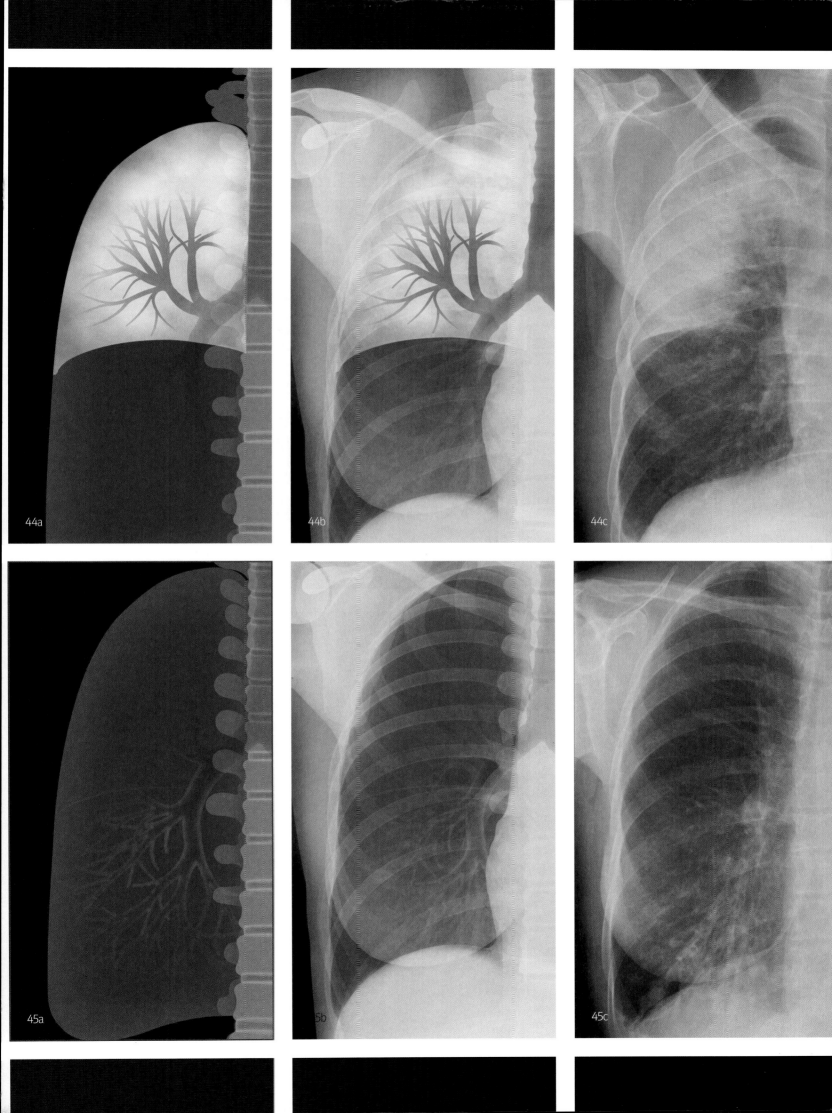

44a

44b

44c

45a

45b

45c

Visual Search of the Trachea & Proximal Bronchi

PA Chest X-ray

1. Start on the right paratracheal (1) region in the lower neck.

2. Follow the outline of the trachea inferiorly and the superior outline of the right mainstem bronchus (2).

3. Follow the inferior outline of the right main stem bronchus (3) to the carina and then the inferior outline of the left main stem bronchus (4).

4. Follow the superior outline of the left main stem bronchus (5) to the trachea.

5. Follow the outline of the trachea superiorly (6).

Complete the visual search by checking the radiodensity of the trachea and proximal bronchi from top to bottom.

Lateral Chest X-ray

1. Start anterior to the trachea in the neck (1).

2. Follow the outline of the trachea inferiorly to below the carina (2).

3. Follow the posterior outline of the trachea (3) to the thoracic inlet.

Complete the visual search by checking the radiodensity of the trachea from top to bottom.

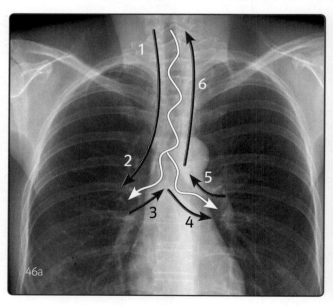

46a

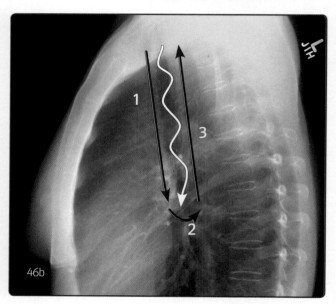

46b

Trachea & Proximal Bronchi Radiological Analysis Checklist

To confidently state that the trachea and proximal bronchi are normal, all parts of the checklist should indicate a normal appearance.

GRAYSCALE

1 Is the grayscale of the trachea altered?

If **YES**, then describe.
Too white/too black.

POSITION

2 Is the trachea deviated?

If **YES**, then describe.
Right/left.
Anterior/posterior.

3 Is the carina angle greater than 90 degrees?

If **YES**, then describe.
Give angle measurement.

SHAPE

4 Is the shape of the trachea narrowed?

If **YES**, then describe.
Focal/diffuse.

5 Is there a visible mass deviating/narrowing the trachea?

If **YES**, then describe.
Size/position.

OTHER

6 Are there any radiological signs related to the trachea present?

If **YES**, then describe.
Air bronchogram.
Tram line.

7 Is there any evidence of previous surgery to the trachea and/or bronchi?

If **YES**, then describe.
Type of surgery and location.
Compare to previous CXR.

8 Are there any lines or tubes in the trachea?

If **YES**, then describe.
Give location of each relative to the carina.

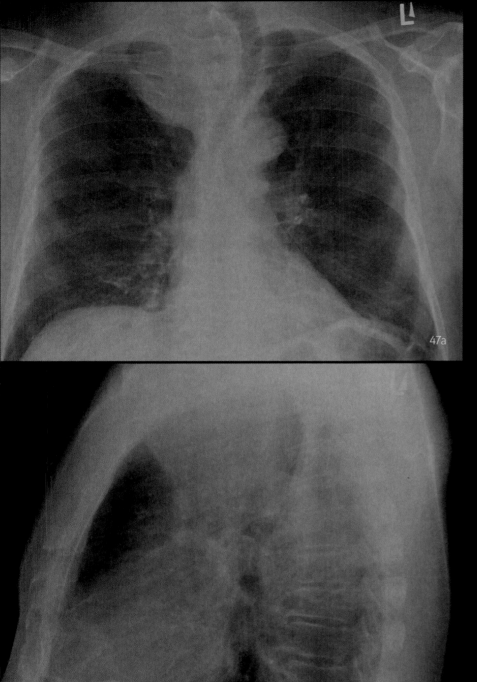

47a

47b

What are
your findings?

You are the intern on call in the emergency department and you are called in to see a 70-year-old male patient who presents with stridor. You try to take a history from the patient, but she is very distressed and cannot communicate properly. On physical examination, you feel a large, firm mass in the lower neck region. Many differential diagnoses run through your mind and you decide that you need a chest x-ray to help eliminate some of them from your list. You order PA and lateral chest x-rays (Fig. 47a,b).

216

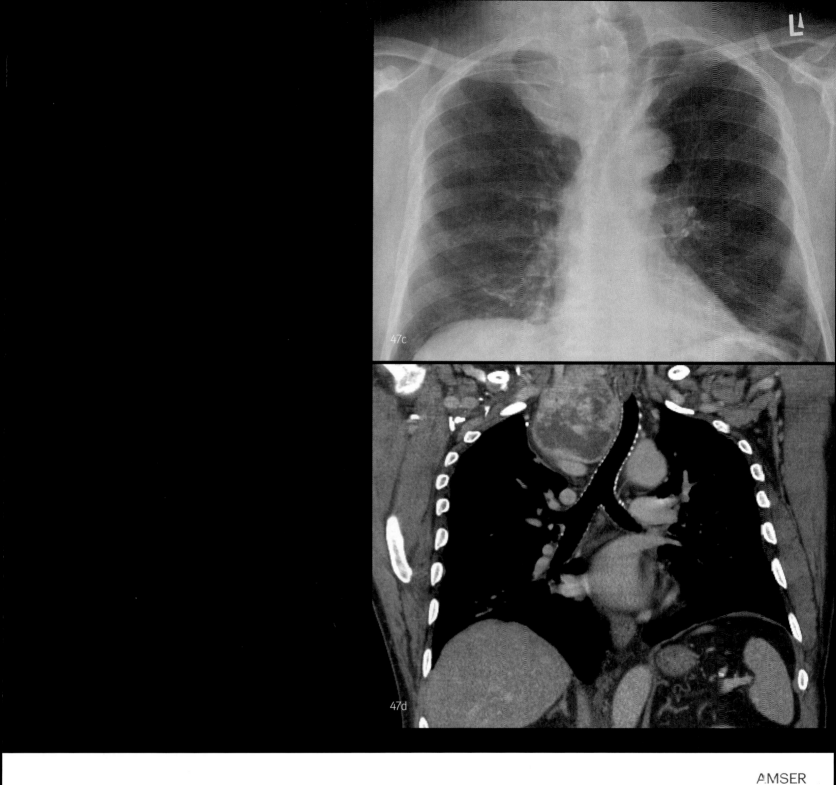

47c

47d

Soft tissue mass in the upper thorax, deviating and narrowing the trachea (Fig. 47a,b,c,d). The differential diagnosis will include mass lesions originating from the anterior superior mediastinum, such as thyroid goiter, tumor, or thymoma.

Based on the findings, the diagnosis is the presence of a large intrathoracic goiter.

48a

48b

48c

48d

48e

This series of images highlights the variability in the radiological appearance of the trachea.

THE SWEEPING TRACHEA

References:

1. Lewis, P.J., Shaffer, K., & Donovan, A. (Eds.). (2012). AMSER National Medical Student Curriculum in Radiology. http://aur.org/Secondary-Alliances.aspx?id=141.

2. Lewis, P.J., & Shaffer, K. (2005). Developing a national medical student curriculum in radiology. *Am. Coll. Radiol. 2*(1):8-11.

3. Holbert, J.M., & Strollo, D.C. (1995). Imaging of the normal trachea. *J. Thorac. Imaging, 10*(3):171-179

4. Haskin, P.H., & Goodman, L.R. (1982). Normal tracheal bifurcation angle: a reassessment. *AJR Am. J. Roentgenol., 139*(5):879-882.

5. Tahir, N., Ramsden, W.H., & Stringer, M.D. (2009). Tracheobronchial anatomy and the distribution of inhaled foreign bodies in children. *Eur. J. Pediatr., 168*(3):289-295.

6. Gibbs, J.M., Chandrasekhar, C.A., Ferguson, E.C., & Oldham, S.A. (2007). Lines and stripes: where did they go?--From conventional radiography to CT. *Radiographics, 27*(1):33-48.

7. McComb, B.L. (2002). The chest in profile. *J. Thorac. Imaging, 17*(1):58-69.

8. Wu, J.W., White, C.S., Meyer, C.A., et al. (1999). Variant bronchial anatomy: CT appearance and classification. *AJR Am. J. Roentgenol., 172*(3):741-744.

9. Yildiz, H., Ugurel, S., Soylu, K., et al. (2006). Accessory cardiac bronchus and tracheal bronchus anomalies: CT-bronchoscopy and CT-bronchography findings. *Surg. Radiol. Anat., 28*(6):646-649.

10. Remy, J., Smith, M., Marache, P., & Nuyts, J.P.(1997). [Pathogenetic left tracheal bronchus. A review of the literature in connection with four cases (author's transl)]. *J. Radiol. Electrol. Med. Nucl., 58*(10):621-630.

11. Jardin, M., & Remy, J. (1986). Segmental bronchovascular anatomy of the lower lobes: CT analysis. *AJR Am. J. Roentgenol., 147*(3):457-468.

12. Sussmann, A.R., & Ko, J.P. (2010). Understanding chest radiographic anatomy with MDCT reformations. *Clin. Radiol., 65*(2):155-166.

13. Gray, H. (2008). *Gray's Anatomy: The Anatomical Basis of Medicine and Surgery.* 38th Ed. New York, NY: Churchill Livingstone.

14. Greene, R., & Lechner, G.L. (1975). "Saber-Sheath" trachea: A clinical and functional study of marked coronal narrowing of the intrathoracic trachea. *Radiology, 115*(2):265-268.

15. Goh, R.H., Dobranowski, J., Kahana, L., & Kay, N. (1995). Dynamic computed tomography evaluation of tracheobronchomegaly. *Can. Assoc. Radiol. J., 46*(3):212-215.

16. Marom, E.M., Goodman, P.C., & McAdams, H.L. (2001). Diffuse abnormalities of the trachea and main bronchi. *AJR Am. J. Roentgenol., 176*(3):713-717.

17. Freitag, L., Ernst, A., Unger, M., et al. (2007). A proposed classification system of central airway stenosis. *Eur. Respir. J., 30*(1):7-12.

18. Murray, J.G., Brown, A.L., Anagnostou, E.A., & Senior, R. (1995). Widening of the tracheal bifurcation on chest radiographs: value as a sign of left atrial enlargement. *AJR Am. J. Roentgenol., 164*(5):1089-1092.

19. Marom, E.M., Goodman, P.C., & McAdams, H.L. (2001) Focal abnormalities of the trachea and main bronchi. *AJR Am. J. Roentgenol., 176*(3):707-711.

20. Fleischner, F.G. (1948). The visible bronchial tree; a roentgen sign in pneumonic and other pulmonary consolidations. *Radiology, 50*(2):184-189.

CHAPTER 8
The HILUM
(the hilar zone)

importance

The hilum on the chest x-ray is a challenging area to master, especially on the lateral x-ray. A lack of knowledge of the radiological anatomy of the hila is one of the main reasons why many medical students (and practising physicians) shy away from the lateral chest x-ray, finding more comfort in the PA projection.

On the PA x-ray, we see the contour of the heart and the two lungs in the orientation similar to how one would view oneself in the mirror if the chest wall happened to be transparent. On the lateral x-ray, the lungs, heart, and vessels all overlap into a confusing grayscale conglomerate. This central white area is the biggest source of confusion, and is the main focus of discussion in this chapter.

Understanding the radiological appearance of the hilum unlocks the understanding of the lateral chest x-ray, and is vital to interpreting the lateral chest x-ray accurately. This chapter will give you the knowledge to feel comfortable identifying landmarks and pathology within the hilum.

objectives

Skills

You will identify

- the proximal right pulmonary artery and proximal left pulmonary artery, on the PA and lateral chest x-rays.

- the branches of the pulmonary arteries on the PA and lateral chest x-rays.

- the pulmonary veins on the PA and lateral chest x-rays.

- pathology within the hilum (distinguishing between enlarged hilar vessels and a hilar mass).

- the important radiological signs related to the hila.

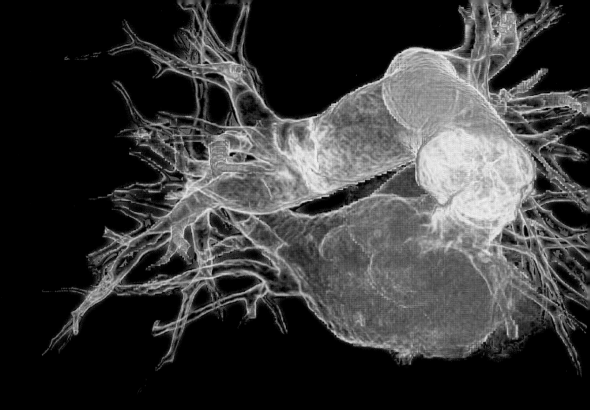

Knowledge:

You will review and understand

- the definition, and working use, of the term hilum.

- the radiological anatomy of the hilar blood vessels (major vessels and branches).

- the important differences between the right and left pulmonary arteries.

- the relationship of the anatomical structures in "the root of the lungs".

- the normal appearance of the hila on the PA and lateral chest x-rays.

- pathology that can involve the hila, and why pathology changes the radiological appearance of the hila.

associated resources

This chapter maps to the following AMSER curriculum content (1,2).

1. Normal radiological anatomy of the hilum
    Pulmonary outflow track
    Pulmonary veins
    Right and left main pulmonary arteries
    Aorto-pulmonary (AP) window

2. Pathological conditions affecting the hilum
    Pulmonary hypertension
    Pulmonary embolism

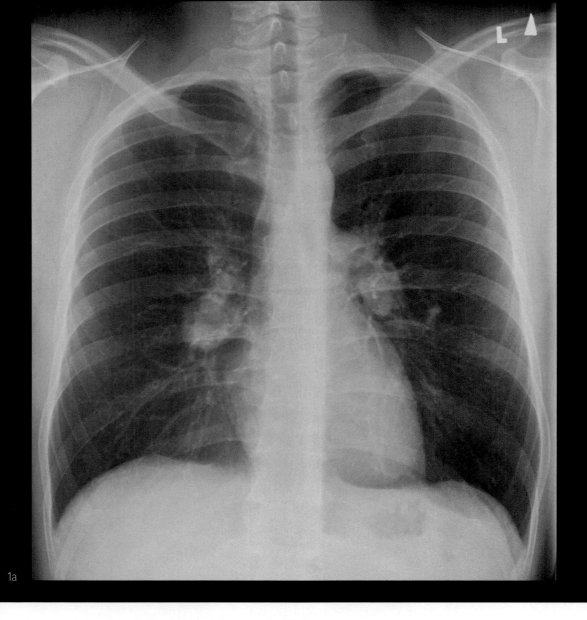

1a

CASE STUDY

A 35-year-old male presents with the recent appearance of red bumps on the skin, swollen glands in the neck and armpits, and redness of both eyes. The patient has also experienced mild shortness of breath on exertion. On physical examination, the patient is found to have enlarged lymph nodes in the neck, axilla and groin. The liver and spleen are also mildly enlarged. You suspect the patient may have intrathoracic adenopathy, and you order chest x-rays (Fig. 1a,b). You examine the x-rays and are asked to report your findings to the staff physician.

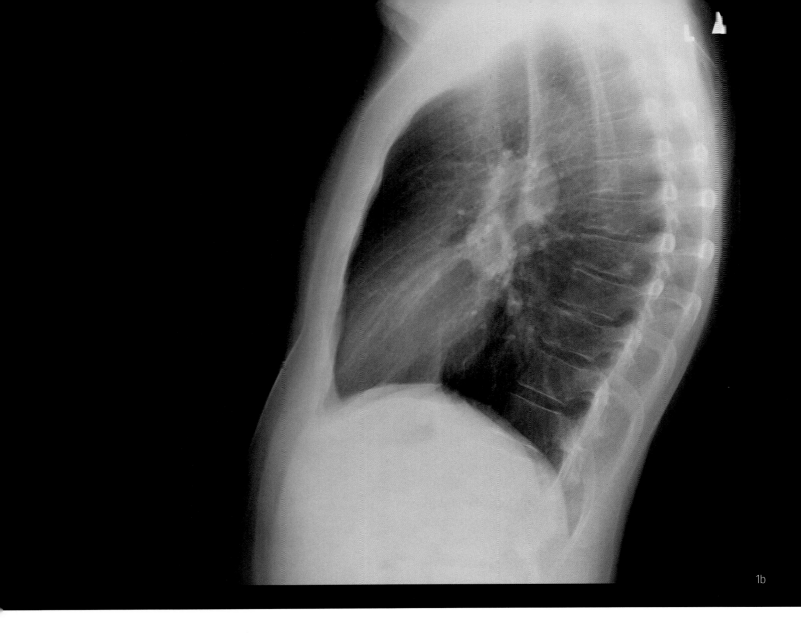

1b

How would you describe the abnormalities to the staff physician?

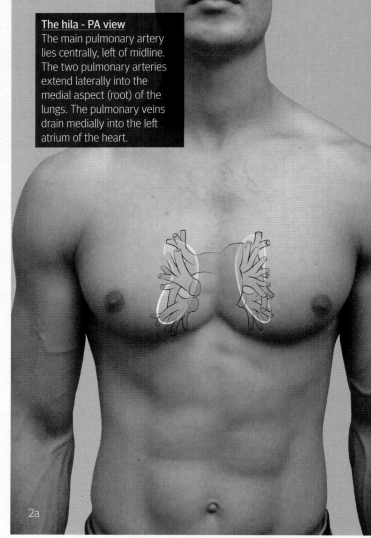

2a

WHAT IS THE HILUM?

What is the meaning of the term "root of the lung"? Is the term "hilar shadow" the same as "the hilum"?

All of these terms are, in fact, used in reference to the hilum. Therefore, some clarification is needed to explain exactly what the term "hilum" means.

The word *hilum* is taken from Latin, and means "a depression, a pit, a little something". In anatomy texts, the hilum is defined as "that part of an organ through which the vessels and nerves enter" (3). The hilum, defined this way, encompasses a large area extending from the upper edge of the pulmonary arteries to the lower edge of the inferior pulmonary veins (Fig. 2a,b).

The Fleishner society defines the hilum as "the composite shadow at the root of each lung produced by bronchi, arteries and veins, lymph nodes, nerves, bronchial vessels and associated alveolar tissue" (4). By this definition, the hilum is not the indentation through which these important structures pass, but the x-ray shadow produced by these structures.

However, these anatomical structures produce not one, but two distinct shadows. The upper hilar shadow is predominantly created by the pulmonary

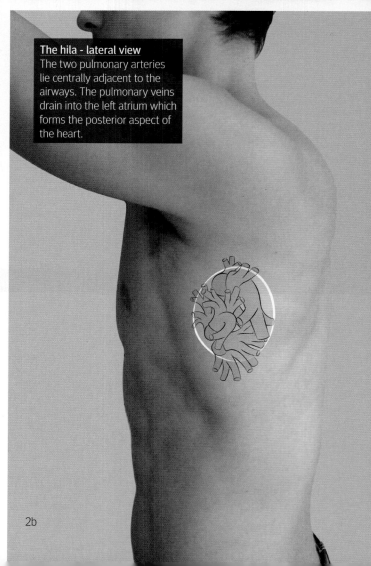

The hila - lateral view
The two pulmonary arteries lie centrally adjacent to the airways. The pulmonary veins drain into the left atrium which forms the posterior aspect of the heart.

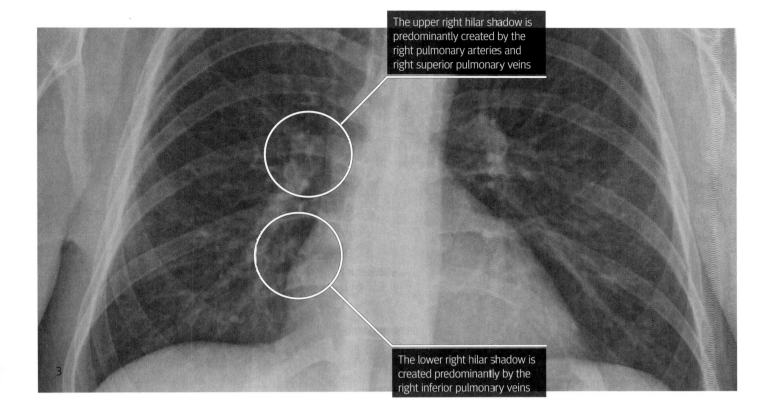

The upper right hilar shadow is predominantly created by the right pulmonary arteries and right superior pulmonary veins

The lower right hilar shadow is created predominantly by the right inferior pulmonary veins

arteries and the superior pulmonary veins, and a lower shadow is predominantly created by the inferior pulmonary veins (Fig. 3).

Because the upper hilar shadow is more easily identified on a chest x-ray, discussion about the hilum is commonly restricted to discussion about the pulmonary arteries and superior pulmonary veins. In the classic British Authors text (5), it is stated that the inferior pulmonary veins enter the heart well below the hilum and, not as classical anatomy teaches, at the level of the hilum. This leads to some confusion because a mass found just above the inferior pulmonary vein may be described as being *infrahilar* (below the hilum) by some, and being within the *inferior hilar* (lower hilum) region by others. Some descriptions of the hilum, such as Heitzman's (6), consider the hilum as part of the mediastinum – and not a region unto itself.

Much of this confusion arises from the use of anatomical terms to denote radiological features. A more appropriate, and less confusing, description of the contents of the hilum is the "root of the lung" or "radix". However, while this term is very descriptive and appropriate to radiology, it is not often used in clinical practice.

The term hilum is not exclusive to the lungs, as a hilum is also found in the spleen, liver, kidneys and lymph nodes.

AUTHOR RECOMMENDATION:
Use the Fleishner Society definition.

The Fleishner society defines the hilum as "the composite shadow at the root of each lung produced by bronchi, arteries and veins, lymph nodes, nerves, bronchial vessels and associated alveolar tissue" (4).

Figure 2. Surface anatomy localization of the hilum. a, frontal perspective, b, lateral perspective.

Figure 3. Hilar shadows. Two distinct hilar shadows are seen on the right of the PA chest x-ray above.

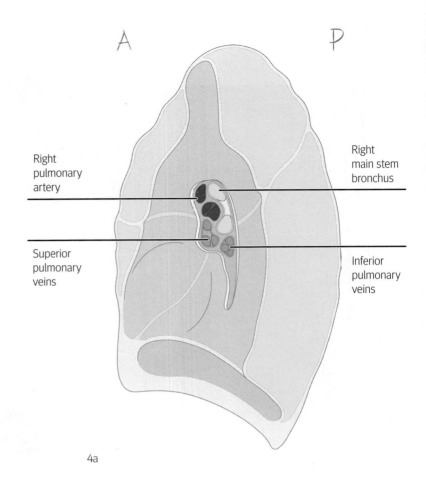

Right
pulmonary
artery

Right
main stem
bronchus

Superior
pulmonary
veins

Inferior
pulmonary
veins

4a

THE HILA -
THE ROOTS OF THE LUNGS

Right Root

The most superior structure of the right hilum (Fig. 4a,b) is the right main stem bronchus. Anterior and medial to the bronchus lies the RPA. Adjacent and anterior to the pulmonary artery is the superior pulmonary vein. The inferior pulmonary vein lies inferiorly.

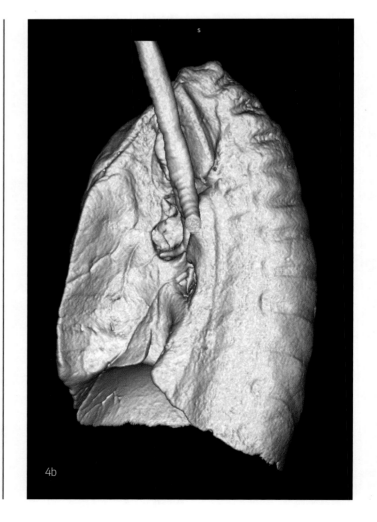

4b

Figure 4. Root of the right lung. a, illustration of the root of the right lung highlighting the components of the right hilum b, CT 3D reconstruction with isolated right lung.

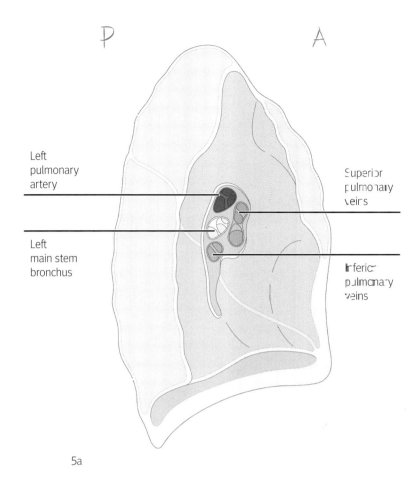

Left pulmonary artery

Left main stem bronchus

Superior pulmonary veins

Inferior pulmonary veins

5a

Left Root

The most superior structure of the left hilum (Fig. 5a,b) is the left pulmonary artery (LPA). Inferior to the LPA lies the left main stem bronchus. Anterior to the LPA is the superior pulmonary vein. The inferior pulmonary vein lies inferiorly.

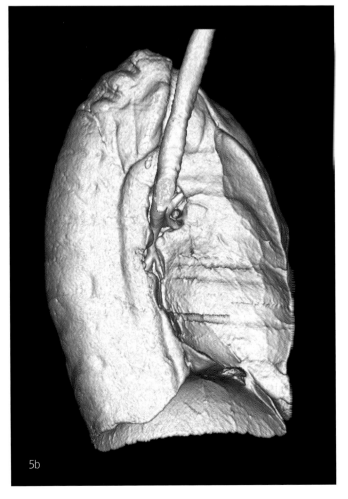

5b

Figure 5. Root of the left lung. a, illustration of the root of the left lung highlighting the components of the left hilum b, CT 3D reconstruction with isolated left lung.

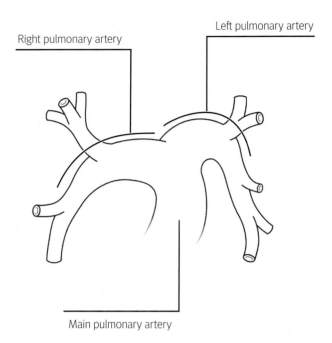

Right pulmonary artery

Left pulmonary artery

Main pulmonary artery

6a

THE PULMONARY ARTERIES

The main pulmonary artery (MPA, or pulmonary trunk) is a short, wide vessel, about 6 cm in length and 3 cm in diameter (7) (Fig. 6a,b). It extends from the conus arteriosum (right ventricular outflow tract) of the right ventricle, and forms a segment of the left heart border. The MPA lies on the left side of the body, and courses obliquely upwards and posteriorly; lying first in front of, and then to the left of, the ascending aorta.

At the undersurface of the aortic arch, at the level of the carina, and slightly to the left of the mid-line, the MPA divides into the right and left pulmonary arteries. The two arteries have almost equal diameters, 19 mm +/- 2 mm (8), but differ significantly in their anatomical course relative to the airways. Understanding this difference will help in identifying the arteries on the chest x-ray.

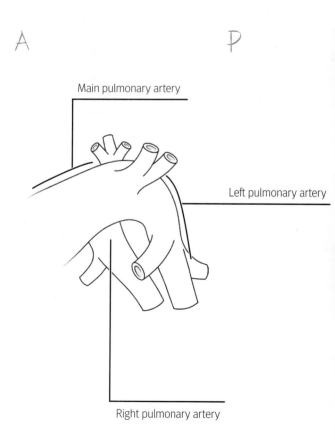

Main pulmonary artery

Left pulmonary artery

Right pulmonary artery

6b

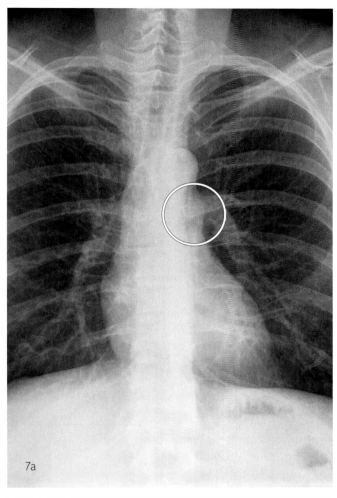

7a

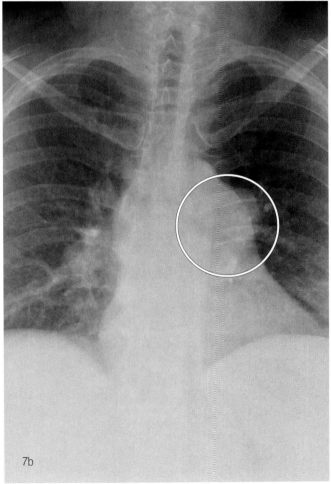

7b

Figure 6. Anatomy of the main pulmonary artery (MPA) and its branches. Illustrations of the main pulmonary artery. a, frontal perspective, b, lateral perspective.

Figure 7. Main pulmonary artery (MPA). a, PA chest x-ray with a normal MPA (circle), b, PA chest x-ray with a prominent MPA (circle).

The Right Pulmonary Artery (RPA)

The RPA is a long vessel. The RPA is long because it must course from the left side of the body to the right, in order to enter into the right lung. The RPA courses horizontally, and lies posterior to the ascending aorta and the SVC, but stays anterior to the anterior border of the lower trachea and the main stem bronchi (Fig. 8a,b).

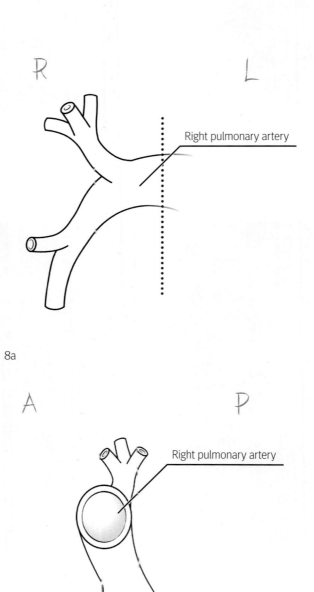

Figure 8. Anatomy of the right pulmonary artery (RPA). Illustrations of the RPA, a, frontal perspective, b, lateral perspective.

Figure 9. Anatomy of the left pulmonary artery (LPA). Illustrations of the LPA,. a, frontal perspective, b, lateral perspective.

230

Left pulmonary artery

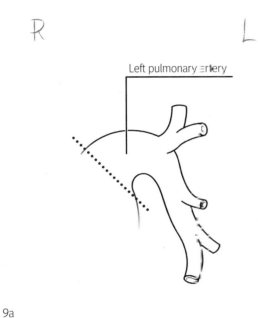

9a

A   P

Main
pulmonary
artery   Left pulmonary artery

9b

In the pediatric population these measurements are smaller and vary more considerably. **!**

The Left Pulmonary Artery (LPA)

The LPA is a shorter vessel compared to the RPA. Shorter because it only has to travel a short distance (from where it begins to the left of midline) to enter into the left lung. The LPA courses from anterior to posterior, and must arch over the left main stem bronchus in order to enter into the left lung (Fig. 9a,b).

	RPA	LPA
Length	Long	Short
Diameter	19 mm +/- 2 mm	19 mm +/- 2 mm
Radiological shape on lateral	Circle	Arch
Relationship to airways	Anterior	Sits on top of left main stem bronchus
Visibility on PA x-ray	Proximal portion is hidden within the mediastinum	Clearly visible
Visibility on lateral x-ray	Clearly visible	Clearly visible

Table 8.1
Comparing the right pulmonary artery (RPA) and left pulmonary artery (LPA)

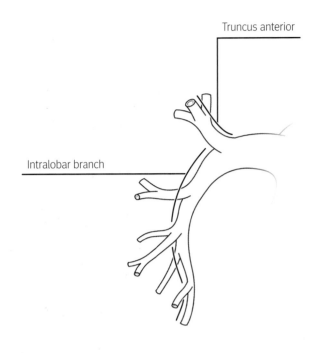

Truncus anterior

Intralobar branch

10a

The Proximal Pulmonary Artery Branches

The RPA divides into two branches within the pericardium, *before* reaching the root of the right lung (Fig. 10a,b). The first branch courses vertically upwards and is called the truncus anterior, while the second branch passes vertically downwards and is called the intralobar, or descending, branch. Simply stated, one of the branches courses upwards and the second branch courses downwards. The descending branch on the right is frequently seen lying adjacent to the right border of the heart.

The LPA divides *after* entering into the left lung (Fig. 11a,b). Like the RPA, one branch of the LPA courses vertically downwards and is called the intralobar or descending branch. However, unlike on the right side, the LPA divides into two or more separate branches destined for the LUL, instead of forming a single common upper lobe trunk. The descending branch on the left is seen behind the heart.

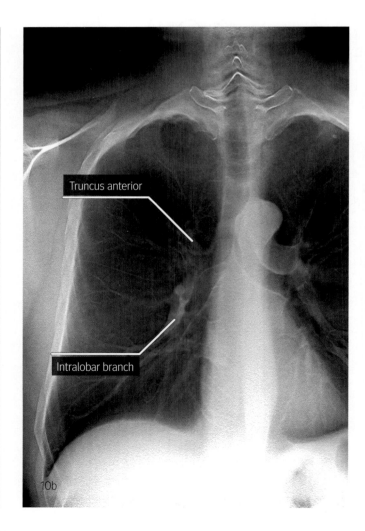

Truncus anterior

Intralobar branch

10b

R   L

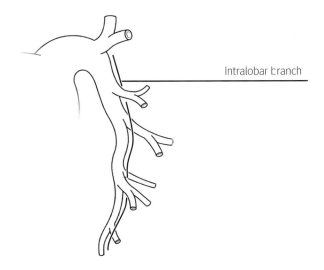

Intralobar branch

11a

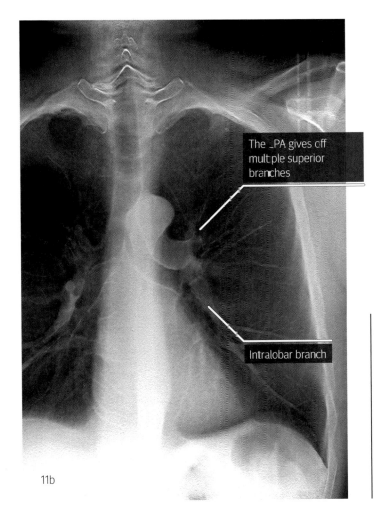

The LPA gives off multiple superior branches

Intralobar branch

11b

Frequency of Visualization on the Lateral X-ray (9)

RPA 96%
LPA 86%

 fv

Although the RPA and LPA are easily seen on the lateral x-ray, the main branches are more difficult to identify because they overlap with the pulmonary veins.

!

Figure 10. Anatomy of the proximal branches of the right pulmonary artery (RPA) from the frontal perspective. a, illustration of the proximal branches of the RPA from the frontal perspective, b, chest tomogram with RPA branches highlighted.

Figure 11. Anatomy of the proximal branches of the left pulmonary artery (LPA) from the frontal perspective. a, illustration of the proximal branches of the LPA from the frontal perspective, b, chest tomogram with LPA branches highlighted.

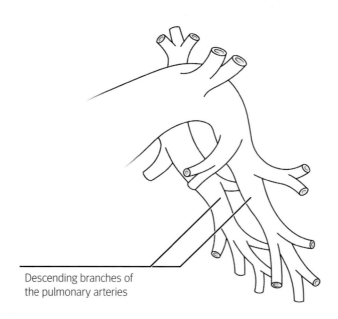

Descending branches of
the pulmonary arteries

12a

The descending branches of the pulmonary arteries course
from their origin centrally, inferiorly and posteriorly. This is
best appreciated on the lateral x-ray where the descending
branches will appear as continuations of the proximal
pulmonary artery coursing obliquely, inferiorly and posteriorly
(Fig. 12a,b). The obliquity is approximately 45 degrees from
the horizontal line.

The arterial branches will gradually become smaller
peripherally. At the level of the secondary lobule (**Ch. 12,
Pg. 451**), a small arterial branch lies centrally within the
lobule adjacent to the airway – whereas the vein lies in
the periphery of the lobule (Fig. 13). These small vessels at
the periphery of the lungs can be identified on a CT scan,
but they are too small to be seen on the chest x-ray.

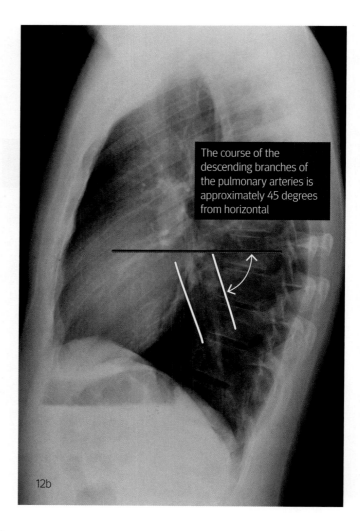

The course of the
descending branches of
the pulmonary arteries is
approximately 45 degrees
from horizontal

12b

Branching vessels extend to the distal one-third of the lung.

!

Two important structures that are vertically oriented on the chest x-ray are the descending branches of the pulmonary arteries, and the right heart border.

!

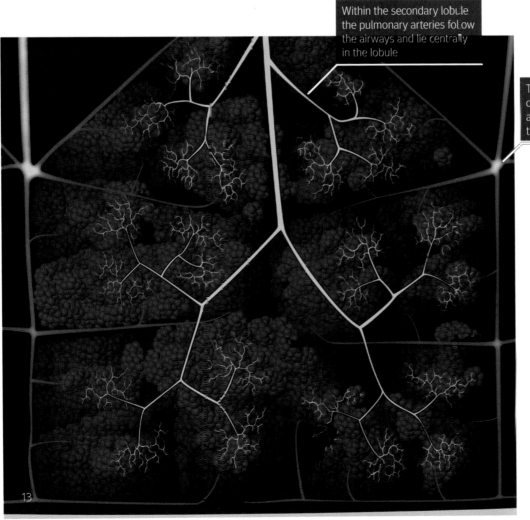

Within the secondary lobule the pulmonary arteries follow the airways and lie centrally in the lobule

The pulmonary veins course in the interstitium around the periphery of the secondary lobule

13

Figure 12. Anatomy of the proximal branches of the pulmonary arteries from the lateral perspective. a, illustration of the RPA from the lateral perspective, b, lateral chest x-ray with the proximal branches of the RPA highlighted.

Figure 13. The anatomy of the arteries and veins of the peripheral lung. Illustration of the secondary lobule of the lung highlighting the path of the blood vessels; the arteries lies centrally and the veins lie peripherally

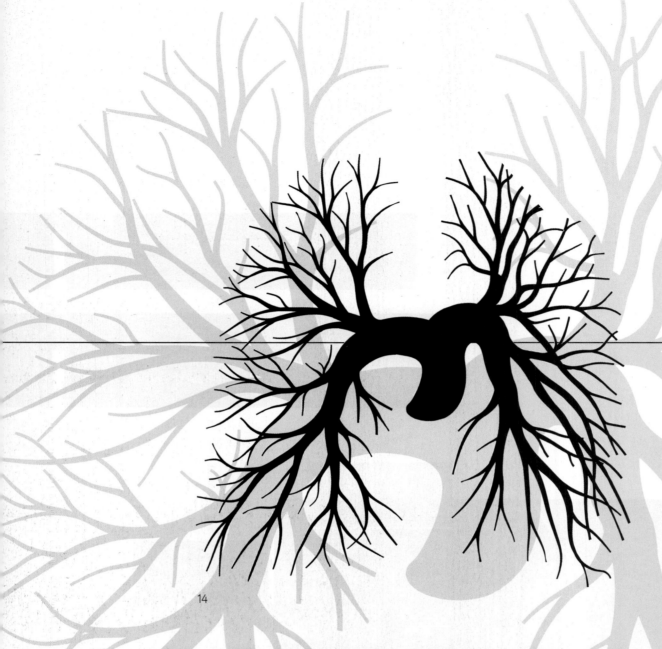

14

The peripheral branches of the pulmonary arteries (Fig. 14)

The truncus anterior divides into apical, anterior ascending, anterior descending, posterior ascending and posterior descending branches destined for the right upper lobe segments. The right middle lobar artery arises from the intralobar branch, and subsequently divides into lateral and medial branches. The intralobar supplies the right lower lobe with superior, sub-superior, medial basal, anterior basal, lateral basal and posterior basal branches.

The superior branches of the LPA are the apical, anterior and posterior (ascending and descending) branches. A lingular branch further divides into superior and inferior branches. The left lower lobe branches are the same as in the right lung.

Figure 14. The peripheral arterial branches. Illustration of the peripheral arterial branches in the lung depicting the gradual decrease in size peripherally.

236

Radiological Shape and Grayscale of the Blood Vessels

In the chapter on the mediastinum, there is a discussion of the radiological appearance of the interfaces between the soft tissues and the lungs (Ch. XX, Pg. XX).

The pulmonary vessels can be seen as separate structures because they create an interface with the lungs (Fig. 15a). An edge will be seen where a blood vessel touches the lung. If the vessel courses parallel to the x-ray beam, it will be seen as a white circle (Fig. 15b). If the vessel courses perpendicular to the direction of the x-ray beam, it will look like a white rectangle (Fig. 15c).

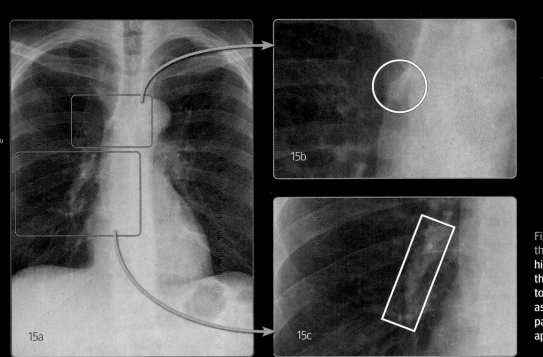

15a

15b

15c

Figure 15. Radiological anatomy of the blood vessels. a, PA chest x-ray highlighting the blood vessels, b, if the blood vessels lie perpendicular to the x-ray beam they will appear as white circles, c, if the vessels lie parallel to the x-ray beam they will appear as white rectangles.

On the PA x-ray, the RPA is hidden in the mediastinum; we can only see the proximal branches coursing superiorly and inferiorly (Fig. 16a,b,c).

The RPA is visible on the lateral x-ray. Since the artery courses from left to right horizontally, one can predict that this vessel will have a circular shape, because, in this profile, the vessel is seen end-on (Fig. 17a,b,c).

Figure 16. Radiological anatomy of the right pulmonary artery (RPA) from the frontal perspective. **a,** PA chest x-ray with the RPA outlined, **b,** PA chest x-ray with grayscale illustration of the RPA overlay, **c,** PA chest x-ray cropped to highlight the RPA.

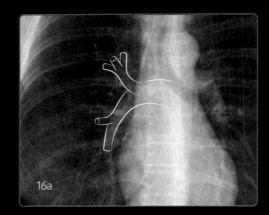

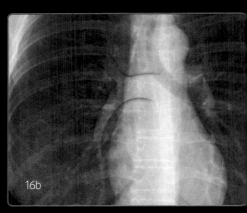

Figure 17. Radiological anatomy of the right pulmonary artery (RPA) from the lateral perspective. **a,** lateral chest x-ray with the RPA outlined, **b,** lateral chest x-ray with grayscale illustration of the RPA overlay, **c,** lateral chest x-ray cropped to highlight the RPA.

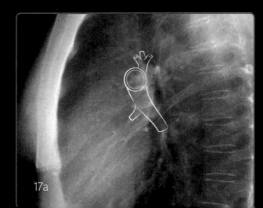

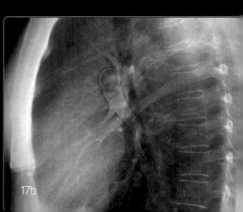

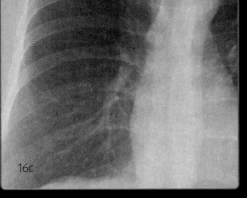

The shadow of the RPA lies more inferiorly than the shadow of the LPA (because it does not arch over the bronchus), and is more difficult to clearly identify on the PA x-ray as it is partially obscured by the shadows of the mediastinum.

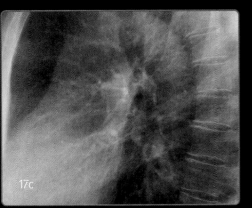

The density (whiteness) of the RPA on the lateral x-ray is usually greater than the density of the heart, and greater than the density of the LPA.

How to identify the RPA on the PA x-ray

It is important to identify the RPA on a PA x-ray in order to distinguish between the normal RPA and pathology that can be found in the right hilar region.

STEP 1
Confirm the patient is midline and not rotated (Ch. 1, Pg. 32).

STEP 2
Focus your vision on the inferior part of the right side of the hilar zone (Fig. 18).

STEP 3
Find a big vessel orientated vertically, lying adjacent and parallel to the right heart border. This is the descending branch of the RPA (Fig. 19).

STEP 4
Follow this vessel superiorly until it curves medially and joins a group of central vascular shadows. The RPA lies at this level, and extends medially (Fig. 20).

STEP 5
Cross-reference the position of the RPA with the position of the LPA, which lies more superiorly, and with the position of the carina (Fig. 21).

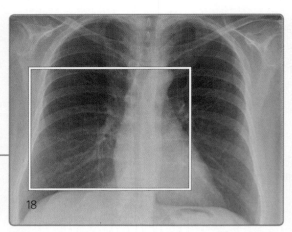

18

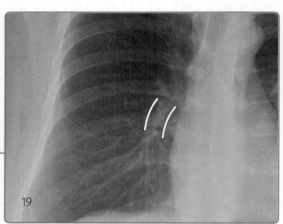

19

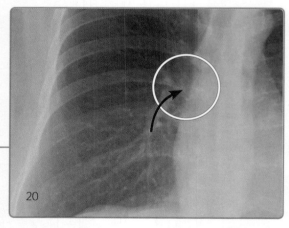

20

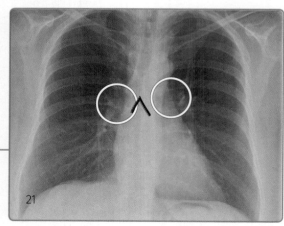

21

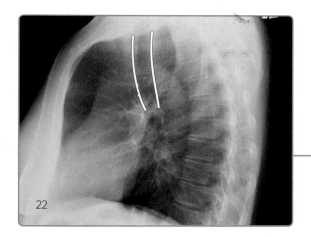

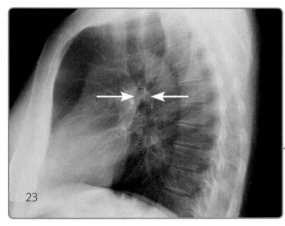

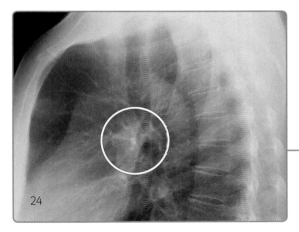

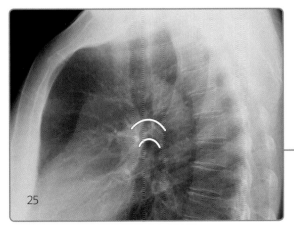

How to identify the RPA on the lateral x-ray

It is important to identify the RPA on a lateral x-ray in order to distinguish between the normal RPA and pathology that can be found in the right hilar region.

STEP 1
Identify the trachea (Ch. 7, Pg. 183)(Fig. 22).

STEP 2
Locate the carina (Ch. 7, Pg. 199)(Fig. 23).

STEP 3
Searching the region anterior to the trachea, visually scan the grayscale from the top of the trachea, inferorly. At approximately the level of the carina the grayscale will change – a white oval will be visible. This is the RPA seen end-on (Fig. 24). The oval of the RPA seen end-on will be one of the whitest structures on the lateral x-ray.

STEP 4
Cross reference the position of the RPA with the position of the LPA – the LPA can be seen as a white arch extending from the superior aspect of the RPA, below the level of the aortic arch (Fig. 25).

On the PA x-ray, the LPA is also partially hidden in the mediastinum; the LPA will produce a white shadow positioned on top of the left main stem bronchus (Fig. 26a,b,c).

The LPA arches over the left main stem bronchus, therefore we can predict that the shape of the LPA on the lateral x-ray will be similar to the aortic arch (an elongated curved structure sitting on the left main stem bronchus) (Fig. 27a,b,c). The grayscale of the LPA is similar, or slightly less white than that of the aorta.

Figure 26. Radiological anatomy of the left pulmonary artery (LPA) from the frontal perspective. **a, PA chest x-ray with the LPA outlined, b, PA chest x-ray with grayscale illustration of the LPA overlay, c, PA chest x-ray cropped to highlight the LPA.**

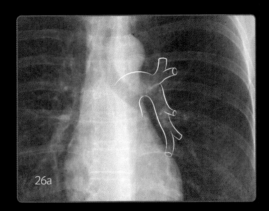
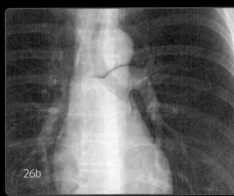

Figure 27. Radiological anatomy of the left pulmonary artery (LPA) from the lateral perspective. **a, lateral chest x-ray with the LPA outlined, b, lateral chest x-ray with grayscale illustration of the LPA overlay, c, lateral chest x-ray cropped to highlight the LPA.**

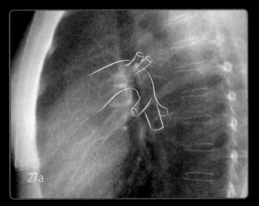
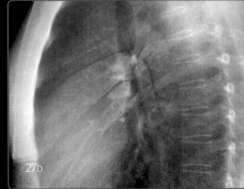

The Aorto-Pulmonary (AP) win

The portion of the lung seen between the superior
the LPA and the aortic arch is called the aorto-pulmo
window (Fig. 28).

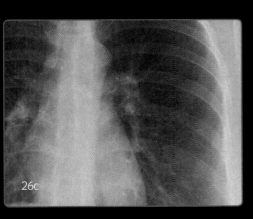

26c

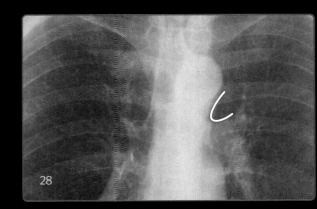

28

Figure 28. The aorto-pulmonary (AP)
window. A PA chest x-ray cropped to
show the AP window (highlighted).

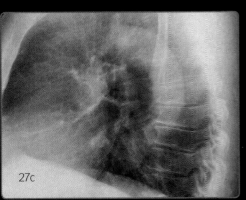

27c

How to identify the LPA on the PA x-ray

It is important to identify the LPA on a PA x-ray in order to distinguish between the normal LPA and pathology that can be found in the left hilar region.

STEP 1
Confirm the patient is midline and not rotated (Ch. 1, Pg. 32).

STEP 2
Focus your vision on the left side of the hilar zone (Fig. 29).

STEP 3
Identify the trachea and the left main stem bronchus (Fig. 30).

STEP 4
The LPA is the white opacity sitting on the left main stem bronchus – the superior edge of the left main stem bronchus corresponds to the inferior edge of the LPA (Fig. 31).

STEP 5
Starting with the inferior border of the LPA, follow the opacity of the LPA superiorly and laterally (at approximately a 45 degree angle), until the opacity ends abruptly. This is the superior border of the artery (Fig. 32).

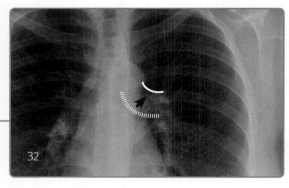

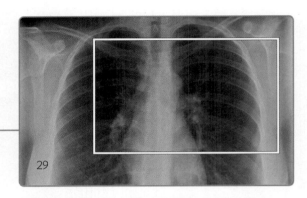

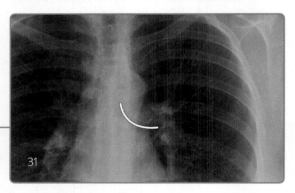

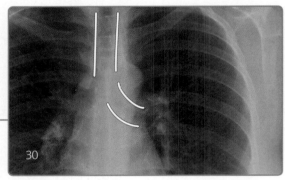

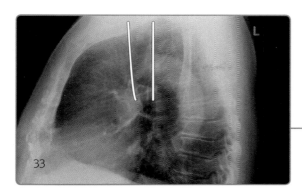

33

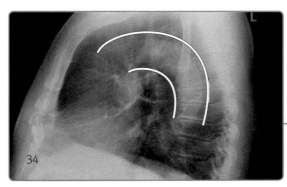

34

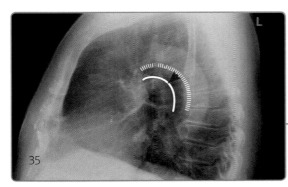

35

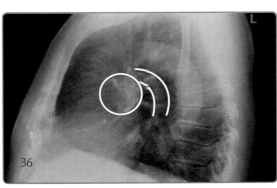

36

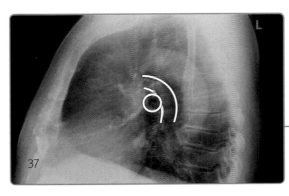

37

How to identify the LPA on the lateral x-ray

It is important to identify the LPA on a lateral x-ray in order to distinguish between the normal LPA and pathology that can be found in the left hilar region.

STEP 1
Identify the trachea (Ch. 7, Pg. 183) (Fig. 33)

STEP 2
Locate the aortic arch (Ch. 9, Pg. 288) (Fig. 34).

STEP 3
Below the inferior edge of the arch is a black area called the aorto-pulmonary (AP) window. Follow this inferiorly until you reach the superior edge of a white arch extending from anterior to posterior. This is the top of the LPA (Fig. 35).

STEP 4
Cross-reference the position of the LPA with the position of the RPA (Fig. 36).

The location of the LPA can also be verified by identifying the left main stem bronchus end-on (Ch. 7, Pg. 183) (Fig. 37).

How to measure the size of the pulmonary arteries

Measuring the caliber of the pulmonary arteries is important for establishing pulmonary artery enlargement, secondary to pulmonary hypertension.

STEP 1
Confirm the patient is midline and not rotated (Ch. 1, Pg. 32).

STEP 2
Identify the descending branch of the RPA (Fig. 38).

STEP 3
Identify the bronchus intermedius (Fig. 39).

STEP 4
Measure the width of the descending branch, at the level where the superior pulmonary vein crosses over the descending artery (Fig. 40).

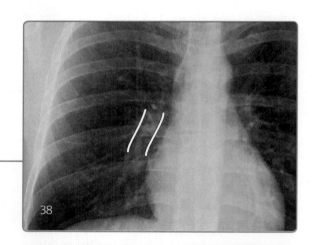

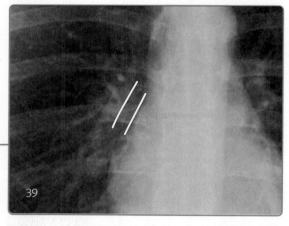

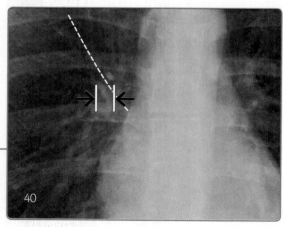

THE H-SIGN

The shape formed by the pulmonary arteries and their vertically-orientated branches, as seen on the PA x-ray, is similar to the shape of the letter "H" (Fig. 41).

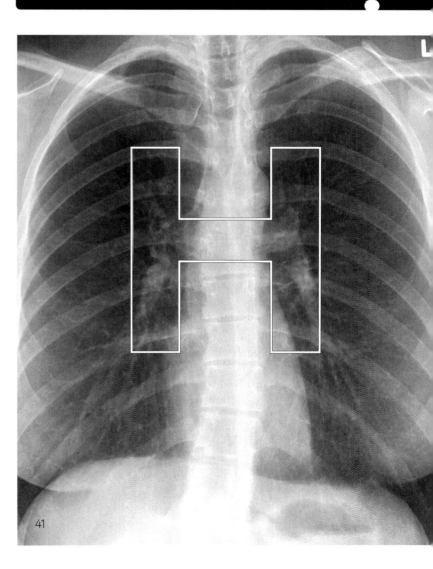

Figure 41. The H-sign. The combined radiological shadows of the main pulmonary arteries and the main branches have the appearance of the letter H.

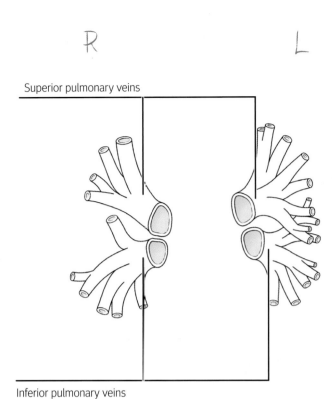

Superior pulmonary veins

Inferior pulmonary veins

R   L

42a

THE PULMONARY VEINS

Each lung has two pulmonary veins – the superior and inferior pulmonary veins – that lie anterior, and medial to the corresponding arteries (Fig. 42a,b). The superior pulmonary veins start superiorly and course inferiorly and medially, draining into the superior lateral part of the left atrium of the heart. (The left atrium is positioned in the thorax, within the middle to lower third of the mediastinum **(Ch. 10, Pg. 346)**).

The heart and the left atrium are structures that lie in the inferior aspect of the thorax. Therefore, the inferior pulmonary veins, which drain the lower portions of the lungs, will course horizontally in order to drain into the left atrium (10).

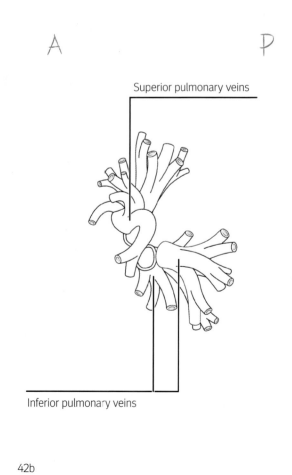

A   P

Superior pulmonary veins

Inferior pulmonary veins

42b

Figure 42. Anatomy of the pulmonary veins. Illustrations of the pulmonary veins, a, frontal perspective, b, lateral perspective.

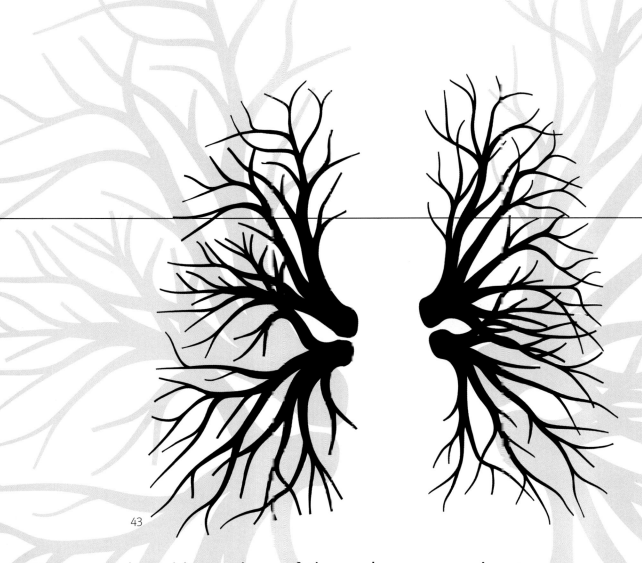

The peripheral branches of the pulmonary veins (Fig. 43)

The right superior pulmonary vein is formed by the union of apical, anterior, posterior and middle lobe branches. The right inferior pulmonary vein is formed by the union of a common basal vein with the superior (apical) vein. The common basal vein is formed by the joining of the RLL superior and inferior basal branches. The left superior pulmonary vein is formed by the union of the apicoposterior, anterior and lingular branches. The left inferior pulmonary vein is formed the same as the right.

Figure 43. The peripheral venous branches. Illustration of the peripheral venous branches in the lung depicting the gradual decrease in size peripherally.

Radiological Shape and Grayscale of the Pulmonary Veins

The pulmonary veins will have the same radiodensity as the pulmonary arteries. Distinguishing between the artery and vein above the level of the heart is difficult because the vessels are in close proximity to each other, and their spatial orientation is similar (Fig. 44a,b,c).

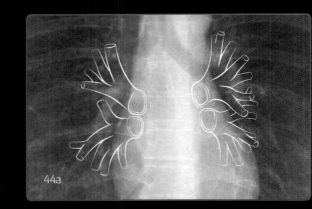

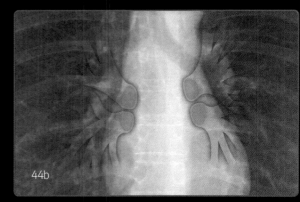

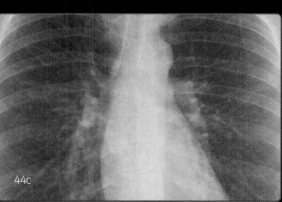

Figure 44. Radiological anatomy of the pulmonary veins from the frontal perspective. a, PA chest x-ray with the pulmonary veins outlined, b, PA chest x-ray with grayscale illustration of the pulmonary veins overlay, c, PA chest x-ray cropped to highlight the pulmonary veins.

The superior pulmonary veins are difficult to distinguish from the arteries. They course from superior and anterior to inferior and posterior. The shape of the superior pulmonary veins is similar to that of a deer's antlers (Fig. 45).

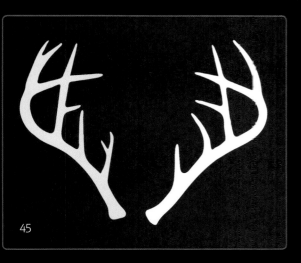

The inferior pulmonary veins can be distinguished from the arteries because they course horizontally and, therefore, perpendicular to the course of the arteries (Fig. 46).

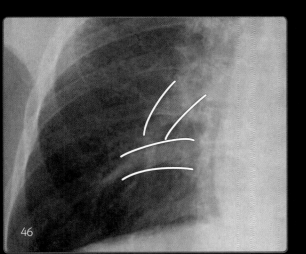

46

Figure 45. Radiological anatomy of the superior pulmonary veins. **Illustration of deer's antlers as a representation of the shape of the superior pulmonary veins.**

Figure 46. Radiological anatomy of the inferior pulmonary veins. **PA chest x-ray with the path of the right inferior veins highlighted.**

How to identify the pulmonary veins on the PA x-ray

The pulmonary veins are important to identify on the PA x-ray in order to distinguish the normal veins from possible hilar pathology.

STEP 1
Confirm the patient is midline and not rotated (Ch. 1, Pg. 32).

STEP 2
Identify the auricle of the left atrium (Fig. 47) (Ch. 10, Pg. 348).

STEP 3
Draw an oval from the auricle across the midline, with the right border of the oval just short of the right heart border. The superior border is below the carina and the inferior border is above the diaphragms. This gives a general outline of the position of the left atrium (Fig. 48). (You can also use the inferior left atrium point (Pg. 253) that can be found on the lateral x-ray, and extrapolate this point to the PA.)

STEP 4
The inferior pulmonary veins are white horizontal branching structures, in the lower one-third of the thorax. They course medially across the descending branches of the pulmonary artery, toward the inferior aspect of the left atrium (Fig. 49).

STEP 5
The superior veins course from superior lateral to inferior medial, to enter into the left atrium (Fig. 50).

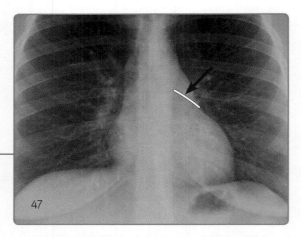

47

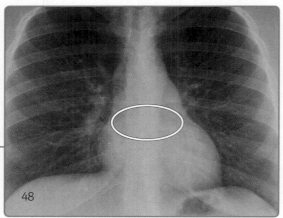

48

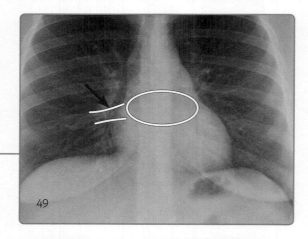

49

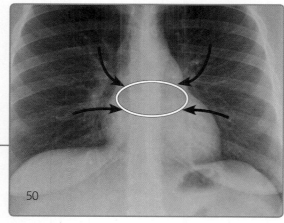

50

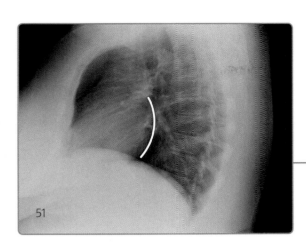

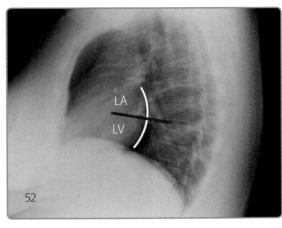

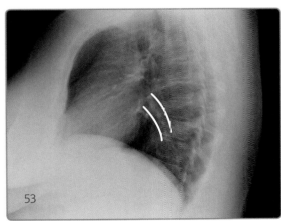

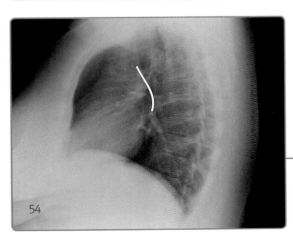

How to identify the pulmonary veins on the lateral x-ray

The pulmonary veins are important to identify on the lateral x-ray in order to distinguish the normal veins from possible hilar pathology.

STEP 1
Identify the posterior border of the cardiac contour (Fig. 51).

STEP 2
Bisect the posterior cardiac contour. The upper half is the left atrium, and the lower half is the left ventricle (Fig. 52). This bisection point is called the inferior left atrium point.

STEP 3
The inferior veins course from posterior lateral to medial, horizontally, and form some of the white rectangles that extend into the inferior aspect of the left atrium (Fig. 53).

STEP 4
The superior veins course from superior lateral to inferior medial, to enter into the superior aspect of the left atrium (Fig. 54).

THE RADIOLOGICAL LOCATION OF THE HILA

Pathology in the thorax can cause a change in the position of the hilum. In order to determine if the hila are too high or too low (displaced) on the PA chest x-ray, we need to first understand their normal position (Fig. 55a,b).

Determining the normal hilar position on the left is easier because we can identify the LPA, sitting on the left main stem bronchus. If the left main stem bronchus is elevated, the left hilum will inevitably be elevated as well.

On the right, the pulmonary artery shadow is difficult to differentiate from the superior pulmonary vein. A reference point that defines the position of the hilum, called the hilar point, can be established (Fig. 56). The right hilar point is at the intersection of the right superior pulmonary vein and the descending branch of the RPA.

The LPA is clearly identifiable on a PA x-ray, and therefore a left hilar point is unnecessary, but a left hilar point can also be determined.

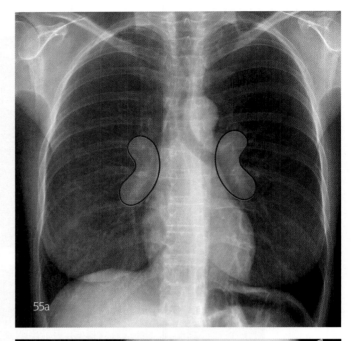

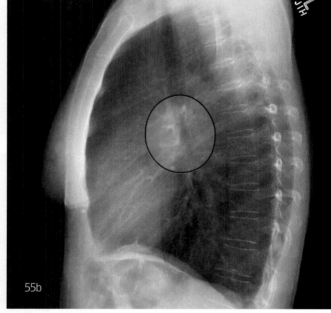

Figure 55. The hilar zone. The position of the radiological hila can be considered as a zone, the hilar zone, on chest x-rays. a, PA chest x-ray with the hilar zone highlighted, b, lateral chest x-ray with the hilar zone highlighted.

Figure 56. Hilar point. The hilar point is a reference point that can be used to determine the position of the right hilum. PA chest x-ray with the right hilar point highlighted.

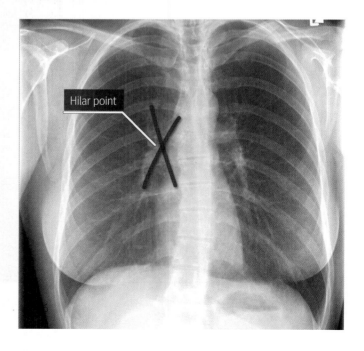

ANATOMICAL RELATIONSHIPS OF THE ROOTS OF THE LUNGS

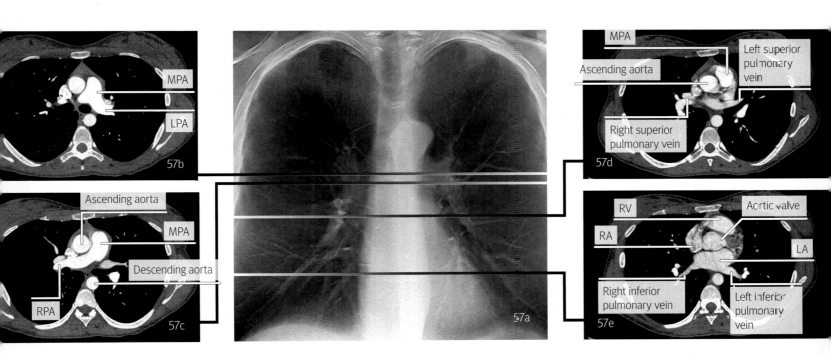

Comprised of many structures, the hilum forms many relationships - both within and external to, its boundaries. The hilar structures can be found between the ascending and descending aorta, extending laterally into the lungs. In the most superior aspect of the hilum, just below the carina (Fig. 57b), the main pulmonary artery and the left pulmonary artery are identifiable. More inferiorly (Fig. 57c) the right pulmonary artery becomes visible to the right of and posterior to the ascending aorta. The medial superior pulmonary vein begins to appear in Figure 57d. At the level of the left atrium (Fig. 57e) the horizontal aspects of the inferior pulmonary veins become visible.

Figure 58. Spatial relationship of the hila with other thoracic anatomical structures. a, Tomographical image of chest showing levels of cross sectional slices, b, slice 1 just below the carina highlighting the main pulmonary artery (MPA) and left pulmonary artery (LPA), c, slice 2 highlighting the MPA, right pulmonary artery (RPA), and the ascending and descending aorta, d, slice 3 highlighting the superior pulmonary veins, ascending and descending aorta and MPA, e, slice 4 highlighting the inferior pulmonary veins and left and right atrium. LA, left atrium, LPA, left pulmonary artery, MPA, main pulmonary artery, RA, right atrium, RPA, right pulmonary artery, RV, right ventricle.

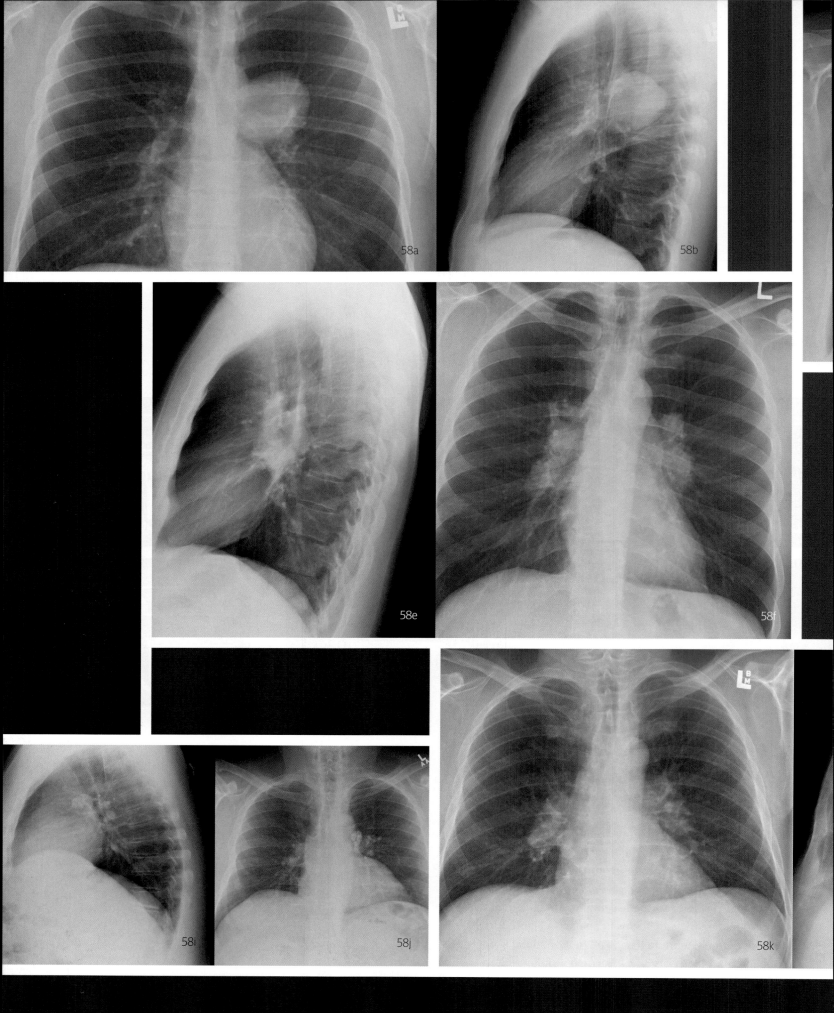

58a

58b

58e

58f

58i

58j

58k

PATHOLOGY OF THE HILUM

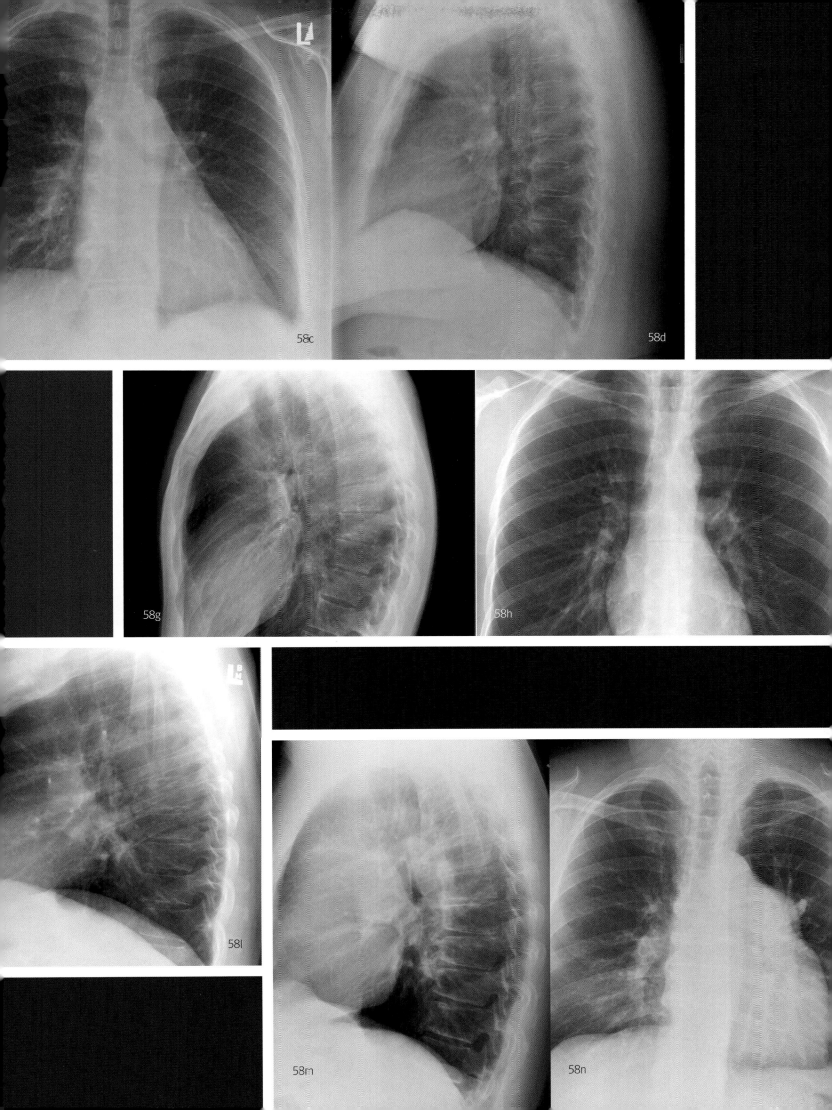

58c

58d

58g

58h

58l

58m

58n

THE ABNORMAL HILUM

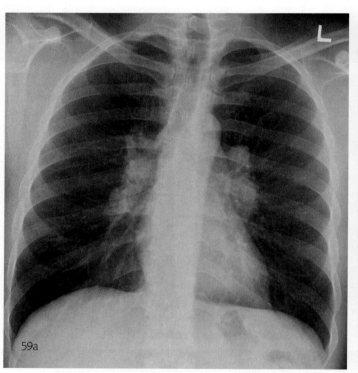

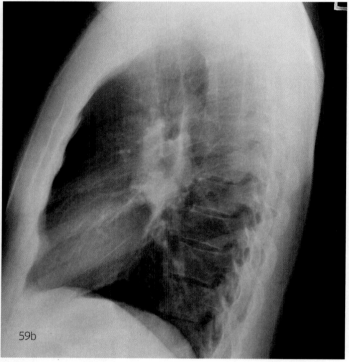

The Radiological Hilum Will Be Abnormal When

1) The grayscale of the hilum is too white (i.e., the density of the hilum is increased).
2) The size of the hilar shadow is enlarged or reduced.
3) The position of the hilum is shifted.
4) The shape of the hilum is distorted.
5) Special Case: The hilar boundaries become ill-defined (hilar haze).

Since there is a right and left hilum, each of these described pathologies can occur unilaterally or bilaterally.

Figure 59. Hilar adenopathy. Pathology can cause a shift in grayscale to too white. a, PA chest x-ray from a patient with adenopathy showing an increase in hilar radiodensity with an increase in size, b, lateral chest x-ray of the same patient.

Figure 60. Hilar lymph node calcification. Pathology can cause a shift in grayscale to too white. a, PA chest x-ray from a patient with calcified hilar lymph nodes showing an increase in hilar radiodensity without an increase in size, b, lateral chest x-ray from the same patient.

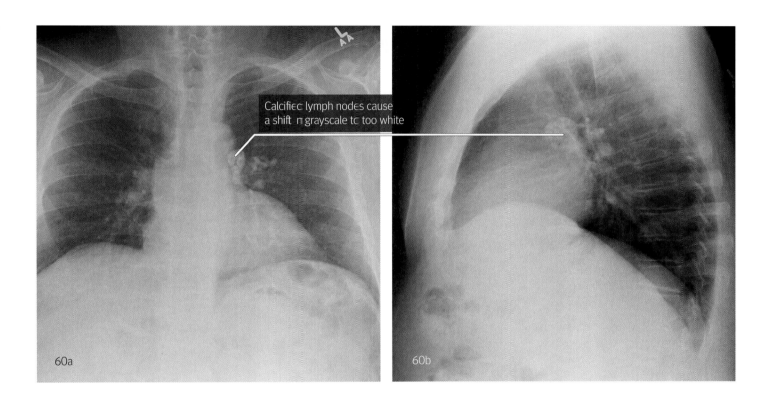

Calcified lymph nodes cause a shift in grayscale to too white

60a

60b

1. Pathology that affects the hilum and shifts the grayscale to 'Too White': the "Too Dense" hilum

The grayscale appearance of the hilum is caused by the summation of densities. Therefore, when there is too much soft tissue in the hilum, the hilum will appear too dense. Enlarged vessels, a tumor, and/or enlarged lymph nodes will all cause the grayscale of the hilum to increase (Fig. 59a,b). If the underlying pathology is small, the hilar density can increase without obvious hilar enlargement on the x-ray.

In addition, calcification in the soft tissues (especially the lymph nodes) can cause the hilar regions to look too white (Fig. 60a,b).

Did you catch the examples on pages 256–257?
Fig. 58c,d – Right hilar mass
Fig. 58i,j – Left hilar calcification

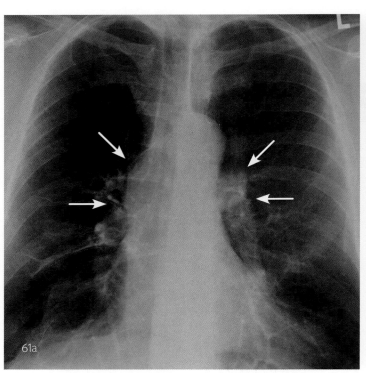

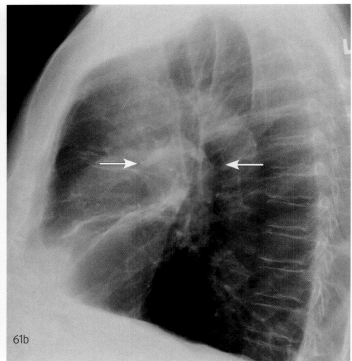

61a

61b

2. Pathology that alters the size of the hilum

Bilateral hilar enlargement

Bilateral hilar enlargement can occur with enlargement of the pulmonary arteries (as seen with pulmonary arterial hypertension) or with bilateral hilar lymph node enlargement.

AMSER | In pulmonary arterial hypertension, the shape of the right and left pulmonary arteries is maintained, but the arteries are enlarged – the large H–sign (Fig. 61a,b).

If hilar lymph nodes are enlarged, the hila will have a lobulated irregular shape (Fig. 62a,b), and the distinction of the pulmonary arteries on the PA and lateral x-rays will be lost – the indistinct H–sign (11). Bilateral hilar adenopathy can be seen with neoplastic disease (lymphoma, metastasis), sarcoidosis, silicosis, and occasionally, with infections.

Figure 61. Large H-sign. Pathology can change the size of the hila. a, PA chest x-ray from a patient with pulmonary hypertension causing an enlargement of the hila (arrows), b, lateral chest x-ray of the same patient.

Figure 62. Indistinct H-sign. Pathology can change the shape of the hila. a, PA chest x-ray from a patient with hilar adenopathy (arrows) causing the hila to have an irregular appearance, b, lateral chest x-ray from same patient.

260

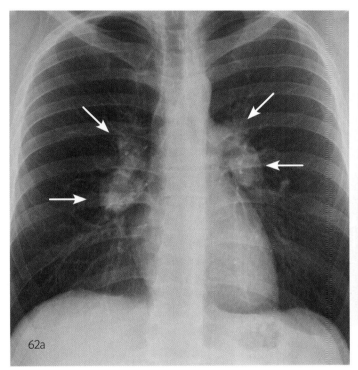

62a

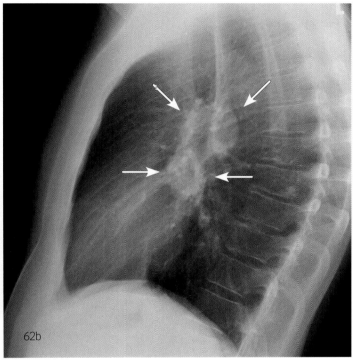

62b

Did you catch the examples on pages 256–257?
Figs. 58e,f and 58k,l – Bilateral hilar enlargement
Fig. 58m,n – Pulmonary hypertension

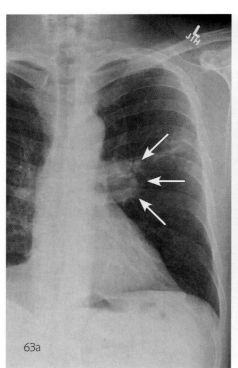

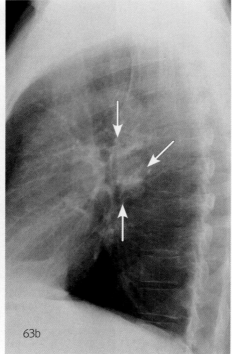

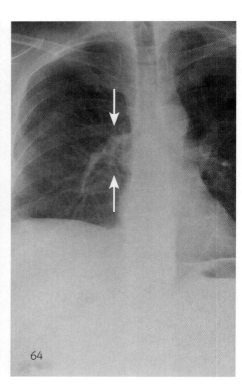

63a

63b

64

Unilateral hilar enlargement

Unilateral hilar enlargement is caused by the presence of a tumor, enlarged nodes, or it may be due to vascular causes (Fig. 63a,b). Unilateral lymph node enlargement is most commonly caused by a tumor (either primary lung cancer, carcinoid, or metastasis), or infections (tuberculosis, fungal, viral). Vascular causes include pulmonary embolism, pulmonary artery aneurysm and/or post-stenotic dilatation in pulmonary artery stenosis (12,13).

Small hilum

A small hilum can be seen following lobectomy, or with lobar collapse (Fig. 64).

AMSER

Figure 63. Unilateral hilar enlargement. Pathology can change the size of the hila. a, PA chest x-ray from a patient with lung cancer resulting in an enlarged right hilum (arrows), b, lateral chest x-ray of the same patient.

Figure 64. Small hilum. Pathology can change the size of the hila. a, PA chest x-ray from a patient with previous right lobectomy resulting in a small left hilum, b, lateral chest x-ray from the same patient.

Figure 65. Altered hilar position due to previous surgery. Pathology can shift the position of the hila. PA chest x-ray from a patient with a post-surgical loss of volume causing a shift in the position of the left hilum.

Figure 66. Altered hilar position secondary to scarring. Pathology can shift the position of the hila. PA chest x-ray from a patient with COPD and previous TB causing a shift in the position of the hila due to scarring.

262

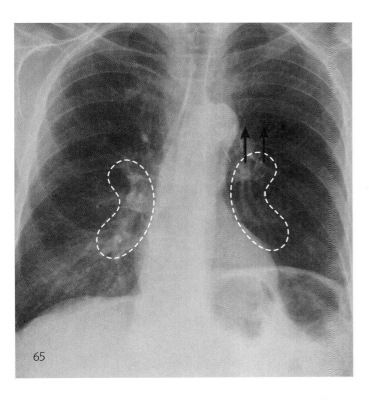

65

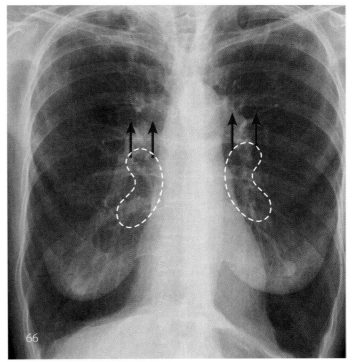

66

3. Pathology that alters the position of the hilum

The hilar position can be elevated, depressed or shifted medially or laterally. A lateral shift will occur when something "pushes" the hilum, such as a large pneumothorax or a large pleural effusion. The position of the hilum will also shift with volume loss, associated with lobar collapse, or previous surgery. In this case, the hilum is pulled in the direction of the pathology (Fig. 65). In the case of a previous pneumonectomy, the position of the normal hilum will shift to the side of the surgery.

Another common cause of position change is retraction of the hilum, secondary to parenchymal scarring (Fig. 66). In this scenario, the hilum will shift in the direction of the scarring.

Did you catch the example on pages 256–257?
Fig. 58a,b – Suprahilar mass

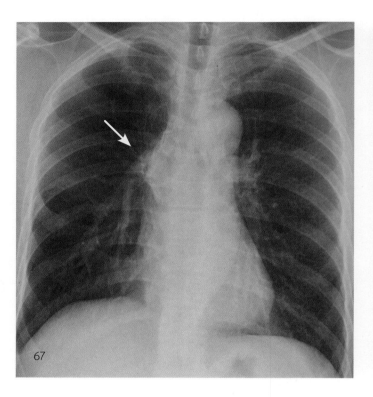

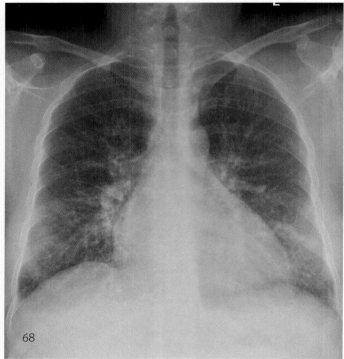

4. Pathology that alters the shape of the hilum

The H-shape can be altered by previous surgery (Fig. 67), or because of underlying pathology. Less commonly, the H-shape can be altered with congenital abnormalities of the pulmonary arteries, such as a hypoplastic pulmonary artery or scimitar syndrome, or by aberrant venous drainage.

5. Special Case: Hilar Haze

Lung interstitium surrounds the normal bronchovascular structures. With pulmonary venous hypertension, fluid leaks into this interstitial space and will cause the outline of the vessels to lose their sharp interface and look hazy (**Ch. 10, Pg. 368**). When this occurs in the hilar and perihilar regions, it is known as hilar haze (Fig. 68).

Figure 67. Altered hilar shape due to surgery. Pathology can alter the shape of the hila. PA chest x-ray from a patient post-surgery, resulting in an altered shape of the right hilum (arrow).

Figure 68. Hilar haze. In pulmonary venous hypertension, fluid leaks into the interstitial space and causes the vessels to look hazy. PA chest x-ray from a patient with pulmonary venous hypertension resulting in the appearance of hilar haze.

SUMMARY OF RADIOLOGICAL CHANGES TO THE HILUM

RADIOLOGICAL CHANGES		ASSOCIATED FINDINGS, DISEASES AND CONDITIONS
1. Too white		• Pulmonary hypertension • Adenopathy (due to: lymphoma, metastasis, sarcoidosis, silicosis, infection) • Calcification of soft tissues (e.g., lymph nodes) • Pulmonary vessel tumor (rare)
2. Size altered	Bilateral enlargement	• Pulmonary arterial hypertension • Bilateral adenopathy (due to: lymphoma, metastasis, sarcoidosis, silicosis, infection)
	Unilateral enlargement	• Lung cancer • Unilateral adenopathy (due to: primary lung cancer, carcinoid, metastasis, infection) • Pulmonary embolism • Pulmonary artery aneurysm • Post-stenotic dilatation following pulmonary artery stenosis • Pulmonary vessel tumor (rare)
	Decreased	• Lobectomy • Lobar collapse
3. Position shifted (elevated/depressed, medially/laterally)		• Pneumothorax • Pleural effusion • Lobar collapse • Parenchymal scarring
4. Shape distorted		• Surgery • Adenopathy • Congenital abnormalities (e.g., hypoplastic pulmonary artery, scimitar syndrome, aberrant venous drainage) • Pulmonary vessel tumor (rare)
5. Special case: Hilar haze		• Pulmonary venous hypertension

Table 8.2
Summary of Radiological Changes to the Hilum

RADIOLOGICAL SIGNS RELATED TO THE HILA

Hilar Convergence Sign

The hilar convergence sign (Fig. 69a,b) is used to distinguish between a perihilar mediastinal mass and a mass in the hilar vascular structures (14). When the pulmonary artery branches converge towards the mass rather than towards the heart, this implies that the mass represents an enlarged pulmonary artery. When the pulmonary artery branches converge towards the heart, rather than the mass, this indicates that the mass represents an extravascular mediastinal mass.

Hilar Overlay Sign

The hilar overlay sign also helps determine whether a mass lies within the mediastinum or hilum. When a mass arises from the hilum, the pulmonary vessels are in contact with the mass and will silhouette with the mass. If the mass lies anterior or posterior to the hilum, the hilar vessels will be visible through the mass. This is the hilar overlay sign (Fig. 70).

H-Sign

The shape formed by the normal pulmonary arteries and their vertically-orientated branches, as seen on the PA x-ray, is similar to the shape of the letter "H" (described by author Dr. J. Dobranowski) (Fig. 71a). In pulmonary hypertension, the H is enlarged but maintained (Fig. 71b), whereas with a bilateral hilar adenopathy, the H-shape is lost (Fig. 71c).

Figure 69. The hilar convergence sign. a, PA chest x-ray with an example of the hilar convergence sign, b, lateral chest x-ray from the same patient. Here, the pulmonary artery branches converge toward the heart, indicating the mass is not hilar in origin.

Figure 70. The hilar overlay sign. A PA chest x-ray with an example of the hilar overlay sign. Notice how the hilar vessels are seen through the mass, indicating the mass is within the mediastinum and not the hilum.

Figure 71. The H-sign. The hila normally resemble an H on the PA chest x-ray; pathology can alter or obliterate this H shape. a, PA chest x-ray with an example of a normal H, b, PA chest x-ray with an example of an enlarged H, c, PA chest x-ray in which the H is obliterated.

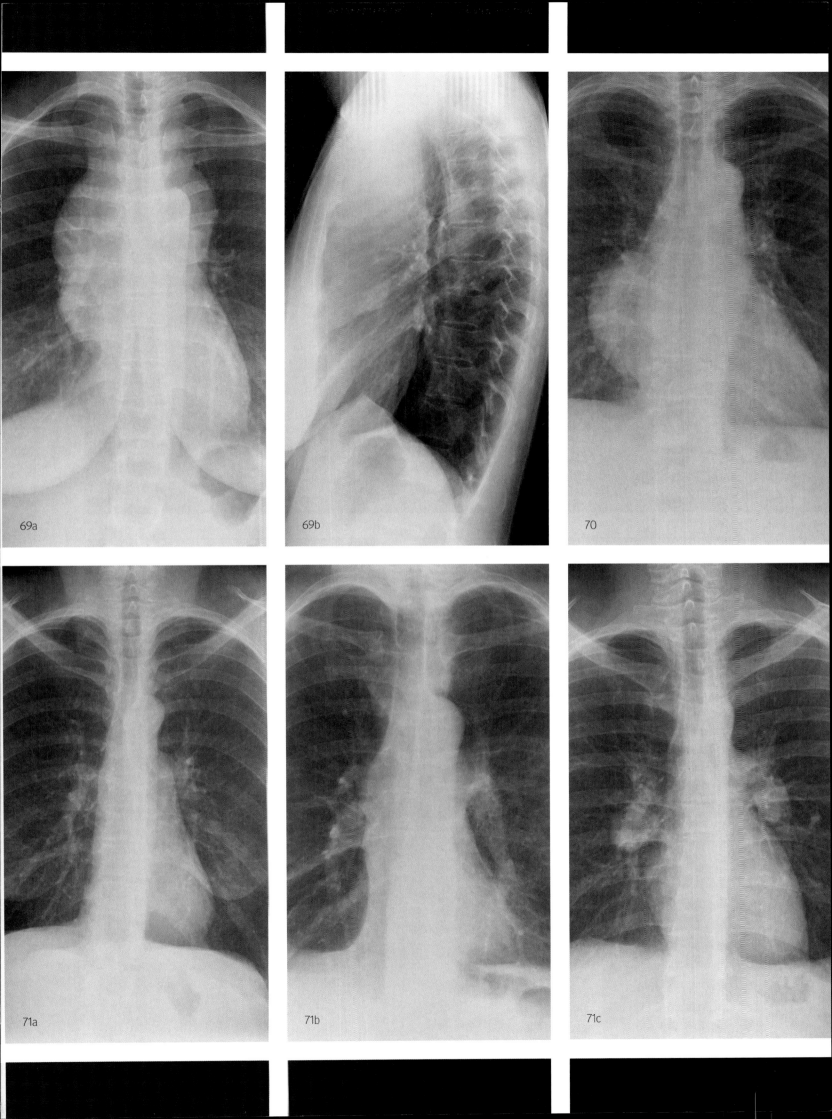

69a

69b

70

71a

71b

71c

Visual Search of the Hilum

PA Chest X-ray

1. Start at the top of the right hilum (1).

2. Follow the lateral outline of the hilum inferiorly to the lower heart level (2).

3. Follow the medial outline of the right hilum superiorly (3).

4. Follow the same instructions on the left.

Complete the visual search by checking for any density changes across the hilum.

Lateral Chest X-ray

1. Start at the mid-trachea (1).

2. Follow from the top (2) of the right pulmonary artery to the bottom (3).

3. Follow the outline of the left pulmonary artery from anterior (4) to posterior.

Complete the visual search by checking for any density changes across the hilum.

VS

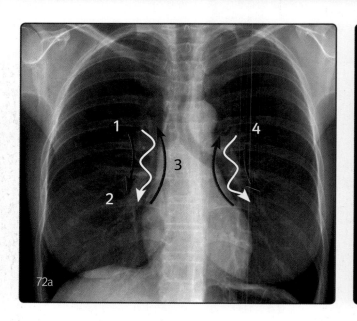

72a

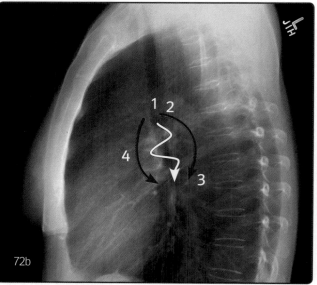

72b

Hilum Radiological Analysis Checklist

GRAYSCALE

1   Is the grayscale of the hilum altered?

If **YES**, then describe.
Too white (too dense)
Right/left/bilateral.

SIZE

2   Is the size of the hilum altered?

If **YES**, then describe.
Too big/too small.
Right/left/bilateral.

POSITION

3   Is the position of the hilum shifted?

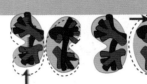

If **YES**, then describe.
Elevated/depressed.
Medial/lateral.
Anterior/posterior.
Right/left/bilateral.

SHAPE

4   Is the H-shape of the hila distorted on the PA x-ray?

If **YES**, then describe.
Lobulated/irregular.
Right/left/bilateral.

5   Are one or both of the arches distorted on the lateral x-ray?

If **YES**, then describe.
Aorta narrowed/distended.
LPA narrowed/distended.

OTHER

6   Is the AP window normal?

If **NO**, then describe.
Blurred/obscured.
Too big/too small.

7   Are there any radiological signs related to the hilum present?

If **YES**, then describe.
Hilar convergence.
Hilar overlay.
H-sign.

8   Is there any evidence of previous surgery to the hilum?

If **YES**, then describe.
Type of surgery and location.
Compare to previous CXR.

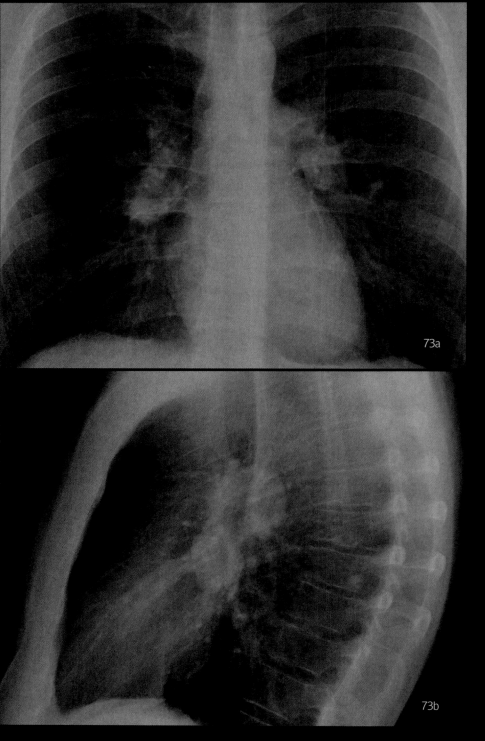

73a

73b

How would you
describe the
abnormalities?

CASE STUDY

A 35-year-old male presents with the recent appearance of red bumps on the skin, swollen glands in the neck and armpits, and redness of both eyes. The patient has also experienced mild shortness of breath on exertion. On physical examination, the patient is found to have enlarged lymph nodes in the neck, axilla and groin. The liver and spleen are also mildly enlarged. You suspect the patient may have intrathoracic adenopathy and you order a chest x-ray (Fig. 73a,b). You examine the x-rays and are asked to report your findings to the staff physician.

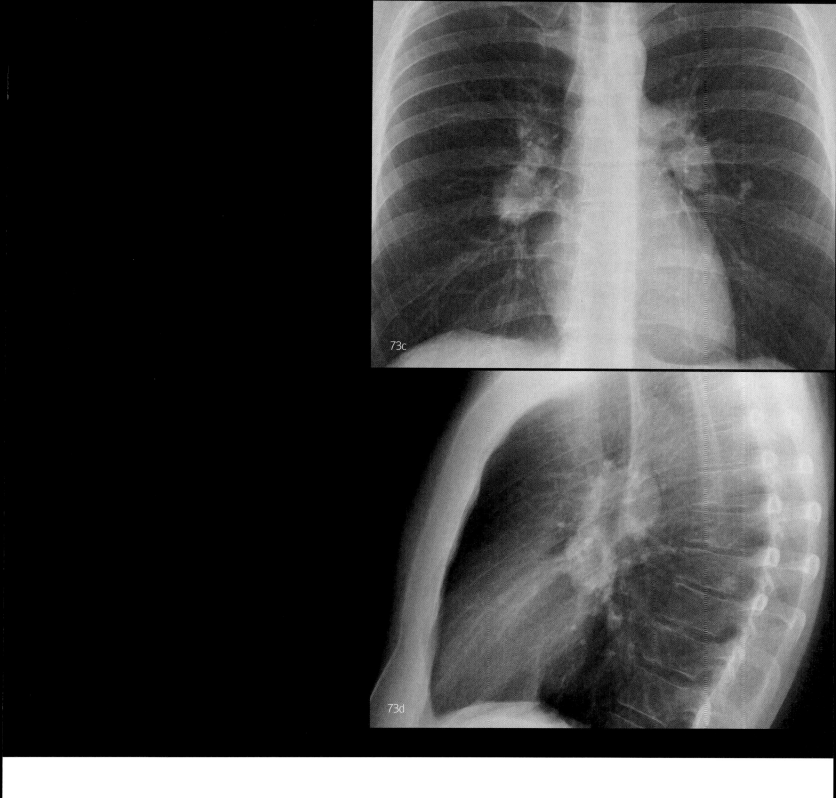

73c

73d

The chest x-ray shows bilateral lobulated enlargement of the hila (Fig. 73c,d). This lobulated appearance is consistent with enlarged lymph nodes.

The patient was diagnosed with sarcodosis after further testing.

References:

1. Lewis, P.J., Shaffer, K., & Donovan, A. (Eds.). (2012). AMSER National Medical Student Curriculum in Radiology. http://aur.org/Secondary-Alliances.aspx?id=141.

2. Lewis, P.J., & Shaffer, K. (2005). Developing a national medical student curriculum in radiology. *Am. Coll. Radiol., 2*(1):8–11.

3. Haubrich, W.S. (2003). *Medical meaning- a glossary of word origins*, 2nd ed. Philadelphia, PA: ACP Press.

4. Tuddenham, W.J. (1984). Glossary of Terms for Thoracic Radiology: recommendations of the Nomenclature Committee of the Fleischner Society. *AJR Am. J. Roentengol., 143*: 509–517.

5. Shanks, S.C., & Kerley, P. (Eds.). (1970). *A Textbook of X-ray Diagnosis. By British Authors.,* 4th ed. London, UK: H.K. Lewis & Co., Ltd.

6. Heitzman, E.R. (1977). *The Mediastinum: Radiologic Correlations with Anatomy and Pathology.* University of Michigan, MI: Mosby.

7. Gray, H. (2008). *Gray's Anatomy: The Anatomical Basis of Medicine and Surgery,* 40th ed. New York, NY: Churchill Livingstone.

8. Kuriyama, K., Gamsu, G., Stern, R.G., et al. (1984). CT-determined pulmonary artery diameters in predicting pulmonary hypertension. *Invest. Radiol., 19*(1):16–22.

9. Proto, A.V. & Speckman, J.M. (1979). The left lateral radiograph of the chest. Part 1. *Med. Radiogr. Photogr., 55*(2):29–74.

10. Budorick, N., McDonald, V., Flisak, M., & Moncada, R. (1989). The pulmonary veins. *Sem. Roentgenol., 24*(2):127–140.

11. Kanemoto, N., Furuya, H., Etoh, T., et al. (1979). Chest roentgenograms in primary pulmonary hypertension. *Chest, 76*(1):45–49.

12. Nguyen, E.T., Silva, C.I.S., Seely, J.M., et al. (2007). Pulmonary artery aneurysms and pseudoaneurysms in adults: findings at CT and radiography. *AJR Am. J. Roentgenol., 188*(2):W126–W134.

13. Khan, A., Cann, A.D., & Shah, R.D. (2004). Imaging of acute pulmonary emboli. *Thorac. Surg. Clin., 14*(1):113–124.

14. Felson, B. (1973). *Chest Roentgenology.* Philadelphia, PA: W.B. Saunders Co.

CHAPTER 9

The MEDIASTINUM
(the mediastinal zone)

importance

The mediastinum is the region of the thorax that lies between the two lungs. This mid-portion of the chest x-ray contains many key structures and landmarks and, therefore, it is important that you understand the anatomical relationships within the mediastinum.

Much like the hilum, the mediastinum is a complex area that is difficult to understand and interpret, on both the PA and lateral chest x-rays. Understanding the radiological appearance of the mediastinum unlocks the understanding of the mid-portion of the chest x-ray. The grayscale of the mediastinum is heterogeneous because of the overlap of multiple anatomical structures. Mastering an appreciation for the relationships between these anatomical structures and how they contribute to the grayscale of the mediastinum is essential for the identification and localization of mediastinal disease. In this chapter, you will learn that the lateral x-ray is key to disease identification and localization within the mediastinum.

Pathology within the mediastinum is often missed because it can easily be hidden by the shadows of overlapping anatomical structures. The accurate localization of pathology is important for the formulation of a differential diagnosis, and for communicating your findings to the patient and other members of the healthcare team. This chapter will provide you with the tools for identifying the structures, the edges and the pathology that can exist within the mediastinum.

objectives

Skills

You will identify

- the landmarks needed to classify the components of the mediastinum.

- the right paratracheal stripe, the paraaortic stripe, the paraspinal stripe, the aorto-pulmonary window and the azygoesophageal recess on a PA chest x-ray.

- the edges of the mediastinum (and their names).

- common mediastinal pathology.

- a mass within the mediastinum, and provide a differential diagnosis based on its location.

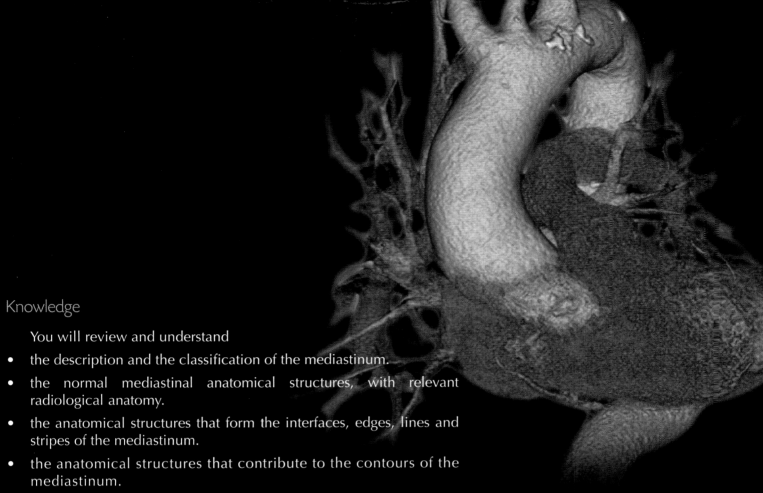

Knowledge

You will review and understand

- the description and the classification of the mediastinum.

- the normal mediastinal anatomical structures, with relevant radiological anatomy.

- the anatomical structures that form the interfaces, edges, lines and stripes of the mediastinum.

- the anatomical structures that contribute to the contours of the mediastinum.

- why, and how, pathology changes the radiological appearance of the mediastinum.

associated resources

This chapter maps to the following AMSER curriculum content (1,2).

1. Normal radiological anatomy of the mediastinum
   Aorta
   Aortic knob (arch)
   Superior vena cava (SVC)
   Carotid and subclavian vessels
   Azygos vein
   Azygoesophageal recess (line)
   Aorto-pulmonary (AP) window
   Right paratracheal stripe (line)

2. Common normal variants
   Mediastinal lipomatosis

3. Pathological conditions affecting the mediastinum
   Pneumomediastinum
   Adenopathy
   Lymphoma
   Sarcoidosis
   Anterior mediastinal mass
   Pleural effusion
   Tumor
   Atelectasis

4. Vascular abnormalities
   Recognition and differential diagnosis of a dilated aorta - aneurysm
   Appearance of great vessel ectasia

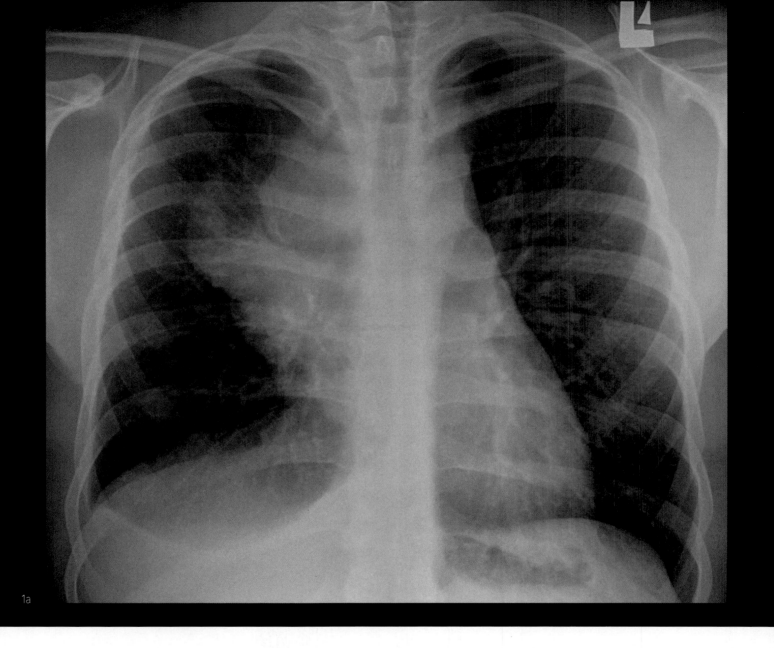

1a

You are working on call in the emergency department. A 50 year old male presents with weight loss, shortness of breath and chest pain. You order a chest x-ray (Fig. 1a,b).

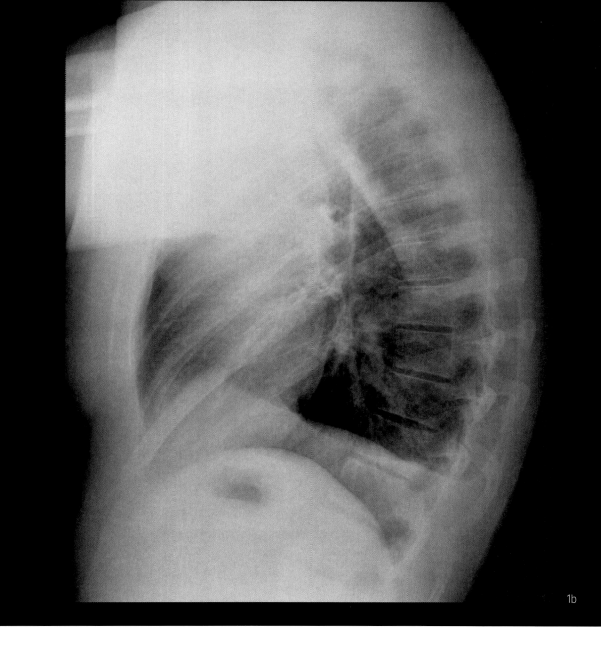

1b

What are
your findings?

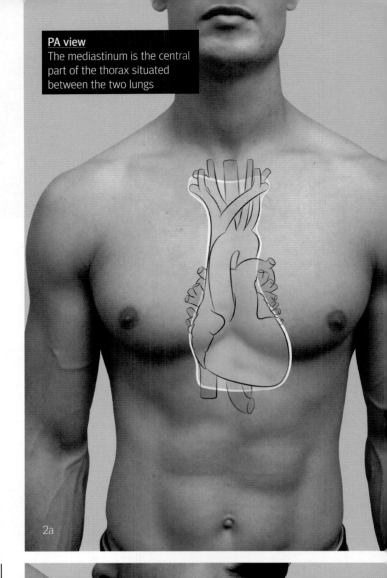

THE MEDIASTINUM

The word mediastinum is derived from the Latin words *medius* meaning "middle", and *stare* meaning "to stand". The anatomical mediastinum is a partition that "stands in the middle" of the thorax, and is bounded by the two pleural cavities medially, the sternum anteriorly, the spine posteriorly, the thoracic inlet superiorly, and the diaphragms inferiorly (Fig. 2a,b).

The mediastinal zone, as described in Chapter 5, is one of the largest zones and it overlaps the lung, pleural, and hilar zones.

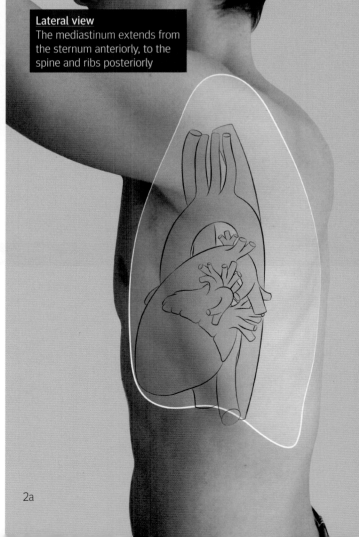

Figure 2. Surface anatomy localization of the mediastinum. a, frontal perspective, b, lateral perspective.

Classification of the Mediastinum

There are no concrete anatomical boundaries for the mediastinum and, therefore, several different descriptions of what constitutes the mediastinum are found in the medical literature and in clinical practice. This lack of a consistent classification of the mediastinum causes confusion regarding the description of the localization of mediastinal pathology. Localization varies depending on the classification used. For example, pathology described as originating in the middle mediastinum using one classification system, may be described as lying in the anterior or posterior, and NOT the middle mediastinum, according to another classification (Fig. 3).

? Anterior mediastinum
? Middle mediastinum
? Posterior mediastinum

Figure 3. Confusing classifications of the mediastinum. The round lesion can be localized to anterior, middle or posterior mediastinum depending on which classification is used. The various lines used in the classification systems are superimposed on this image.

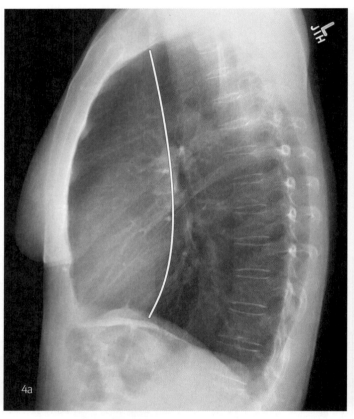
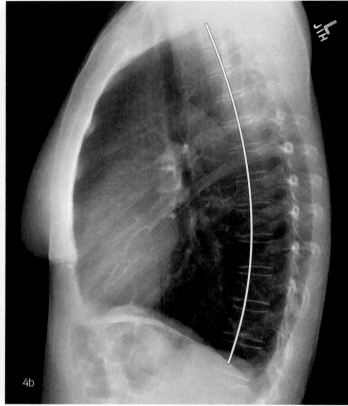

Felson classification

Benjamin Felson introduced a classification system that has broad acceptance in the radiology community (3). In this classification, the mediastinum is divided into anterior, middle and posterior compartments. This is convenient because the literature describes mediastinal pathology as existing in an anterior, middle or posterior location.

The lateral chest x-ray is the most useful tool when considering the anterior-posterior orientation within the thorax, and Felson uses the lateral projection as the basis for his classification. According to his classification, the mediastinum is divided conceptually, using two lines. One line extends along the anterior wall of the trachea, continuing down over the posterior aspect of the

Figure 4. Felson's classification of the mediastinum - PART I. Felson's classification of the mediastinum employs two lines to divide the mediastinum. These lateral chest x-rays illustrate the positioning of the lines according to Felson. a, line 1 runs along the posterior border of the trachea and the posterior border of the heart, b, line 2 runs parallel to the vertebral bodies one centimeter posterior to the anterior border of the vertebral bodies.

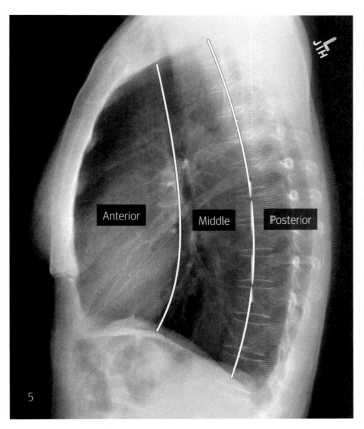

5

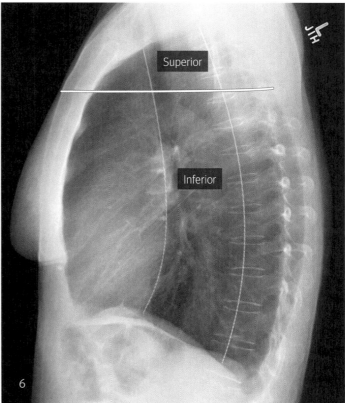

6

pericardium to the diaphragm (Fig. 4a). The second line connects points drawn one centimeter posterior to the anterior aspect of the thoracic vertebral bodies (Fig. 4b).

Structures anterior to the first line are within the anterior mediastinum, while those posterior to the second line lie within the posterior mediastinum. Structures between the two lines are within the middle mediastinum (Fig. 5).

This classification can be modified by adding a third line, which extends from the angle of Louis to the inferior end-plate of the fourth thoracic vertebrae (T4) (Fig. 6). This line further divides the mediastinum into superior and inferior compartments.

Figure 5. Felson's classification of the mediastinum - PART II. Felson's classification of the mediastinum employs two lines to divide the mediastinum into compartments. This lateral chest x-ray illustrates the use of the division lines according to Felson to divide the mediastinum into anterior, middle and posterior compartments.

Figure 6. Felson's classification of the mediastinum - PART III. Felson's classification can be modified by adding a third line to divide the mediastinum into superior and inferior compartments. A lateral chest x-ray is shown using the third line to make this division.

MEDIASTINUM Chapter 9 SECTION II

281

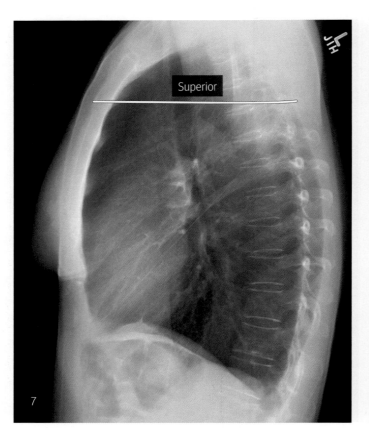

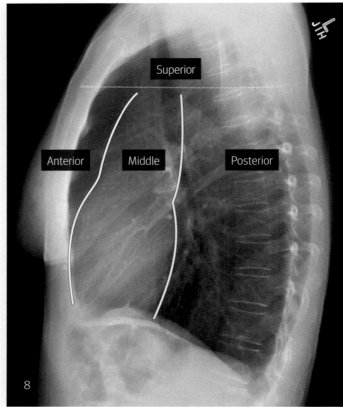

Classical anatomical classification

The classical anatomical classification divides the mediastinum into four compartments (Fig. 7) (4). The superior compartment lies above the line joining the angle of Louis to the inferior border of T4.

Below this line the mediastinum is further divided into the anterior, middle and posterior compartments (Fig. 8). The anterior compartment is anterior to the pericardium and posterior to the sternum. The posterior compartment is posterior to the pericardium. The middle compartment is between the anterior and posterior compartments.

Figure 7. Classical anatomical classification of the mediastinum - PART I. A line that extends from the angle of Louis to the inferior end plate of T4 divides the mediastinum into superior and inferior compartments.

Figure 8. Classical anatomical classification of the mediastinum - PART II. The lines of the classical classification system divide the mediastinum into anterior, middle and posterior compartments, as shown in this lateral chest x-ray.

Other Classifications
of the Mediastinum

Another useful classification that follows the great vessels in the thorax, divides the mediastinum into pre-vascular, vascular, and post-vascular compartments (Fig. 9)(5).

A more in-depth classification has been proposed by Heitzman, in which the mediastinum is divided into seven regions: the thoracic inlet, anterior mediastinal compartment, supra-aortic area, infra-aortic area supra-azygos area, infra-azygos area, and the hila (6).

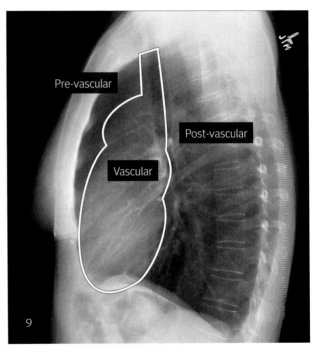

Figure 9. The vascular-based division. In some cases it may be useful to divide the mediastinum into pre-vascular, vascular, and post-vascular compartments as shown in this lateral chest x-ray.

AUTHOR RECOMMENDATION:
Use the Felson classification.

Felson's classification uses two lines to divide the mediastinum into anterior, middle and posterior compartments.
Line 1: anterior trachea and posterior pericardium.
Line 2: 1 cm posterior to anterior edge of vertebral column.

THE ANATOMICAL STRUCTURES
OF THE NORMAL MEDIASTINUM
ACCORDING TO FELSON'S CLASSIFICATION

ANTERIOR	MIDDLE
Thymus* Vessels: Internal mammillary Lymph nodes/lymphatics Nerves Fat	Esophagus Tracheobronchial tree (Ch. 7) Vessels: Aorta, SVC, IVC Lymph nodes/lymphatics Nerves: Phrenic Fat

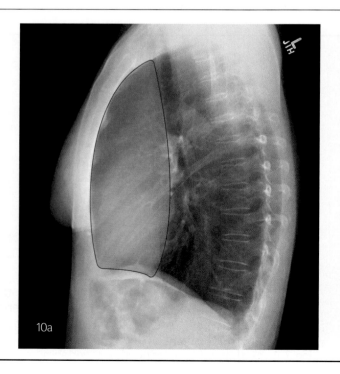

10a

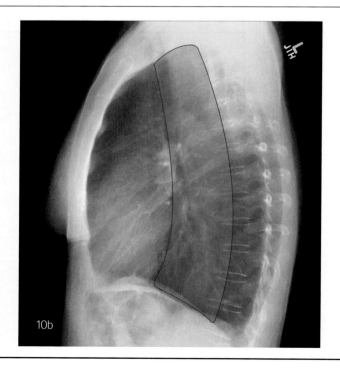

10b

POSTERIOR

Vessels: Azygos
Lymph nodes/lymphatics (thoracic duct)
Nerves: Sympathetic chain and intercostals
Fat

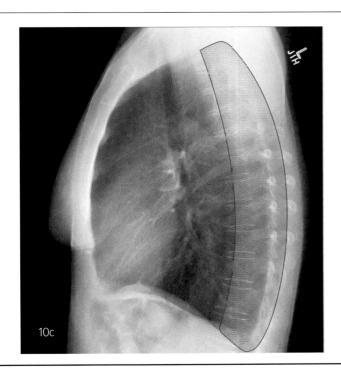

10c

Figure 10. The anatomical structures of the normal mediastinum according to Felson's Classification. Lateral chest x-ray with the three Felson classification compartments highlighted: a, the anterior mediastinum, b, the middle mediastinum, c, the posterior mediastinum. *not usually seen in adults unless abnormal, IVC, inferior vena cava, SVC, superior vena cava.

MEDIASTINUM **Chapter 9** SECTION II

The Aorta

The word aorta is new Latin, from the Greek word *aorte*, from *aeirein* meaning "to lift". As the main artery leading from the heart, the aorta provides oxygenated blood to the circulatory system.

The aorta originates from the right superior aspect of the heart (7,8,9). The aorta extends superiorly, posteriorly and to the left, arches 180 degrees, and then extends inferiorly to the diaphragmatic hiatus and into the abdominal cavity. The thoracic aorta has four components: the aortic root, the ascending aorta, the transverse aorta (the aortic arch), and the descending aorta (Fig. 11a,b).

1. Aortic Root – This segment is composed of the aortic annulus, the ventriculo-aortic junction and the sinotubular junction.

2. Ascending Aorta – This section extends from the root to the level of the origin of the brachiocephalic artery.

3. Aortic Arch – The superior edge of the aortic arch lies at the level of the fourth or fifth thoracic vertebra (T4-T5). The arch gives rise to the brachiocephalic artery (from which the right subclavian artery and the right common carotid artery originate), the left common carotid and the left subclavian arteries.

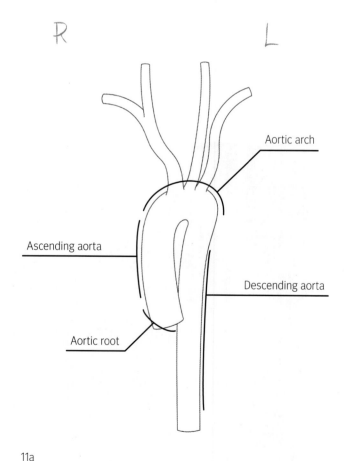

R   L

Aortic arch

Ascending aorta

Descending aorta

Aortic root

11a

286

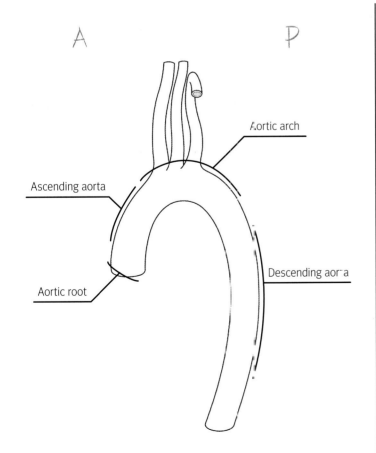

A   P

Aortic arch

Ascending aorta

Aortic root

Descending aorta

11b

4. Descending Aorta – This portion extends into the abdomen through the aortic hiatus within the diaphragm.

The normal diameter of the thoracic aorta is less than or equal to 3 cm. A dimension between 3 and 4 cm is known as ectasia, and greater than 4 cm is an aneurysm.

NORMAL VARIANTS

Some normal variants in the development of the aorta are:
- Left-sided arch with an aberrant right subclavian artery.
- Right-sided arch.
- Cervical arch.
- Common trunk for brachiocephalic artery and the left common carotid.
- Direct origin of the left vertebral artery from the aortic arch.

Figure 11. Anatomy of the aorta.
Illustrations of the aorta, a, frontal perspective, b, lateral perspective.

Radiological Shape and Grayscale of the Aorta

On the PA x-ray, the aortic root is part of the cardiac density superiorly on the right (Fig. 12a,b,c). The aortic root lies posterior and to the left of the superior vena cava (SVC). The ascending aorta is usually not seen directly because its right lateral edge lies, like the aortic root, medial to the right lateral edge of the SVC and is, therefore, hidden within the mediastinum. The aortic arch forms part of the mediastinal contour on the left, above the left pulmonary artery (LPA) (Fig. 12d). This part of the mediastinal contour is sometimes referred to as the aortic knob, and represents the transition from the aortic arch to the descending aorta. The descending aorta appears as the inferior continuation of the arch. It courses inferiorly and medially on PA x-rays. The lateral left border of the descending aorta forms an interface with the lung and is visible as the left paraaortic stripe.

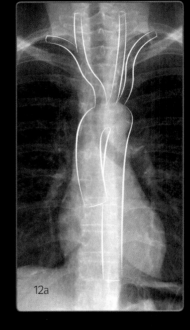

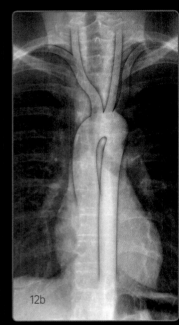

Figure 12. Radiological anatomy of the aorta from the frontal perspective. a, PA chest x-ray with the aorta outlined, b, PA chest x-ray with grayscale illustration of the aorta overlay, c, PA chest x-ray cropped to highlight the aorta, d, magnification of the PA chest x-ray to highlight the BIG ARCH (the aorta) and the LITTLE ARCH (the left pulmonary artery).

12a

12b

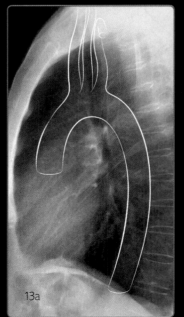

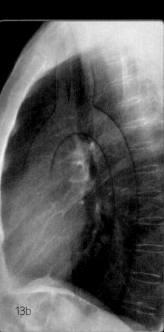

Figure 13. Radiological anatomy of the aorta from the lateral perspective. a, lateral chest x-ray with the aorta outlined, b, lateral chest x-ray with grayscale illustration of the aorta overlay, c, lateral chest x-ray cropped to highlight the aorta with the aortic arch highlighted.

13a

13b

When viewed on a lateral x-ray (Fig. 13a,b,c), the aorta lies in the upper half of the thorax and courses from anterior to posterior in the shape of an arch (the big arch), above the superior edge of the LPA (the little arch). On the lateral x-ray, the most easily identified part of the aorta is the aortic arch; its top is usually found at the level of the fourth or fifth thoracic vertebra (T4-T5). From the posterior portion of the arch, the descending aorta continues inferiorly, following the contour of the spine. At the level of the diaphragm, the aorta lies posterior to the heart and inferior to the vena cava.

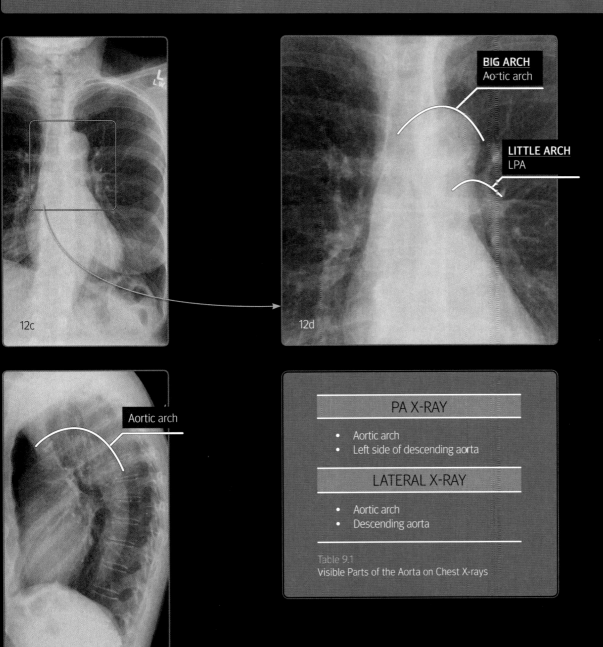

12c

12d

BIG ARCH
Aortic arch

LITTLE ARCH
LPA

Aortic arch

13c

PA X-RAY
• Aortic arch • Left side of descending aorta

LATERAL X-RAY
• Aortic arch • Descending aorta

Table 9.1
Visible Parts of the Aorta on Chest X-rays

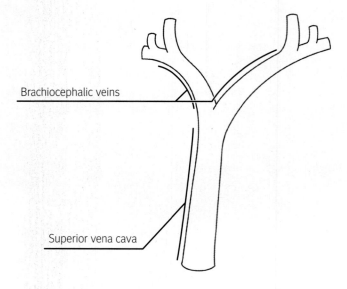

Brachiocephalic veins

Superior vena cava

14a

The Superior Vena Cava

The *venae cavae* are the two largest veins of the body; their name derived from the words *vena* meaning "vein", and *cava*, derived from the Latin word *cavus* meaning "hollow". The superior vena cava (SVC), as its name suggests, is the more superior of the two major veins, lying in the upper thorax. The SVC drains the blood from the head and the upper extremities.

The SVC forms at the point where the two brachiocephalic veins join, at approximately the level of the sternal angle (the second costal cartilage on the right) (Fig. 14a,b). The SVC descends inferiorly on the right side of the aorta. It receives the azygos vein at the level of the superior border of the right main stem bronchus. The SVC drains into the right atrium, just below the level of the carina.

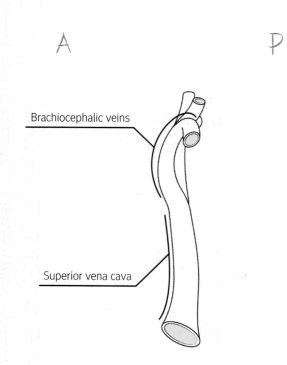

A   P

Brachiocephalic veins

Superior vena cava

Figure 14. Anatomy of the superior vena cava (SVC). Illustrations of the SVC, a, frontal perspective, b, lateral perspective.

14b

Radiological Shape and Grayscale of the SVC

On the PA x-ray (Fig. 15a,b,c), the SVC (together with the right brachiocephalic vein) forms the right superior edge of the mediastinum (10,11,12). This edge extends vertically from the right heart border superiorly, into the thoracic inlet.

From the lateral perspective, the SVC descends from the thoracic outlet superiorly, lying anterior to the trachea and the RPA, and eventually drains into the right atrium. Because of this positioning, the SVC is not seen as a distinct structure on the lateral x-ray.

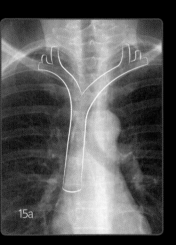
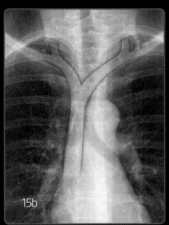
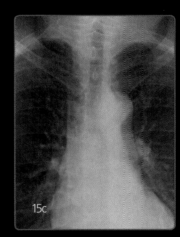

Figure 15. Radiological anatomy of the superior vena cava (SVC) from the frontal perspective. a, PA chest x-ray with the SVC outlined, b, PA chest x-ray with grayscale illustration of the SVC overlay, c, PA chest x-ray cropped to highlight the SVC.

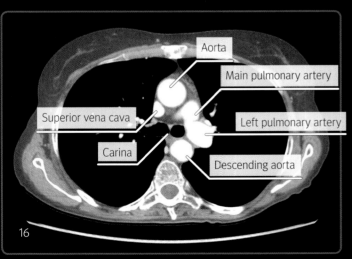

Figure 16. Superior vena cava (SVC) cross-sectional relationships. A chest CT scan depicting the relationship of the SVC with other thoracic structures.

The Inferior Vena Cava

The inferior vena cava (IVC) is the second of the two major veins. As the more inferior of the two, it is located medially in the lower thorax travelling along the spine. The IVC drains the venous blood from the abdomen and lower extremities.

The IVC begins in the abdomen at the level of the fifth lumbar vertebra (L5), with the junction of the two common iliac veins (Fig. 17a,b). The IVC enters the thorax through the hiatus in the center tendon of the diaphragm. Within the thorax, the IVC enters the right atrium, inferiorly.

R   L

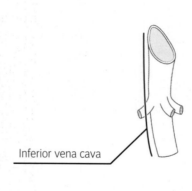

Inferior vena cava

17a

A   P

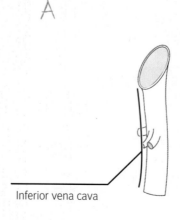

Inferior vena cava

17b

Figure 17. Anatomy of the inferior vena cava (IVC). Illustrations of the IVC, a, frontal perspective, b, lateral perspective.

Radiological Shape and Grayscale of the IVC

The IVC is only rarely seen on the PA chest x-ray – when it is seen, t is usually in patients with hyperinflated lungs (Fig. 18a,b,c).

On the lateral chest x-ray, the posterior edge of the IVC can frequently be seen as a vertical edge extending inferiorly from the posterior inferior aspect of the heart border (Fig. 19).

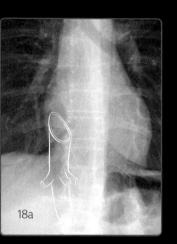
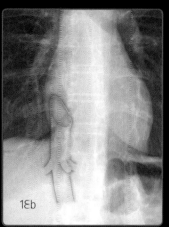
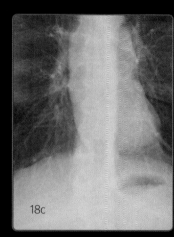

18a

18b

18c

Figure 18. Radiological anatomy of the inferior vena cava (IVC) from the frontal perspective. a, PA chest x-ray with the IVC outlined, b, PA chest x-ray with grayscale illustration of the IVC overlay, c, PA chest x-ray cropped to highlight the IVC.

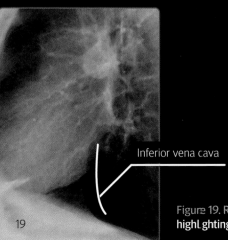

Inferior vena cava

19

Figure 19. Radiological anatomy of the inferior vena cava (VC) from the lateral perspective. A lateral chest x-ray highLghting the IVC.

The Vascular Pedicle

The superior mediastinum can be thought of as a vascular pedicle, with a vein (the SVC) on the right side and the left subclavian artery on the left (12,13).

When a patient changes from an erect to a supine position, there is an increase in the central venous pressure, with an enlargement of the SVC. The distance between the edge of the SVC and the spinous processes increases; whereas, the distance between the spinous processes and subclavian artery edge remains unchanged. The measurement of this ratio can be useful in evaluating central venous pressure and fluid status (particularly in comparison with previous x-rays) in patients with chronic obstructive airways disease, where parenchymal vascular changes such as upper lobe vascular redistribution (pulmonary venous hypertension) may not be evident (Fig. 20).

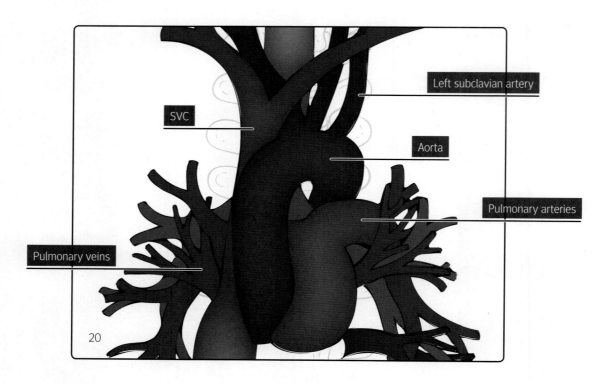

Figure 20. Vascular pedicle. An illustration of the vascular pedicle. The superior mediastinum can be thought of as a vascular pedicle with the superior vena cava on the right and the left subclavian artery on the left.

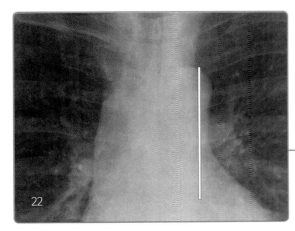

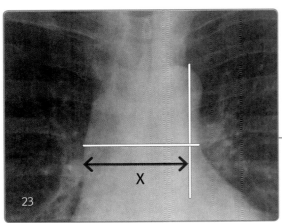

How to measure the width of the vascular pedicle

The measurement of the vascular pedicle can be useful in evaluating central venous pressure and fluid status.

STEP 1
Confirm that the patient is midline and is not rotated (Ch. 1, Pg. 32).

STEP 2
Focus your vision on the superior part of the mediastinum at the level of the aortic arch (Fig. 21).

STEP 3
Draw a first line extending inferiorly from the point that the left subclavian artery exits the aortic arch (Fig. 22).

STEP 4

Draw a horizontal line from the point where the SVC crosses the right main stem bronchus to intersect with the first line (Fig. 23).

The width of the vascular pedicle is the length of the second line to the point of intersection (X).

The normal vascular pedicle measures 48 +/- 5 mm on the upright PA x-ray, and increases to 58 to 64 mm on the supine AP x-ray (12,13).

R   L

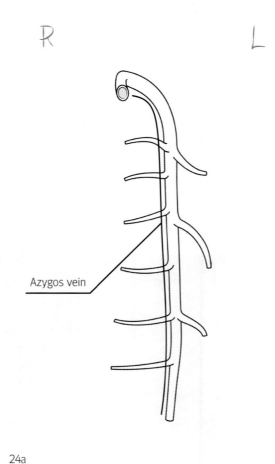

Azygos vein

24a

The Azygos Vein

Normally lying just to the right of the spine, the azygos vein drains the deoxygenated blood from the walls of the thorax and abdomen into the SVC.

The word azygos is derived from the Greek words *a* and *zygon* (a-zygon), meaning "not a pair". The azygos vein is so named because it has no true symmetrical equivalent on the left side of the body (the hemiazygos and its accessory on the left side are considered tributaries rather than the left counterpart of a pair).

The azygos vein starts in the abdomen at the level of the first or second lumbar vertebra (L1-L2), as the continuation of the ascending lumbar vein (Fig. 24a,b). It enters into the thorax through the aortic hiatus in the diaphragm, and courses vertically along the anterior lateral right side of the vertebral column. At the level of the fourth thoracic vertebra (T4), the azygos vein courses anteriorly, arching over the hilar structures to empty into the SVC.

A   P

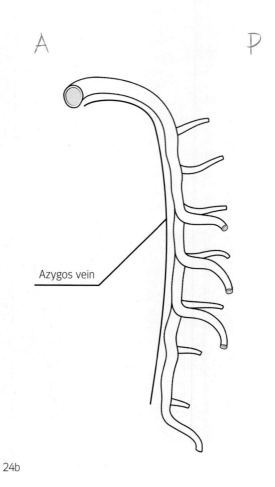

Azygos vein

Figure 24. Anatomy of the azygos vein.
Illustrations of the azygos vein, a, frontal perspective, b, lateral perspective.

24b

Radiological Shape and Grayscale of the Azygos Vein

The only portion of the azygos vein that is seen directly, and consistently, on the PA chest x-ray is the azygos arch as it approaches the SVC (14,15) (Fig. 25a,b,c). Because the azygos vein courses anteriorly to enter into the SVC, it will be seen end-on on the PA x-ray: the azygos vein can be identified as a white oval sitting on the right main stem bronchus. Superior to this oval, and continuous with the oval, is the right paratracheal stripe (Ch. 7, Pg. 186).

Together with the esophagus the azygos vein contributes to the white edge of the azygoesophageal recess (Ch. 9, Pgs. 299, 306; Ch. 11 Pg. 394).

The size of the azygos vein varies and will depend on the position of the patient during the examination. The vein will be larger on supine examinations.

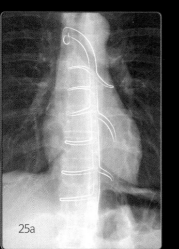
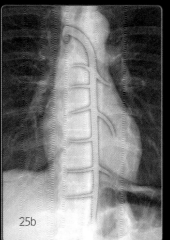
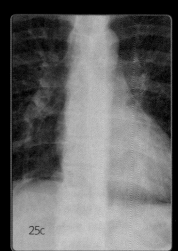

25a

25b

25c

Figure 25. Radiological anatomy of the azygos vein from the frontal perspective. a, PA chest x-ray with the azygos vein outlined, b, PA chest x-ray with grayscale illustration of the azygos vein overlay, c, PA chest x-ray cropped to highlight the azygos vein.

R   L

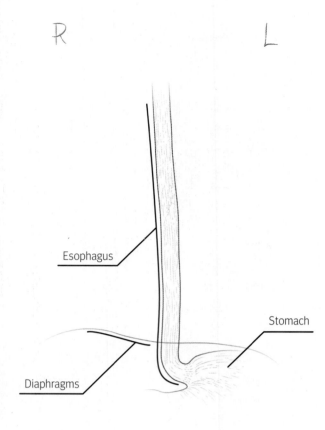

Esophagus

Stomach

Diaphragms

26a

> **!** The normal esophagus is not visible on the lateral x-ray.

The Esophagus

The word esophagus is derived from the Greek words *oise*, the future imperative of *pherein* meaning "to bear or carry", and *phagein* meaning "to eat or devour" (16).

The esophagus extends from the lower part of the pharynx to the stomach (Fig. 26a,b). The esophagus is approximately 25 to 30 cm long (about the length of your forearm). Within the thorax, the esophagus lies first behind the trachea and then behind the heart. Superiorly, the esophagus lies in the midline, but below the main stem bronchi, it starts to deviate to the left. It extends through the diaphragm at the level of the eleventh or twelfth thoracic vertebra (T11-T12).

A   P

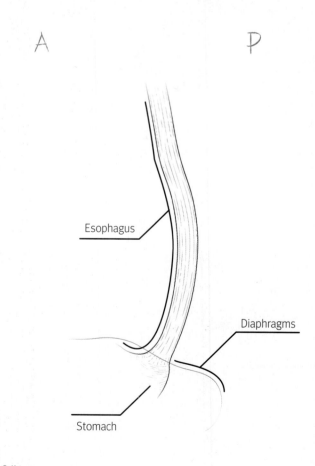

Esophagus

Diaphragms

Stomach

26b

Figure 26. Anatomy of the esophagus. Illustrations of the esophagus, a, frontal perspective, b, lateral perspective.

Radiological Shape and Grayscale of the Esophagus

The outline of the esophagus is difficult to establish on standard x-rays, especially superiorly. Under normal circumstances, the lumen is empty. If, however, there is air in the esophagus at the time of the x-ray examination, this air will mark the position of the lumen of the esophagus (17). Within the mediastinum inferiorly, posteriorly and just to the left of the midline, the esophagus and azygos vein together form an interface with the right lung called the azygoesophageal recess (14) (Fig. 27a,b,c,d).

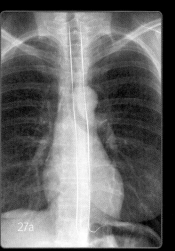

27a

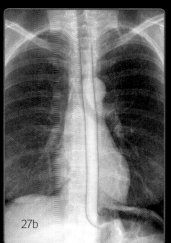

27b

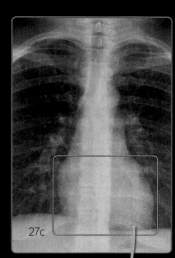

27c

Figure 27. Radiological anatomy of the esophagus from the frontal perspective. a, PA chest x-ray with the esophagus outlined, b, PA chest x-ray with grayscale illustration of the esophagus overlay, c, PA chest x-ray cropped to highlight the esophagus, d, magnification of the PA chest x-ray to highlight the azygoesophageal recess.

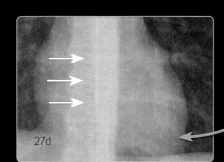

27d

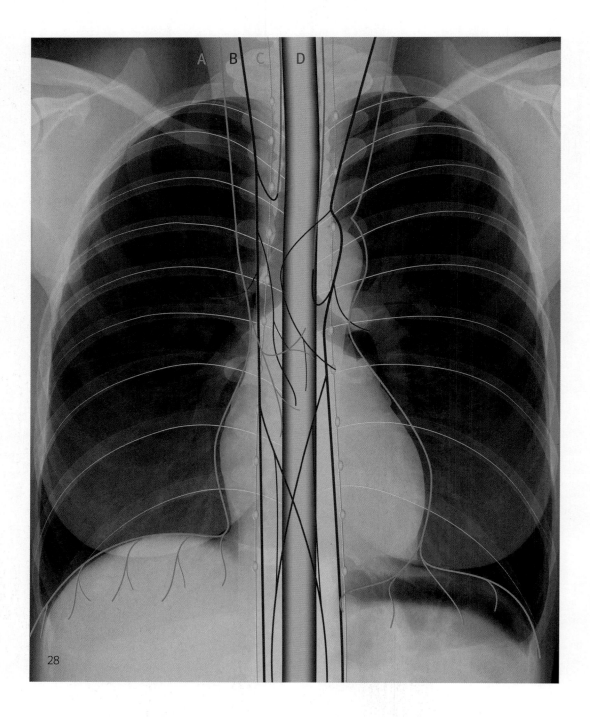

A B C D

28

The Nerves

The nerves within the thorax are not visible on the PA or lateral x-rays because of their size and position deep within the mediastinum (Fig. 28) (18). However, knowledge of the anatomical course of the nerves is important because tumors involving the nerves should be considered in the differential diagnosis of mediastinal tumors.

Figure 28. Mediastinal nerves. Illustration of the mediastinal nerves superimposed on a PA chest x-ray. A, phrenic nerve, B, vagus nerve, C, sympathetic chain, D, spinal cord.

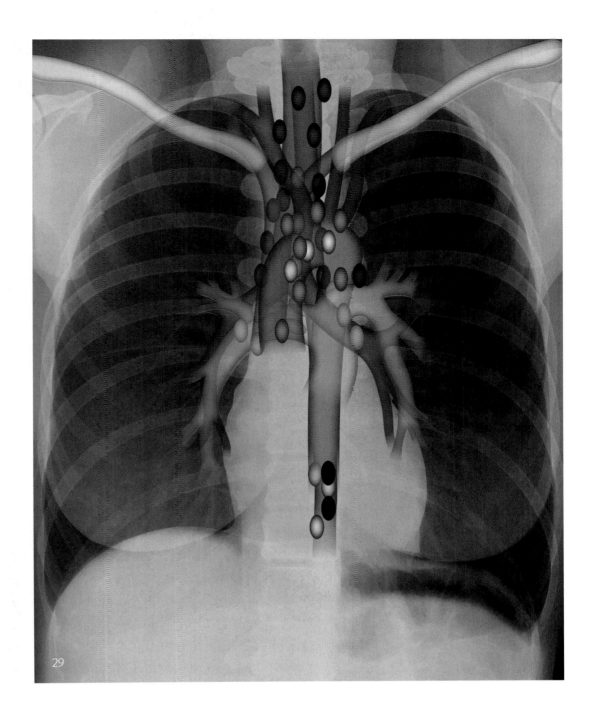

29

The Lymph Nodes

Lymph nodes are found throughout the mediastinum within all of the compartments. General awareness of the presence of these nodes is important because abnormal mediastinal lymph nodes on an x-ray may be the first evidence of cancer, infection or sarcoidosis (Fig. 29).

Figure 29. Classification of mediastinal lymph nodes. Illustration of all of the mediastinal lymph nodes superimposed on a PA chest x-ray.

Classification of Mediastinal Lymph Nodes

A classification of the mediastinal lymph nodes has been accepted, and describes fourteen nodal stations within the mediastinum (19).

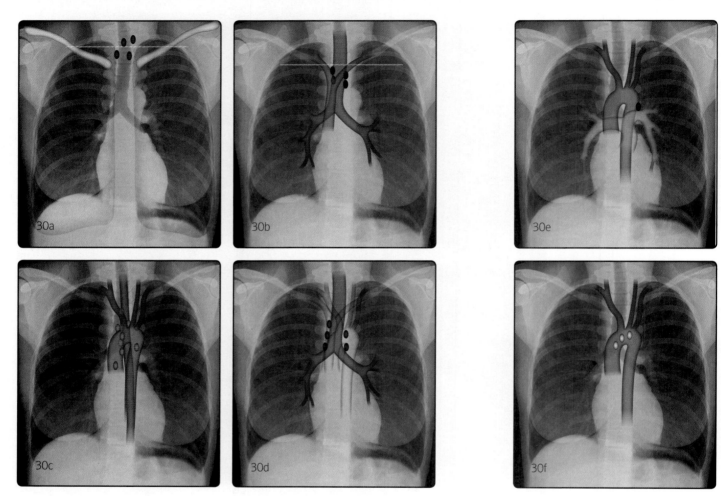

Superior mediastinal nodes

1. Highest mediastinal nodes: the nodes lying above a horizontal line at the upper rim of the brachiocephalic (left innominate) vein, where it ascends to the left, crossing in front of the trachea at its midline (Fig. 30a).
2. Upper paratracheal nodes: the nodes lying above a horizontal line drawn tangential to the upper margin of the aortic arch, and below the inferior boundary of the highest mediastinal nodes (Fig. 30b).
3. Prevascular and retrotracheal nodes (Fig. 30c).
4. Lower paratracheal nodes: the lower paratracheal nodes on the right lie to the right of the midline of the trachea, between a horizontal line drawn tangential to the upper margin of the aortic arch and a line extending across the right main stem bronchus at the upper margin of the (right upper lobe) RUL bronchus, and are contained within the mediastinal pleural envelope; the lower paratracheal nodes on the left lie to the left of the midline of the trachea, between a horizontal line drawn tangential to the upper margin of the aortic arch and a line extending across the left main stem bronchus at the level of the upper margin of the LUL bronchus, medial to the ligamentum arteriosum, and are contained within the mediastinal pleural envelope (Fig. 30d).

Aortic nodes

5. Subaortic (aorto-pulmonary window): the subaortic nodes are lateral to the ligamentum arteriosum (or the aorta, or the LPA), and proximal to the first branch of the LPA, and lie within the mediastinal pleural envelope (Fig. 30e).

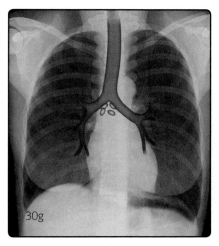

30g

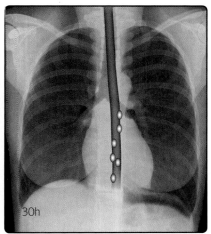

30h

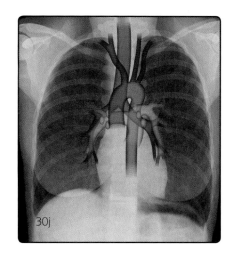

30j

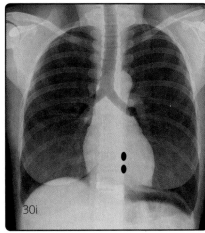

30i

6. Para-aortic nodes (ascending aorta or phrenic): the nodes lying anterior, and lateral, to the ascending aorta and the aortic arch (or the innominate artery), beneath a line tangential to the upper margin of the aortic arch (Fig. 30f).

Inferior mediastinal nodes

7. Subcarinal nodes: the nodes lying caudal to the carina of the trachea, but not associated with the lower lobe bronchi or arteries within the lung (Fig. 30g).
8. Paraesophageal nodes (below carina): the nodes lying adjacent to the wall of the esophagus, and to the right or left of the midline, excluding the subcarinal nodes (Fig. 30h).
9. Pulmonary ligament nodes: the nodes lying within the pulmonary ligament, including those in the posterior wall and lower part of the inferior pulmonary vein (Fig. 30i).

Intra-pulmonary nodes

10. Hilar (Fig. 30j).
11. Interlobar.
12. Lobar.
13. Segmental.
14. Subsegmental.

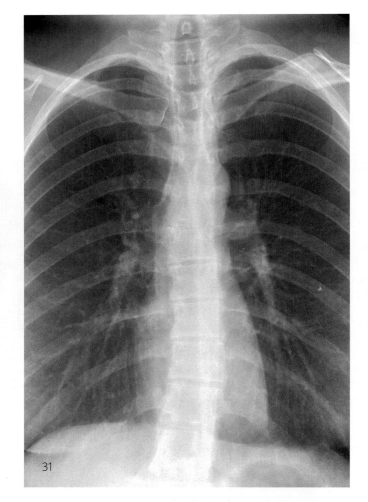

31

MEDIASTINAL INTERFACES

The general concept of radiological interfaces is presented in detail in **Chapter** 2.

Briefly, an x-ray interface requires two significantly different radiological densities to be touching. The mediastinal anatomical structures lie between the two lungs and create various different interfaces – the lung-mediastinal interfaces (Fig. 31). Furthermore, the air within the trachea allows for additional – tracheal-mediastinal interfaces. Interfaces can also form between the two lungs and the adjacent pleura.

In discussion of the mediastinum and these interfaces, terms such as "line", "stripe" and "edge" are frequently used, and these terms need further clarification (20).

The term line refers to an extended longitudinal shadow in the lung or mediastinum, no greater than 2 mm in width (Fig. 32a).

A stripe is a line that measures 2 to 5 mm in width (Fig. 32b).

An edge is formed when a structure interfaces with the lung to create a border that does not qualify as a line or stripe.

The lung-mediastinal interfaces can be further subdivided into peripheral and central.

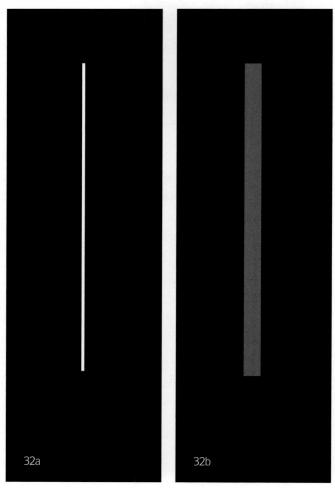

32a   32b

304

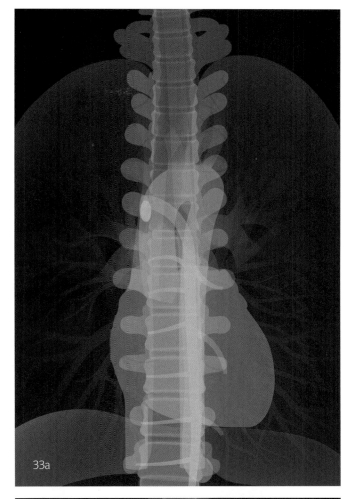

33a

Central Mediastinal Interfaces

If one could somehow remove the heart from the chest x-ray image, leaving everything else intact, the chest x-ray would clearly show the relationship between the lungs and the remaining mediastinal structures that form the central lung-mediastinum interfaces (Fig. 33a,b).

Figure 31. Mediastinal interfaces on the PA chest x-ray. The mediastinal structures lie between the two lungs, and therefore they create various interfaces, as shown in this PA chest x-ray.

Figure 32. Mediastinal interfaces creating lines and stripes. Illustation of, a, line, b, stripe.

Figure 33. Central mediastinal interfaces. Grayscale illustration of the mediastinal structures. a, with the heart, b, without the heart. When the heart is removed the relationship between the lungs and the remaining mediastinal structures is clear.

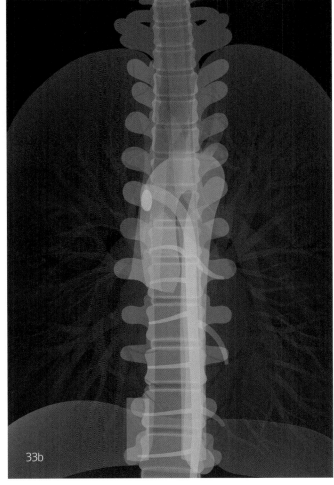

33b

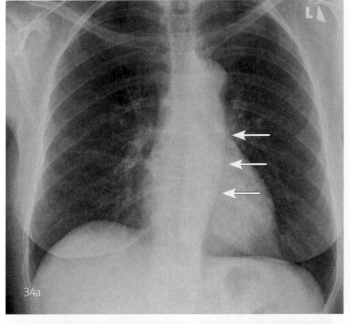

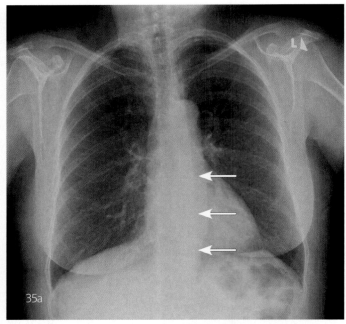

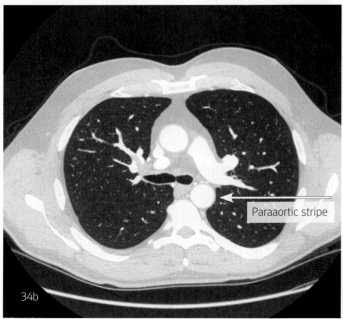

Paraaortic stripe

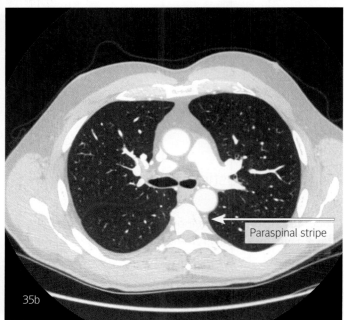

Paraspinal stripe

There are four important central lung-mediastinum interfaces that you should be able to identify confidently.

1. Lung-mediastinum interface related to the aorta – the paraaortic stripe (**Ch.11, Pg.394**) (Fig. 34a,b).

2. Lung-mediastinum interface related to the paraspinal soft tissues – the left paraspinal stripe (**Ch.11, Pg.394**) (Fig. 35a,b).

AMSER 3. Lung-mediastinum interface related to the esophagus and the azygos vein – the azygoesophageal recess (**Ch.9, Pgs.297, 299; Ch11, Pg. 394**) (Fig. 36a,b).

AMSER 4. Lung-mediastinum interface related to the aorta and the LPA – the aorto-pulmonary (AP) window (**Ch.8, Pg.243**) (Fig. 37a,b) (21).

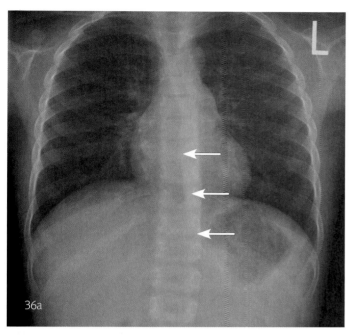

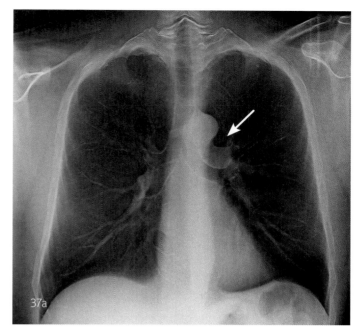

36a

37a

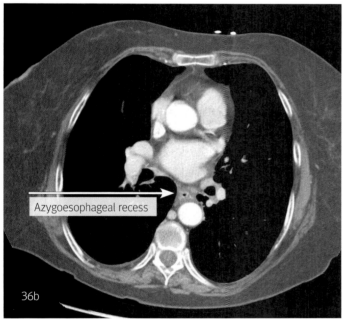

Azygoesophageal recess

36b

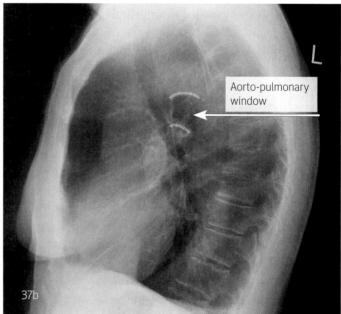

Aorto-pulmonary window

37b

Figure 34. The paraaortic stripe. The location of the paraaortic stripe on, a, a PA chest x-ray, b, a chest CT scan.

Figure 35. The left paraspinal stripe. The location of the paraspinal stripe on, a, a PA chest x-ray, b, a chest CT scan.

Figure 36. The azygoesophageal recess. The location of the azygoesophageal recess on, a, a PA chest x-ray, b, a chest CT scan.

Figure 37. The aorto-pulmonary (AP) window. The location of the AP window on, a, PA chest tomogram, b, lateral chest x-ray.

Additional lung-mediastinal interfaces include (22):

Right paraaortic stripe
Right paraspinal stripe
Right paraesophageal stripe
Left paraesophageal stripe
Preaortic recess
Supraaortic recess
Supraazygos recess
Aortic nipple

Peripheral Lung-Mediastinal Interfaces – The Lateral Edges of the Mediastinum

The peripheral lung-mediastinal interfaces form the radiological borders, or edges, of the mediastinum. These are the most lateral aspects of the mediastinum.

On the PA chest x-ray, when looking at the central portion of the chest, you can easily identify the cardiac shadow, as well as a soft tissue density extending from the heart in a superior direction. On the right side, in the superior thorax, the mediastinal edge is formed by the SVC (Fig. 38a). More inferiorly, the right atrium interfaces with the lung.

The most superior part of the left mediastinal border (Fig. 38b), is formed by an arterial structure – the left subclavian artery (as opposed to a venous structure, as on the right). Below the subclavian artery lies the aortic arch, from which the left subclavian artery originates. Below the aortic arch are the pulmonary outflow tract/ main pulmonary artery (MPA) and the auricle of the left atrium. The auricle of the left atrium usually forms a straight, rather than convex, margin. Below the auricle, the mediastinal edge is formed by the left ventricle.

The right ventricle does not contribute to the mediastinal contours on the PA x-ray, as it lies anteriorly, and is not a border-forming structure.

NORMAL VARIANTS
Common normal variations in the mediastinal edges include (23,24,25) the following.
- Dextrocardia – the heart shadow is reversed (Fig. 39a).
- Situs inversus – all of the thoracic structures are reversed (Fig. 39b).
- Right-sided aortic arch (Fig. 39c).
- Cervical aortic arch.
- Double aortic arch (Fig. 39d).
- Aberrant (anomalous) right subclavian artery (Fig. 39e).
- Left superior vena cava.

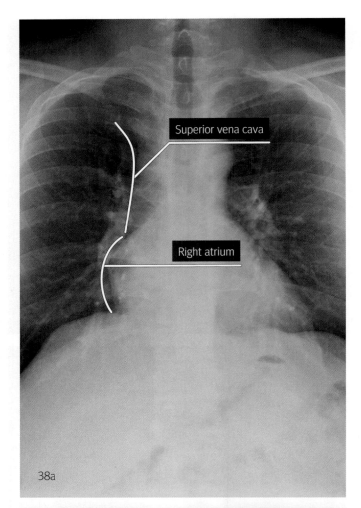

Superior vena cava

Right atrium

38a

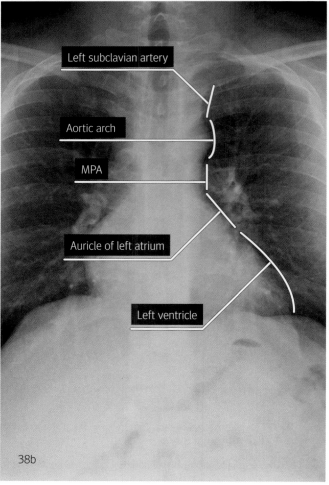

Left subclavian artery

Aortic arch

MPA

Auricle of left atrium

Left ventricle

38b

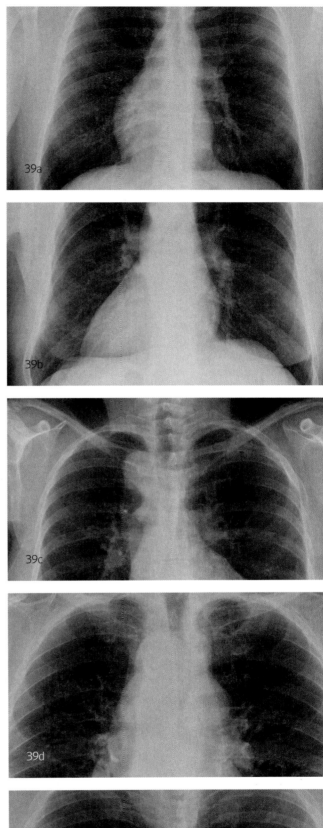

Figure 38. Mediastinal borders. Because of the interfaces created by the relationship of the mediastinal structures to the lungs, the lateral edges, or borders of the mediastinum, are visible. a, PA chest x-ray with the right mediastinal borders highlighted, b, PA chest x-ray with the left mediastinal borders highlighted.

Figure 39. Variations of the supporting mediastinal edges. In the normal population variations to the mediastinal edges can be seen on x-rays, and are not considered pathological. Series of PA chest x-rays with examples of the following normal variants: a, dextrocardia, b, situs inversus c, right aortic arch, d, double aortic arch, e, aberrant right subclavian artery.

The Lung-Lung Interfaces

The lung-lung interfaces are created when one lung and adjacent pleura touches the contralateral lung and adjacent pleura.

The anterior junction line (Figs. 40a,b,c,d and 41a,b) is produced by four layers of pleura – the visceral and parietal pleural layers on both the right and left – coming together between the aerated lungs, anterior to the great vessels. Where the four layers of pleura come together, a line is formed, which is almost vertical in orientation and measures approximately 1 mm in width. Because of the position of the lungs in the anterior part of the chest, this line can never extend higher than the suprasternal notch (26).

Similarly, the posterior junction line forms where the same four pleural layers touch each other posteriorly, between the aerated lungs (Figs. 41a,b and 42a,b,c,d). This usually occurs between the esophagus and the spinal column. Unlike the anterior junction line, this line does extend above the level of the suprasternal notch on the PA x-ray, and can be up to 2 mm wide. It ends inferiorly at the superior margin of the aortic arch, where the right and left pleural layers split to accommodate the aorta. As there is no density interface with the lungs below this point, the pleural edges are silhouetted by the aorta and, therefore, are not visible (27).

Figure 40. The anterior junction line. The position of the anterior junction line on, a, PA chest x-ray, b, coronal chest CT scan, c, horizontal chest CT scan (mediastinal algorithm), d, horizontal chest CT scan.

Figure 41. The anterior and posterior junction lines. 3D reconstruction of the pleura showing the anterior and posterior junction lines from, a, the frontal perspective, b, the horizontal perspective.

Figure 42. The posterior junction line. The position of the posterior junction line on, a, PA chest x-ray, b, coronal chest CT scan, c, horizontal chest CT scan (mediastinal algorithm), d, horizontal chest CT scan.

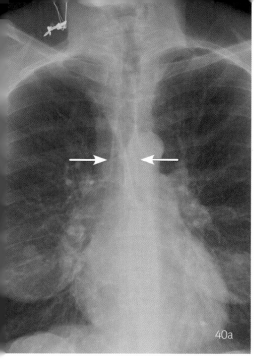

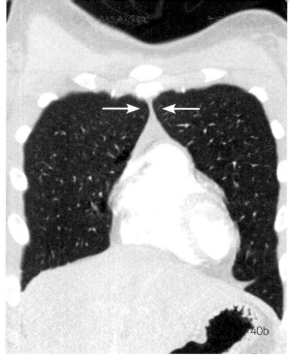

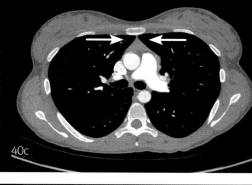

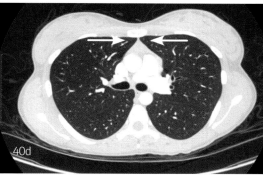

40a

40b

40c

40d

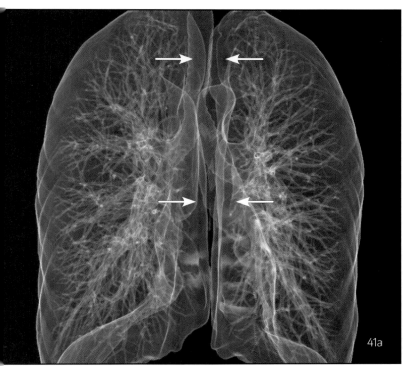

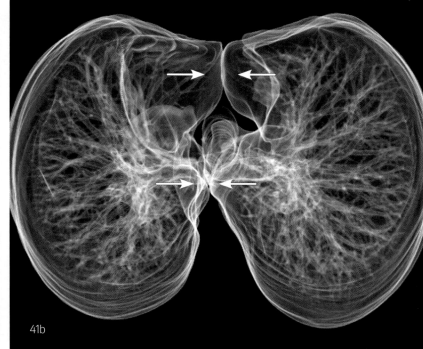

41a

41b

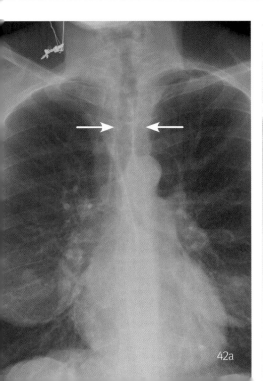

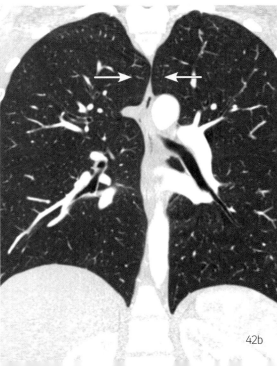

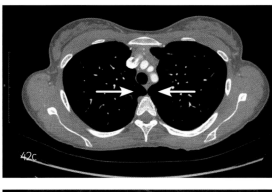

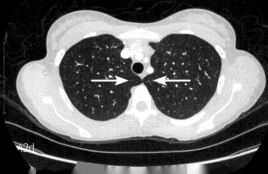

42a

42b

42c

42d

Trachea - Mediastinal Interfaces

The right paratracheal stripe is a vertically-oriented density measuring approximately 1 to 3 mm in width, that extends from the thoracic inlet to the right tracheobronchial angle, as seen on the PA chest x-ray (Fig. 43a). The right tracheobronchial angle is created where the right edge of the trachea intersects the medial superior edge of the right main stem bronchus.

The right paratracheal stripe is formed by the right tracheal wall, the contiguous mediastinal interstitial tissues, and the adjacent pleura (Fig. 43a,b). The azygos vein lies at the inferior extent of the paratracheal stripe, nestled in the tracheobronchial angle, but is distinct from the stripe.

Mediastinal Interfaces on the Lateral X-ray

On the lateral x-ray, the mediastinum extends posteriorly from the front of the chest to the spine and posterior ribs (Fig. 44). As such, there are no distinct edges to the mediastinum on the lateral x-ray.

What can be seen, however, are

- Borders of the heart.
- Border of the IVC.
- Border of the aorta.

Figure 43. The paratracheal stripe. The position of the paratracheal stripe on, a, PA chest x-ray, b, chest CT scan.

Figure 44. Mediastinal interfaces on the lateral chest x-ray. Given that the mediastinum extends from the front of the chest to the spine, there are no distinct edges to the mediastinum on the lateral chest x-ray. A few borders that can be seen are identified on this lateral x-ray (the borders of the heart, inferior vena cava (IVC) and aorta).

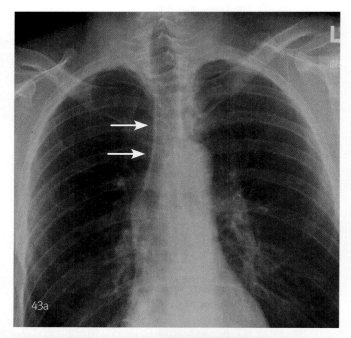

43a

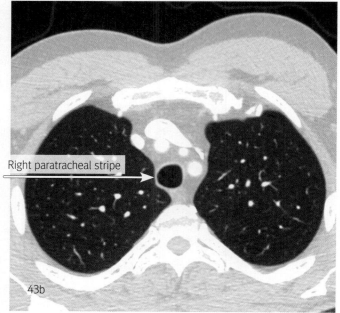

Right paratracheal stripe

43b

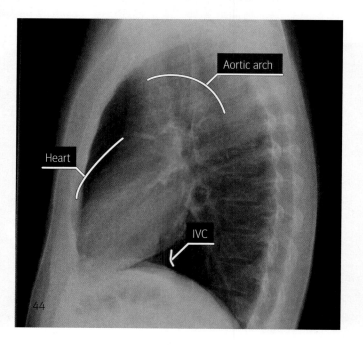

Aortic arch

Heart

IVC

44

Frequency of Visualization of Mediastinal Interfaces on the PA X-ray (28,29,30)

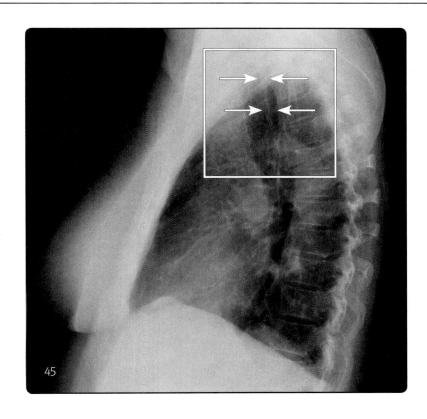

45

Additional trachea-mediastinal interfaces

The posterior paratracheal stripe is seen on the lateral x-ray (Fig. 45), and ranges in width from 2 to 5 mm. It extends from the thoracic inlet to the tracheal bifurcation, and is formed by the posterior wall of the trachea and the contiguous mediastinal interstitial tissues.

Figure 45. The posterior paratracheal stripe. The location of the posterior paratracheal stripe on the lateral chest x-ray (arrows).

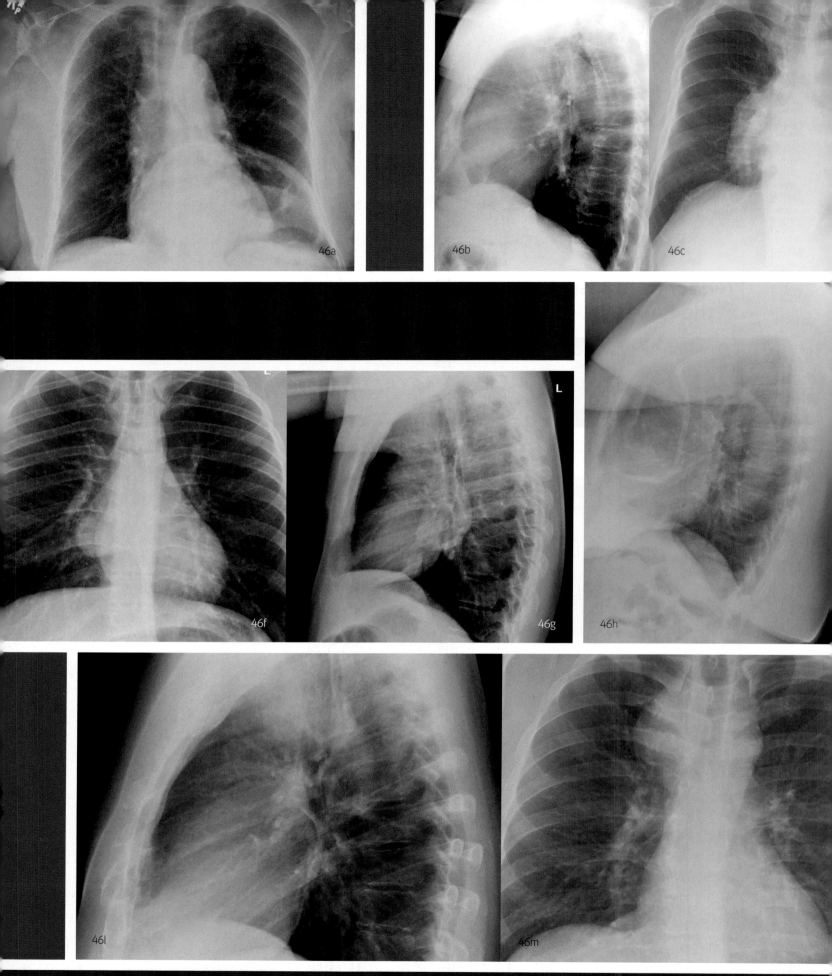

46a

46b

46c

46f

46g

46h

46l

46m

PATHOLOGY OF THE MEDIASTINUM

Examples images of diseases and conditions that affect the mediastinum.

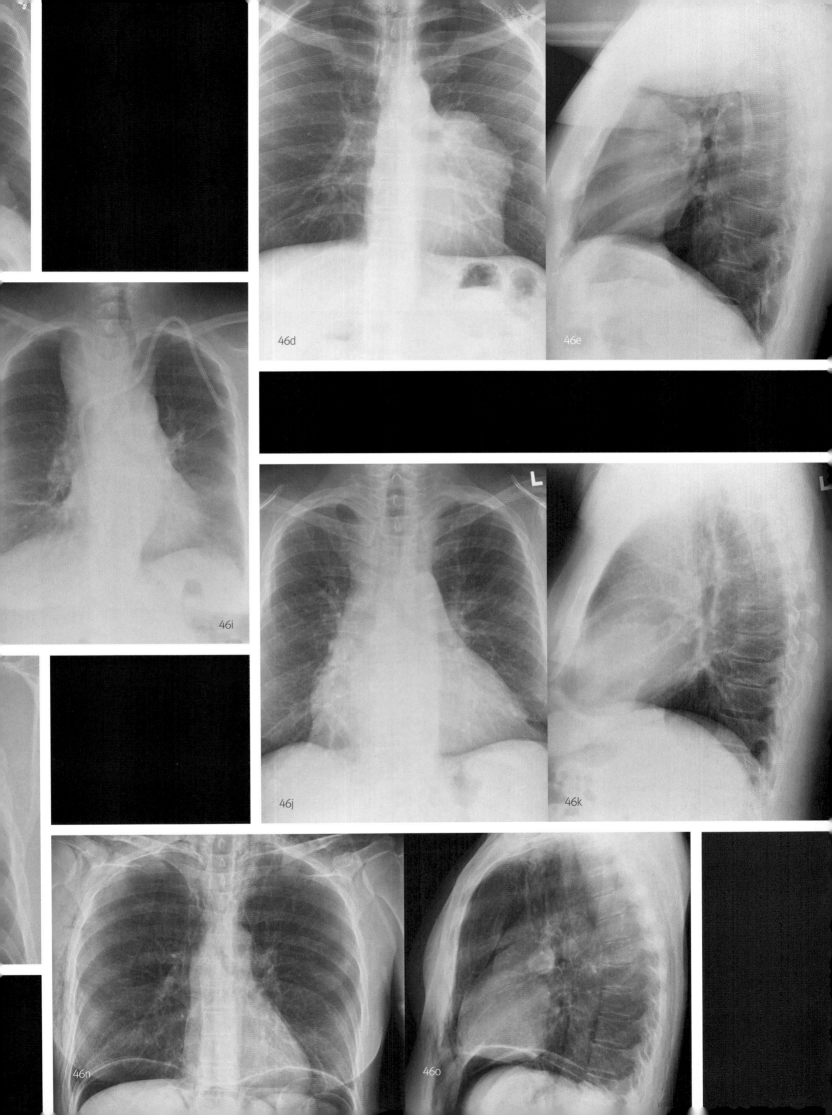

46d

46e

46i

46j

46k

46n

46o

THE ABNORMAL MEDIASTINUM

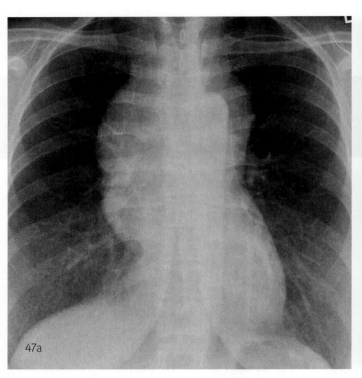

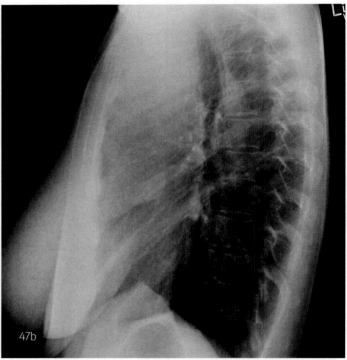

The Radiological Mediastinum will be Abnormal When

1) The grayscale of the mediastinum is too white or too black.
2) The size or shape of the mediastinum is altered.
3) The position of the mediastinum is shifted.

1a. Pathology that affects the mediastinum and shifts the grayscale to 'Too White'

Most pathology involving the mediastinum will cause the mediastinum to look whiter (too white). For example, the grayscale of the mediastinum will change to too white with calcification (Fig. 47a,b).

Figure 47. Mediastinal calcification. Pathology can shift the grayscale of the mediastinum to too white. a, PA chest x-ray from a patient with calcification of the mediastinum, causing it to appear too white, b, lateral chest x-ray from the same patient.

Figure 48. Lipomatosis. The mediastinum can also appear too white under normal conditions. a, PA chest x-ray from a patient with lipomatosis in which the mediastinum is too white due to excessive adipose tissue, b, CT scan from the same patient. Note the large amounts of subcutaneous adipose tissue (arrows) and excessive adipose tissue within the mediastinum (arrow heads).

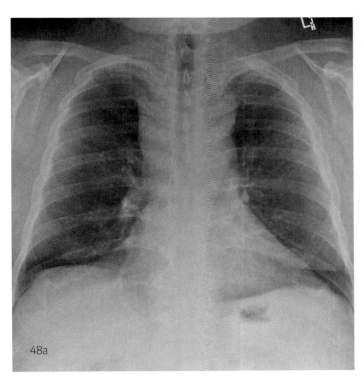

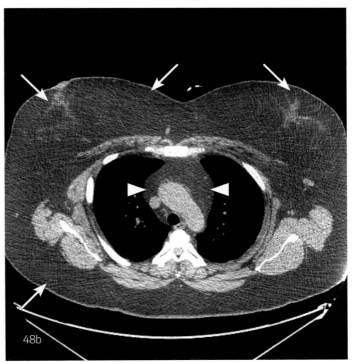

48a

48b

When the mediastinum is too white, but normal

The mediastinum can look too white (and enlarged) when there is excessive adipose tissue, such as in individuals with mediastinal lipomatosis (Fig. 48a,b). This can occur in patients on long-term steroid therapy.

Did you catch the example on pages 315–315?
Fig. 46j,k – Lipomatosis

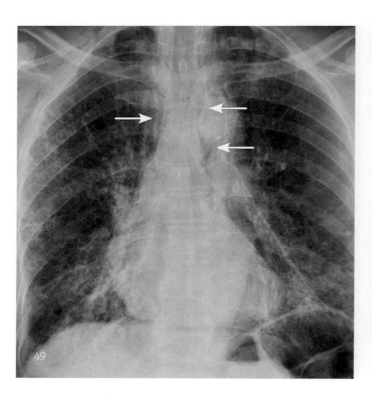

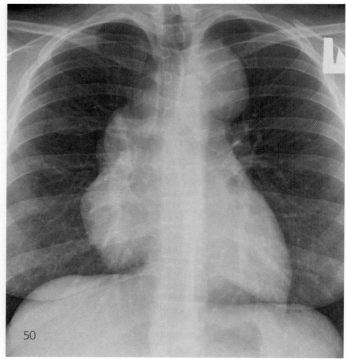

1b. Pathology that affects the mediastinum and shifts the grayscale to 'Too Black'

AMSER Air within the mediastinum (e.g., pneumomediastinum) will cause the grayscale to shift to too black (Fig. 49). Air in the mediastinum usually appears as black lines, sometimes outlining anatomical structures.

2. Pathology that alters the size and shape of the mediastinum

Mediastinal enlargement

Pathology involving the mediastinum, such as anterior mediastinal tumors and the enlarged lymph nodes (adenopathy) associated with sarcoidosis, will commonly enlarge the contours of mediastinum (Fig. 50).

Figure 49. Pneumomediastinum. Pathology can shift the grayscale of the mediastinum to too black such as in this PA chest x-ray from a patient with a pneumomediastinum where the mediastinum (arrows) appears too black due to the abnormal accumulation of air.

Figure 50. Mediastinal enlargement. Pathology can change the size of the mediastinum such as in this PA chest x-ray from a patient with a mass located centrally in the thorax causing enlargement of the mediastinum.

Figure 51. Pneumothorax causing shift in mediastinum. Pathology can shift the position of the mediastinum, such as in this PA chest x-ray from a patient with a large pneumothorax of the right lung causing the mediastinum to shift to the left.

Figure 52. Unfolded aorta. With age, the elongation of the aorta can cause a prominent bowed appearance as seen in this PA chest x-ray.

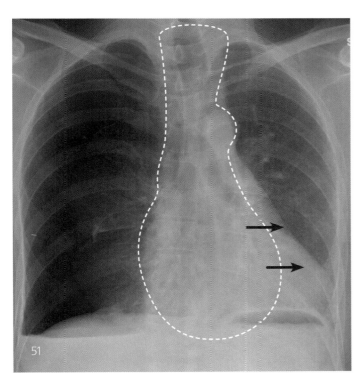

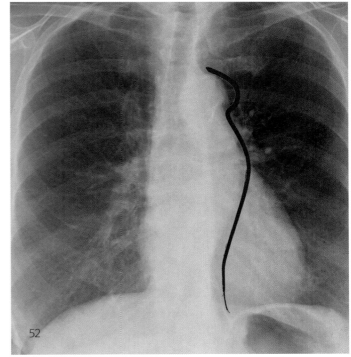

51

52

3. Pathology that alters the position of the mediastinum

A change in mediastinal position most commonly occurs when the mediastinum is displaced because of a mass effect related to a large pneumothorax, a large pleural effusion or a large tumor. In each case, the mediastinum is displaced away from the pathology (Fig. 51).

On the other hand, if there is volume loss with one lung, either because of collapse or surgery, the mediastinum will be displaced toward the pathology.

What is an Unfolded Aorta?

Unfolded is a term used to describe age-related changes involving the aorta (8). With age, the length of the aorta increases. This elongation explains the prominent and commonly bowed appearance of the arch and the descending aorta in the aging population (31) (Fig. 52).

Did you catch the examples on pages 314–314?
Figs. 46b,c and 46d,e – Anterior mediastinal mass
Fig. 46f,g – Middle mediastinal mass
Fig. 46h,i – Goiter
Fig. 46l,m – Right paratracheal mass
Fig. 46n,o – Pneumomediastinum

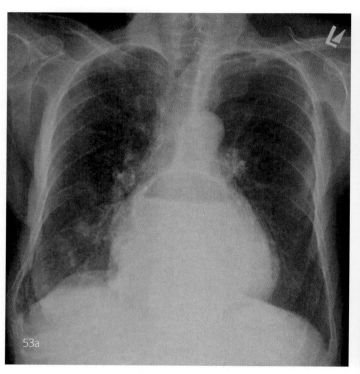 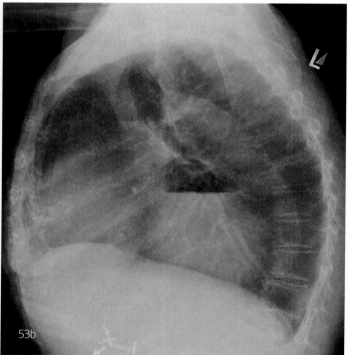

The Many Faces of Hiatus Hernia

There are two types of hiatus hernia: sliding and paraesophageal (Fig. 53a,b). If small, both types may not be visible on a chest x-ray. Larger hiatus hernias can be seen as an air-containing soft tissue density in the lower aspect of the middle mediastinum.

Occasionally, the entire stomach can enter into the thoracic cavity. In order for this to occur, the stomach must rotate on its long axis, resulting with the greater curvature lying more cranial to the lesser curvature. This extreme form of hiatus hernia is called intrathoracic gastric volvulus (Fig. 53c,d), and can lead to vascular compromise and superior mesenteric artery infarction.

Figure 53. Hiatus hernia. There are many appearances of a hiatus hernia. a, PA chest x-ray from a patient with a hiatus hernia, b, lateral chest x-ray from the same patient, c, an extreme form of hiatus hernia, gastric volvulus, on a PA chest x-ray, d, lateral chest x-ray from the same patient.

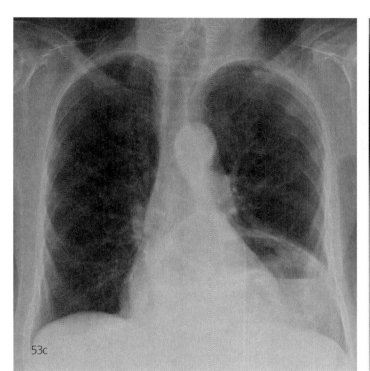

53c

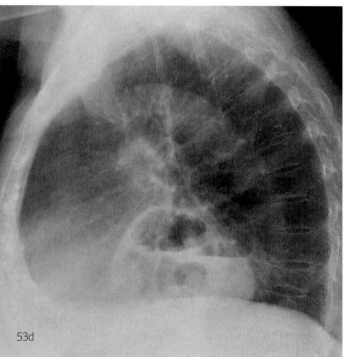

53d

Did you catch the example on pages 314–315?
Fig. 46a – H atus hernia

DIFFERENTIAL DIAGNOSIS BASED ON LOCATION WITHIN the MEDIASTINUM

AMSER

The type of pathology that can occur in the mediastinum will depend in part from which compartment the pathology originated.

If the abnormality originates from the anterior mediastinum (Fig. 54a,b), think "4T"s! (32,33)

1. thyroid – goiter, thyroid tumor
2. thymoma
3. teratoma
4. testicular carcinoma metastases

Also consider aneurysm of the ascending aorta, lymphoma, and mediastinal lipomatosis.

If the abnormality originates from the middle mediastinum (Fig. 55a,b), think "anatomical structures"!

1. nodes (adenopathy) – related to sarcoidosis, lymphoma, infection, metastatic disease
2. bronchi – bronchogenic tumour, carcinoid, carcinoma
3. esophagus – leiomyoma, carcinoma
4. aorta – aneurysm, ectasia
5. great vessels - aneurysm, ectasia
6. hernia – hiatus hernia

If the abnormality originates from the posterior mediastinum (Fig. 56a,b), think "nerves"!

1. nerves – neuroma, ganglioneuroma
2. nodes (adenopathy) – related to sarcoidosis, lymphoma, infection, metastatic disease
3. vascular – aortic aneurysm
4. paraspinal / spinal abnormalities – abscess, metastatic disease

Figure 54. Pathology in the anterior mediastinum. An example of pathology in the anterior mediastinum. a, PA chest x-ray with a large thymoma (arrows), b, lateral chest x-ray from the same patient.

Figure 55. Pathology in the middle mediastinum. An example of pathology in the middle mediastinum. a, PA chest x-ray with a bronchogenic cyst (arrows), b, lateral chest x-ray from the same patient.

Figure 56. Pathology in the posterior mediastinum. An example of pathology in the posterior mediastinum. a, PA chest x-ray with a neural tumor (arrows), b, lateral chest x-ray from the same patient.

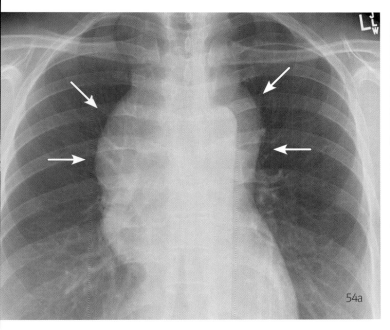

54a

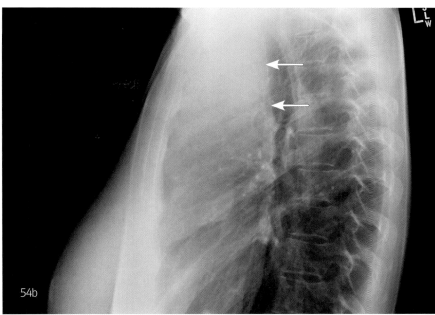

54b

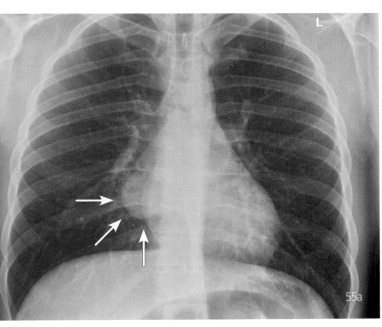

55a

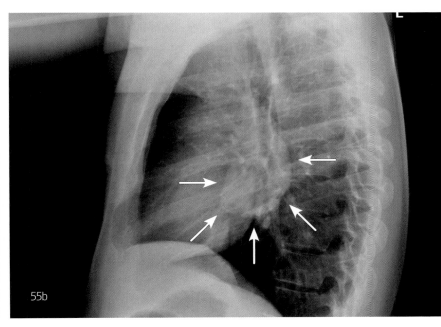

55b

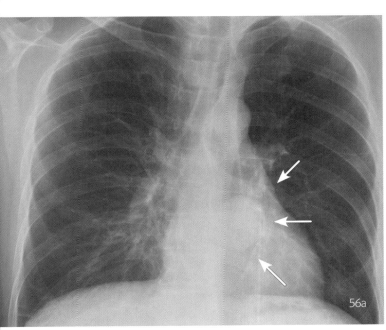

56a

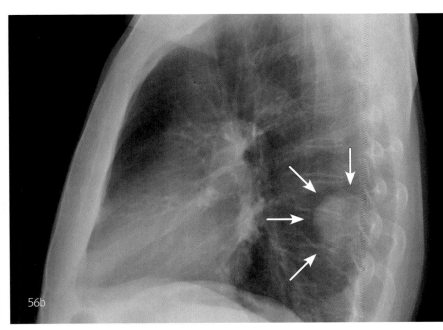

56b

323

LOCALIZATION OF MEDIASTINAL PATHOLOGY

In trying to localize pathology to the mediastinum, as opposed to the pleura or to the lung parenchyma, it is useful to evaluate the interface created between the mediastinal pathology and the lung. Pathology arising from the mediastinum will be separated from the lung tissue by the pleura and will maintain a smooth contour; whereas pathology arising from the lung itself may have a spiculated, ill-defined border (Fig. 57a,b). Pathology arising from the mediastinum will displace the pleura in such a way that the mediastinal pathology will maintain obtuse angles with the lung.

Perhaps the easiest method of localizing pathology to the mediastinum is by the mass effect of the pathology on other mediastinal structures, such as displacement of the trachea or displacement of the great vessels.

A number of indirect radiological signs are available to help localize mediastinal pathology. One of these signs is the silhouette sign (Fig. 58)(**Pg. XX**).

The localization of pathology to the mediastinum is simplified with the use of cross-sectional imaging. However, in some instances – such as tumors related to the pleura – even with cross-sectional imaging, the exact point of origin of the pathology cannot be determined.

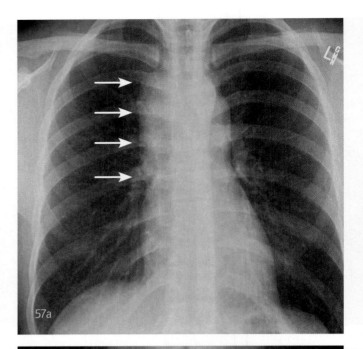

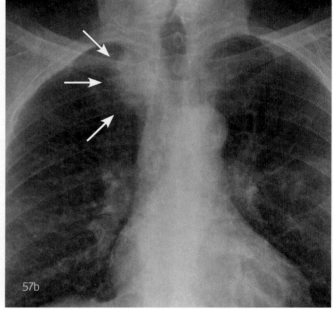

Figure 57. Localization of mediastinal pathology. The borders of a tumor can be used to localize its origin. a, PA chest x-ray with a tumor with smooth defined contours, originating in the mediastinum, b, PA chest x-ray with a tumor with a spiculated, ill-defined border originating in the lung.

Figure 58. The silhouette sign. The silhouette sign can be used to localize mediastinal pathology. PA chest x-ray with a tumor causing a loss of the right inferior border of the mediastinum – the silhouette sign.

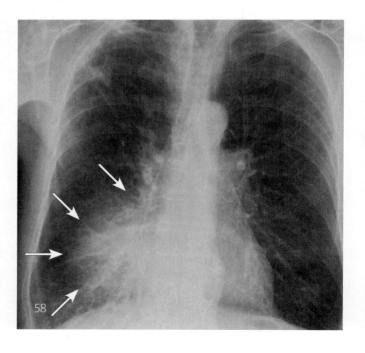

SUMMARY OF RADIOLOGICAL CHANGES TO THE MEDIASTINUM

RADIOLOGICAL CHANGES		ASSOCIATED FINDINGS, DISEASES AND CONDITIONS
1. Change in grayscale	Too white	• Calcification • Hiatus hernia • Mediastinal lipomatosis
	Too black	• Pneumomediastinum • Hiatus hernia (with air)
2. Change in size and/or shape		• Tumors (anterior, middle and posterior) • Adenopathy (due to: lymphoma, sarcoidosis) • Goiter • Aneurysm (ascending aorta) • Unfolded (ectatic) aorta
3. Change in position		• Mass effect (due to: pneumothorax, pleural effusion, atelectasis (collapse), surgery or tumor)

Table 9.2
Summary of Radiological Changes to the Mediastinum

RADIOLOGICAL SIGNS
RELATED TO THE MEDIASTINUM

1,2,3 Sign

The 1,2,3 sign refers to the characteristic pattern of lymph node enlargement in sarcoidosis, which includes (1) the right paratracheal, (2) the right hilar, and (3) the left hilar nodes (Fig 59).

Hilar Overlay Sign

The hilar overlay sign helps distinguish if a mass lies within the mediastinum or hilum. When a mass arises from the hilum, the pulmonary vessels are in contact with the mass and will silhouette with the mass. If the mass lies anterior or posterior to the hilum, the hilar vessels will be visible through the mass. This is the hilar overlay sign (Fig. 60).

Iceberg Sign

If a paraspinal opacity gets wider as it gets close to the diaphragm, this usually indicates that there will be significant associated abdominal disease. An example may be a paraspinal abscess that can have thoracic as well as abdominal portions (Fig. 61). This is called the iceberg or thoracoabdominal sign (34).

The Silhouette Sign

The silhouette sign occurs whenever two structures of similar radiological density are touching each other. When this occurs on an x-ray, the two will appear as one structure (i.e., the interface between them is lost) (Fig. 62).

Figure 59. The 1, 2, 3 sign. PA chest x-ray with an example of the 1,2,3 sign with characteristic pattern of adenopathy in sarcoidosis, 1, right paratracheal, 2, right hilar and, 3, left hilar lymph node enlargement.

Figure 60. The hilar overlay sign. PA chest x-ray with an example of the hilar overlay sign. The proximal right pulmonary artery (arrows) is clearly seen through the density of the mediastinal mass.

Figure 61. The iceberg sign. PA chest x-ray with an example of the iceberg sign in a patient with a hiatus hernia. Arrows show the soft tissue mass extending inferiorly to the diaphragm suggesting that the lesion extends into the abdomen.

Figure 62. The silhouette sign. PA chest x-ray with an example of the silhouette sign at the right edge of the mediastinum.

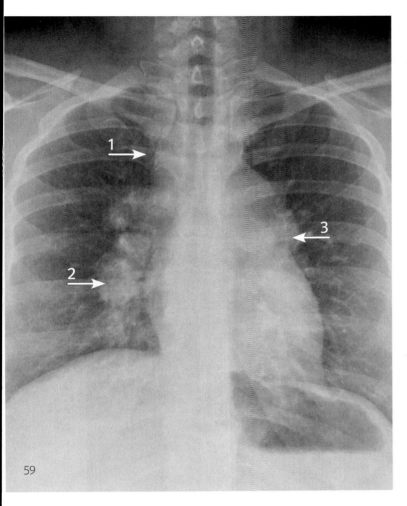

59

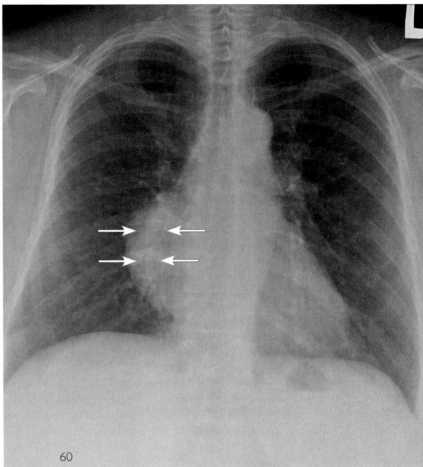

60

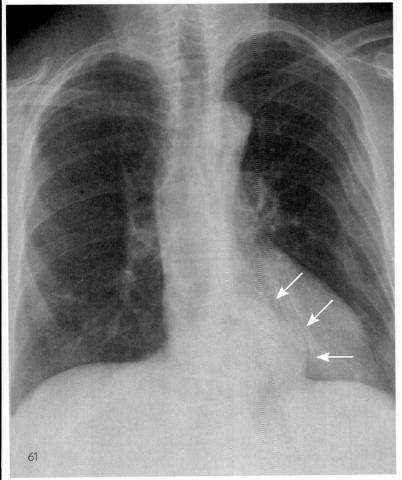

61

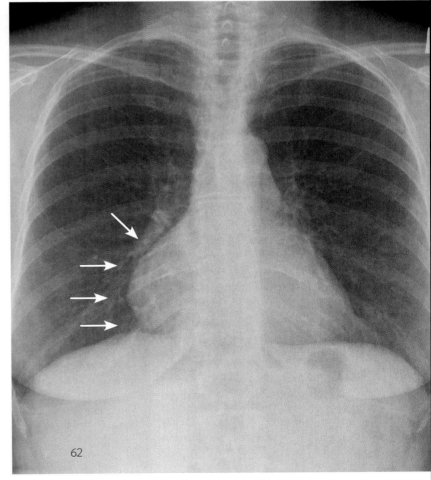

62

Visual Search of the Mediastinum

PA Chest X-ray

1. Start with the right superior mediastinal edge (SVC) (1) at the level of the clavicles.

2. Follow this edge inferiorly to the right cardiac border (2).

3. Follow the right heart edge inferiorly to the diaphragm (3).

4. Follow the left heart edge superiorly to the aorta (4).

5. Follow the aorta superiorly to the right superior mediastinal edge (left subclavian artery) (5).

6. Follow the left superior mediastinal edge superiorly to the level of the clavicles (6).

7. Identify the following
   • Right paratracheal stripe.
   • Azygoesophageal recess.
   • Paraaortic stripe.
   • Left paraspinal stripe.
   • Aorto-pulmonary window.

Complete the visual search by checking for any density changes across the mediastinum from top to bottom.

VS

Lateral Chest X-ray

1. Start from the neck (1).

2. Scan across the thorax from front to back from superior to inferior, looking for any abnormal densities (2).

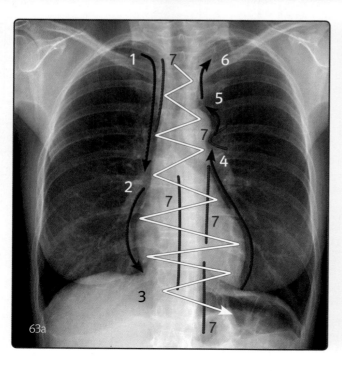

63a

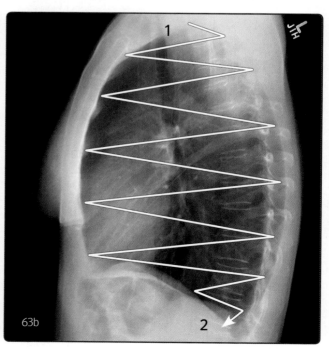

63b

Mediastinum Radiological Analysis Checklist

To confidently state that the mediastinum is normal, all parts of the checklist should indicate a normal appearance.

GRAYSCALE

1 Is the grayscale of the mediastinum altered?

If **YES**, then describe.
Too white/too black.
Pathology/lipomatosis.

SIZE

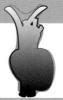

2 Is the size of the mediastinum altered?

If **YES**, then describe.
Too big.
Right/left.
Anterior/middle/posterior compartment.

SHAPE

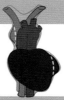

3 Are the mediastinal contours abnormal?

If **YES**, then describe.
Right/left.
Distorted/missing/additional.

POSITION

4 Is the position of the mediastinum shifted?

If **YES**, then describe.
Right/left.
Anterior/posterior.

OTHER

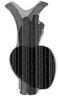

5 Is the AP window normal?

If **NO**, then describe.
Blurred, obscured.
Too big/too small.

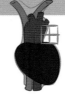

6 Are the lines and stripes normal?

If **NO**, then describe.
Too wide/irregular/missing.

7 Are there any radiological signs related to the mediastinum present?

If **YES**, then describe.
123.
hilar overlay.
Iceberg.
Silhouette.

8 Is there any evidence of previous surgery to the mediastinum?

If **YES**, then describe.
Type of surgery and location.
Compare to previous CXR.

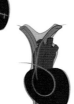

9 Are there any lines or tubes in the mediastinum?

If **YES**, then describe.
Give location of each relative to the carina and SVC.

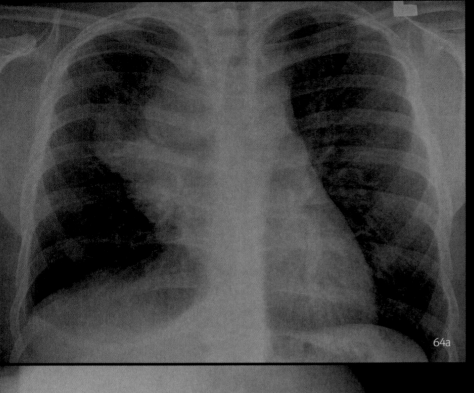

64a

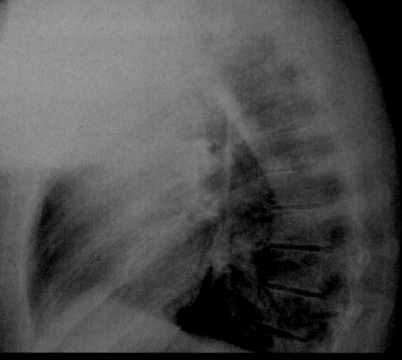

64b

What are your findings?

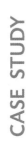

You are working on call in the emergency department. A 50 year old male presents with weight loss, shortness of breath and chest pain. You order a chest x-ray (Fig. 64a,b).

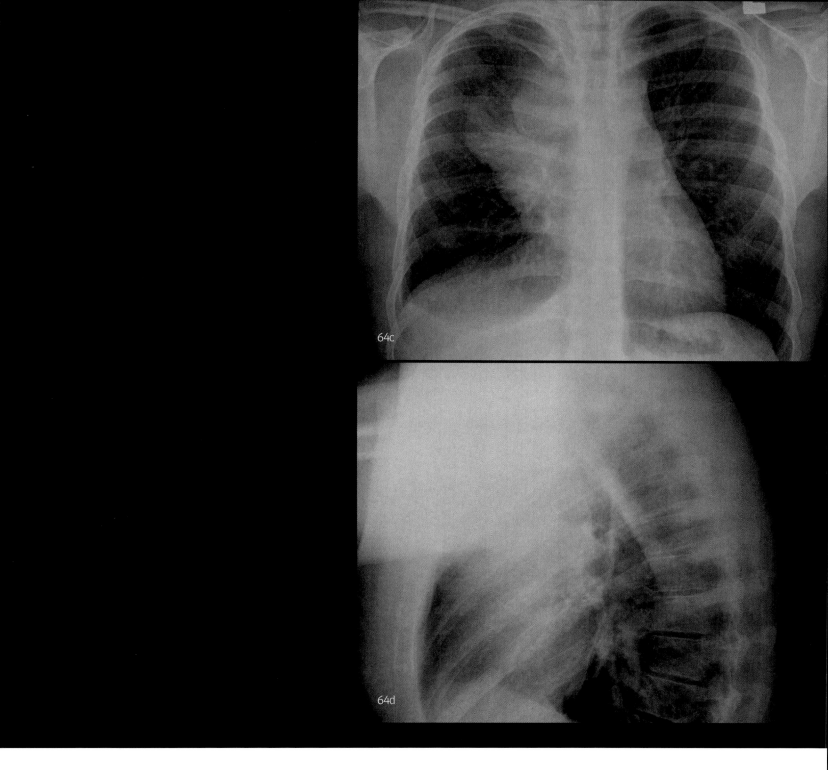

64c

64d

Using the techniques described in this chapter, make sure to examine all of the normal mediastinal structures. You will notice that the mediastinum is enlarged (Fig. 64c,d). The outer contours of the mediastinum are lobulated. There is mass effect on the airways with the trachea being narrowed and displaced to the left. There is no calcification. The abnormality lies within the anterior mediastinum. The patient also has a right pleural effusion.

Summary: Anterior mediastinal mass.

Differential diagnosis: Thyroid, thymoma, teratoma, testicular metastases, lymphoma.

Based on the findings, the diagnosis is malignant thymoma.

DISCUSSION

This series of images highlights the variability in the radiological appearance of the thoracic aorta.

THE SWAYING AORTA

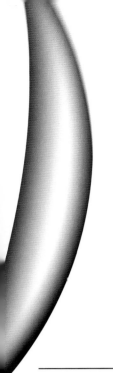

References

1. Lewis, P.J., Shaffer, K., & Donovan, A. (Eds.). (2012). AMSER National Medical Student Curriculum in Radiology. http://aur.org/Secondary-Alliances.aspx?id=141.

2. Lewis, P.J., & Shaffer, K. (2005). Developing a national medical student curriculum in radiology. Am. Coll. Radiol., 2(1):8–11.

3. Felson, B. (1973). Chest Roentgenology. Philadelphia, PA: W.B. Saunders Co.

4. Gray, H. (2008). Gray's Anatomy: The Anatomical Basis of Medicine and Surgery, 40th ed. New York, NY: Churchill Livingstone.

5. Zylak, P.J., Pallie, W., & Jackson, R. (1982). Correlative anatomy and computed tomography" a module on the mediastinum. Radiographics, 2:555–592.

6. Heitzman, E.R. (1977). The mediastinum: radiologic correlations with anatomy and pathology. University of Michigan, MI: Mosby.

7. Alexander, S.A., & Rubin, G.D. (2009). Imaging the thoracic aorta: anatomy, technical considerations, and trauma. Sem. Roentgenol., 44(1):8–15.

8. Anderson, R.H. (2000). Clinical anatomy of the aortic root. Heart (Br. Card. Soc.), 84(6):670–673.

9. O'Rourke, M., Farnsworth, A., & O'Rourke, J. (2008). Aortic dimensions and stiffness in normal adults. JACC. Cardiovasc. Imaging, 1(6):749–751.

10. Bennett, W.F., Altaf, F., & Deslauriers, J. (2011). Anatomy of the superior vena cava and brachiocephalic veins. Thorac. Surg. Clinics., 21(2):197–203.

11. Albrecht, K. (2004). Applied anatomy of the superior vena cava--the carina as a landmark to guide central venous catheter placement. Br. J. Anaesthesia, 92(1):75–77.

12. Milne, E.N.C., Pistolesi, M., Miniati, M., et al. (1985). The vascular pedicle of the heart and the vena azygos. Part I. The normal subject. Radiology, 152:1–158.

13. Miller, R.R., & Ely, E.W. (2006). Radiographic measures of intravascular volume status: the role of vascular pedicle width. Curr. Opin. Crit. Care., 12(3):255–262.

14. Ravenel, J.G., & Erasmus, J.J. (2002). Azygoesophageal recess. J. Thorac. Imaging, 2:219–226.

15. Fleischner, F.G., & Udis, S.W. (1952). Dilatation of the azygos vein; a roentgen sign of venous engorgement. Am. J. Roentgenol. Radium Ther. Nucl. Med., 67: 569–575.

16. Haubrich, W.S. (2003). Medical meaning - a glossary of word origins, 2nd ed. Philadelphia, PA: ACP press.

17. Proto, A.V., & Lane, E.J. (1977). Air in the esophagus: a frequent radiographic finding. AJR Am. J. Roentgenol., 129(3):433–440.

18. Aquino, S.L., Duncan, G.R., & Hayman, L.A. (2001). Nerves of the thorax: atlas of normal and pathologic findings. Radiographics, 21(5):1275–1281.

19. Suwatanapongched, T., & Gierada, D.S. (2006). CT of thoracic lymph nodes. Part I: anatomy and drainage. Br. J. Radiol., 79(947):922–928.

20. Tuddenham, W.J. (1984). Glossary of Terms for Thoracic Radiology: recommendations of the Nomenclature Committee of the Fleischner Society. *AJR Am. J. Roentengol., 143*: 509–517.

21. Parkinson, J., & Bedford, D. (1936). The aortic triangle: radiological landmark in the left oblique projection. *Lancet, 2*:909–911

22. Gibbs, J.M., Chandrasekhar, C.A., Ferguson, E.C., & Oldham, S.A. (2007). Lines and stripes: where did they go? From conventional radiography to CT. *Radiographics, 27*(1):33–48.

23. Maldonado, J.A., Henry, T., & Gutiérrez, F.R. (2010). Congenital thoracic vascular anomalies. *Radiol. Clin. North Am., 48*(1):85–115.

24. Gildenhorn, H.L., Rubenstein, L.H., & Snider, G.L. (1956). Dextroposition of the descending thoracic aorta. *Radiology., 67*(3):333–338.

25. Felson, B. (1989). The superior vena cava: conventional projections. *Sem. Roentgenol., 24*(2):91–95.

26. Proto, A.V., Simmons, J.D., & Zylak, C.J. (1983). The anterior junction anatomy. *Crit. Rev. Diagn. Imaging, 19*(2):111–173.

27. Proto, A.V., Simmons, J.D., & Zylak, C.J. (1983). The posterior junction anatomy. *Crit. Rev. Diagn. Imaging, 20*:121–173.

28. Woodring, J.H., & Daniel, T.L. (1986). Mediastinal analysis emphasizing plain radiographs and computed tomograms. *Med. Radiogr. Photogr., 62*:1-48.

29. Paling, M.R., & Pope, T.L. Jr. (1987). The variable nature of the mediastinal contour lines: CT/Chest radiography correlation. *J. Computed Tomography, 11*:254–260.

30. Proto, A.V. (1987). Mediastinal anatomy: emphasis on conventional images with anatomic and computed tomographic correlations. *J. Thorac. Imaging, 2*:1–48.

31. Suguwara, J., Hayashi, K., Yokoi, T., & Tanaka, H. (2008). Age-associated elongation of the ascending aorta in adults. *J. Am. Coll. Cardiol. Img., 1*:739–748.

32. Tomaszek, S., Wigle, D.A., Keshavjee, S., & Fischer, S. (2009). Thymomas: review of current clinical practice. *Annals Thorac. Surg., 87*(6):1973–1980.

33. Priola, S.M., Priola, A.M., Cardinale,L., et al. (2006). The anterior mediastinum: anatomy and imaging procedures. *La Radiologia Medica., 111*(3):295–311.

34. Felson, B. (1969). The mediastinum. *Semin. Roentgenol., 4*:41–58.

CHAPTER 10

The HEART & PERICARDIUM (the cardiac zone)

importance

Historically, chest x-rays have played an important role in the diagnosis of cardiac disorders. Today, traditional x-ray imaging for cardiac disease has largely been replaced by other imaging modalities, especially echocardiography. However, standard chest x-rays continue to provide valuable information about the heart and related pathologies (1).

This chapter explains how to identify the normal heart and its borders on a standard chest x-ray, and describes the grayscale appearance of the heart in various clinical conditions. The features of a failing heart on an x-ray are very important to identify, and must be memorized by all students and doctors. The rapid and accurate interpretation of pathology related to the heart and pericardium on the PA and lateral chest x-rays is vital in emergency situations.

A full review of the heart and pericardium is beyond the scope of this text; this chapter will discuss the heart and pericardium as they relate to the radiological image.

objectives

Skills

You will identify

- the four cardiac chambers, and their location, on PA and lateral x-rays.
- the anatomical structures that form the borders of the heart on PA and lateral x-rays.
- the position of the cardiac valves, within the cardiac shadow, on the PA and lateral x-rays.
- cardiac enlargement.
- the radiological features of cardiac failure.

Knowledge

You will review and understand

- the spatial localization of the heart chambers.
- the spatial localization of the heart valves.

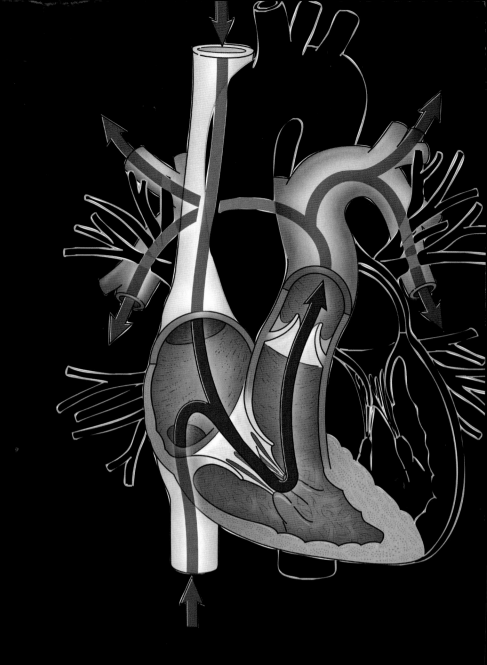

associated resources

This chapter maps to the following AMSER curriculum content (2,3).

1) Normal radiological anatomy of the heart and pericardium.
    Right ventricle (RV)
    Right atrium (RA)
    Left ventricle (LV)
    Left atrium (LA)
    Pericardium
    Position of heart valves
    Common normal variants: Pericardial fat pads

2. Pathological conditions affecting the heart and pericardium.
    Aortic, mitral valve, and annulus calcifications
    Cardiomegaly: individual chamber enlargement, and generalized
        cardiomegaly
    Cardiac failure: pulmonary venous hypertension, interstitial
        edema, and alveolar edema

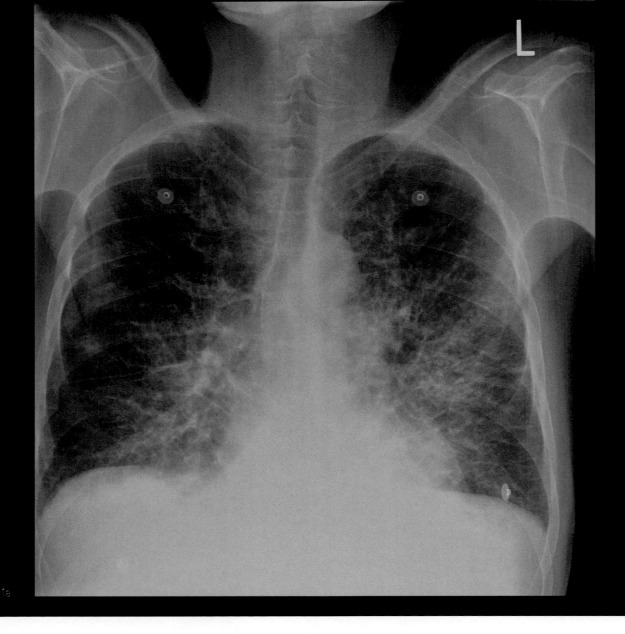

CASE STUDY

During one of your overnight on-call shifts, a 60-year-old post-operative male patient suddenly complains of shortness of breath. He does not have any associated chest pain, palpitations, sweating or nausea. The patient is gasping for each breath and you sit him up from his recumbent position and start him on high-flow oxygen. He feels a bit better at this time, and you set off to investigate possible causes of his shortness of breath. You suspect that the patient is suffering from congestive heart failure and you order a chest x-ray, stat (Fig. 1a,b). The staff physician on duty calls you from a dinner party and demands to know immediately what the chest x-ray shows... there is no time to wait for a formal report from a radiologist.

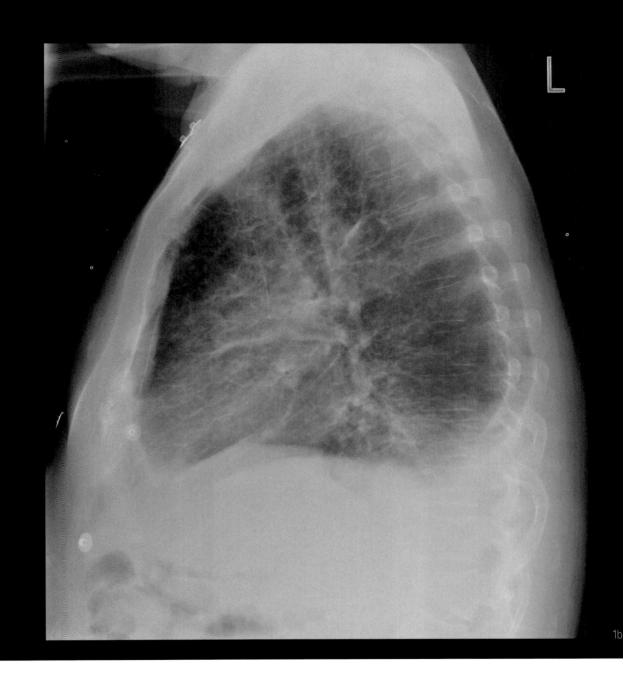

1b

How would you describe
your findings to the staff physician?

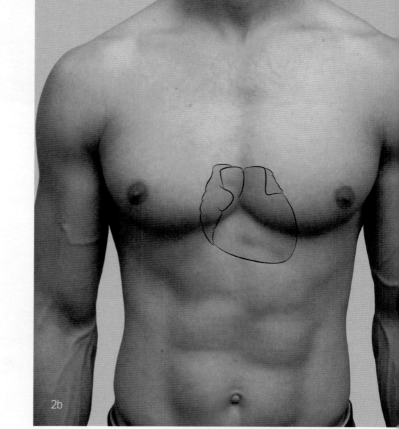

THE HEART & PERICARDIUM

A muscular organ that pumps blood through the body, the heart is central to the circulation of blood through the lungs, as well as to all vital organs and the periphery of the body. The heart and its associated pericardium are positioned centrally in the thorax, nestled underneath the sternum, lying slightly left of midline (Fig. 2a,b).

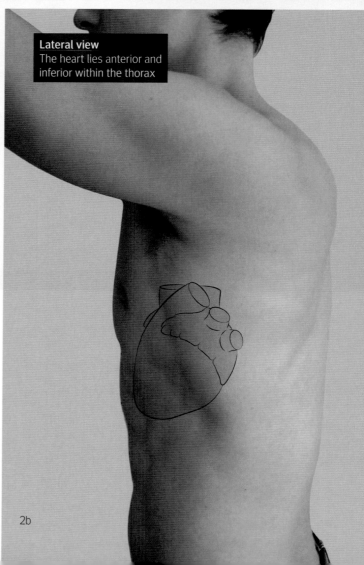

Lateral view
The heart lies anterior and inferior within the thorax

Figure 2. Surface anatomy localization of the heart and pericardium. a, frontal perspective, b, lateral perspective.

2b

2b

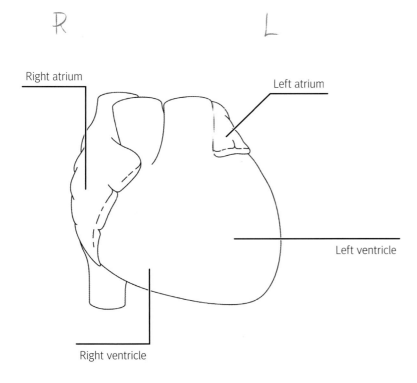

Right atrium

Left atrium

Left ventricle

Right ventricle

3a

The Heart

The heart (derived from the old English word *heorte*) is a conical-shaped muscular organ, comprised of two ventricles and two atria (Fig. 3a,b)(4). Atrium is taken from the Latin word *atrium* meaning "an open area in a house", and the word ventricle is derived from the Latin word *ventriculus* meaning "a little belly".

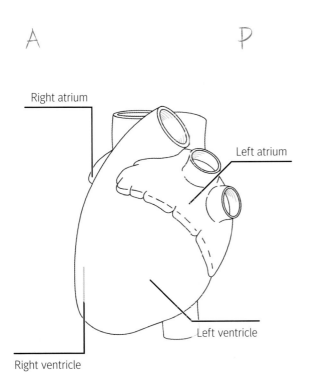

Right atrium

Left atrium

Left ventricle

Right ventricle

3b

Figure 3. Anatomy of the heart.
Illustrations of the heart, a, frontal perspective, b, lateral perspective.

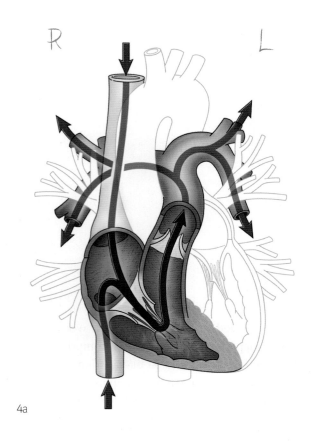

4a

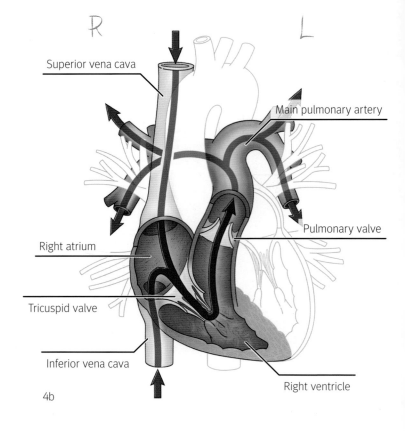

Superior vena cava

Main pulmonary artery

Pulmonary valve

Right atrium

Tricuspid valve

Inferior vena cava

Right ventricle

4b

Venous deoxygenated blood arrives at the right atrium via the superior and inferior *venae cavae* and the coronary sinus. The blood is pumped through the tricuspid valve into the right ventricle, then through the pulmonary valve into the pulmonary outflow tract and the pulmonary arteries (Fig. 4a,b).

Figure 4. Right blood circulation.
a, illustration of the right circulation, b, illustration of the right circulation, annotated.

Figure 5. Left blood circulation.
a, illustration of the left circulation, b, illustration of the left circulation, annotated.

R   L   R   L

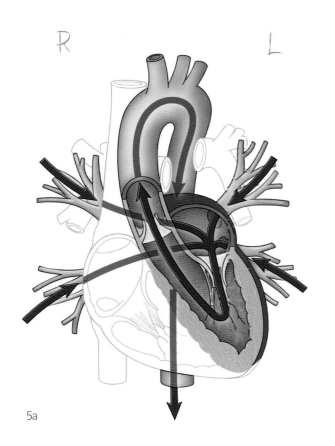

5a

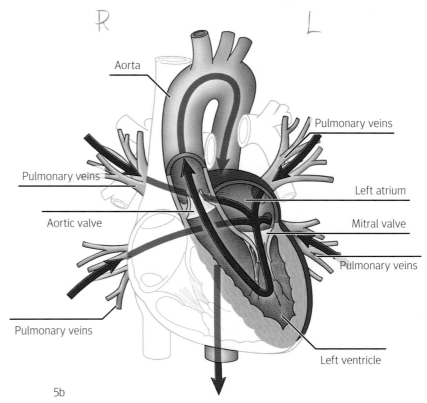

Aorta

Pulmonary veins

Pulmonary veins

Left atrium

Aortic valve

Mitral valve

Pulmonary veins

Pulmonary veins

Left ventricle

5b

Oxygenated blood arrives at the left atrium via four pulmonary veins. The blood travels through the mitral valve into the left ventricle, then through the aortic valve into the aorta, and into the systemic circulation (Fig. 5a,b).

Radiological Shape and Grayscale of the Heart

On the PA view, the heart lies centrally in the mediastinum, normally with two-thirds of its bulk located to the left of the midline (Fig. 6a,b,c)(5). On the PA x-ray, the grayscale of the heart resembles a cone with sternocostal, diaphragmatic and pulmonary surfaces. The long axis of this cone extends from the right shoulder to the left hypochondrium, with the apex lying at the fifth interspace, in the midclavicular line.

On the lateral x-ray, the heart lies within the inferior aspect of the anterior half of the thorax (Fig. 7a,b,c), and as on the PA x-ray, has a conical shape. The long axis of the cone is directed from anterior and inferior to superior and posterior.

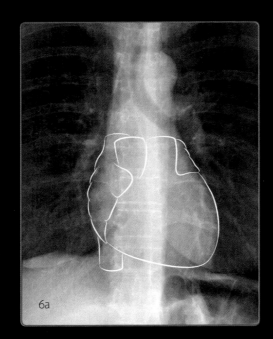

6a

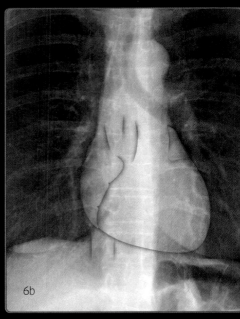

6b

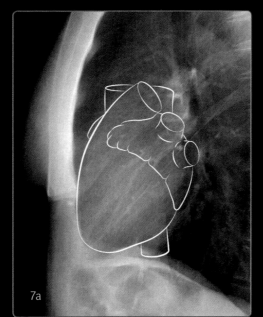

7a

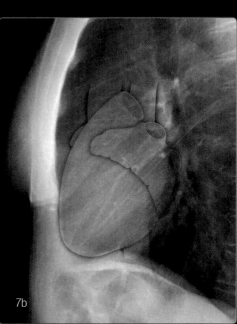

7b

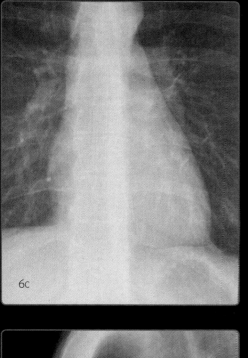

6c

Figure 6. Radiological anatomy of the heart from frontal perspective. a, PA chest x-ray with the heart outlined, b, PA chest x-ray with grayscale illustration of heart overlay, c, PA chest x-ray cropped to highlight the heart.

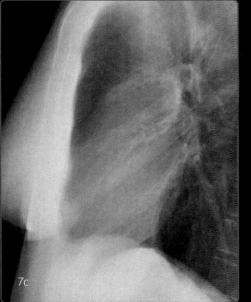

7c

Figure 7. Radiological anatomy of the heart from the lateral perspective. a, lateral chest x-ray with the heart outlined, b, lateral chest x-ray with grayscale illustration of the heart overlay, c, lateral chest x-ray cropped to highlight the heart.

The Position of the Atria and Ventricles

The atria and ventricles are usually described as "right" and "left" to differentiate the right and left circulatory systems. Anatomically, the right atrium (RA) lies anterior and on the right; the right ventricle (RV) lies anteriorly; the left ventricle (LV) lies on the left; and the left atrium (LA) lies posteriorly (Fig. 8a,b).

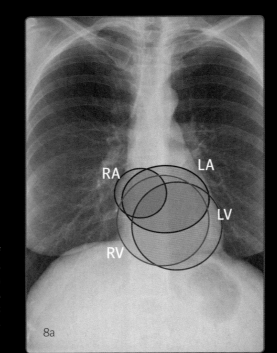

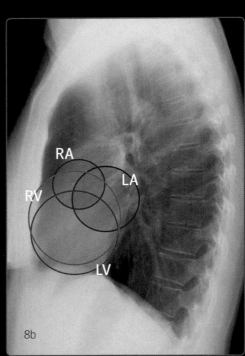

Figure 8. Radiological anatomy of the atria and ventricles. **Chest x-rays highlighting the spatial localization of the atria and ventricles. a, PA chest x-ray, b, lateral chest x-ray; RA, right atrium, RV, right ventricle, LA, left atrium, LV, left ventricle.**

The Position of the Heart Valves

The most superior cardiac valve is the pulmonary valve (PV) (Fig. 9a,b). The pulmonary valve lies on the left side of midline at the level of the auricle of the left atrium. The mitral valve (MV) is vertically-oriented, and lies below the level of the pulmonary valve (6). The aortic valve (AV) is connected to the mitral valve, but is horizontally-oriented, and overlies the spine. The most inferior valve, the tricuspid valve (TV), lies on the right, below the aortic valve.

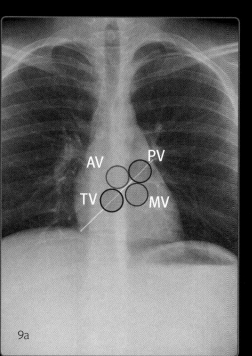

9a

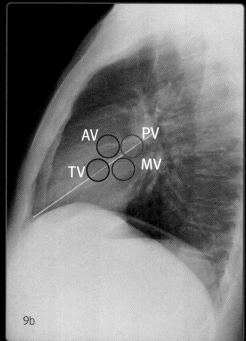

9b

Figure 9. Radiological anatomy of the heart valves. **Chest x-rays highlighting the spatial localization of the heart valves. a, PA chest x-ray, b, lateral chest x-ray. AV, aortic valve, MV, mitral valve, PV, pulmonary valve, TV, tricuspid valve.**

How to identify the location of the aortic and mitral valves on the PA x-ray

Knowing the location of the valves is useful in assessing proper positioning of tubes and lines entering the heart.

STEP 1
Confirm that the patient is midline and not rotated (Ch. 1, Pg. 32).

STEP 2
Identify the auricle of the left atrium (Fig. 10).

STEP 3
Draw a line from the auricle of the left atrium to the point where the right atrium intersects with the diaphragm (Fig. 11). The aortic valve (AV) lies above, and the mitral valve (MV) lies below, this line (Fig. 12).

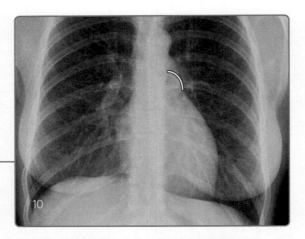

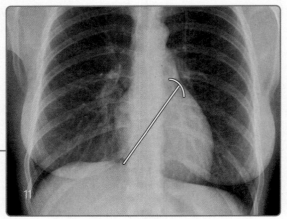

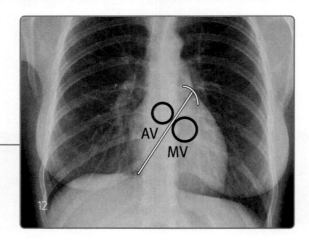

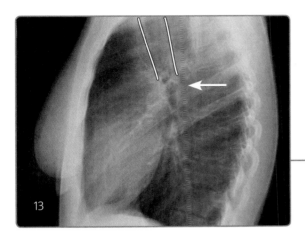

13

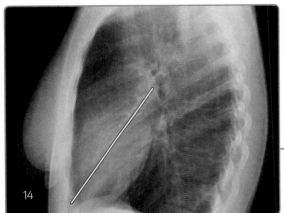

14

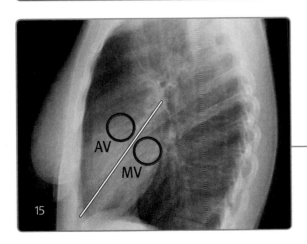

AV

MV

15

How to identify the location of the aortic and mitral valves on the lateral x-ray

Knowing the location of the valves is useful in assessing proper positioning of tubes and lines entering the heart.

STEP 1
Identify the trachea and carina (Fig. 13) (Ch. 7, Pg. 199).

STEP 2
Draw a line from the carina to the anterior costophrenic angle (Fig. 14). The aortic valve (AV) lies above, and the mitral valve (MV) lies below, this line (Fig. 15).

?

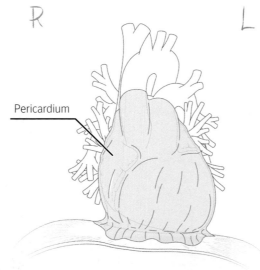

16a

The Pericardium

The word pericardium is the Latinized form of the Greek word *perikardion* meaning "membrane around the heart", derived from the Greek word for heart, *kardia*, and *peri*, meaning "around, near or about".

The pericardium is a fibrous sac that surrounds the heart consisting of two layers: the (inner) visceral pericardium and the (outer) parietal pericardium (Fig. 16a,b,c)(9). A layer of epicardial fat lies beneath the visceral pericardium. The visceral pericardium, or epicardium, covers the heart and extends for a short distance along the pulmonary veins, the superior vena cava (SVC), the inferior vena cava (IVC), the ascending aorta and the main pulmonary artery, before folding upon itself to become the parietal pericardium (akin to the relationship between the visceral and parietal pleura; Ch. 11, Pg. XX).

The pericardial cavity (Fig. 16c) is similar to the pleural cavity, in that it represents a potential space that can accumulate fluid or air. In the normal population, the pericardial space contains approximately 15 to 50 ml of clear fluid that reduces the friction between the two pericardial layers.

The main function of the pericardium is to contain the heart and limit cardiac motion within the mediastinum. The pericardium also protects the heart from local inflammatory disease (e.g., pneumonia), and limits acute enlargement of the heart chambers that can occur with increased preload.

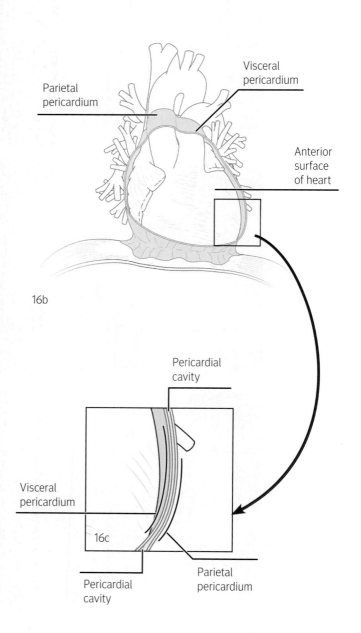

Figure 16. Anatomy of the pericardium. Illustrations of the pericardium, a, frontal perspective, b, frontal perspective cut away, c, highlighting the pericardial cavity.

Radiological Shape and Grayscale of the Pericardium

The pericardium is normally very thin and is, therefore, not visualized on PA chest x-rays – the lateral contour of the cardiac shadow also represents the lateral margin of the parietal pericardium (10). Because the myocardium cannot be distinguished with certainty from the pericardium on the PA x-ray, the term cardiopericardial silhouette is a more accurate name for the heart shadow.

Occasionally, on the lateral chest x-ray, the normal pericardium may be seen as a 1 to 2 mm thick, curved stripe, anterior to the heart, set between the more radiolucent mediastinal fat anteriorly and the epicardial fat posteriorly.

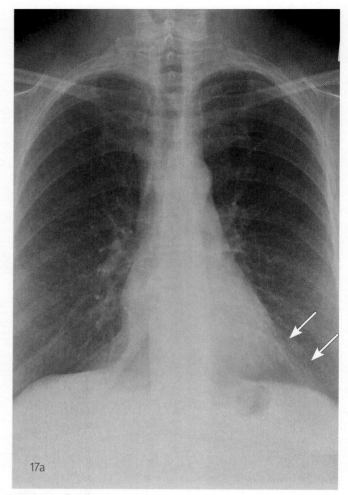

17a

The Cardiac/Epicardial Fat Pad

AMSER Between the lung and the parietal pericardium, there may be a layer of mediastinal fat, known as the cardiac/epicardial fat pad. The epicardial fat is a normal finding and is seen most commonly in the left cardiophrenic angle. Composed of adipose tissue, the fat pads are less radiopaque than the adjacent left ventricle. This difference in density causes the left heart border to fade away inferiorly and laterally on the PA x-ray (Fig. 17a).

The epicardial fat pad typically has a triangular shape and can be readily seen on the lateral x-ray. The triangle lies in the anterior left cardiophrenic angle, with its apex pointing posteriorly and superiorly (Fig. 17b).

A prominent fat pad can make assessment of the heart size difficult, and can sometimes mimic cardiac enlargement (Fig. 18a,b) (11).

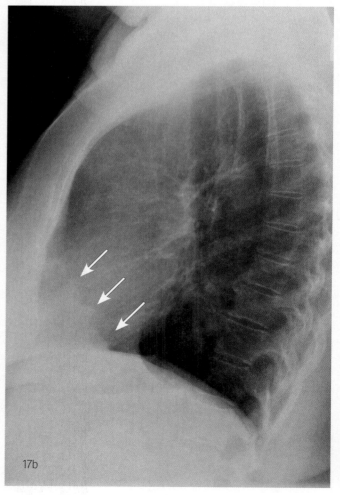

17b

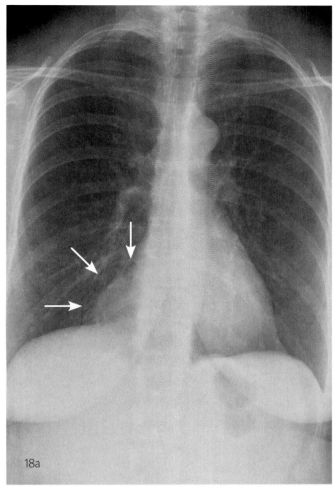

18a

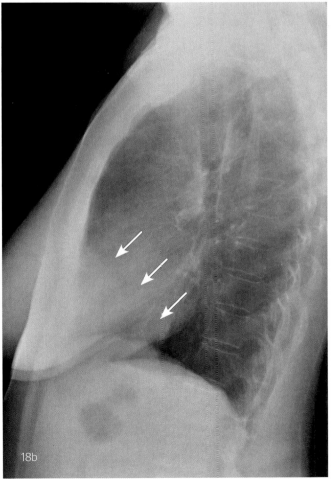

18b

Frequency of Visualization of the Epicardial Fat Pad

32% of normal patients will have a fat pad visible on the lateral chest x-ray (12).

Figure 17. The epicardial fat pad. The epicardial/cardiac fat pad is a normal finding on the chest x-ray. a, PA chest x-ray highlighting a normal epicardial fat pad (arrows) in the left cardiophrenic angle, b, lateral chest x-ray from the same case, highlighting the epicardial fat pad (arrows). Note the typical triangular appearance in the anterior left cardiophrenic angle.

Figure 18. A prominent epicardial fat pad. A prominent epicardial fat pad can cause difficulties assessing heart size, and can mimic cardiac hypertrophy. a, PA chest x-ray highlighting a prominent epicardial fat pad (arrows), b, lateral chest x-ray from the same case, highlighting the prominent fat pad (arrows).

INTERFACES RELATED TO THE HEART & PERICARDIUM

Cardiac – Lung Interfaces (13)

On the PA chest x-ray (Fig. 19a), on the right, the cardiac contour is created superiorly by the SVC and inferiorly by the right atrium. In some patients, below the right atrium, the suprahepatic portion of the IVC can be seen. On the left, the cardiac contour is created inferiorly by the left ventricle, and more superiorly, by the auricle of the left atrium. Above the auricle of the LA lies the main pulmonary artery (which lies just below the aortic arch). The right ventricle (an anterior structure) does not contribute to the cardiac contour on the PA x-ray.

On the lateral x-ray (Fig. 19b), the anterior cardiac contour is formed by the right ventricle. The posterior contour is formed by the left atrium superiorly, and the left ventricle inferiorly. The posterior border of the IVC can be seen at the level of the diaphragm, creating the most inferior cardiac contour.

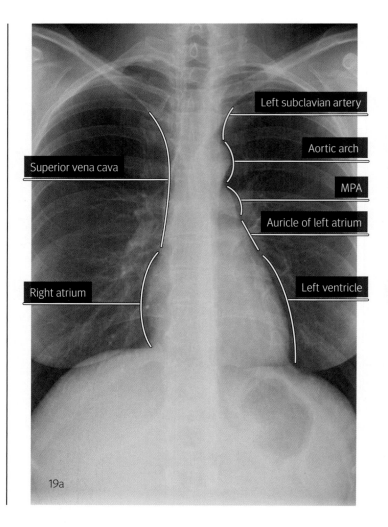

Left subclavian artery

Aortic arch

MPA

Auricle of left atrium

Superior vena cava

Left ventricle

Right atrium

19a

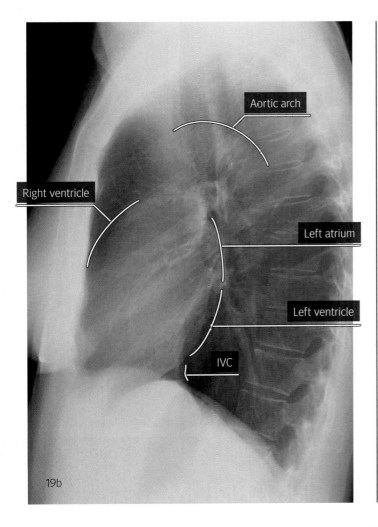

SEGMENT OF CARDIAC CONTOUR	Corresponding Anatomical Structure on the PA
Right – superior	SVC
Right – inferior	Right atrium
Left – superior	Aortic arch
Left – below knob	Pulmonary outflow tract/MPA
Left – below outflow tract	Auricle of left atrium
Left – inferior	Left ventricle

SEGMENT OF CARDIAC CONTOUR	Corresponding Anatomical Structure on the Lateral
Anterior	Right ventricle
Posterior – superior	Left atrium
Posterior – inferior	Left ventricle
Inferior	IVC

Table 10.1
Cardiopericardial Silhouette Contour Segments. IVC, inferior vena cava; MPA, main pulmonary artery, SVC, superior vena cava.

Figure 19. Cardiac-lung interfaces.
A number of interfaces are related to the heart and pericardium. a, PA chest x-ray highlighting the various cardiac contour segments seen on a PA chest x-ray, b, lateral chest x-ray highlighting the various cardiac contour segments seen on a lateral chest x-ray.

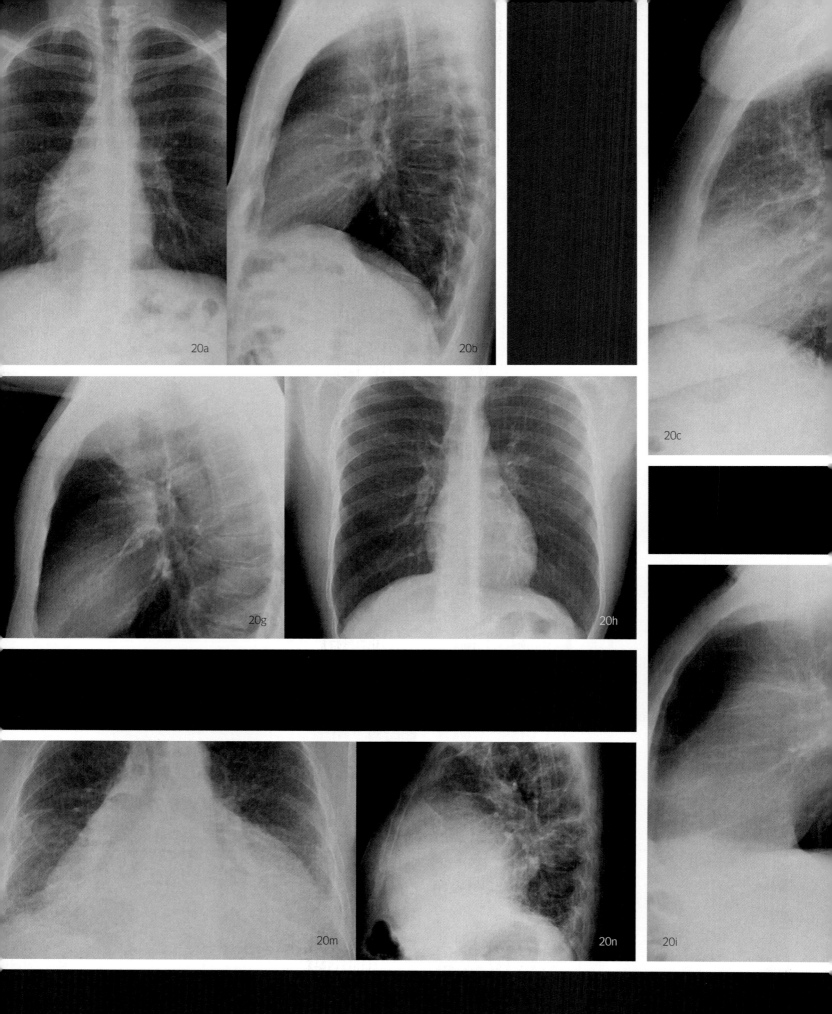

20a

20b

20c

20g

20h

20m

20n

20i

PATHOLOGY OF THE HEART & PERICARDIUM

Example images of diseases and conditions that affect the heart and pericardium

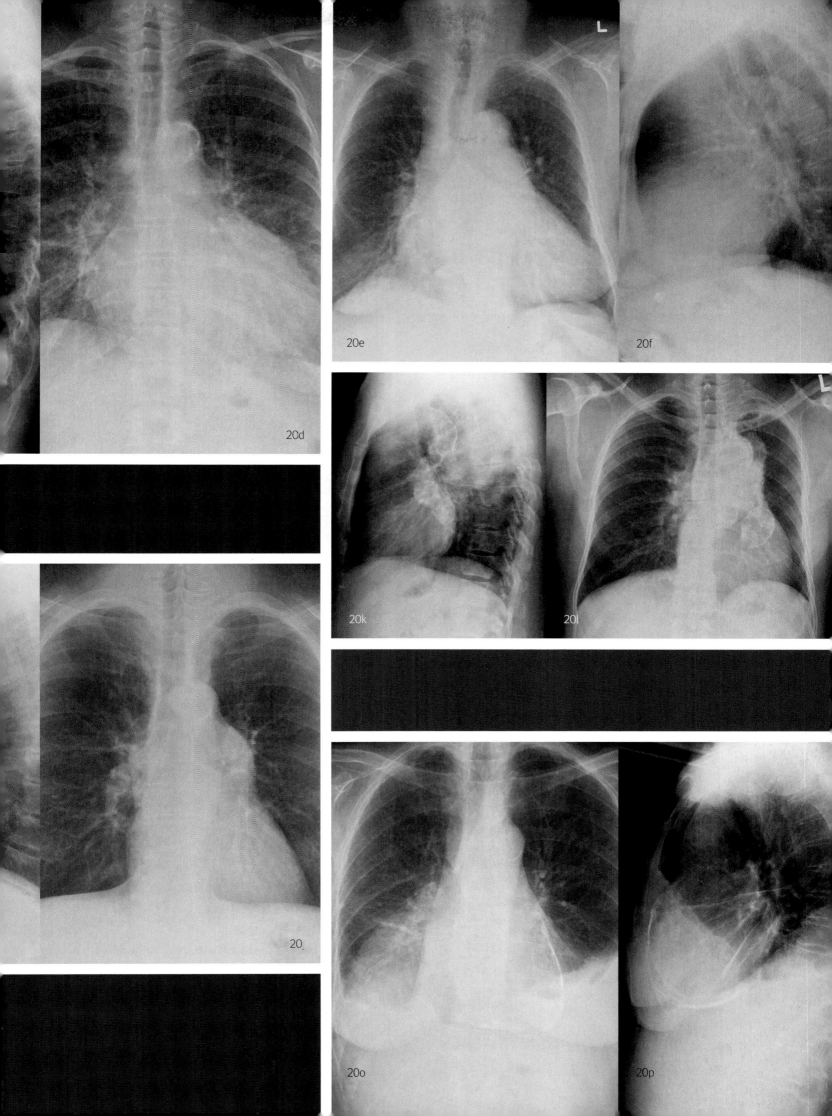

20d

20e

20f

20k

20l

20

20o

20p

THE ABNORMAL HEART

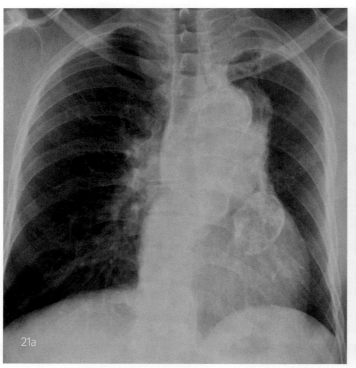

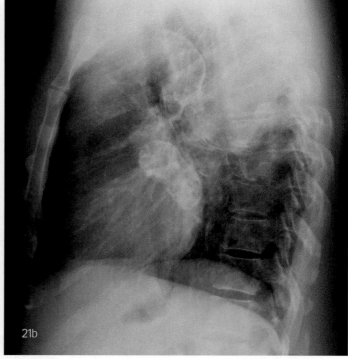

The Radiological Cardiopericardial Silhouette Will Be Abnormal When

1) The grayscale of the cardiopericardial silhouette is too white.

2) The size of the cardiopericardial silhouette is enlarged.

3) The shape of the cardiopericardial silhouette is distorted (focal enlargement of specific cardiopericardial silhouette contours).

4) The position of the cardiopericardial silhouette is shifted.

5) Special case: the Failing Left Heart – Congestive Heart Failure (CHF).

Figure 21. Cardiac calcification. Pathology can cause the grayscale of the heart to appear too white. a, PA chest x-ray in which the heart appears too white due to extensive aortic and cardiac calcification, b, lateral chest x-ray from the same patient.

Figure 22. Left ventricle aneurysm calcification. a, PA chest x-ray from a patient with a calcified left ventricle aneurysm, b, lateral chest x-ray from the same patient.

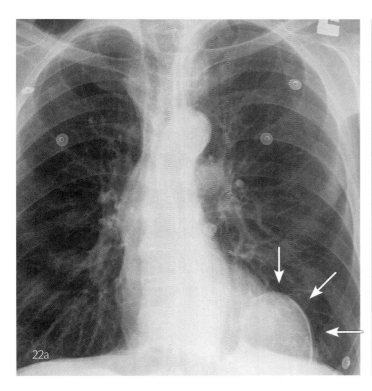

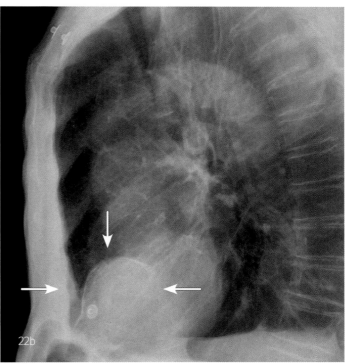

1. Pathology that affects the heart and shifts the grayscale of the cardiopericardial silhouette to 'Too White' - cardiac calcification

Cardiac calcification can involve the endocardium, the myocardium or the pericardium (see the Abnormal Pericardium, **Pg. 374**), as well as the valves and the coronary arteries (14,15). Cardiac calcification can be seen in patients with previous rheumatic heart disease, and in patients following cardiac infarction (Figs. 21a,b and 22a,b).

AMSER

Did you catch the example on pages 356–357?
Fig. 20k,l – Left atrium calcification

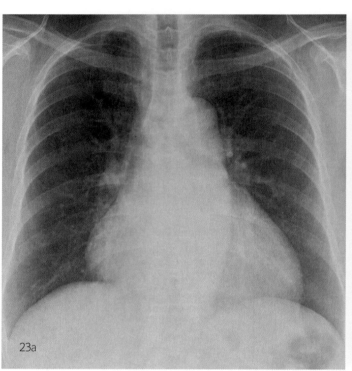

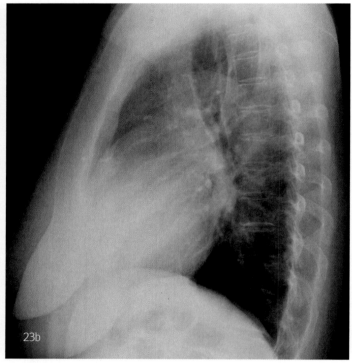

2. Pathology that alters the size of the cardiopericardial silhouette

Cardiac enlargement (Cardiomegaly)

The cardiac silhouette is enlarged if the cardiothoracic ratio exceeds 60% (Pg. 363)(13).

In cases of cardiac enlargement, it is difficult to pinpoint which cardiac chamber is involved. The exception to this is left atrial enlargement, because of its characteristic x-ray features.

An enlarged left atrium will produce a second vertical cardiac contour on the right side of the cardiac shadow, medial to the right cardiac edge (Fig. 23a)(16). The left atrium enlarges from side to side, but also posteriorly. This posterior enlargement will cause splaying of the carinal angle on the PA chest x-ray.

Figure 23. Enlarged heart. Pathology can cause the heart to change in size. a, PA chest x-ray in which the heart looks too big (cardiomegaly), b, lateral chest x-ray from the same case.

Figure 24. Pectus excavatum. Under certain conditions the heart can appear too big, but be normal. a, PA chest x-ray from a patient with pectus excavatum causing the heart to appear too big, and the cardiothoracic (CT) ratio to increase; b, lateral chest x-ray from the same patient. In this case, the enlargement of the heart and CT ratio does not indicate pathology.

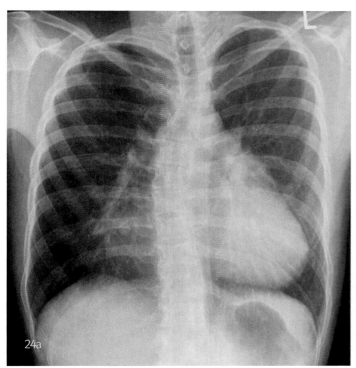

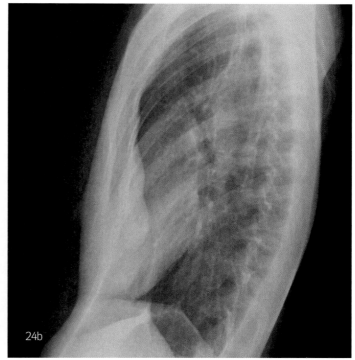

On the lateral view, a prominent opacity may be seen protruding from the posterior border of the heart, just below the level of the carina (T4) (Fig. 23b).

When the cardiopericardial silhouette is enlarged, but normal

The normal heart may appear enlarged on a chest x-ray for various reasons. One cause of apparent cardiac enlargement relates to the technique of the x-ray examination. The heart is an anterior structure. Because of magnification effects (**Ch. 2, Pg. 74**), the heart will look larger on an AP x-ray than on a PA x-ray. The heart will also appear enlarged if the patient has not taken a good inspiration. In addition, the heart appears enlarged in patients with a pectus excavatum deformity of the chest (Fig. 24a,b), because of flattening of the heart between the sternum and the spine – the pinching effect. The heart can also appear enlarged in patients with an absent pericardium.

Did you catch the example on pages 356–357?
Fig. 20e,f – Cardiomegaly

> On x-rays, it may be impossible to differentiate cardiac enlargement from pericardial effusion (Fig. 25a,b,c,d) (16).

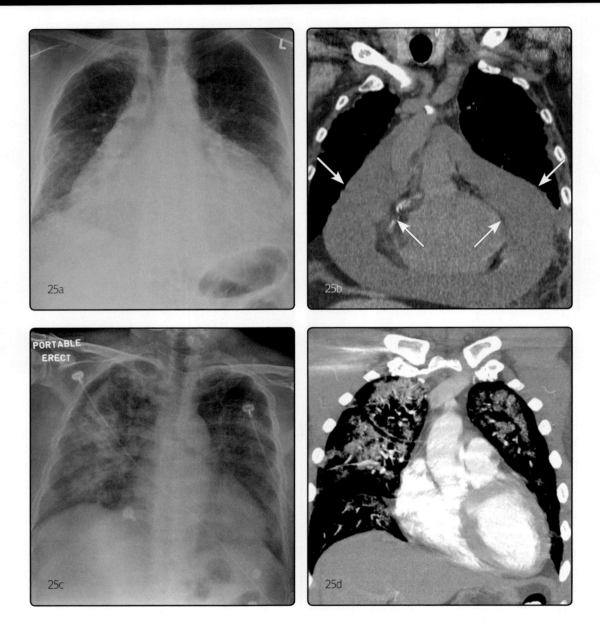

Figure 25. Cardiac enlargement versus pericardial effusion. In some cases it may be difficult to differentiate between cardiac enlargement and pericardial effusion on chest x-rays; in these cases a CT scan is helpful. a, PA chest x-ray with a pericardial effusion, b, CT scan with a pericardial effusion (arrows), c, PA chest x-ray with cardiac enlargement, d, CT scan with cardiac enlargement.

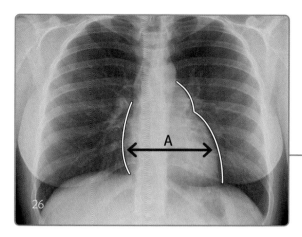

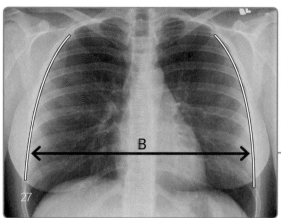

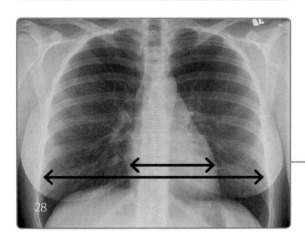

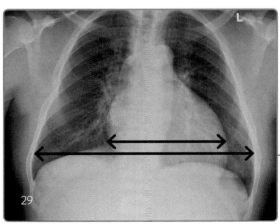

How to measure the cardiothoracic ratio

The cardiothoracic ratio is an important tool for establishing cardiac enlargement.

STEP 1
Confirm that the patient is midline and not rotated (Ch 1, Pg. 32).

STEP 2
Identify the most lateral edges (right and left) of the cardiopericardial silhouette, and measure the distance between them – distance "A" (Fig. 26).

STEP 3
Measure the distance from the lateral edge of one lung to the lateral edge of the other lung – distance "B" (Fig. 27).

STEP 4
Calculate the cardiothoracic ratio (CR). CR = distance A/distance B. In a normal adult, the cardiothoracic ratio should be less than 0.6 (Fig. 28). In cases where the heart is enlarged the cardiothoracic ratio will be >0.6 (Fig. 29).

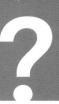

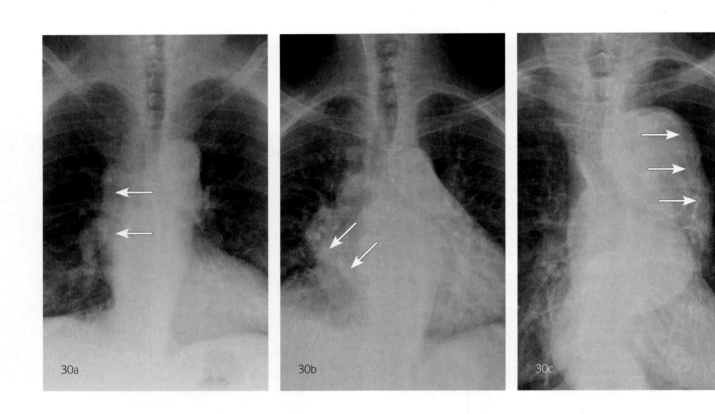

30a

30b

30c

3. Pathology that affects the shape of the cardiopericardial silhouette - abnormalities of specific segments of the cardiac contour

Specific segments of the cardiac contour can enlarge and cause the following x-ray changes.

A dilated ascending aorta will create a bulge, involving the right superior cardiac contour. Instead of the edge of the mediastinum being created by the SVC, it is created by the right edge of the aorta (Fig. 30a).

The lower right cardiac edge can become prominent with right or left atrial enlargement (Fig. 30b).

The aortic arch edge on the left will become prominent with aneurysms (Fig. 30c).

Figure 30. Abnormal cardiac contours. Pathology can alter the shape of the cardiopericardial silhouette; specific segments of the cardiac contour can enlarge due to various pathologies. a, PA chest x-ray with an altered right superior cardiac contour due to a dilated ascending aorta, b, PA chest x-ray with a prominent lower right cardiac edge due to left atrial (LA) enlargement, c, PA chest x-ray with a prominent aortic arch edge due to an aortic aneurysm, d, PA chest x-ray with a prominent main pulmonary artery due to pulmonary hypertension, e, PA chest x-ray with a prominent LA and left atrial appendage (arrows) due to mitral valve disease, f, PA chest x-ray with a prominent left ventricle contour due to a left ventricular (LV) enlargement (LV aneurysm).

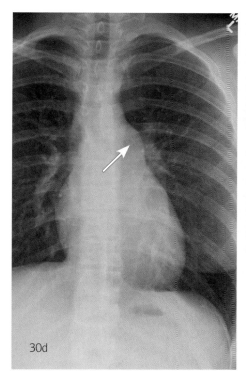

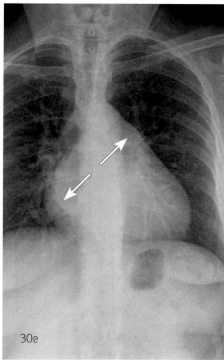

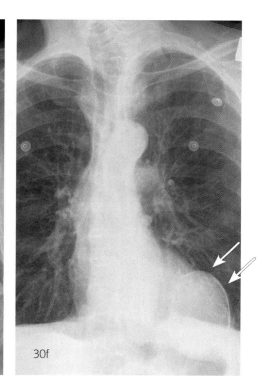

30d

30e

30f

A prominent main pulmonary artery is seen in normal young adults, especially females, but will become very prominent with pulmonary hypertension (Fig. 30d).

The auricle of the left atrium will be prominent with left atrial enlargement (Fig. 30e).

The left ventricle contour becomes prominent with right or left ventricular enlargement (Fig. 30f)

When the shape of the cardiopericardial silhouette is altered, but is normal

On some chest x-rays, the radiological silhouette of the heart may appear abnormal, and yet may not reflect any pathology. For example, in some individuals the heart is pointed toward the right side of the chest instead of the left. This congenital condition is referred to as dextrocardia.

Did you catch the example on pages 356–357?
Fig. 20a,b – Dextrocardia

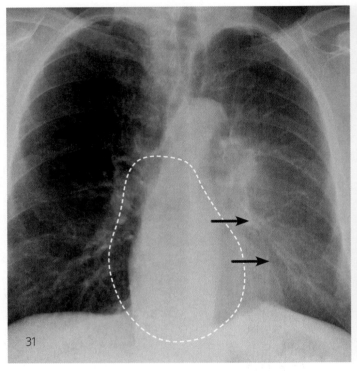

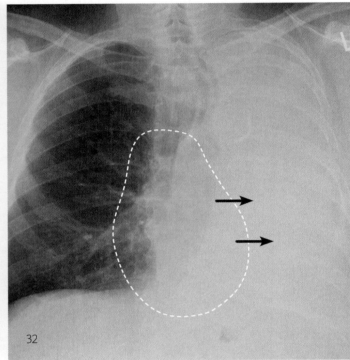

4. Pathology that affects the position of the cardiopericardial silhouette

The position of the cardiopericardial silhouette can change if there is volume loss (e.g., collapse, post-operative) within a lung, causing the mediastinum and the cardiopericardial silhouette to shift towards the involved side (Figs. 31 and 32).

The position of the cardiopericardial silhouette will also shift in cases where there is a large mass, a pleural effusion, or a pneumothorax. In these cases the cardiopericardial silhouette will shift away from the abnormality (Figs. 33 and 34).

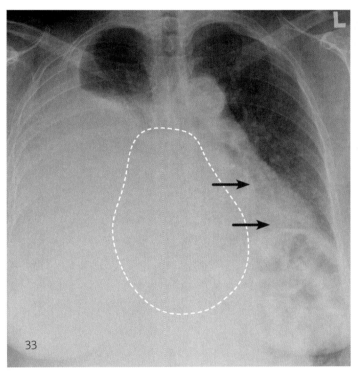

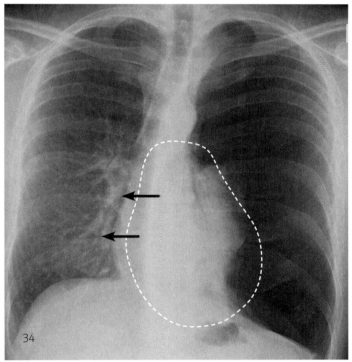

Figure 31. Cardiopericardial silhouette displacement due to left upper lobe collapse. Pathology can cause the position of the cardiopericardial silhouette to shift. PA chest x-ray from a patient with left upper lobe collapse causing the cardiopericardial silhouette to shift to the left, towards the collapse.

Figure 32. Cardiopericardial silhouette displacement due to previous pneumonectomy. Pathology can cause the position of the cardiopericardial silhouette to shift. PA chest x-ray in which the cardiopericardial silhouette is shifted to the left due to a previous left lung pneumonectomy.

Figure 33. Cardiopericardial silhouette displacement due to pleural effusion. Pathology can cause the position of the cardiopericardial silhouette to shift. PA chest x-ray from a patient with a massive pleural effusion in the right hemithorax, causing the cardiopericardial silhouette to be pushed to the left away from the effusion.

Figure 34. Cardiopericardial silhouette displacement due to pneumothorax. Pathology can cause the position of the cardiopericardial silhouette to shift. PA chest x-ray from a patient with a pneumothorax in the left hemithorax causing the cardiopericardial silhouette to be pushed to the right, away from the pneumothorax.

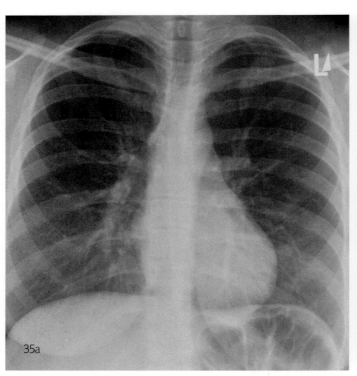

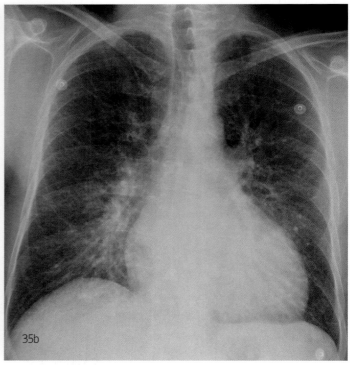

35a

35b

5. SPECIAL CASE: The failing left heart (Congestive Heart Failure, CHF)

The radiological features of the failing left heart involve the heart and the lungs (17,18).

The failing heart can enlarge, causing an increase in the cardiothoracic ratio.

As the ability of the heart to pump blood deteriorates, characteristic chest x-ray features can be anticipated. These are divided into three stages.

STAGE 1

First, there is enlargement of the pulmonary veins. Normally, the lower lobe veins are larger in caliber than similar veins in the upper lobes. With CHF, the upper lobe veins are more prominent, are seen more peripherally, have more visible peripheral branches, and the caliber of the upper lobe veins can become greater than the lower lobe veins (Fig. 35a,b).

STAGE 2

With an increase in hydrostatic pressure, fluid starts leaking into the interstitial spaces (interstitial edema) . Fluid within the bronchovascular interstitium will manifest as bronchial wall cuffing (Fig. 36a). To see bronchial wall cuffing, you need to identify a bronchus on the PA x-ray, which is oriented so it is seen end-on. A normal bronchus will have a very thin border. Bronchial wall cuffing is seen when the border of the bronchus becomes thickened (i.e., cuffed). Fluid within the interstitium surrounding the blood vessels will make the vessels appear blurry - hilar haze.

Fluid accumulating in the interlobular septae will manifest as Kerley B lines. These are thin, distinct, 1 to 2 cm lines that are in the periphery of the lungs and extend to the

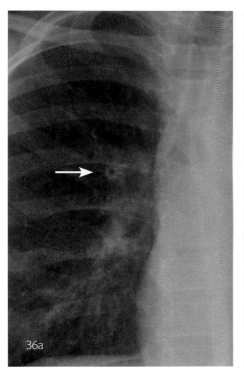

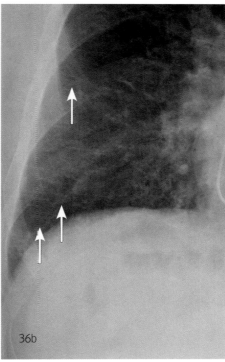

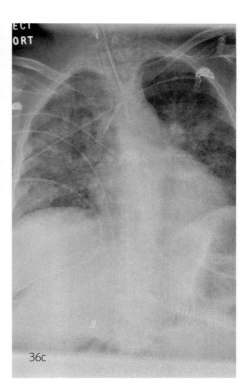

36a   36b   36c

pleura (Fig. 36b). Kerley B lines are most frequently seen on the PA x-ray peripherally and inferiorly, and on the lateral x-ray in the retrosternal airspace.

Fluid accumulating in the more central interstitium will manifest as Kerley A lines. These are thicker, longer (2 to 3 cm) lines, that course across the lungs centrally.

STAGE 3

With further increase in hydrostatic pressure, fluid starts accumulating in the alveolar spaces (alveolar edema). When this happens, ill-defined opacities start appearing on the chest x-ray, first peripherally, but quickly involving all of the lung segments (Fig. 36c). At this point, the patient is very ill and in most cases, only portable x-rays can be performed.

Fluid can also start accumulating in the pleural spaces. When this happens, the pleural fluid first accumulates on the right, and later, on the left.

Did you catch the examples on pages 356–357?
Fig. 20e,f – Cardiomegaly
Fig. 20i,j – Prominent pulmonary outflow tract

Figure 35. Congestive heart failure (CHF) - Stage 1. In the first stage of CHF the upper lobe veins become larger in caliber than the lower lobe veins. a, Normal PA chest x-ray; note the larger size of the lower lobe veins, b, PA chest x-ray from patient with CHF; note the larger upper lobe veins.

Figure 36. Congestive heart failure (CHF) - Stages 2&3. Pulmonary edema is the major feature of CHF in the latter stages, and manifests in different ways. a, PA chest x-ray with bronchial cuffing (arrow), b, PA chest x-ray with Kerley B lines (arrows), c, PA chest x-ray with alveolar edema.

HEART & PERICARDIUM **Chapter 10** SECTION II

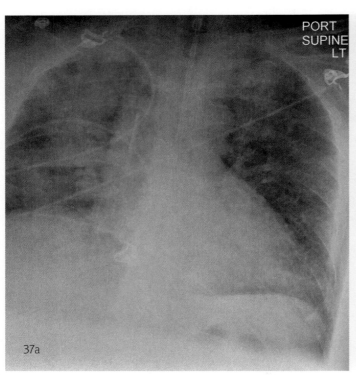

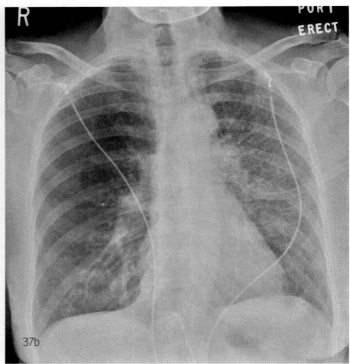

The Abnormal Pulmonary Vasculature

Understanding the radiological features of a failing heart requires an understanding of the normal, and the abnormal, appearance of the pulmonary vasculature (19,20,21). A detailed description of the pulmonary vasculature is found in **Chapter 8**. Included in this chapter is only a brief discussion about changes to the vasculature, specifically relating to the failing heart.

Engorgement of the Pulmonary VEINS

Pulmonary venous hypertension

The pulmonary veins can get engorged in pulmonary venous hypertension. The upper lobe vessels are equal or larger than the lower lobe vessels, and the descending branch of the RPA is normal in size (less than 17 mm).

Enlargement of the Pulmonary ARTERIES

Pulmonary arterial hypertension

The pulmonary arteries can enlarge in pulmonary arterial hypertension. The descending branch of the right pulmonary artery is less than 17 mm, and the upper lobe vessels are smaller than the lower lobe vessels. There is pruning of the peripheral vessels.

Shunt vascularity

Enlargement of the pulmonary arteries can also increase in situations where the circulation to the lungs is increased, as in shunt vascularity. Similar to pulmonary arterial hypertension, the descending branch of the right pulmonary artery is less than 17 mm. However, in cases of shunt vascularity, the upper lobe vessels are equal or larger than the lower lobe vessels.

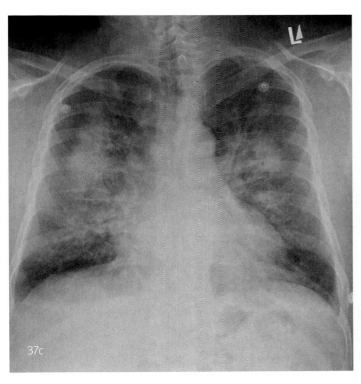

37c

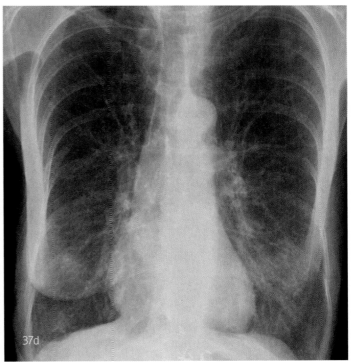

37d

In cases of cardiac failure, the radiological pulmonary vasculature will be abnormal when the size of the upper lobe vessels is enlarged – this is called vascular redistribution.

The Many Faces of Cardiac Failure

Rarely, pulmonary edema can occur in one lung – unilateral pulmonary edema (Fig. 37a,b). This has been documented in patients who develop pulmonary edema following thoracocentesis, or in patients with cardiac failure, who lie continuously on one side.

Pulmonary edema occurring in some anuric patients (i.e., those in renal failure) can manifest with alveolar edema accumulating predominantly in the perihilar regions. This is referred to as Bat Wing Edema (Fig. 37c).

Pulmonary edema (Fig. 37d), occurring in patients with emphysema can have an unusual distribution of both the interstitial and alveolar edema.

Did you catch the example on pages 356–357?
Fig. 20c,d – Cardiac failure

Figure 37. Variations in the appearance of pulmonary edema. Pulmonary edema can have different appearances on an x-ray, a,b, PA chest x-rays from patients with unilateral pulmonary edema, c, PA chest x-ray from a patient with Batwing edema. c, PA chest x-ray from a patient with edema with COPD, d, PA chest x-ray from a patient with pulmonary edema with emphysema.

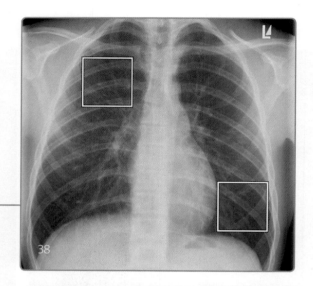

How to assess for vascular redistribution

Assessing for vascular redistribution is important for determining patient fluid status and diagnosing congestive heart failure.

STEP 1
Make sure that the examination was taken in the erect position, and with good inspiration.

STEP 2
Identify a 3 X 3 cm area in the RUL, below the clavicles, lateral to the SVC, and above the hilum (Fig. 38).

STEP 3
Within this area, identify individual blood vessels and note their caliber (Fig. 39).

STEP 4
Now identify a similar size area in the RLL, and note the caliber of the vessels (Fig. 40).

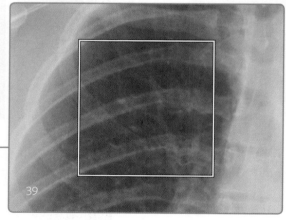

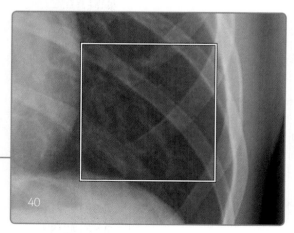

In the normal population, on an erect examination with full inspiration, the upper lobe vessels are smaller in caliber than the vessels of the lower lobes. This is because the blood flow is greater in the lower lobes. This does not hold true on **SUPINE** x-rays in which the upper lobe vessels can be the same size as the lower lobe vessels.

Vascular redistribution may be impossible to identify on chest x-rays in patients with chronic obstructive pulmonary disease (COPD), because the hyperinflated lungs characteristic of COPD will not allow the vessels to enlarge.

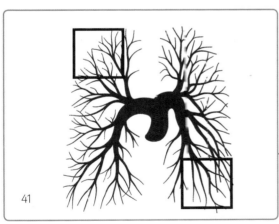

41

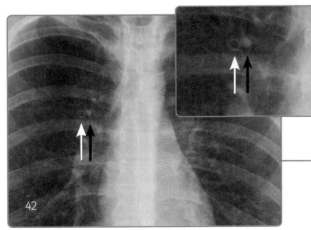

42

STEP 5
Compare the caliber of the vessels in the upper lung zone to the caliber of the vessels in the lower lung zone. Normally, the upper zone vessels are smaller than the lower zone vessels (Fig. 41).

STEP 6
Compare the caliber of the vessels to the adjacent bronchi. In the normal patient, the diameters should be the same (Fig. 42).

THE ABNORMAL PERICARDIUM

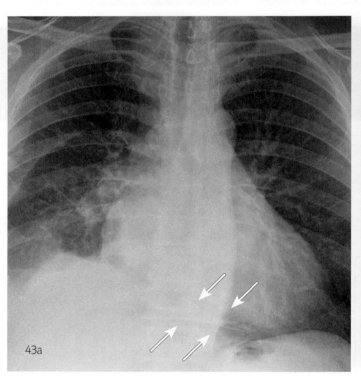

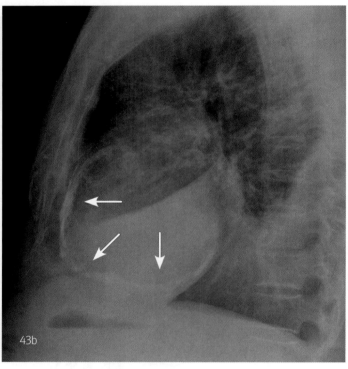

The Radiological Pericardium Will be Abnormal When

1) The grayscale of the pericardium is too white or too black.

2) The size of the pericardium is too big or too small.

1a. Pathology that affects the pericardium and shifts the grayscale to 'Too White'

The pericardium can calcify. If the calcification is tangential to the x-ray beam, it will be seen on PA and lateral x-rays as curvilinear white opacities, outlining the cardiac contours (Fig. 43a,b). Pericardial calcification occurs predominantly on the right, over the anterior and diaphragmatic aspects of the heart (15).

1b. Pathology that affects the pericardium and shifts the grayscale to 'Too Black'

Air within the pericardial sac (i.e., pneumopericardium) will cause the grayscale to shift to too black. The air will outline the exterior of the heart medially and the pericardium laterally (Fig. 44).

2. Pathology that alters the size of the cardiopericardial silhouette

Enlarged pericardium – pericardial effusion and tamponade

The pericardium, similar to the pleura, can accumulate fluid; referred to as a pericardial effusion (22).

If the accumulation of fluid is slow, the cardiopericardial silhouette will enlarge and will have a rounded appearance

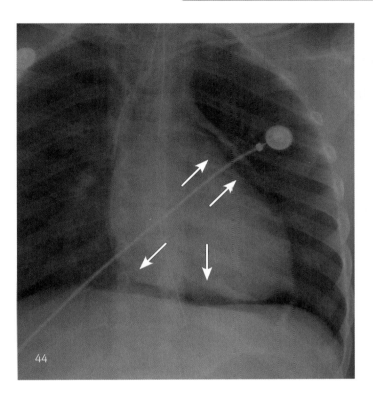

44

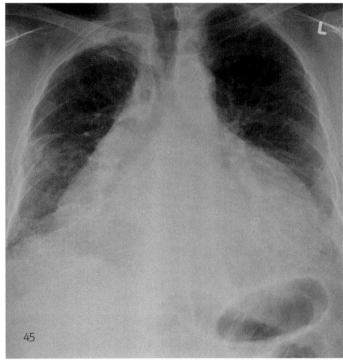

45

(Fig. 45). Displacement of the pericardial fat pad can occasionally be seen.

When the accumulation of fluid is rapid, such as in a hemorrhage into the pericardial sac, the accumulated fluid can restrict the return of blood to the heart and cause acute cardiac tamponade.

Instead of fluid, air can enter into the pericardial sac causing a pneumopericardium. Rapid accumulation of pericardial air can also lead to acute tamponade.

Did you catch the examples on pages 356–357?
Fig. 20m,n – Pericardial effusion
Fig. 20o,p – Pericardial calcification

Figure 43. Pericardial calcification. Pathology can cause the grayscale of the pericardium to appear too white. a, PA chest x-ray in which the pericardium appears too white due to pericardial calcifications, b, lateral chest x-ray from the same patient. Note the region of too white in the pericardium (arrows).

Figure 44. Pneumopericardium. Pathology can cause the grayscale of the pericardium to appear too black. PA chest x-ray in which the pericardium appears too big due to air in the pericardial sac (arrows), a pneumopericardium.

Figure 45. Enlarged pericardium. Pathology can cause the pericardium to appear too big. PA chest x-ray in which the pericardium appears too big due to a pericardial effusion.

Pathology That Alters the Size of the Pericardium and Distorts the Cardiopericardial Silhouette

Absent pericardium

Congenital absence of the pericardium is rare, and occurs as the result of agenesis of the left common cardiac vein, and abnormal development of the pleuropericardial membrane (23). These congenital pericardial defects can occur alone, or in association with other congenital anomalies. The most common form is complete absence of the left pericardium. When this occurs, the apex of the heart may be displaced and the cardiac silhouette will appear more horizontal (Fig. 46).

The pericardium may also be absent due to clinical intervention. This occurs when the pericardium is invaded by tumor and is partially removed during thoracic surgery.

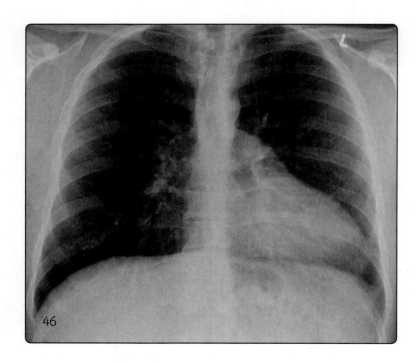

Figure 46. Absent pericardium. Congenitally absent pericardium causing a shift in the apex of the heart, and as a result, a change in the shape of the cardiopericardial silhouette.

SUMMARY OF RADIOLOGICAL CHANGES
TO THE HEART & PERICARDIUM

RADIOLOGICAL CHANGES TO THE...		HEART	PERICARDIUM
1. Change in grayscale	Too white	• Calcification (endocardium, myocardium, valves, coronary arteries) (due to: rheumatic heart disease, post-cardiac infarction)	• Calcification
	Too black	---	• Air (post-op) trauma • Pneumopericardium
2. Change in size	Too big	• Cardiac enlargement (general) (Cardiomegaly) • Left atrial enlargement	• Pericardial effusion • Pneumopericardium
	Too small	• COPD (hyperinflation of lungs makes heart look smaller)	
3. Change in shape		• Dilated ascending aorta • Atrial enlargement • Aneurysm • Ventricular enlargement • Pulmonary hypertension • Dextrocardia	• Congenital absence of pericardium
4. Change in position		• Pneumothorax • Pleural effusion • Tumor • Lung collapse • Surgery	• Congenital absence of pericardium
4. Special Case: CHF		• Interstitial edema • Bronchial wall cuffing • Kerley A lines • Kerley B lines • Alveolar edema • Pleural fluid • Bat-wing edema	----

Table 10.2
Summary of Radiological Changes to the Heart & Pericardium. COPD, chronic obstructive pulmonary disease, CHF, congestive heart failure.

Visual Search of the Heart & Pericardium

PA Chest X-ray

1. Start on the right superiorly at the level of the SVC (1).

2. Follow the lateral outline of the heart inferiorly to the right cardiophrenic angle (2).

3. Follow the inferior outline of the heart medially to the left cardiophrenic angle (3).

4. Follow the left outline of heart superiorly to above the aorta (4).

Complete the visual search by checking for any density changes across the heart from top to bottom.

Lateral Chest X-ray

1. Start at the top anterior to the trachea (1).

2. Follow the anterior outline of the heart inferiorly to the anterior diaphragm (2).

3. Follow the inferior outline of the heart posteriorly to the posterior cardiac edge (3).

4. Follow posterior outline of heart superiorly to the thoracic inlet (4).

Complete the visual search by checking for any density changes across the heart from top to bottom.

VS

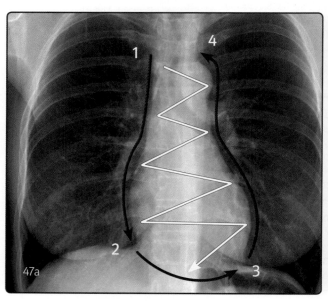

47a

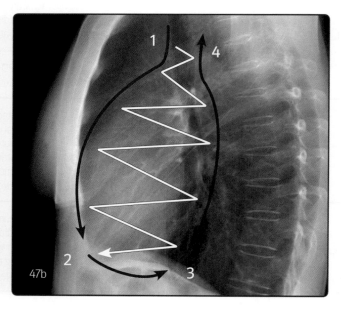

47b

Heart & Pericardium Radiological Analysis Checklist

To confidently state that the heart and pericardium are normal all parts of the checklist should indicate a normal appearance.

GRAYSCALE

1 Is the grayscale of the cardiopericardial silhouette altered?

If **YES**, then describe.
Too white/too black.

SIZE

2 Is the size of the cardiopericardial silhouette altered?

If **YES**, then describe.
Too big/too small.
Pathological/magnification effect/pectus excavatum.

POSITION

3 Is the position of the cardiopericardial silhouette shifted?

If **YES**, then describe.
Up/down.
Right/left.
Anterior/posterior.

SHAPE

4 Is the shape of the cardiopericardial silhouette distorted?

If **YES**, then describe.
Name specific contour.
Pathological/normal variant.

OTHER

5 Is there any evidence of previous surgery to the heart or pericardium?

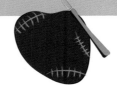

If **YES**, then describe.
Type of surgery and location.
Compare to previous CXR.

CONGESTIVE HEART FAILURE

6 Are there signs of vascular redistribution?

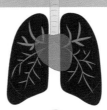

If **YES**, then describe.
Pulmonary venous hypertension/
pulmonary arterial hypertension /
shunt vascularity.

7 Are there signs of edema?

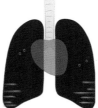

If **YES**, then describe.
Interstitial/alveolar.
Kerley A/Kerley B/cuffing.

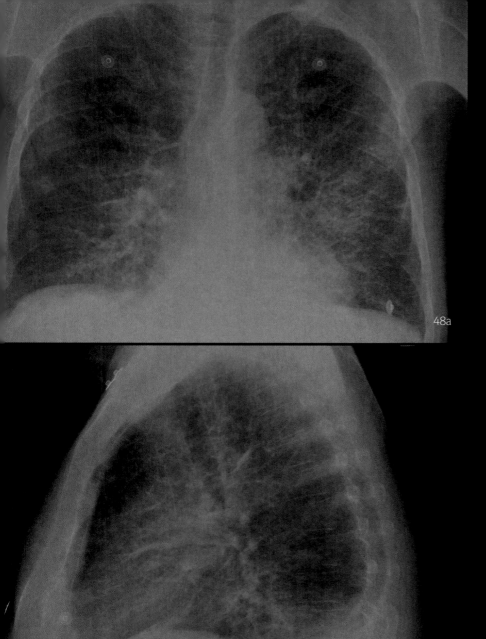

48a

48b

How would you
describe your findings
to the staff physician?

CASE STUDY

During one of your overnight on-call shifts, a 60-year-old post-operative male patient suddenly complains of shortness of breath. He does not have any associated chest pain, palpitations, sweating or nausea. The patient is gasping for each breath and you sit him up from his recumbent position and start him on high-flow oxygen. He feels a bit better at this time and you set off to investigate possible causes of his shortness of breath. You suspect that the patient is suffering from congestive heart failure and you order a chest x-ray, stat (Fig. 48a,b). The staff physician on duty calls you from a dinner party and demands to know immediately what the chest x-ray shows... there is no time to wait for a formal report from a radiologist. What do you tell the staff physician?

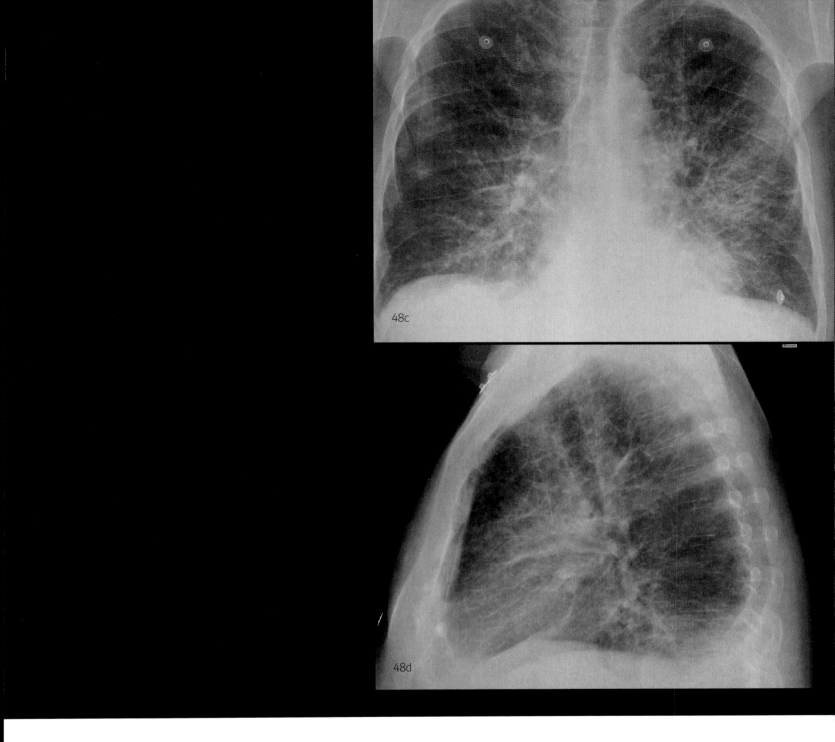

48c

48d

Recognizing a failing heart on a chest x-ray is a crucial skill to master. As you have read in this chapter, the features of a failing heart on a chest x-ray involve both the heart and lungs. Figures 48c and 48d show the following features. The heart is mildly enlarged. There is prominence of the upper lobe vessels, perihilar haze, bronchial cuffing, and increased interstitial and alveolar densities. Kerley B lines are evident. The patient has bilateral pleural effusions.

Based on the findings, the diagnosis is interstitial and alveolar pulmonary edema.

1. Rose, C.P., & Stolberg, H.O. (1983). The limited utility of the plain chest film in the assessment of left ventricular structure and function. *Invest. Radiol.,* *17*:139–144.

2. Lewis, P.J., Shaffer, K., & Donovan, A. (Eds.). (2012). AMSER National Medical Student Curriculum in Radiology. http://aur.org/Secondary-Alliances.aspx?id=141.

3. Lewis, P.J., & Shaffer, K. (2005). Developing a national medical student curriculum in radiology. *Am. Coll. Radiol., 2*(1):8–11.

4. Anderson, R.H., Razavi, R., & Taylor, A.M. (2004). Cardiac anatomy revisited. *J. Anat., 205*:159-177.

5. Anderson, R.H., & Loukas, M. (2008). The importance of attitudinally appropriate description of cardiac anatomy. *Clin. Anat., 22*:47–51.

6. Muresian, H. (2009). The clinical anatomy of the mitral valve. *Clin. Anat., 22*(1):85–98.

7. Romero, R.C., & Boxt, L.M. (1999). Plain-film evaluation of valvular heart disease. *Semin. Roentgenol., 34*(3):216–227.

8. Coulden, R., & Lipton, M.J. (1994). Radiological examination in valvular heart disease. In: Zaibag, M.A., & Duran, C. (Eds.). *Valvular heart disease.* New York, NY: Marcel Dekker.

9. Broderick, L.S., Brooks, G.N., & Kuhlman, J.E. (2005). Anatomic pitfalls of the heart and pericardium. *RadioGraphics, 25*:441–453.

10. Hipona, F.A., & Paredes, S. (1976). The radiology of pericardial disease. *Cardiovasc. Clin., 7*:91–124.

11. Paling, M.R., & Pope, T.L. Jr. (1987). The variable nature of the mediastinal contour lines: CT/Chest radiography correlation. *J. Computed Tomography, 11*:254–260.

12. Carsky, E.W., Mauceri, R.A., & Azimi, F. (1980). The epicardial fat pad sign: analysis of frontal and lateral chest radiographs in patients with pericardial effusion. *Radiology, 137*(2):303–308.

13. Baron, M.G. (2000). The cardiac silhouette. *J. Thorac. Imag., 15*(4):230–242.

14. Ferguson, E.C., & Berkowitz, E.A. (2010). Cardiac and pericardial calcifications on chest radiographs. *Clin. Radiol., 65*(9):685–694.

15. MacGregor, J.H., Chen, J.T., Chiles, C., et al. (1987). The radiographic distinction between pericardial and myocardial calcifications. *AJR Am. J. Roentgenol., 148*(4):675–677.

16. Arendt, J. (1948). Radiological differentiation between pericardial effusion and cardiac dilatation. *Radiology, 50*(1):44–51.

17. Pistolesi, M., Miniati, M., Milne, E.N.C., et al. (1985). The chest roentgenogram in pulmonary edema. *Clin. Chest Med., 6*:315–344.

18. Ely, E.W., & Haponik, E.F. (2002). Using the chest radiograph to determine intravascular volume status: the role of vascular pedicle width. *Chest, 121*:942–950.

19. Tops, L.F., van der Wall, E.E., Schalij, M.J., & Bax, J.J. (2007). Multi-modality imaging to assess left atrial size, anatomy and function. *Heart, 93*(11):1461–1470.

20. McHugh, T.J., Forrester, J.S., Adler, L., et al. (1972). Pulmonary vascular congestion in acute myocardial infarction: Hemodynamic and radiologic correlations. *Ann. Intern. Med., 76*:29–33.

21. Woodring, J.H. (1991). Pulmonary artery-bronchus ratios in patients with normal lungs, pulmonary vascular plethora, and congestive heart failure. *Radiology, 179*:115–122.

22. Mellins, H.Z., Kottmeier, P., & Kiely, B. (1959). Radiologic signs of pericardial effusion; an experimental study. *Radiology, 73*(1):9–16.

23. Abbas, A.E., Appleton, C.P., Liu, P.T., & Sweeney, J.P. (2005). Congenital absence of the pericardium: case presentation and review of literature. *Int. J. Cardiol., 98*:21–25

CHAPTER 11
The PLEURA
(the pleural zone)

importance

The pleura is involved in many disease processes, and a systematic examination of the pleura on the PA and lateral chest x-rays is an important habit to develop. The pleura and the pleural spaces are not directly visualized on standard x-rays; however, this chapter provides the tools to identify the pleural zone, and to rapidly check for pathology. Understanding the concept of the potential pleural space is essential to understanding the radiological appearance of pathology that can affect this radiological zone.

The accurate localization of pathology to the pleura is important for differential diagnoses, and for communicating your findings to the patient and other members of the healthcare team. Pathology involving the pleura can be life-threatening and requires accurate, prompt detection. You will learn how to identify a pneumothorax and other potentially fatal conditions that involve the pleura. You do not want to miss a life-threatening pneumothorax!

objectives

Skills

You will identify

- the normal radiological appearance of the pleura, the borders of the pleural space, and the location of the pleura on the PA and lateral chest x-rays.

- the pleural fissures on the PA and lateral chest x-rays.

- the azygous fissure (accessory fissure) and lobe on the PA and lateral chest x-rays.

- important radiological signs related to the pleura.

- common pathology localized to the pleura and pleural space, and determine the degree of pathology involving the pleura.

You will provide

- a systematic approach for the review of the pleura.

- a differential diagnosis for pleural abnormalities.

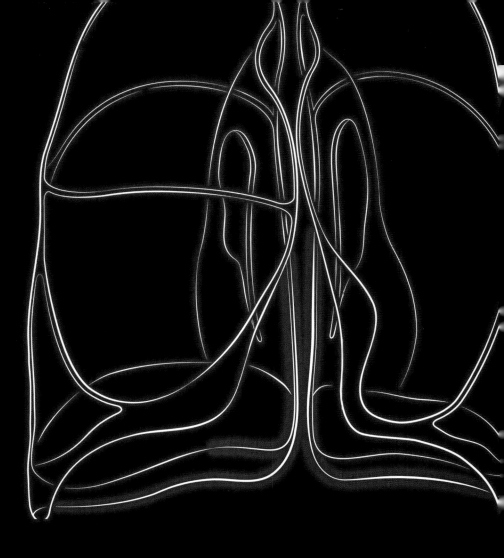

Knowledge

You will review and understand

- the definition of the pleura, and its relationship to the lungs and thoracic cavity.
- the normal anatomy of the pleura and fissures.
- why pathology changes the radiological appearance of the pleural space.

associated resources

This chapter maps to the following AMSER curriculum content (1,2).

1) Normal radiological anatomy of the pleura.
    Costophrenic and cardicphrenic angles
    Minor and major fissures
    Azygos lobe

2) Pathological conditions affecting the pleura.
    Pleural effusion: small, large, importance of subpulmonic, decubitus, supine and upright x-rays
    Pneumothorax: small, large, tension, importance of supine, upright, decubitus and expiratory x-rays
    Pneumomediastinum
    Empyema
    Pleural thickening and calcifications (asbestos exposure)
    Pseudotumor

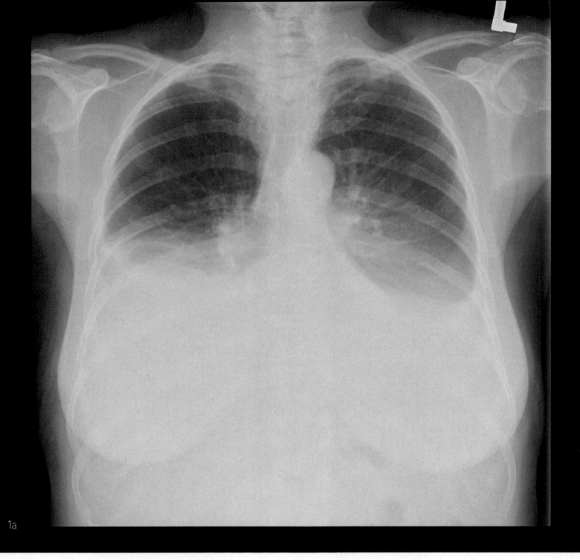

1a

You are called to the ward to see a 58-year-old female patient who has been admitted with a two-week history of shortness of breath, a productive cough, and fever. The nurse claims that her dyspnea has been getting worse throughout the day. You examine the patient and find that there is stony dullness on percussion of the lung bases, and decreased breath sounds bilaterally. You request PA and lateral chest x-rays (Fig. 1a,b).

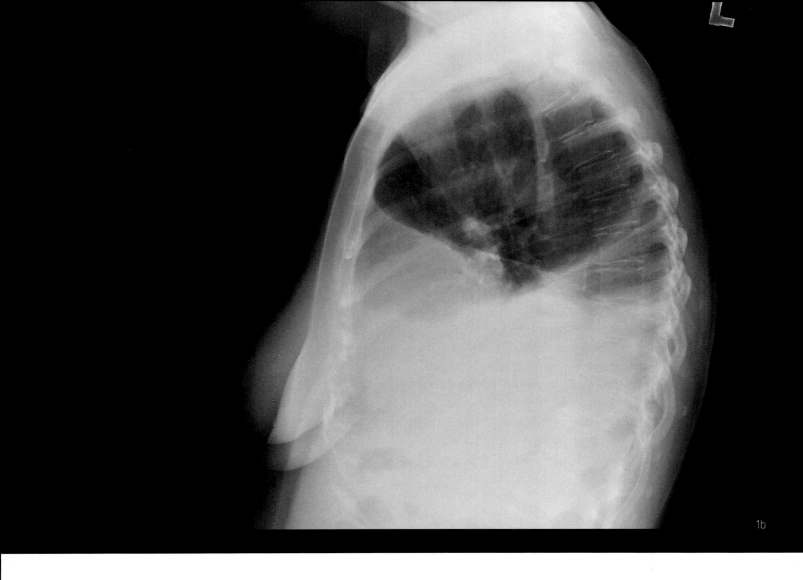

1b

What do you see
on the chest x-rays?

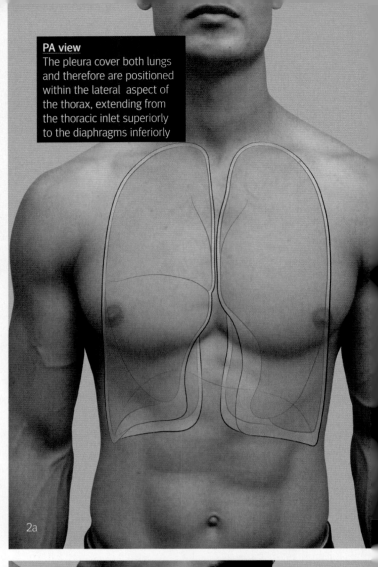

2a

WHAT IS THE PLEURA
(THE PLEURAL ZONE) ?

Lying just beyond the outer edges of the lungs, the pleural zone is roughly defined by the region of the thorax that is occupied by the lungs. The apex of the pleura (and, therefore, of the pleural zone) corresponds to the apex of the lungs, and lies medially, 2.5 cm above the clavicles, and posterior to the sternocleidomastoid muscle (Fig. 2a). The lower limits of the pleura cross the 8th rib in the midclavicular line, the 10th rib in the midaxillary line, and the 12th rib at the lateral border of the spine. During normal respiration, the lower limits of the pleura are usually 5 cm below the lower edge of the lung (Fig. 2b) (3).

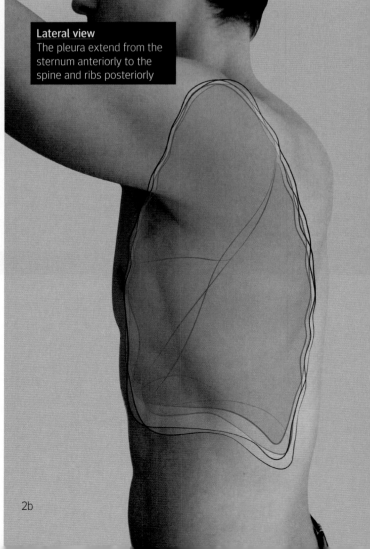

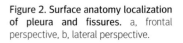

Figure 2. Surface anatomy localization of pleura and fissures. a, frontal perspective, b, lateral perspective.

2b

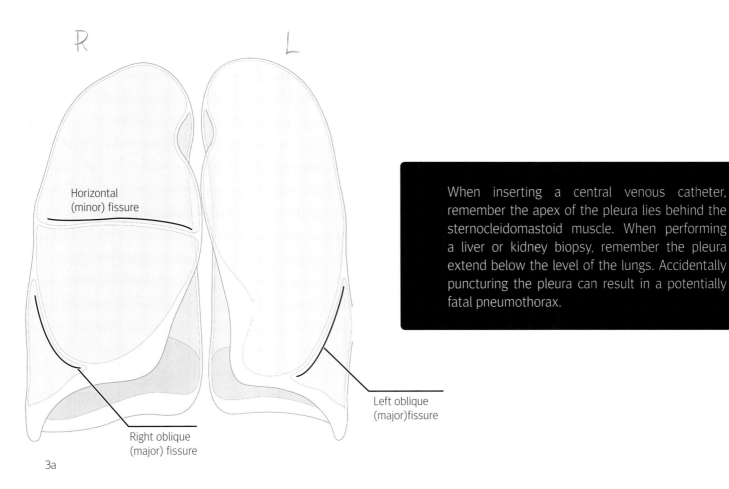

Horizontal
(minor) fissure

Right oblique
(major) fissure

Left oblique
(major)fissure

3a

When inserting a central venous catheter, remember the apex of the pleura lies behind the sternocleidomastoid muscle. When performing a liver or kidney biopsy, remember the pleura extend below the level of the lungs. Accidentally puncturing the pleura can result in a potentially fatal pneumothorax.

Horizontal
(minor) fissure

Oblique
(major) fissures

3b

The Pleura

The word *pleura* is taken from the Greek language, and refers to "the rib", or to "the side of the body wall containing the ribs". The pleura is a thin, double-layered, serous membrane.

A component of the pleura covers the outer surface of the lungs, and this is called the visceral pleura. The visceral pleura also covers the internal surfaces of the lung lobes, creating the fissures (Fig. 3a,b).

Figure 3. Anatomy of the pleura.
Illustration of the pleura, a, frontal perspective, b, lateral perspective.

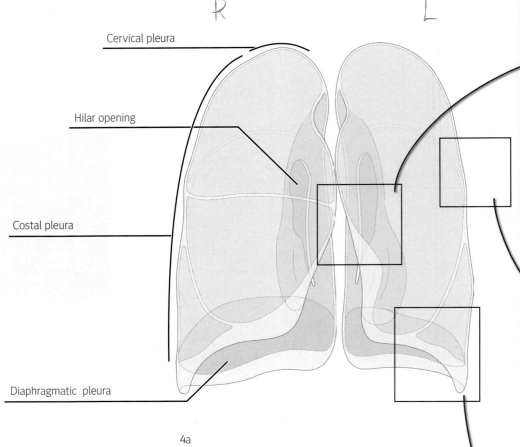

Cervical pleura

Hilar opening

Costal pleura

Diaphragmatic pleura

4a

At the root of each lung, there is an opening in the visceral pleura. Here, the visceral pleura is reflected back on itself to form a double layer, and the visceral pleura continues as the parietal pleura. The parietal pleura (the outer pleural layer) covers the chest wall, pericardium and diaphragms. The parietal pleura is attached to the bony thorax by a layer of fibrous tissue called the endothoracic fascia.

The parietal pleura can be divided into regions, based on the anatomical structures it abuts (Fig. 4a,b).

Costal Pleura – the portion that covers the internal surfaces of the thoracic wall, or the rib cage.

Mediastinal Pleura – the portion that covers the lateral borders of the mediastinum.

Diaphragmatic Pleura – the portion that covers the superior border of the diaphragm on each side of the mediastinum.

Cervical Pleura – the cup-shaped portion that covers the apex of the lungs (also called the cupola).

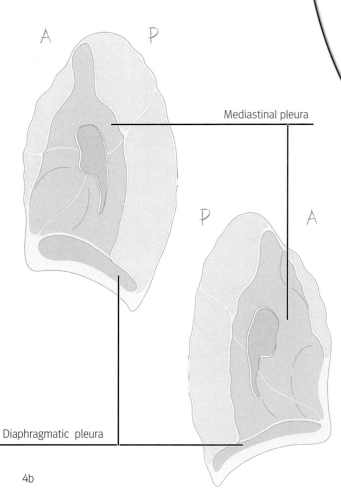

Mediastinal pleura

Diaphragmatic pleura

4b

Figure 4. Regions of the pleura. Illustration of the regions of the parietal pleura, a, frontal perspective, b, lateral perspective.

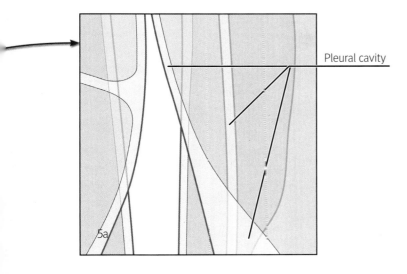

Pleural cavity

5a

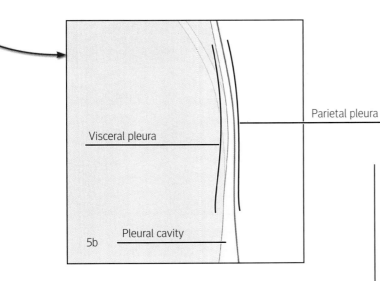

Visceral pleura

Parietal pleura

Pleural cavity

5b

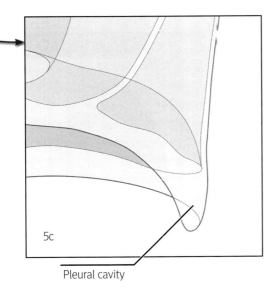

5c

Pleural cavity

The Pleural Cavity / Pleural Space

Between the visceral pleura and the parietal pleura exists a thin space – the pleural space or pleural cavity (Fig. 5a,b,c). Within the pleural space, at any moment, under normal conditions, a thin film of fluid (approximately 7-16 ml) is present. The pleural cavity, therefore, exists as a potential space that can accumulate air or fluid in pathological conditions.

Normally, a balance exists between the total daily production of pleural fluid (approximately 250 ml) and the total daily fluid absorption. Pleural fluid will accumulate in the pleural space when the balance is disrupted; when more fluid is produced or introduced than can be absorbed.

Figure 5. The pleural cavity. Illustration of the pleural cavity, a,b,c, a series of magnifications of the frontal view in Figure 4a highlighting the various aspects of the pleural cavity.

PLEURA **Chapter 11** SECTION II

Radiological Shape and Grayscale of the Pleura (I)

The visceral pleura lies on the surface of the lungs, and the parietal pleura is adherent to the chest wall. However, neither the parietal nor the visceral pleura can be seen on x-rays. They are both too thin to absorb sufficient radiation to form a definable radiological structure. The small amount of fluid normally present within the pleural space is also not enough to be visible on x-rays.

The location of the pleura can be inferred by locating other, clearly visible, anatomical structures, such as the lungs. The superior, lateral, and medial borders of the lungs define the location of respective borders of the pleura. The location of the inferior pleural border is more complex because the inferior reflections of the pleura extend lower than the lowest borders of the lungs, especially posteriorly and posteromedially. Inferiorly and anteriorly, the superior border of the diaphragms corresponds to the inferior border of the pleura (4).

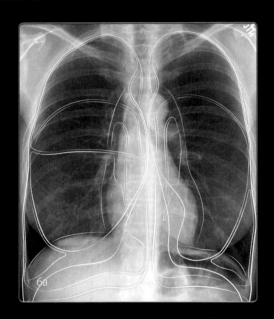

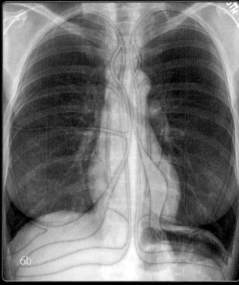

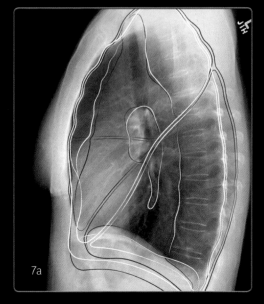

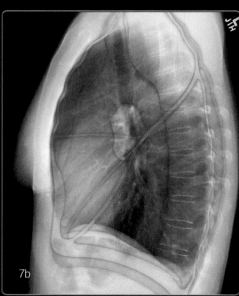

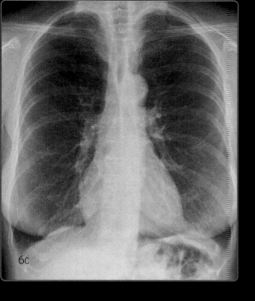

Figure 6. Radiological anatomy of the pleura from the frontal perspective. a, PA chest x-ray with the pleura outlined, b, PA chest x-ray with grayscale illustration of the pleura overlay, c, PA chest x-ray cropped to highlight the pleura.

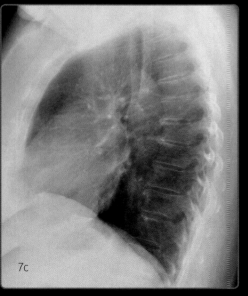

Figure 7. Radiological anatomy of the pleura from the lateral perspective: a, lateral chest x-ray with the pleura outlined, b, lateral chest x-ray with grayscale illustration of the pleura overlay, c, lateral chest x-ray cropped to highlight the pleura.

Radiological Shape and Grayscale of the Pleura (II)

Although we are not able to view the pleura entirely on an x-ray, there are a number of components of the pleura that are visible. Looking at these components, in conjunction with the anatomical reference structures below, helps us to infer the position of the normal pleura, and deduce whether or not the pleura is diseased. These components, on the PA (Fig. 8a) and lateral (Fig. 8b) x-rays, are the following.

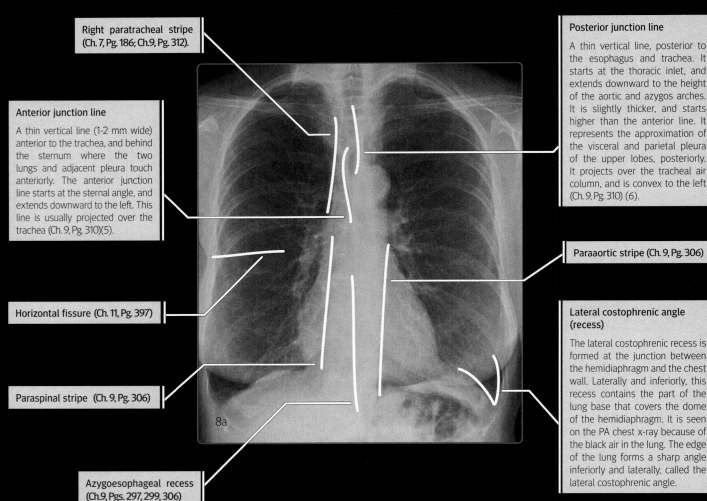

8a

Right paratracheal stripe (Ch. 7, Pg. 186; Ch.9, Pg. 312).

Anterior junction line

A thin vertical line (1-2 mm wide) anterior to the trachea, and behind the sternum where the two lungs and adjacent pleura touch anteriorly. The anterior junction line starts at the sternal angle, and extends downward to the left. This line is usually projected over the trachea (Ch. 9, Pg. 310)(5).

Horizontal fissure (Ch. 11, Pg. 397)

Paraspinal stripe (Ch. 9, Pg. 306)

Azygoesophageal recess (Ch.9, Pgs. 297, 299, 306)

Posterior junction line

A thin vertical line, posterior to the esophagus and trachea. It starts at the thoracic inlet, and extends downward to the height of the aortic and azygos arches. It is slightly thicker, and starts higher than the anterior line. It represents the approximation of the visceral and parietal pleura of the upper lobes, posteriorly. It projects over the tracheal air column, and is convex to the left (Ch. 9, Pg. 310) (6).

Paraaortic stripe (Ch. 9, Pg. 306)

Lateral costophrenic angle (recess)

The lateral costophrenic recess is formed at the junction between the hemidiaphragm and the chest wall. Laterally and inferiorly, this recess contains the part of the lung base that covers the dome of the hemidiaphragm. It is seen on the PA chest x-ray because of the black air in the lung. The edge of the lung forms a sharp angle inferiorly and laterally, called the lateral costophrenic angle.

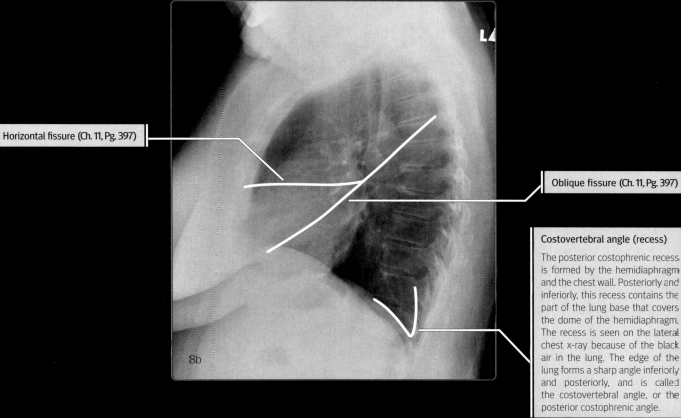

Horizontal fissure (Ch. 11, Pg. 397)

Oblique fissure (Ch. 11, Pg. 397)

Costovertebral angle (recess)

The posterior costophrenic recess is formed by the hemidiaphragm and the chest wall. Posteriorly and inferiorly, this recess contains the part of the lung base that covers the dome of the hemidiaphragm. The recess is seen on the lateral chest x-ray because of the black air in the lung. The edge of the lung forms a sharp angle inferiorly and posteriorly, and is called the costovertebral angle, or the posterior costophrenic angle.

8b

How to establish the location of the pleura

Determining the location of the layers of the pleura is an important step when trying to identify or exclude pleural pathology.

Parietal pleura

STEP 1
Confirm that the patient is midline and not rotated (Ch. 1, Pg. 32).

STEP 2
Identify the inner surface of each rib (Fig. 9).

STEP 3
Connect the dots (Fig. 10). This forms the parietal pleura line, and it defines the position of the parietal pleura.

Visceral pleura

STEP 1
Confirm that the patient is midline and not rotated (Ch. 1, Pg. 32).

STEP 2
Identify the outer surface of each lung (Fig. 11).

STEP 3
Draw a line along the contour of each lung (Fig. 12). This forms the visceral pleura line, and it defines the position of the visceral pleura.

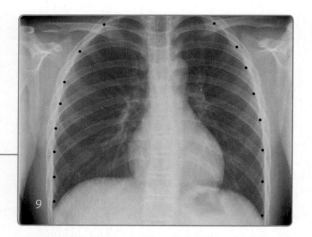

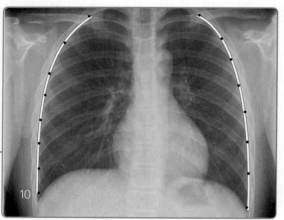

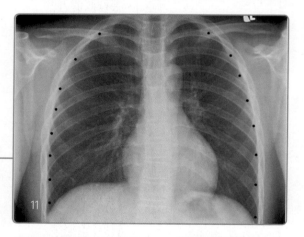

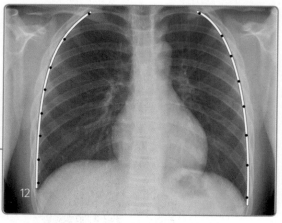

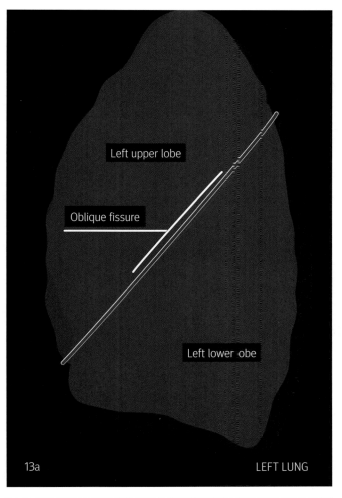

Left upper lobe

Oblique fissure

Left lower lobe

13a   LEFT LUNG

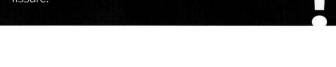

The oblique fissure is also known as the major fissure, and the horizontal fissure is also known as the minor fissure.

!

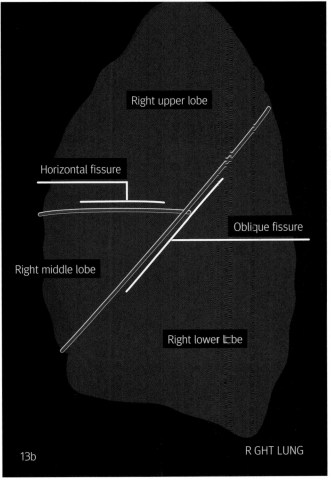

Right upper lobe

Horizontal fissure

Oblique fissure

Right middle lobe

Right lower lobe

13b   RIGHT LUNG

The Fissures

A fissure is a long, narrow opening, a cleft or groove that divides an organ into lobes. Each of the lungs is divided into lobes by structures called fissures (7). The lung fissures consist of two layers of visceral pleura. Fissures are important radiological landmarks, used to help us localize pathology to specific lobes of the lung (Ch. 17).

The left lung is divided into two lobes (upper and lower) by an oblique fissure (Fig. 13a).

The right lung is divided into three lobes (upper, middle and lower) by an oblique and a horizontal fissure (Fig. 13b).

Figure 13. The fissures. Artistic rendition of the fissures of the, a, left lung, b, right lung.

THE OBLIQUE (MAJOR) FISSURES

The oblique fissures are not normally seen on the PA view of the chest.

On the lateral x-ray (Fig. 14), the oblique fissures course obliquely from superior posterior (at the approximate level of the aortic arch), to inferior anterior (to the level of the anterior edge of the diaphragms). The oblique fissures will be seen as thin white lines — either continuous or interrupted — on the lateral x-ray.

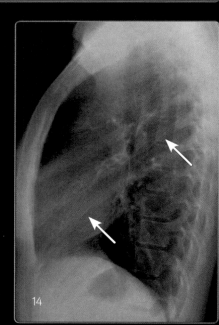

Figure 14. Radiological anatomy of the oblique (major) fissures. **A lateral chest x-ray with the course of the oblique fissures highlighted.**

THE HORIZONTAL (MINOR) FISSURE

The horizontal fissure separates the upper lobe from the middle lobe within the right lung. It courses from the oblique fissure posteriorly to the anterior surface of the lung. It can be seen on the PA x-ray as a thin line extending from the edge of the right lung laterally, towards the right hilum (Fig. 15a).

On the lateral x-ray (Fig. 15b), the horizontal fissure is seen coursing from the oblique fissure at the level of the hila to the anterior edge of the lung.

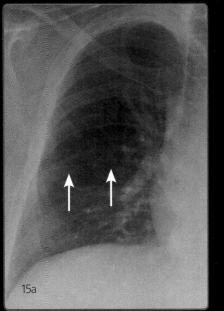

15a

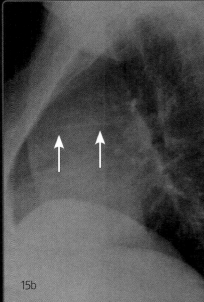

15b

Figure 15. Radiological anatomy of the horizontal (minor) fissure. a, PA chest x-ray with the course of the horizontal fissure highlighted, b, lateral chest x-ray with the course of the horizontal fissure highlighted.

Frequency of Visualization on the PA X-ray (8)

Horizontal (minor) fissure   74.7%
Inferior accessory fissure   7.1%
Superolateral oblique fissure   5.1%

Superomedial oblique fissure   4.7%
Superior accessory fissure   2.9%

Frequency of Visualization on the Lateral X-ray (9)

Oblique (major) fissures   62%
Horizontal (minor) fissure   44%

On a CT scan, the fissures can be easily visualized as vascular-free areas on the axial planes (Fig. 16a), or as thin lines in the sagittal and coronal planes (Fig. 16b,c).

ra

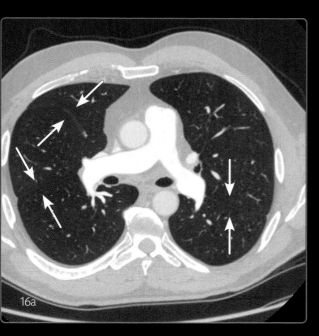

16a

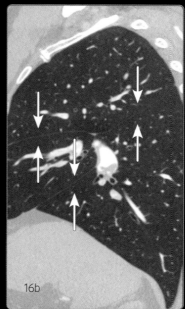

16b

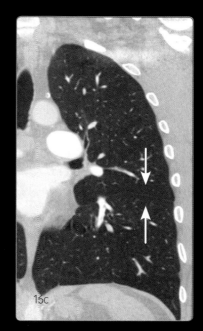

16c

Figure 16. Radiological appearance of the fissures on CT scans. **The appearance of the fissures on CT scans in the, a, axial plane, b, sagittal plane, c, coronal plane.**

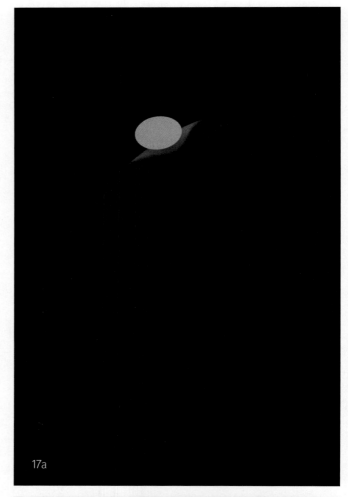

17a

Accessory Fissures

Accessory fissures are identified in the general population as normal variants of the lung fissures (10). The most common is the azygos fissure, which occurs in approximately 1% of the population. This fissure is caused by the azygos vein pulling four layers of pleura through the right lung as it courses to drain into the superior vena cava (SVC) (Figs. 17a,b,c and 18). (The presence of an azygos fissure leads to the creation of an accessory lobe within the right lung, the azygos lobe.)

Accessory fissures can also be found between the apical segment of the lower lobes and the basal segments of the lower lobes.

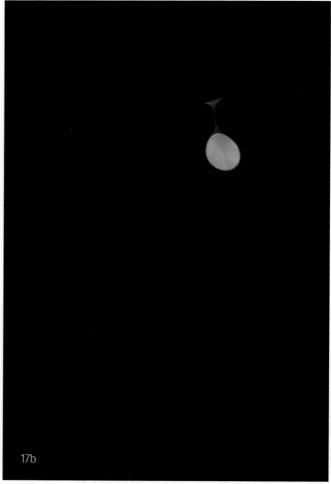

17b

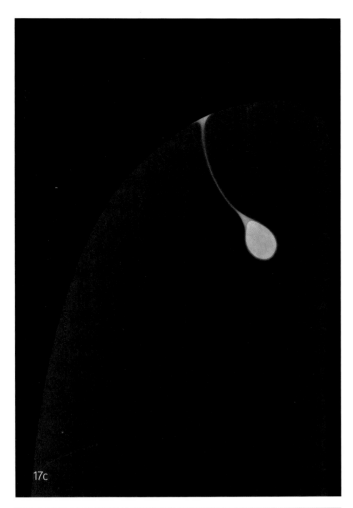

17c

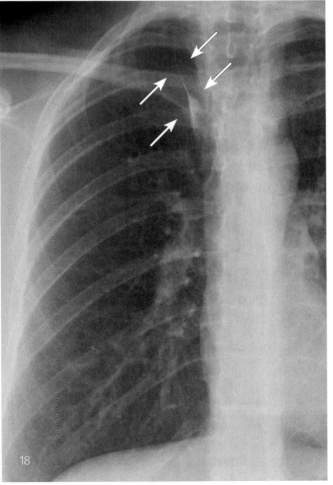

18

FISSURE	LOCATION
Azygos fissure	Right apex
Superior accessory fissure	Between the apical and basal segments of the lower lobes
Left horizontal fissure	Left mid-lung
Inferior accessory fissure	Surrounds the medial basal segment of the lower lobe: between the segments of the middle lobe on the right and the lingula on the left, and the lower lobes

Table 11.1
The Accessory Fissures

Figure 17. The formation of the azygos fissure. Artistic rendition of the formation of the azygos fissure. a, position of the azygos vein outside the pleura, b, the azygos vein as it crosses the pleura into the right lung, c, the azygos vein in the medial aspect of the right lung. The pleura is pulled into the lung creating the fissure and the accessory azygos lobe.

Figure 18. The azygos fissure. PA chest x-ray with the azygos fissure highlighted.

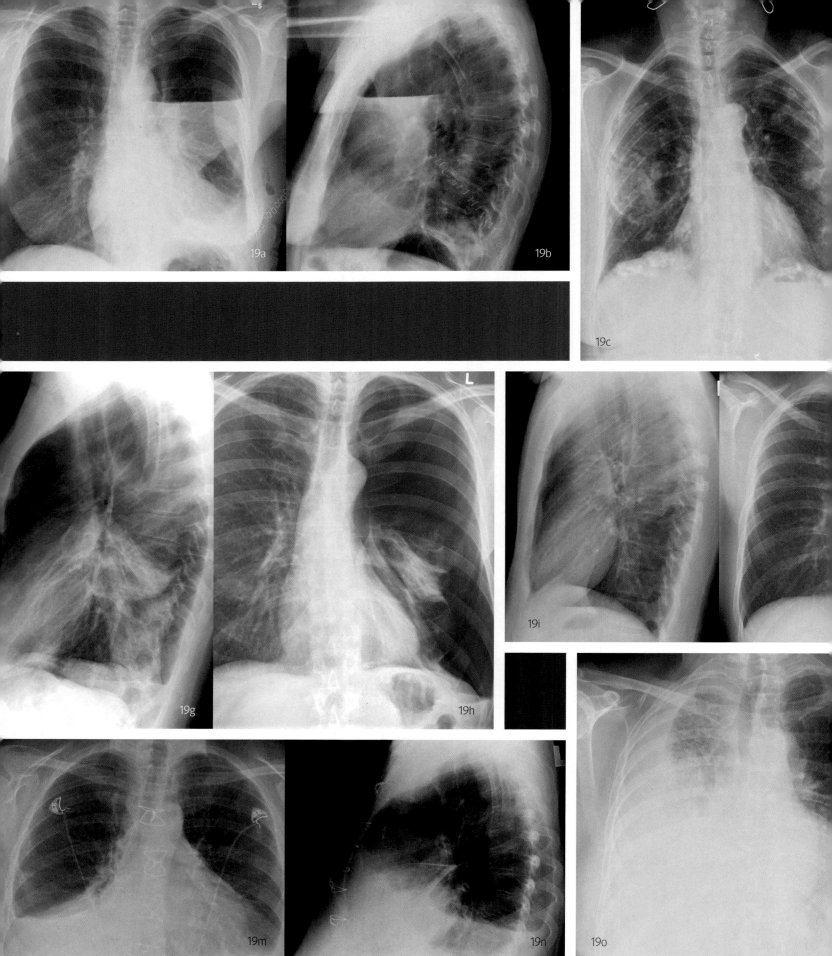

PATHOLOGY OF THE PLEURA

Example images of diseases and conditions that affect the pleura.

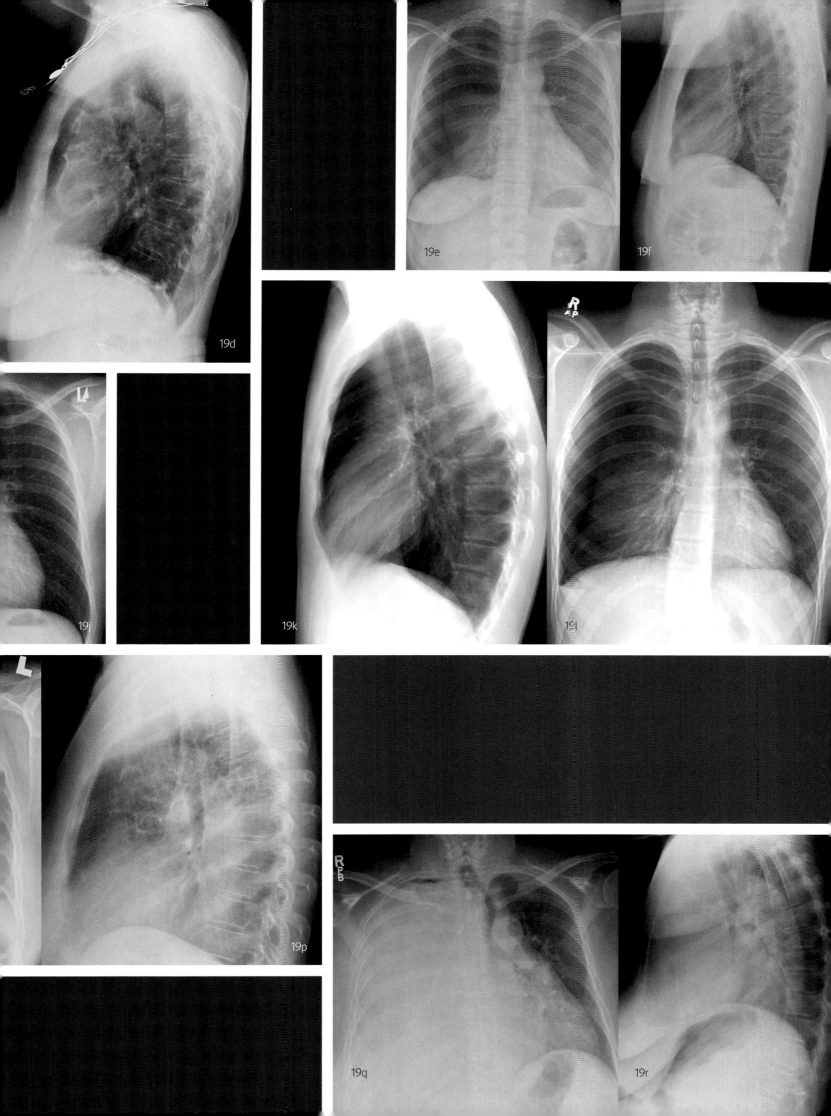

THE ABNORMAL PLEURA

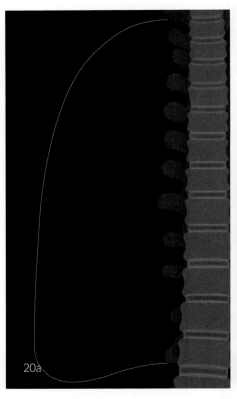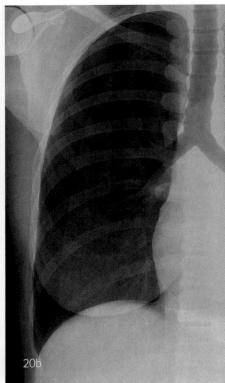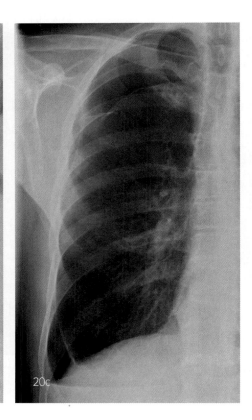

The Radiological Pleura
Will Be Abnormal When

1. The pleural space becomes visible and the grayscale is too black, or too white, or too white AND too black.

1a. Pathology that affects the pleura and shifts the grayscale to 'Too Black'

Pneumothorax

With a pneumothorax, there is a collection of air in the pleural space, which causes the pleura to become visible on the x-ray and look too black.

Air in the pleural space rises to the highest point. Therefore, when a patient with a pneumothorax is sitting in the upright position, air moves to the apex of the lung.

Figure 20. Pneumothorax. Pathology of the pleura can cause the grayscale to shift to too black. a, artistic representation of a pneumothorax, b, artistic representation of a pneumothorax with all thoracic structures, c, PA chest x-ray from a patient with a pneumothorax.

Figure 21. Scapula mimicking a pneumothorax. The edge of the scapula (arrows) can mimic a pneumothorax as seen on this PA chest x-ray.

Figure 22. Pneumothorax on expiration film. A pneumothorax can be seen more clearly on an expiration film. Example images from a patient with a pneumothorax (arrows) on, a, inspiration, b, expiration.

PLEURA **Chapter 11 SECTION II**

406

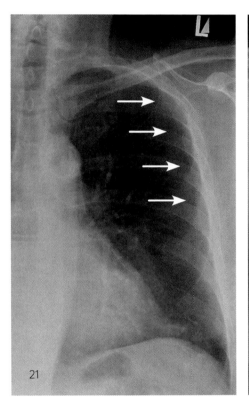

21

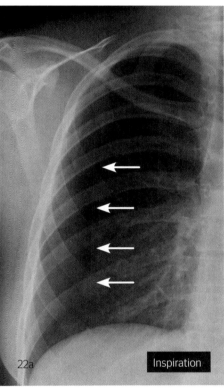

22a — Inspiration

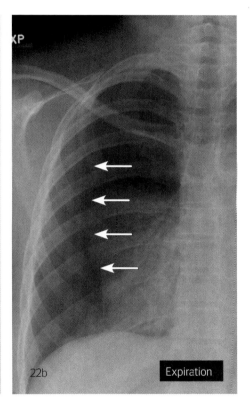

22b — Expiration

When looking for a pneumothorax on an upright x-ray, the first place to look is the upper thorax, bilaterally (for an apical pneumothorax) (Fig. 20a,b,c). The pneumothorax is seen as a peripheral crescent of deep black adjacent to the grayness of the adjacent lungs, delineated by a thin, white line, representing the visceral pleura (because it has been separated from the parietal pleura by the air in the pleural space). This line is very subtle and can often be confused with a rib or the medial edge of the scapula (Fig. 21). In addition, no vascular markings will be seen lateral to this pleural line.

On expiration views, the lungs appear smaller and denser. Since the air in the pleural space (pneumothorax) does not change size or density, it appears relatively larger on the expiration x-ray (Fig. 22a,b). Furthermore, the denser lung will look whiter, making the pneumothorax more obvious.

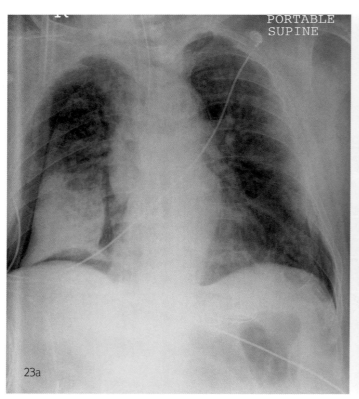

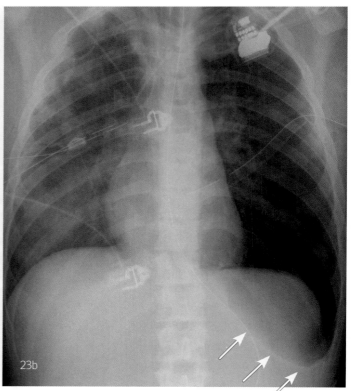

On a supine AP chest radiograph, the pneumothorax is layered horizontally across the anterior aspect of the chest. In this case, the most reliable sign of a pneumothorax is the deep sulcus sign (Fig. 23a,b)(**Pg. 430**)(11,12).

Figure 23. Pneumothorax on a supine chest x-ray. Pathology can shift the grayscale of the pleura to too black. a, supine x-ray from a patient with a pneumothorax on the right, b, AP x-ray with the pneumothorax (arrows) identified by the presence of the deep sulcus sign on the left.

On the normal AP x-ray, the lateral costophrenic angles are sharp. The pleural space, however, reaches quite far inferiorly and when it is full of air, the costophrenic angle on the affected side becomes much deeper and sharper than normal (Fig. 24).

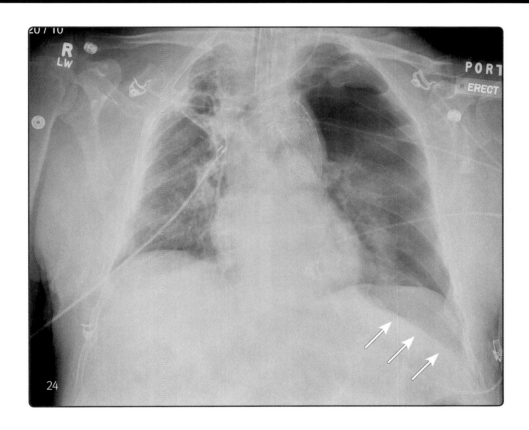

Figure 24. Deep costophrenic angle.
When the costophrenic angle becomes full of air, as with a pneumothorax, the angle becomes much deeper and sharper than normal. AP chest x-ray from a patient with a pneumothorax highlighting a deep and sharp costophrenic angle.

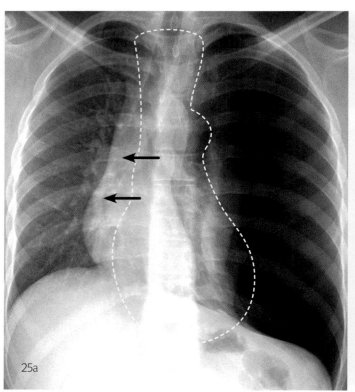
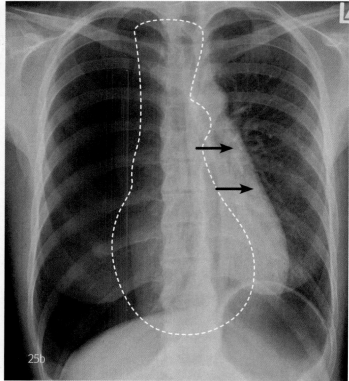

A tension pneumothorax occurs when there is an air leak in the pleura that acts as a one-way valve. This creates persistent, increased, intrapleural pressure that compresses the normal lung. This causes a restrictive ventilatory defect, and a ventilation-perfusion imbalance. A tension pneumothorax is diagnosed on a chest x-ray when the mediastinal structures and the trachea are deviated away from the midline of the body by air within the pleural space (Fig. 25a,b).

Pneumomediastinum

Pneumomediastinum is air within the mediastinum, and is commonly associated with a pneumothorax. Thin, black, usually vertical lines, are seen within the mediastinum, outlining the normally not visible anatomical structures, such as the aorta and heart (Fig. 26a,b).

Figure 25. Tension pneumothorax. A tension pneumothorax is important to recognize immediately on a chest x-ray; it can be identified by the presence of air in the pleural space and a characteristic displacement of mediastinal structures. a, PA chest x-ray from a patient with a tension pneumothorax, b, PA chest x-ray from a second patient with a tension pneumothorax.

Figure 26. Pneumomediastinum. Pathology can cause the grayscale of the pleura to appear too black. Air within the mediastinum is seen as "too black" vertical lines (arrows) within the mediastinum. a, PA chest x-ray from a patient with a pneumomediastinum, b, lateral chest x-ray from the same patient.

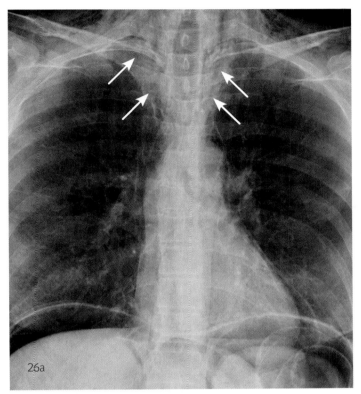

26a

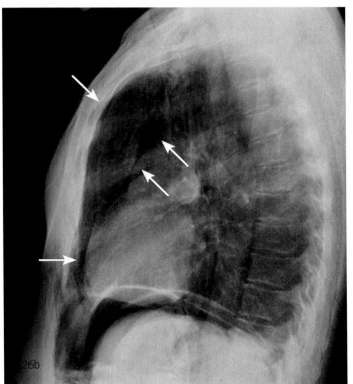

26b

Did you catch the examples on pages 404–405?

Fig. 19e,f – Pneumothorax

Fig. 19g,h – Massive pneumothorax

Fig. 19k,l – Tension pneumothorax

How to identify a pneumothorax on the PA x-ray

The lungs should extend all the way out to the chest wall. If there is air within the pleural space, the air will rise to the most superior aspect of the pleural space. Air outside of the lungs, within the pleural space, will look blacker than the air within the lungs, and allows the visceral pleura to be visualized. (An interface forms between the air in the pleural space, the pleura, and the air in the lungs.) Remember that overlapping soft tissues and ribs can obscure this difference in blackness.

STEP 1
Confirm that the patient is midline and not rotated (Ch. 1, Pg. 32).

STEP 2
Identify how the x-ray was performed – inspiration or expiration (Fig. 27).

STEP 3
Look for an asymmetry of grayscale – a pneumothorax will make the side of the lungs with the pneumothorax look too black (Fig. 28).

STEP 4
If one side is too black – use the steps to establish the location of the pleura (Pg. 396) (Fig. 29).

STEP 5
If the pneumothorax is not immediately obvious, look at the apices – then follow the cortical outline of the 1st, then 2nd, then 3rd, etc. ribs (Fig. 30):

STEP 6
Confirm the pneumothorax

A   By identifying the edge of the visceral pleura line.

B   By the lack of vascular markings adjacent to the visceral pleura.

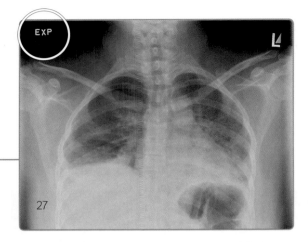

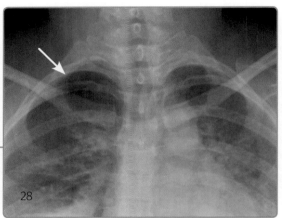

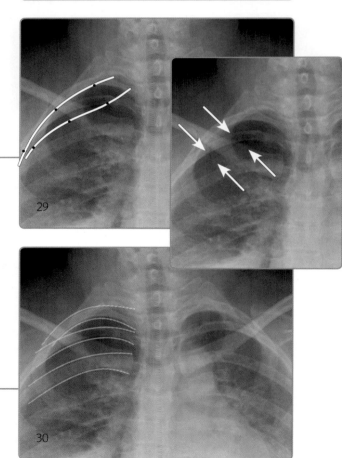

A skin fold may cause a line that appears very similar to a pneumothorax. In order to differentiate, remember:
1) The skin fold often extends beyond the borders of the lungs.
2) A skin fold is often relatively straight, whereas a pneumothorax follows the curve of the rib cage (Fig. 31).

In addition, be careful not to confuse a pneumothorax with a lung cyst or a large bleb!

!

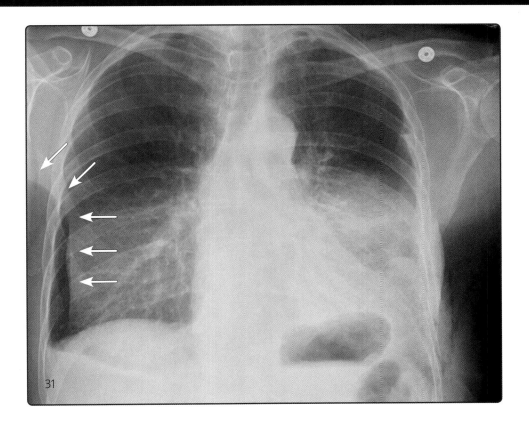

31

Figure 31. Skin fold can mimic a pneumothorax. PA chest x-ray of a patient with a skin fold over the right hemithorax. Notice how the line of the edge extends past the border of the lungs.

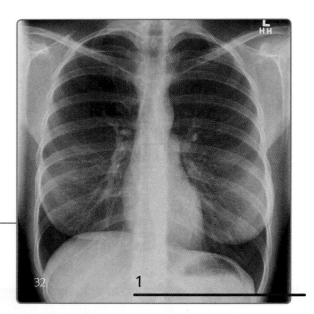

How to calculate the size of a pneumothorax on the PA x-ray(13,14)

Calculating the size of the pneumothorax is important for determining the course of treatment.

STEP 1
Confirm that the patient is midline and not rotated (Ch. 1, Pg. 32).

STEP 2
Identify the lowest edge of the lung on the side of the pneumothorax, point 1 (Fig. 32).

STEP 3
Identify the apex of the hemithorax, point 2 (Fig. 33)

STEP 4
Find the midpoint between points 1 and 2. This is point 3 (Fig. 34).

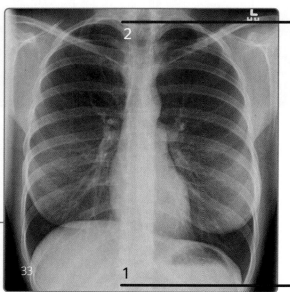

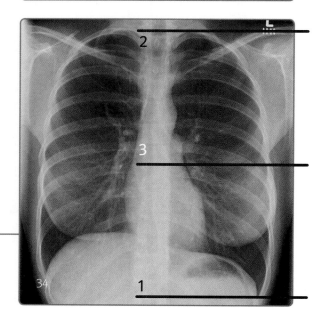

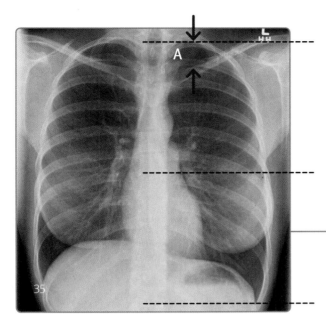

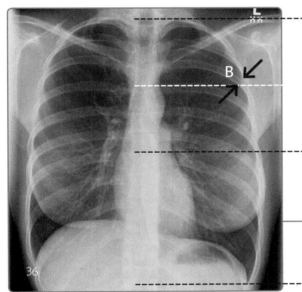

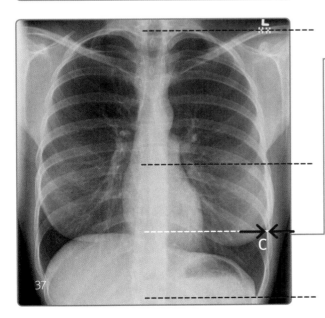

% pneumothorax can also be calculated as % = 4.2 + [4.7 X (A+B+C)](13)

STEP 5
Measure in cm the distance from the apex of the thorax to the apex of the lung, distance A (Fig. 35).

STEP 6
Measure in cm the distance from the wall of the thorax to the lateral edge of the lung, at a point halfway between point 3 and point 2, distance B (Fig. 36).

STEP 7
Measure in cm the distance from the wall of the thorax to the lateral edge of the lung, at a point halfway between point 3 and point 1, distance C (Fig. 37).

STEP 8
The interpleural distance = A+B+C/3, and this closely predicts pneumothorax size.

For example, an average interpleural distance of 3 cm = 30% pneumothorax, 4 cm = 40%, 5 cm = 50%.

> With a pleural effusion, the visceral and parietal pleural lines are separated by a white space.

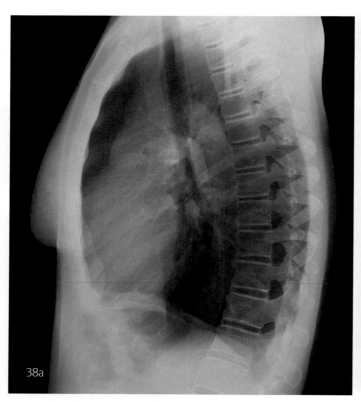

38a

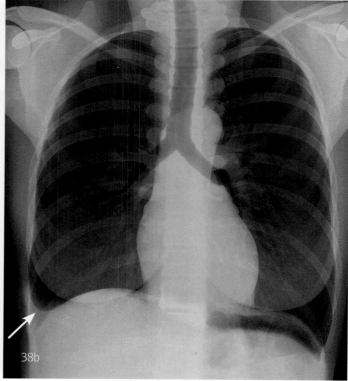

38b

1b. Pathology that affects the pleura and shifts the grayscale to 'Too White'

Pleural effusion

When fluid enters the pleural space, as in cases where there is a pleural effusion, the pleura will become visible and the grayscale will be too white. The radiological appearance of a pleural effusion depends on gravity, the rigidity of the lungs and the ability of the lower lobes to change volume (15). Gravity will cause the fluid to drop to the lowest part of the thorax, which is the posterior costophrenic recess.

Initially, the fluid will only be visible on the lateral chest x-ray, with displacement of the posterior costophrenic recess and adjacent lung. The posterior cardiophrenic angle stays normal.

With further accumulation of fluid, the rigidity of the lungs decreases, the alveoli collapse and the posterior costophrenic angle becomes blunted (Fig. 38a).

As more pleural fluid accumulates, the lateral costophrenic recess will be displaced, and eventually the lateral costophrenic angle will become blunted (Fig. 38b).

On the lateral x ray, approximately 50 ml of fluid is needed to cause blunting (meniscus) of the costovertebral angle. Approximately 200 ml of fluid will cause blunting of the costophrenic angle.

Figure 38. Pleural effusion. Pathology can cause the grayscale of the pleura to appear too white. Artistic representation of pleural effusion. a, blunting of posterior costophrenic angle from the lateral perspective, b, blunting of lateral costophrenic angle from the frontal perspective (arrow).

416

Although more difficult to visualize, a pleural effusion can be seen on a supine film when the fluid collection is greater than 200 ml. In this case, the pleural effusion can be detected as an increased opacity of the hemithorax without the loss of the pulmonary vasculature, or blunting of the costophrenic angles (Fig. 39). If enough fluid is present, the lungs will be displaced medially from the ribs, and the effusion will be seen as a vertical band of white running parallel to the lungs.

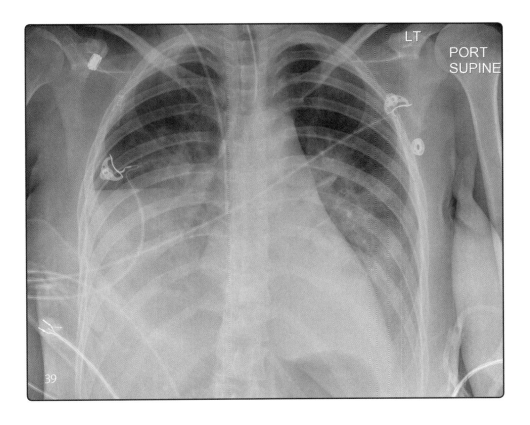

Figure 39. Pleural effusion on a supine chest x-ray. Pleural effusions can be seen on a supine chest x-ray if the fluid collection is greater than 200 ml. Layering of pleural fluid within the most dependent portion of the hemithorax on the right.

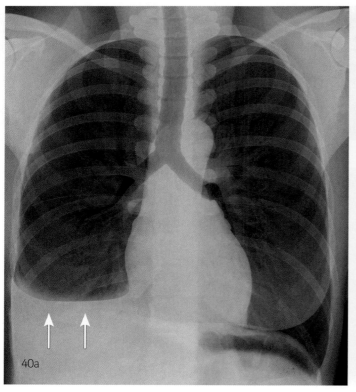
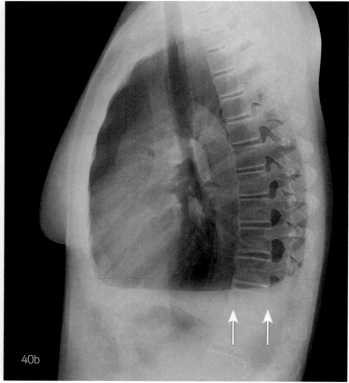

In an erect patient, fluid may collect in the subpulmonic area below the lung. A subpulmonic effusion will mimic the appearance of an elevated hemidiaphragm, because the fluid collection mimics the contour of the diaphragm. This also results in flattening of the medial hemidiaphragm, causing the dome of the diaphragm to appear to be shifted laterally. A subpulmonic effusion can also appear as blunting of the lateral costophrenic angles on the AP view (Fig. 40a), and blunting of the posterior costophrenic angle on the lateral view (Fig. 40b).

A loculated pleural effusion is one in which the buildup of pleural fluid occurs within the fissures, or between defined segments of visceral and parietal layers. In this type of pleural effusion, the fluid is not free-flowing. This will also occur when fluid accumulates in a pleural space that has internal, closed-off, areas due to scarring (Fig. 41a,b).

Figure 40. Subpulmonic pleural effusion. Artistic representation of a subpulmonic pleural effusion. a, frontal perspective, b, lateral perspective. Notice how the fluid collection mimics the appearance of an elevated diaphragm.

Figure 41. Loculated pleural effusion. a, PA chest x-ray from a patient with a loculated pleural effusion, b, lateral chest x-ray from the same patient.

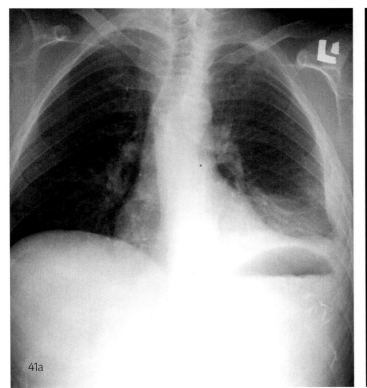

41a

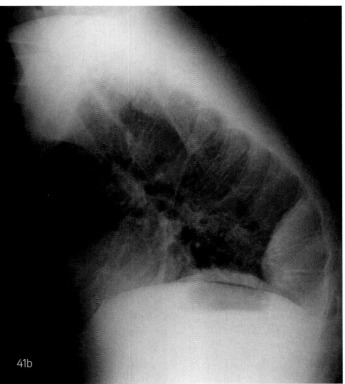

41b

Did you catch the examples on pages 404–405?
Fig. 19m,n – Bilateral pleural effusions
Fig. 19o,p – Massive pleural effusion
Fig. 19q,r – Tension pleural effusion

How to estimate the size of a pleural effusion on PA and lateral x-rays

Estimating the size of a pleural effusion is important for determining the course of treatment, and monitoring response to treatment (15).

STEP 1
Confirm that the patient is midline and not rotated (Ch. 1, Pg. 32).

STEP 2
Identify the costophrenic and costovertebral angles, bilaterally (Fig. 42a,b).

STEP 3
Identify the top of each hemidiaphragm (Fig. 43a,b).

STEP 4
If on one side there is a meniscus of the costovertebral angle, correlate this with the presence or absence of a meniscus of the ipsilateral costophrenic angle.

STEP 5
If a meniscus of the costophrenic angle is present, compare it with the position of the top of the ipsilateral hemidiaphragm.

STEP 6
You can now grade the size of the effusion as grade 0-4 (Pgs. 422-423).

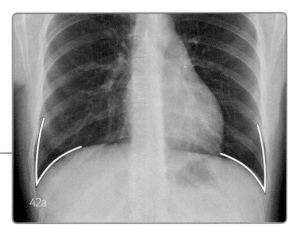

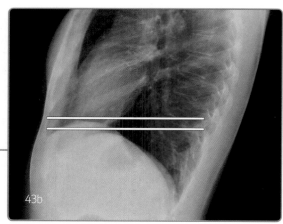

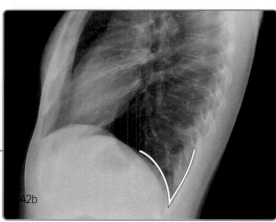

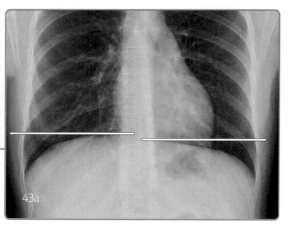

It is important to note that in some adults, there is a collection of fat between the lateral lung border and the ribs. This is called extrapleural fat, and is a normal finding. It should not be mistaken for bilateral pleural effusions (Fig. 44). In order to differentiate, remember it is most likely an extrapleural fat collection if: 1) there are no other signs of a pleural effusion present, 2) it is seen in the upper lung zones, and 3) it does not exceed 3-4 mm in thickness.

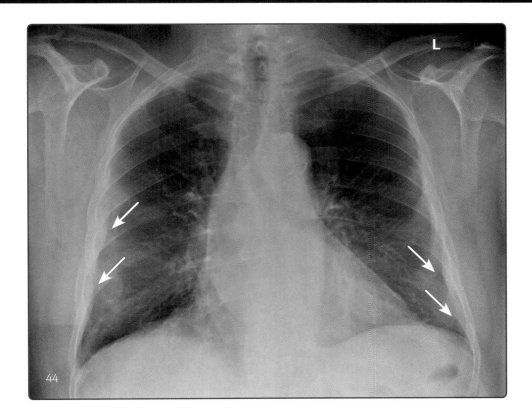

Figure 44. Extrapleural fat. A PA chest x-ray from a patient with an accumulation of fat between the lateral lung border and the ribs, laterally (arrows). When present, care must be taken to not confuse this with pleural effusions.

ESTIMATING THE SIZE OF PLEURAL EFFUSIONS

CHARACTERISTIC	GRADE 0
Costophrenic angle meniscus	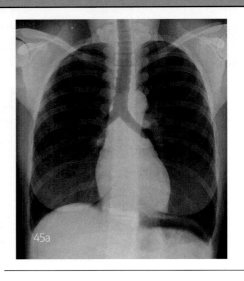 Absent
Costovertebral angle meniscus	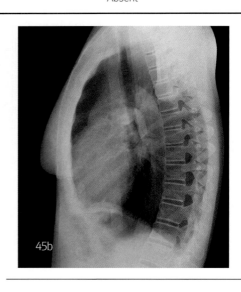 Absent
Volume of pleural fluid (ml)	Nil

Table 11.2
Summary of Estimating the Size of Pleural Effusions

GRADE 1	GRADE 2	GRADE 3

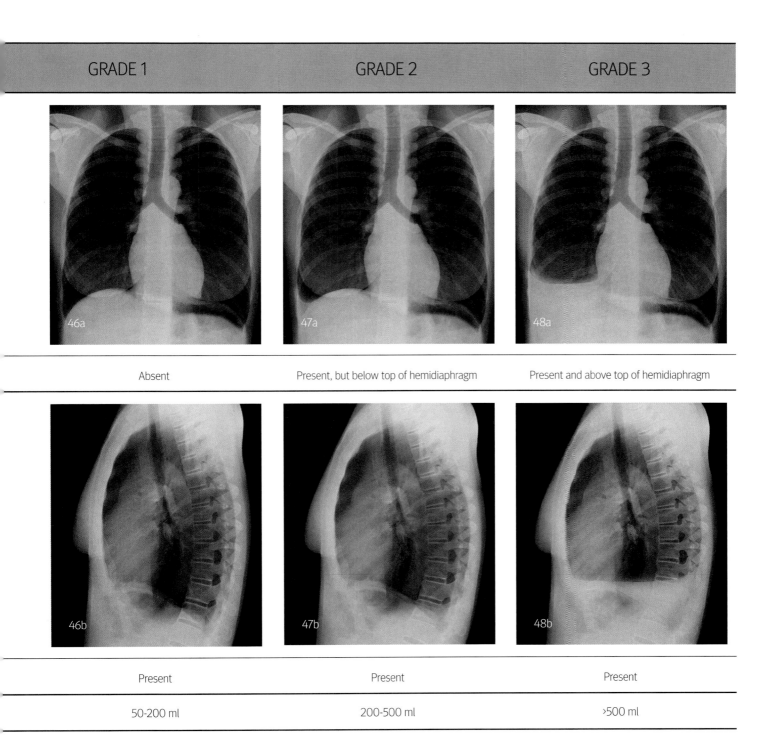

Absent	Present, but below top of hemidiaphragm	Present and above top of hemidiaphragm
Present	Present	Present
50-200 ml	200-500 ml	>500 ml

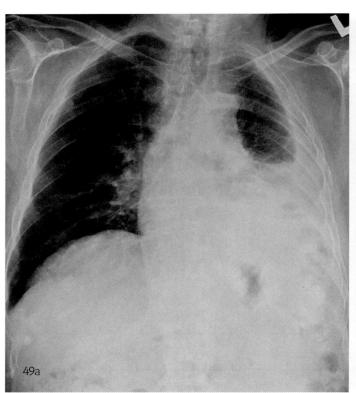 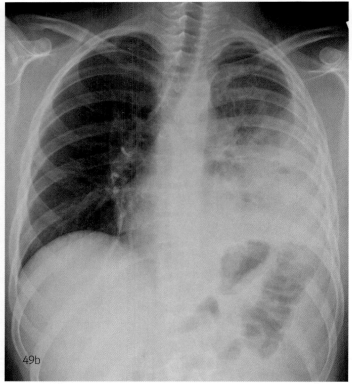

49a 49b

Empyema Pathology

AMSER Empyema is defined as an infected pleural effusion. On the chest x-ray, an empyema can look similar to a pleural effusion, and cause the pleura to look too white (Fig. 49a). The infected pleural fluid or empyema can contain gas, either in the form of an air-fluid level, or as small bubbles. In this case, the 'too white' pleura would have areas of too black (Fig. 49b).

Pleural tumors

Pleural tumors can be benign or malignant (16). Benign pleural tumors include lipomas and fibromas. Pleural tumors on an x-ray will form a sharp interface with the adjacent lung, and will form an obtuse angle with the adjacent chest wall (Fig. 50a). Mesothelioma is an aggressive pleural tumor that can appear as an irregular,

Figure 49. Empyema. Pathology can cause the pleura to look too white. a, PA chest x-ray from a patient with a homogenous empyema in the left lower thorax, b, PA chest x-ray from a patient with an empyema with locules of gas (too white and too black).

Figure 50. Pleural tumor. Pathology can cause the pleura to look too white. a, artistic representation of a pleural tumor, b, PA chest x-ray from a patient with pleural tumors in the left hemithorax.

424

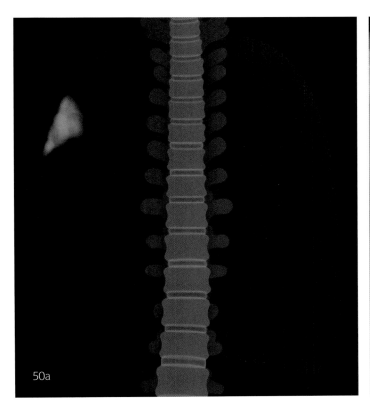

50a

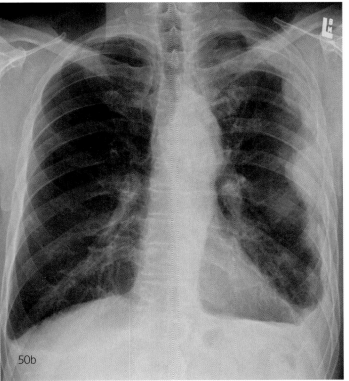

50b

nodular opacity on an x-ray, and is frequently associated with a pleural effusion (Fig. 50b).

Pleural plaques related to asbestos exposure can mimic pleural tumors.

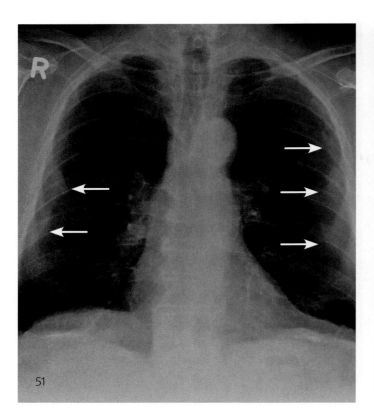

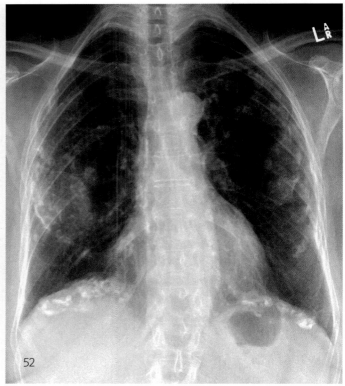

Pleural thickening and calcification

AMSER Pleural thickening results from a fibrotic/scarring reaction involving the pleura. This can occur following pleural infection, inflammation, trauma, surgery, or following exposure to asbestos. The pleural thickening can be diffuse, involving a large area of the pleura, or it can be focal.

Radiologically, the diffuse pleural thickening can mimic a pleural effusion, but typically, it will not change over time and with gravity. Also the pleural involvement can be seen anywhere, not only in the gravity-dependent parts of the thorax.

Focal pleural thickening, or pleural plaques, are irregular, pleural opacities that can involve any part of the pleura (Fig. 51). However, when they are associated with asbestos exposure, the pleural plaques typically involve the diaphragmatic pleura.

Figure 51. Pleural plaques. Pathology can cause the pleura to appear too white as in this PA chest x-ray from a patient with pleural plaques.

Figure 52. Calcified pleural plaques. Pathology can cause the pleura to appear too white as in this PA chest x-ray from a patient with calcified pleural plaques.

Figure 53. Hydropneumothorax. Pathology can cause the pleura to appear too white. a, artistic representation of a hydropneumothorax, b, PA chest x-ray from a patient with a hydropneumothorax.

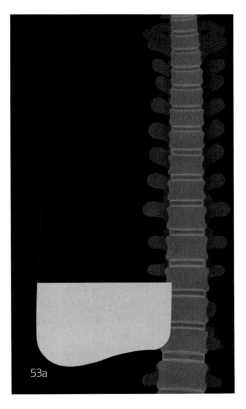

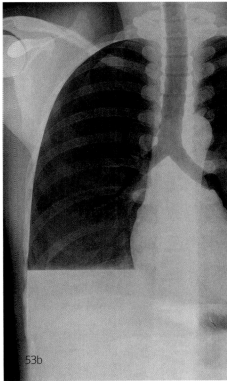

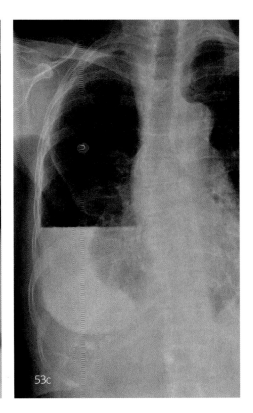

The x-ray appearance of pleural plaques and calcifications can be quite bizarre (Fig. 52), and may require CT scanning for clarification.

1c. Pathology that affects the pleura and shifts the grayscale to 'Too White' AND 'Too Black'

A hydropneumothorax occurs when the pleural space becomes filled with both fluid and air. An abnormal interface will be seen, with 'too black' air forming a straight horizontal edge on top of the 'too white' fluid (the air-fluid level) (Fig. 53a,b,c).

Did you catch the examples on pages 404–405?
Fig. 19a,b – Air-fluid level
Fig. 19c,d – Asbestos plaques

PLEURA **Chapter 11** SECTION II

427

Air in the pleural space rises, and fluid drops

The lateral decubitus view (Ch.1, Pg. 21) is a sensitive tool for recognizing pleural fluid, and can detect an accumulation of as little as 5 ml in volume. In the erect position a pleural effusion is seen as a uniform band of soft tissue density causing blunting of the costophrenic angle (Fig. 54a). In the decubitus position the fluid drops inferiorly and can be seen as a band of soft tissue lying along the chest wall (Fig. 54b). (17).

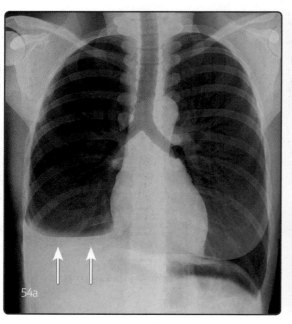
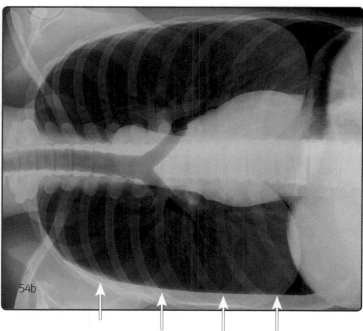

54a

54b

Figure 54. Pleural effusion on the decubitus view. a, artistic representation of a pleural effusion on an erect view, arrows outlining pleural fluid in the inferior aspect of the thorax, b, artistic representation of a pleural effusion on a decubitus view, arrows outline the pleural fluid layering in the most inferior aspect of the hemithorax which is now lateral.

SUMMARY OF RADIOLOGICAL CHANGES TO THE PLEURA

RADIOLOGICAL CHANGES TO THE PLEURA		ASSOCIATED FINDINGS, DISEASES AND CONDITIONS
1. Change in grayscale	Too black	• Pneumothorax • Tension pneumothorax • Pneumomediastinum
	Too white	• Pleural effusion (water, blood) • Subpulmonic pleural effusion • Tension pleural effusion • Empyema • Pleural thickening (scarring) (due to: infection trauma, surgery, or asbestos) • Calcification • Plaques (asbestos) • Tumor (e.g., lipoma, fibroma, mesothelioma) • Pseudotumor
	Too white AND too black	• Hydropneumothorax • Empyema with air

Table 11.3
Summary of Radiological Changes to the Pleura

RADIOLOGICAL SIGNS
RELATED TO THE PLEURA

Pseudotumor Sign (Vanishing Tumor Sign)

The pseudotumor sign is named for a sharply marginated collection of pleural fluid, contained either within an interlobar pulmonary fissure or in a subpleural location, adjacent to a fissure (18). On an x-ray, this collection will have a lenticular, or oval, shape (Fig. 55a,b). Seventy-five percent will develop within the horizontal fissure and will be seen on both the PA and lateral x-rays. If it occurs in the oblique fissure, it may only be seen on the lateral x-ray.

Characteristically, the collection of fluid will diminish with treatment of the underlying clinical problem – hence the name: vanishing tumor.

Deep Sulcus Sign

In the supine position, air in the pleural space will collect in the most anterior part of the thorax, which is in the lower aspect of the chest. The air in this position will make the costophrenic angle appear deepened, producing the deep sulcus sign (Fig. 56) (11,12).

Figure 55. Pseudotumor sign. a, PA chest x-ray from a patient with pleural fluid accumulating in the oblique fissure (arrows) causing the pseudo tumor sign, b, lateral chest x-ray from the same patient.

Figure 56. Deep sulcus sign. AP chest x-ray from a patient with a pneumothorax resulting a deepening of the costophrenic angle (arrows), otherwise known as the deep sulcus sign.

430

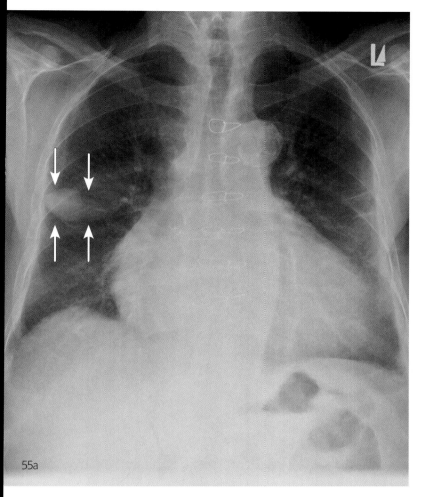

55a

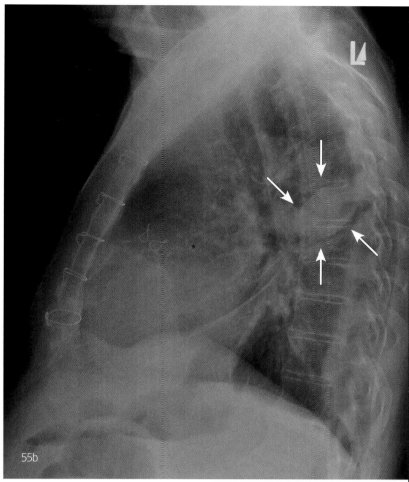

55b

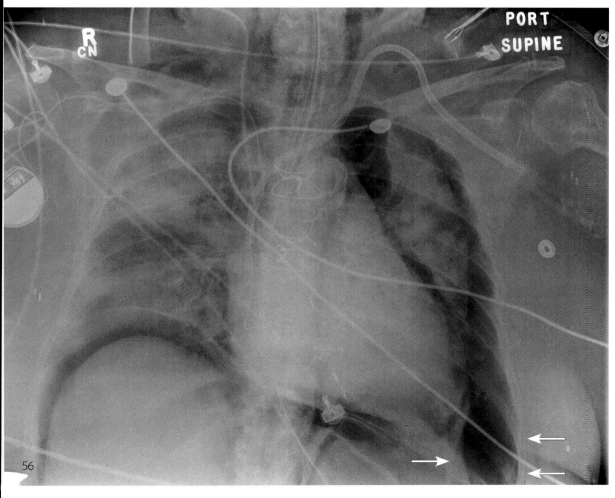

56

Visual Search of the Pleura

PA Chest X-ray

1. Start at the right apex (1).

2. Follow the lateral outline of the pleura inferiorly to the right costophrenic angle (2).

3. Follow the inferior outline of the pleura medially to the mediastinum (3).

4. Follow the medial outline of pleura to the apex.

Complete the visual search by checking for any density changes across the thorax from top to bottom.

Follow the same instructions on the left.

Lateral Chest X-ray

1. Start at the apex anteriorly (1).

2. Follow the outline of the pleura inferiorly to the diaphragm (2).

3. Follow the outline of the pleura posteriorly to the costovertebral angles (3).

4. Follow posterior outline of pleura superiorly to the apex.

Complete the visual search by checking for any density changes across the thorax from top to bottom.

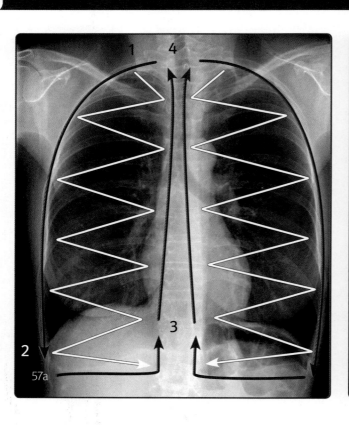

57a

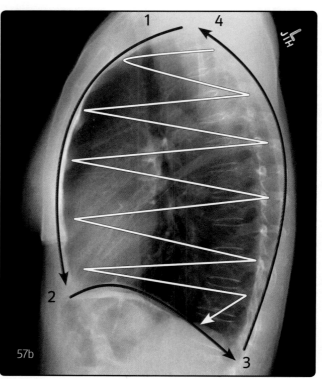

57b

Pleura Radiological Analysis Checklist

To confidently state that the pleura is normal, all parts of the checklist should indicate a normal appearance.

GRAYSCALE

1 Do the lungs extend all the way to the ribs?

> If **NO**, is the grayscale of the pleura altered?

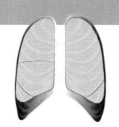

If **YES**, then describe.
Too white/too black/too white AND too black.
Right/left/bilateral.

SIZE

2 Is the size of the pleural space altered?

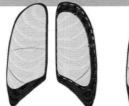
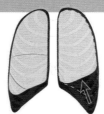

If **YES**, then describe.
Right/left/bilateral.
Give size of pneumothorax or pleural effusion.

POSITION

3 Are the fissures shifted?

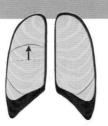

If **YES**, then describe.
Elevated/depressed.
Medial/lateral.

SHAPE

4 Is the shape of the lateral or posterior costophrenic angles altered?

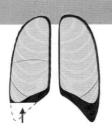
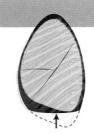

If **YES**, then describe.
Right/left/bilateral.
Blunted.

OTHER

5 Are there any radiological signs related to the pleura?

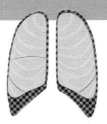

If **YES**, then describe.
Pseudotumor.
Deep sulcus.

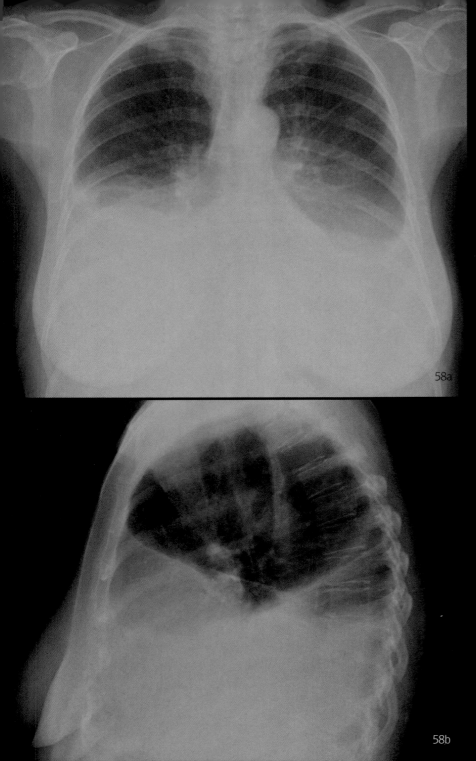

58a

58b

What do you see on the chest x-rays?

CASE STUDY

You are called to the ward to see a 58-year-old female patient that has been admitted with a two-week history of shortness of breath, a productive cough and fever. The nurse claims that her dyspnea has been getting worse throughout the day. You examine the patient and find that there is stony dullness on percussion of the lung bases and decreased breath sounds bilaterally. You request PA and lateral chest x-rays (Fig. 58a,b).

434

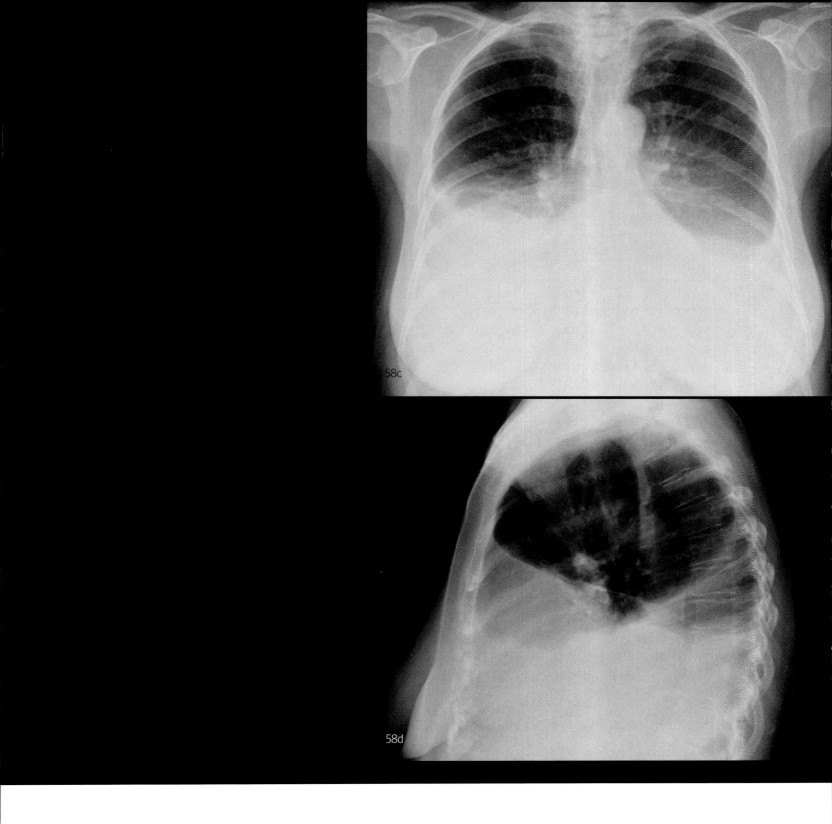

58c

58d

The pleura is commonly affected by pathology, and recognizing pathology localized to the pleura can be vital when forming a list of differential diagnoses. Figure 58c and 58d show bilateral pleural effusions. Look at both the lateral and PA x-rays and you will see a fluid collection within the pleural spaces bilaterally. Since this is a large effusion, you can see the effusion extending up into the inferior aspect of the major fissures. Can you see the fissures on the lateral x-ray? Can you estimate the size of the pleural effusions?

Based on the findings, the diagnosis is malignant bilateral effusions.

DISCUSSION

References

1. Lewis, P.J., Shaffer, K., & Donovan, A. (Eds.). (2012). AMSER National Medical Student Curriculum in Radiology. http://aur.org/Secondary-Alliances.aspx?id=141.

2. Lewis, P.J., & Shaffer, K. (2005). Developing a national medical student curriculum in radiology. *Am. Coll. Radiol., 2*(1):8–11.

3. Bertin, F., & Deslauriers, J. (2011). Anatomy of the pleura: reflection lines and recesses. *Thorac. Surg. Clin., 21*(2):165–171.

4. Genereux, G.P. (1983). The posterior pleural reflections. *AJR Am. J. Roentgenol., 141*(1):141–149.

5. Proto, A.V., Simmons, J.D., & Zylak, C.J. (1983). The anterior junction anatomy. *Crit. Rev. Diagn. Imaging, 19*(2):111–173.

6. Proto, A.V., Simmons, J.D., & Zylak, C.J. (1983). The posterior junction anatomy. *Crit. Rev. Diagn. Imaging, 20*:121–173.

7. Meenakshi, S., Manjunath, K.Y., & Balasubramanyam, V. (2003). Morphological variations of the lung fissures and lobes. *Indian J. Chest Dis. & Allied Sci., 46*(3):179–182.

8. Abiru, H., Ashizawa, K., Hashmi, R., & Hayashi, K. (2005). Normal radiography anatomy of thoracic structures: analysis of 1000 chest radiographs in Japanese population. *Br. J. Radiol., 78*:398–404.

9. Proto, A.V., & Speckman, J.M. (1979). The left lateral radiograph of the chest. Part 1. *Med. Radiogr. Photogr., 55*(2):29–74.

10. Cronin, P., Gross, B.H., Kelly, A.M., et al. (2010). Normal and accessory fissures of the lung: evaluation with contiguous volumetric thin-section multidetector CT. *Eur. J. Radiol., 75*(2):e1–8.

11. Cummin, A.R.C., Smith, M.J., & Wilson, A.G. (1987). Pneumothorax in the supine patient. *Br. Med. J., 295*:591–592.

12. Kong, A. (2003). The deep sulcus sign. *Radiology, 228*(2):415–416.

13. Collins, C.D., Lopez, A., Mathie, A., et al. (1995). Quantification of pneumothorax size on chest radiographs using interpleural distances: regression analysis based on volume measurements from helical CT. *AJR Am. J. Roentgenol., 165*(5):1127–1130.

14. Kelly, A.M., Weldon, D., Tsang, A.Y.L. & Graham, C.A. (2006). Comparison between two methods for estimating pneumothorax size from chest X-rays. *Respir. Med., 100*(8):1356–1359.

15. Blackmore, C.C., Black, W.C., Dallas, R.V., & Crow, H.C. (1996). Pleural fluid volume estimation: a chest radiograph prediction rule. *Academ. Radiol., 3*(2):103–109.

16. Dynes, M.C., White, E.M., Fry, W.A., & Ghahremani, G.G. (1992). Imaging manifestations of pleural tumours. *Radiographics, 12*:1191–1201.

17. Froudarakis, M.E. (2008). Diagnostic work-up of pleural effusions. *Respiration, 75*(1):4–13.

18. Feder, B.H., & Wilk, S.P. (1956). Localized Interlobar effusion in heart failure: Phantom lung tumor. *Dis. Chest, 30*:289–297.

CHAPTER 12

The LUNGS & AIR SPACES (the lung zone)

importance

The lungs are a pair of complex, air-filled organs that occupy a significant part of the thorax. Through the processes of inspiration and expiration, oxygen is delivered into the lungs and carbon dioxide is expelled. The low density of the lungs (due to the air contained within) produces a fantastic black backdrop on x-rays, on which lung pathology can be seen.

On a chest x-ray, many anatomical structures overlap the lungs, and can hide lung pathology. Understanding the grayscale of the lungs, and how disease processes alter the normal lung grayscale, are paramount in identifying pathology. In this chapter, you will learn a systematic approach to evaluating the appearance of the lungs on a chest x-ray – an approach that will help you to better identify all lung pathology.

objectives

Skills

You will identify

- the lobes and segments of the right and left lungs.
- the inferior border of each lung on the PA and lateral chest x-rays.
- the lung regions (zones) on the PA and lateral chest x-rays.
- the borders of the lungs on the PA and lateral chest x-rays.
- lung and air space pathology, using the grayscale method.
- common lung pathology, based on regional localization.
- the common places on the chest x-ray where pathology is often missed.

Knowledge

You will review and understand

- the basic anatomy of the lungs.
- the radiological anatomy of the lungs.
- the important relationship that the lungs have with the mediastinal and hilar structures, and how interfaces are formed.
- the grayscale map of the normal lung.
- important common pathology of the lungs and airspaces.

associated resources

This chapter maps to the following AMSER curriculum content (1,2).

1) Normal radiological anatomy of the lungs.
   Right upper lobe (RUL)
   Right middle lobe (RML)
   Right lower lobe (RLL)
   Left upper lobe (LUL)
   Left lower lobe (LLL)
   Major and minor fissures
   Retrosternal clear space

2) Pathological conditions affecting the lungs and airspaces.
   Masses
   Danger zones for missing tumors
   Atelectasis
   Pneumonia:
       Differential diagnosis of consolidation
       Signs: Silhouette, spine, air bronchogram
       Viral/Atypical patterns, PCP
   Interstitial abnormalities:
       Emphysema

3) Other
   Distinguishing causes of hemithorax opacification
   (effusion vs. atelectasis vs. pneumonia vs. pneumonectomy)

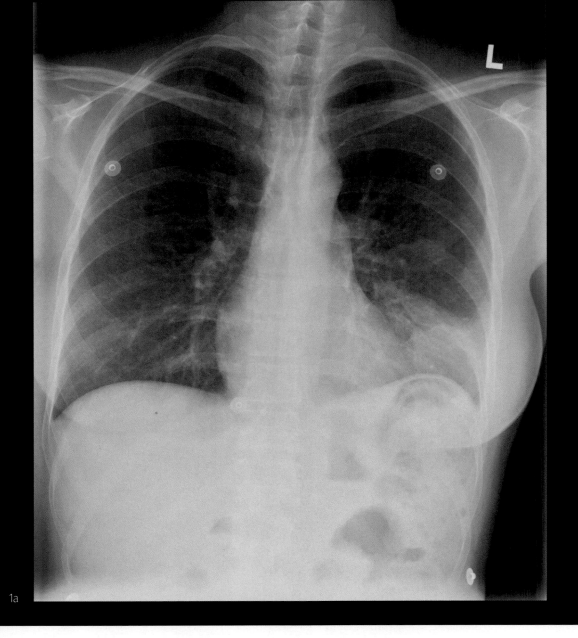

1a

CASE STUDY

You are the intern on call at a rural hospital. Your pager goes off when a 69-year-old female patient presents to the emergency department with a two-week history of flu-like symptoms, productive cough and fever. After a thorough history and examination, you suspect that she has a community-acquired pneumonia, and proceed to investigate with lab work and a chest x-ray (Fig. 1a,b). You call the consultant on call, and proceed to describe the x-ray findings.

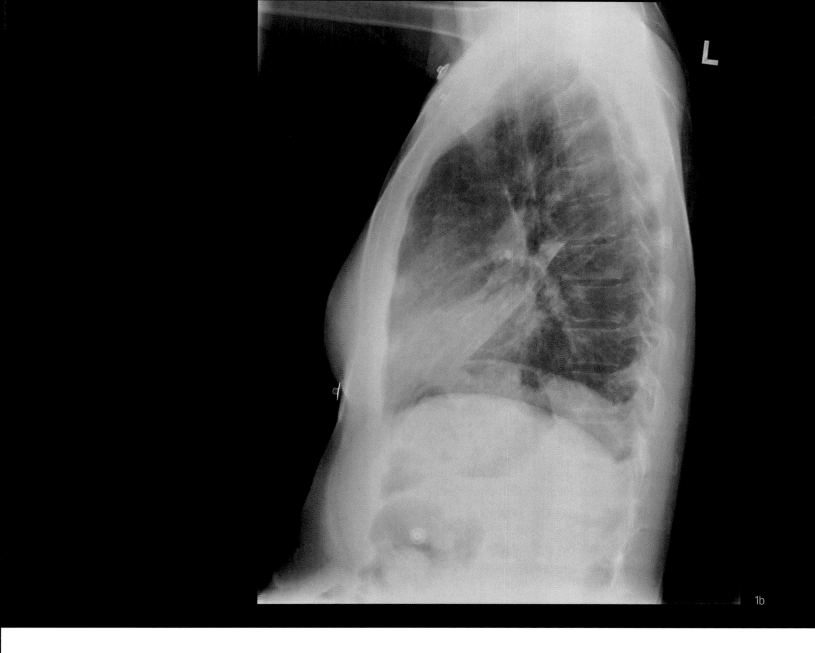

1b

How would you
describe your findings?

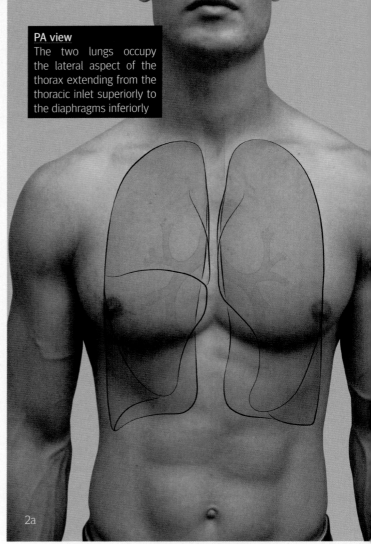

2a

THE LUNGS

The lungs are the major organs of respiration, acting as the site of exchange of carbon dioxide and oxygen. The word lung is thought to originate from the Sanskrit word *langhu* meaning "lightweight", and is used interchangeably with the word pulmonary, derived from the Latin *pulmo* meaning "the lung".

The lungs fill the majority of the space within the thorax (Fig. 2a,b). The lungs are situated with their superior aspects (apices) extending into the base of the neck, and their most inferior portions (bases) lying on the diaphragms. The maximum volume to which the lungs can be expanded with the greatest possible inspiration (total lung capacity) is approximately 6 liters in males, and 4.2 liters in females (3).

The lungs are each the shape of a cone cut vertically in half, with the cut surface facing medially and the top directed cranially (Fig. 3a,b). The right lung is slightly wider than the left, but is shorter in the craniocaudal direction.

The surface of the lungs is covered with visceral pleura, with the exception of the medial aspect where the hilar structures enter the lungs.

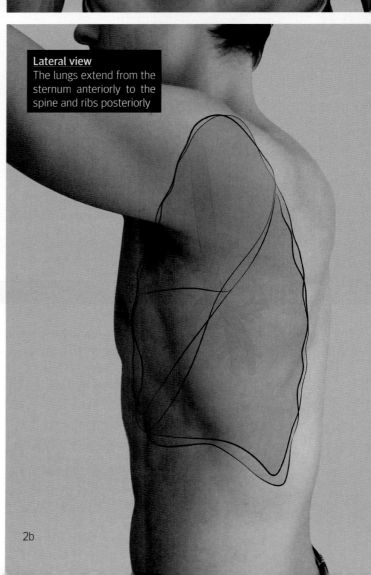

Lateral view
The lungs extend from the sternum anteriorly to the spine and ribs posteriorly

2b

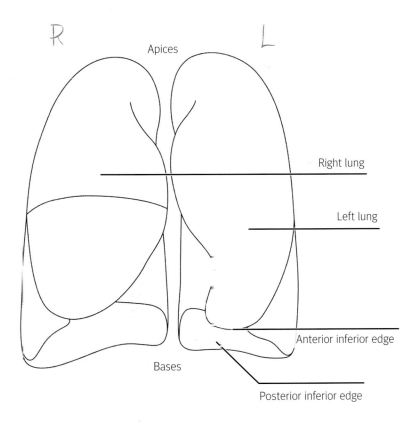

R   L

Apices

Right lung

Left lung

Anterior inferior edge

Bases

Posterior inferior edge

3a

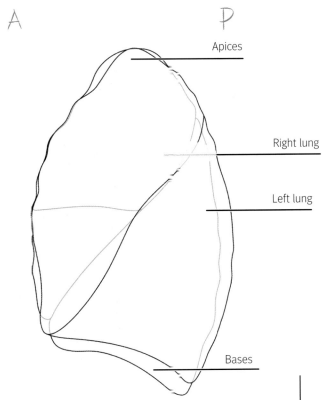

A   P

Apices

Right lung

Left lung

Bases

3b

Figure 2. Surface anatomy localization of the lungs. a, frontal perspective, b, lateral perspective.

Figure 3. The lungs. Illustrations of the lungs, a, frontal perspective, b, lateral perspective.

The Lobes of the Lungs

AMSER Each lung is comprised of lobes: the right lung has three lobes, and the left lung has two lobes (4).

The right lung is divided into the right upper lobe (RUL), the right middle lobe (RML) and the right lower lobe (RLL) (Fig. 4a,b)(5,6). The RLL is separated from the middle and upper lobes by the oblique (major) fissure. The RML is further separated from the RUL by the horizontal (minor) fissure.

The left lung is divided into the left upper lobe (LUL) and the left lower lobe (LLL) (Fig. 4c,d) (5,6). The lower lobe is separated from the upper lobe by the oblique (major) fissure.

Right upper lobe (RUL)

Right middle lobe (RML)

Right lower lobe (RLL)

RIGHT LUNG - LATERAL VIEW

4b

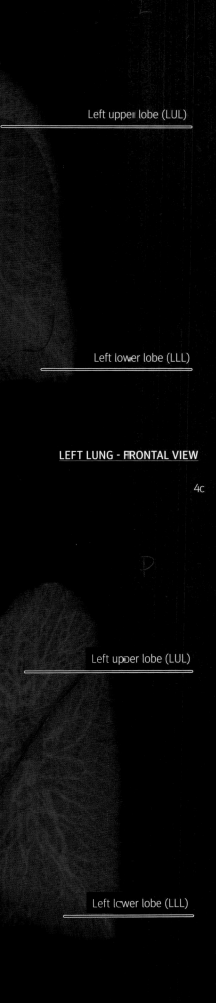

Left upper lobe (LUL)

Left lower lobe (LLL)

LEFT LUNG - FRONTAL VIEW

4c

Left upper lobe (LUL)

Left lower lobe (LLL)

Figure 4. The lobes of the lungs. 3D reconstructed lungs highlighting the lobes. a, right lung from the frontal perspective b, right lung from the lateral perspective, c, left lung from the frontal perspective, d, left lung from the lateral perspective.

LEFT LUNG - LATERAL VIEW

4d

The Segments of the Lungs

The lobes of the lungs, in turn, are made up of anatomical units called the bronchopulmonary segments (4). Each bronchopulmonary segment possesses its own pulmonary artery, pulmonary vein, bronchus and lymphatics. Because these are anatomically distinct, each segment can be involved with pathology without the involvement of neighboring segments. In addition, the individual segments can be removed surgically without interfering with the function of other units.

Each bronchopulmonary segment is shaped like a pyramid with the apex of the pyramid directed toward the pulmonary hilum (Fig. 5). Each segment is surrounded by connective tissue that is continuous with the sub-pleural connective tissue.

The Left Lung Segments

The LUL (Fig. 6a,b) has an anterior segment (similar to the RUL); however, unlike the RUL, the LUL apical and posterior segments are usually fused forming the apicoposterior segment.

The LLL, similar to the RLL, has an apical segment and anterior, posterior, medial and lateral basal segments. (Fig. 6c,d).

The left lung has no middle lobe, but the equivalent of the RML would be the two lingular segments of the LUL. The superior and inferior lingular segments of the LUL lie in approximately the same location as the middle lobe segments on the right (Fig. 6c,d).

Figure 5. The segments of the lungs. Illustration of the segments of the lungs as pyramidal structures meeting at the hilum (root of the lungs).

Figure 6. The bronchovascular segments of left lung. A series of illustrations of the bronchovascular segments of the left lung. LUL from the, a, frontal perspective, b, lateral perspective. LLL from the, c, frontal perspective, d, lateral perspective.

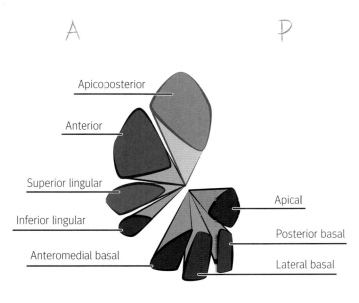

Apicoposterior

Anterior

Superior lingular

Inferior lingular

Anteromedial basal

Apical

Posterior basal

Lateral basal

5

LEFT LUNG - LEFT LATERAL

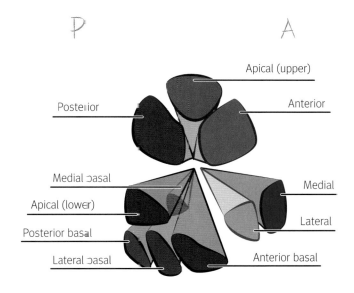

Posterior

Apical (upper)

Anterior

Medial basal

Apical (lower)

Posterior basal

Lateral basal

Medial

Lateral

Anterior basal

RIGHT LUNG - RIGHT LATERAL

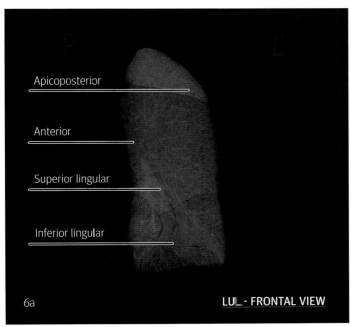

Apicoposterior

Anterior

Superior lingular

Inferior lingular

6a

LUL - FRONTAL VIEW

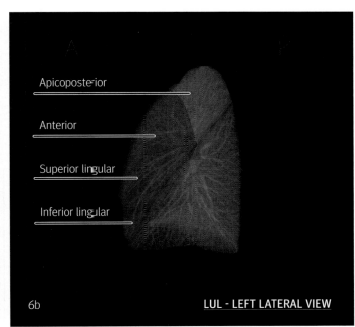

Apicoposterior

Anterior

Superior lingular

Inferior lingular

6b

LUL - LEFT LATERAL VIEW

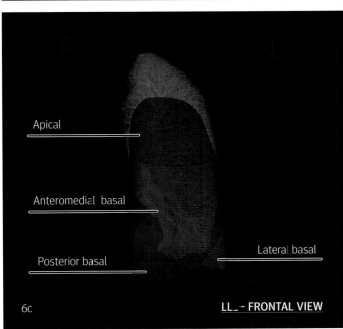

Apical

Anteromedial basal

Posterior basal

Lateral basal

6c

LLL - FRONTAL VIEW

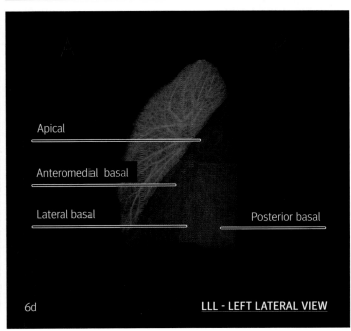

Apical

Anteromedial basal

Lateral basal

Posterior basal

6d

LLL - LEFT LATERAL VIEW

LUNGS **Chapter 12** SECTION II

The Right Lung Segments

The RUL (Fig. 7a,b) has an apical segment, as well as anterior and posterior segments.

The RML (Fig. 7c,d) is divided into medial and lateral segments.

The RLL (Fig. 7e,f) can be compared to a cone or pyramid. The upper part of the cone is formed by a lung segment called the apical segment. If we cut off this apical segment (the top of the cone), we are left with four basal segments. Depending upon the position of these segments relative to the heart, the lateral chest wall, and the front and back of the chest, these are described as the anterior, posterior, medial and lateral basal segments.

LUNG	LOBE	SEGMENT
Right	Upper	Apical
		Anterior
		Posterior
	Middle	Medial
		Lateral
	Lower	Apical
		Medial basal
		Anterior basal
		Lateral basal
		Posterior basal
Left	Upper	Apicoposterior
		Anterior
		Lingula medial
		Lingula lateral
	Lower	Apical
		Anteromedial basal
		Lateral basal
		Posterior basal

Table 12.1
The Segments of the Lungs

Figure 7. The bronchovascular segments of the right lung. A series of illustrations of the bronchovascular segments of the right lung. RUL from the, a, frontal perspective, b, lateral perspective. RML from the, c, frontal perspective, d, lateral perspective. RLL from the, e, frontal perspective, f, lateral perspective.

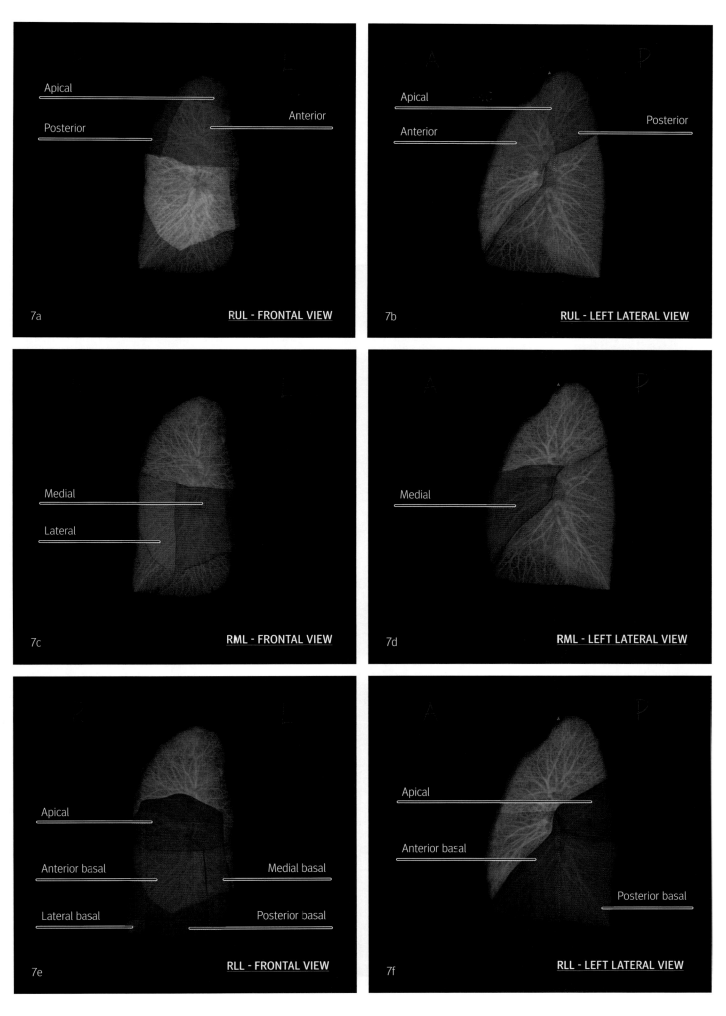

Apical

Posterior

Anterior

7a   **RUL - FRONTAL VIEW**

Apical

Anterior

Posterior

7b   **RUL - LEFT LATERAL VIEW**

Medial

Lateral

7c   **RML - FRONTAL VIEW**

Medial

7d   **RML - LEFT LATERAL VIEW**

Apical

Anterior basal

Medial basal

Lateral basal

Posterior basal

7e   **RLL - FRONTAL VIEW**

Apical

Anterior basal

Posterior basal

7f   **RLL - LEFT LATERAL VIEW**

THE TISSUE COMPONENTS OF THE LUNGS

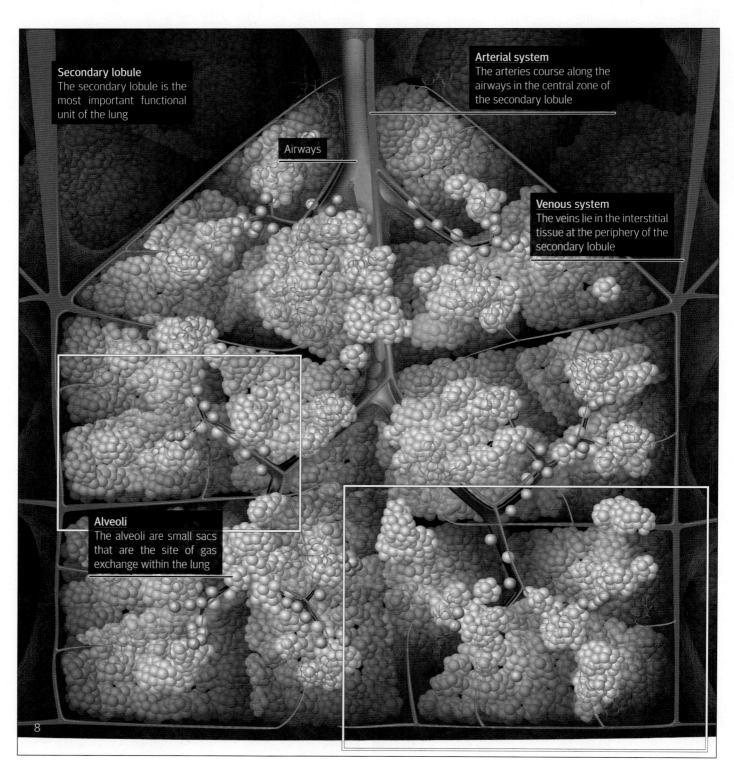

Secondary lobule
The secondary lobule is the most important functional unit of the lung

Arterial system
The arteries course along the airways in the central zone of the secondary lobule

Airways

Venous system
The veins lie in the interstitial tissue at the periphery of the secondary lobule

Alveoli
The alveoli are small sacs that are the site of gas exchange within the lung

8

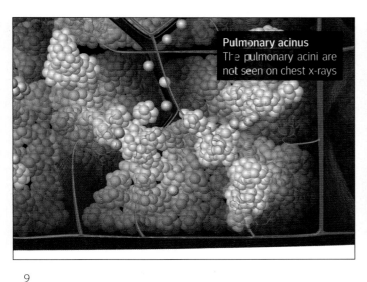

9

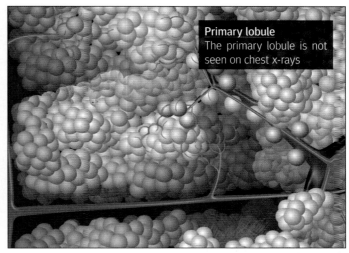

10

The lung tissue is comprised of three distinct components:

1. the airspaces,
2. the interstitium,
3. the blood vessels.

The Airspaces

The airspaces, as the name suggests, contain air and are divided into discrete anatomical units called the secondary lobules, primary lobules, and acini.

The secondary lobule is the most important functional unit of the lungs (7,8). It is defined as the portion of the lung distal to the lobular bronchioles. A single secondary lobule contains 6 to 12 acini, and 30 to 50 primary lobules, surrounded by connective tissue septae - the interlobular septae. The diameter of a secondary lobule measures 1 to 2.5 cm (Fig. 8).

A pulmonary acinus is defined as the portion of lung distal to the terminal bronchiole, and is composed of respiratory bronchioles, alveolar ducts, alveolar sacs and alveoli (Fig.9). Because of their small size, pulmonary acini are not seen on chest x-rays.

The primary pulmonary lobule consists of all the alveolar ducts, alveolar sacs and alveoli, distal to the last respiratory bronchiole with their accompanying blood vessels, nerves and connective tissue) (Fig.10). Primary lobules are also not seen on chest x-rays.

Figure 8. Secondary lobule. Illustration of the secondary lobule of the lung.

Figure 9. Pulmonary acinus. Illustration of a pulmonary acinus.

Figure 10. Primary lobule. Illustration of a primary lobule of the lung.

Radiological Shape and Grayscale of the Lungs

The basic grayscale of the lungs on PA and lateral chest x-rays is dark gray (Fig. 11a,b,c). The air in the airspaces gives the lungs the blackness they exhibit on chest x-rays. Compare the grayscale of the air in the lungs to the grayscale of the air outside of the lungs, seen above the patient's shoulders in the upper, outer parts of the chest x-ray image. The air in the room is much blacker.

On closer inspection, the dark gray of the lungs is not homogeneous. Instead, the lungs are comprised of various shades of gray as a result of multiple interfaces formed between the various tissues making up the air-spaces (e.g., lobules and acini), and the edges of the pulmonary blood vessels (Fig. 11d). Knowing the appearance of the normal pulmonary vessels is vital to deciding whether the lung parenchyma is normal or abnormal (Pg. XX, Ch. XX).

The grayscale appearance of the lungs is further complicated by the overlap of the lungs with many other thoracic structures (Fig. 11e). On the PA x-ray, there are significant portions of the lungs that overlap with abdominal structures. The overlap may make identification of subtle lung pathology difficult.

Figure 12. Radiological anatomy of the lungs from the frontal perspective. a, PA chest x-ray with the lungs outlined, b, PA chest x-ray with a grayscale illustration of the lungs overlay, c, PA chest x-ray cropped to highlight the lungs.

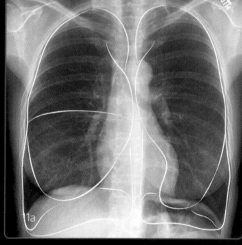

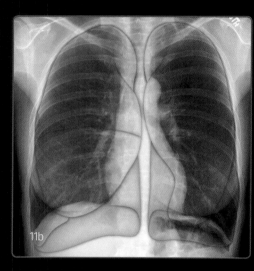

Figure 13. Radiological anatomy of the lungs from the lateral perspective. a, lateral chest x-ray with the lungs outlined, b, lateral chest x-ray with a grayscale illustration of the lungs overlay, c, lateral chest x-ray cropped to highlight the lungs.

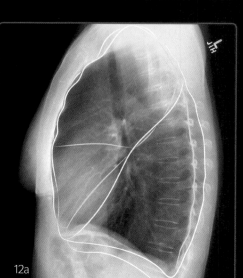

On the lateral x-ray, the grayscale of the posterior lungs will appear more black inferiorly (Fig. 12a,b,c). This normal gradient in grayscale is due to the fact that the lungs are wider and contain more air inferiorly. For this same reason, on the lateral x-ray, the thoracic vertebrae will look more black inferiorly. This forms the basis for the spine sign.

Additionally, on a normal lateral x-ray examination, superior to the heart and anterior to the ascending aorta, there is minimal overlap of soft tissues with the lungs. The lungs in this area are blacker. This area is called the retrosternal airspace, and should not be more than one third of the entire retrosternal region (Fig. 12c) (9).

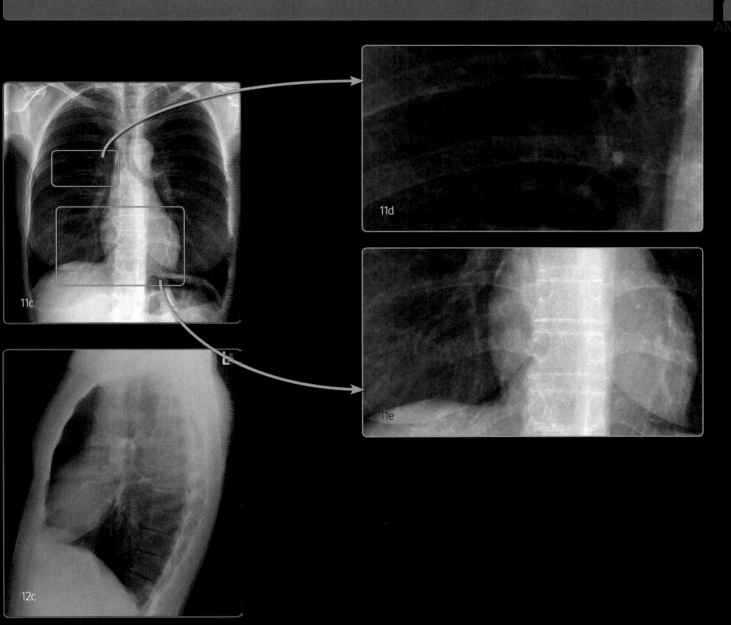

11c

11d

11e

12c

Boundaries of the X-ray Shadow Created by the Lungs

The lungs extend superiorly to the thoracic apex or thoracic inlet. Inferiorly, the lungs terminate at the diaphragms. On the PA x-ray, the superior border of the lungs is clearly identified. However on the PA x-ray, the inferior border of the lungs is frequently wrongly placed at the level of the top of the visible diaphragms. The inferior border of the lungs can, in fact, lie over 15 cm below the level of the top of the diaphragms, as seen on this PA x-ray (Fig. 13a). The most superior and most inferior borders of the lungs are best appreciated on the lateral chest x-ray (Fig. 13b) (10). On the PA x-ray, the lungs extend laterally to the ribs, or chest wall. Medially, the lungs have a more complex appearance, as they border and conform to the shape of the mediastinum and create the mediastinal interfaces (Fig. 13a). The lateral x-ray (Fig. 13b) shows the lungs extending to the sternum anteriorly, and to the posterior ribs and vertebral column posteriorly.

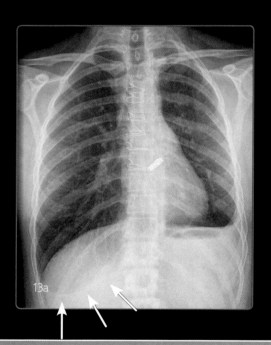
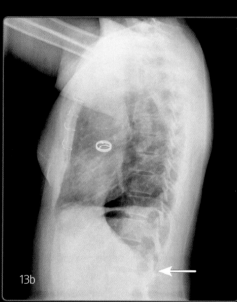

Figure 13. Radiological anatomy of the lungs - the boundaries of the lungs. **Inferior border of the lungs highlighted on, a, PA chest x-ray, b, lateral chest x-ray.**

13a

13b

PRINCIPAL OBSERVATION	RELEVANT CONTRIBUTORS
Lungs will look blacker if there is less overlying soft tissue	• Retrosternal air space • Previous mastectomy
Lungs will look whiter if there is more overlying soft tissue	• Subdiaphragmatic lungs are almost completely white on PA x-ray • Breast shadows
Lungs will look blacker where the blood vessels are smallest	• Periphery of lungs is blacker on the lateral x-ray, the lungs are blacker more inferiorly and posteriorly

Table 12.2
Observations on the Radiodensity of Normal Lungs

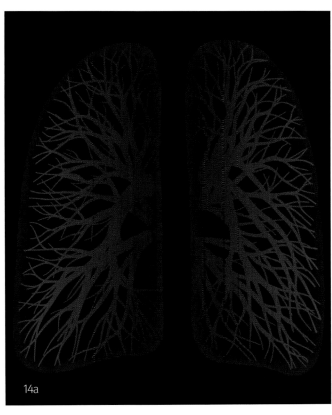

14a

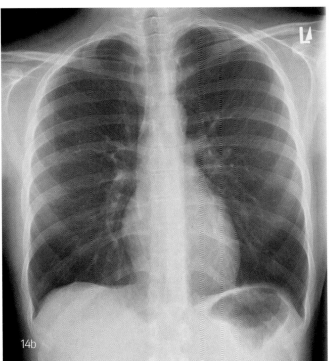

14b

The Interstitium

The interstitium represents the connective tissue scaffolding that holds up the airspaces. The interstitium will be further discussed in Chapter 13.

The Blood Vessels

The vascular markings are visible as white markings on the chest x-ray, and can be distinguished from other structures because they follow a predictable course, are seen to branch, and the width of their shadow decreases gradually from the center of the chest x-ray to the periphery.

The vascular markings are seen throughout the lungs – even peripherally – but are most pronounced centrally (Fig. 14a,b).

Figure 14. Vascular markings on the lungs. a, illustration of the course of the blood vessels as they decrease in size to the periphery of the lungs in te frontal perspective, b, PA chest x-ray highlighting the vascular markings throughout the lungs.

How to locate the inferior border of the lungs on the PA x-ray

Pathology can hide within the inferior portions of the lungs, and can be missed on the PA chest x-ray. This is because these areas overlap with the upper abdominal structures. Therefore, it is important to pay special attention to this portion of the lungs.

You will need to look at both the lateral and PA x-rays.

STEP 1
Start with the lateral x-ray. Identify the top-most point of the right hemidiaphragm (Fig. 15).

STEP 2
Draw a horizontal line extending from this point, posteriorly (Fig. 16).

STEP 3
Identify the most inferior aspect of the right lung (costovertebral angle) (Fig. 17).

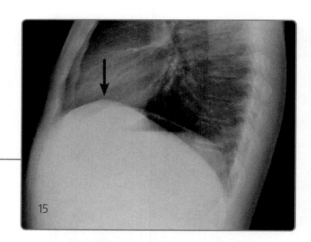

15

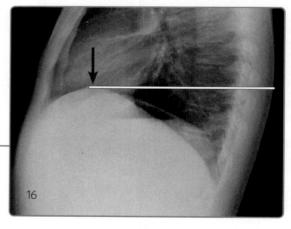

16

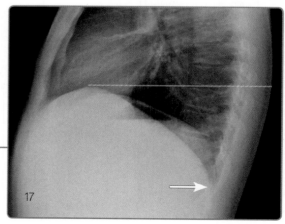

17

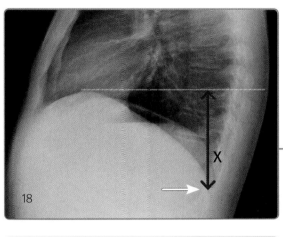

18

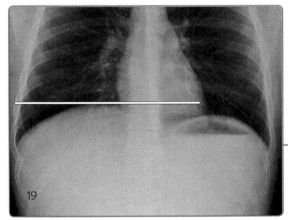

19

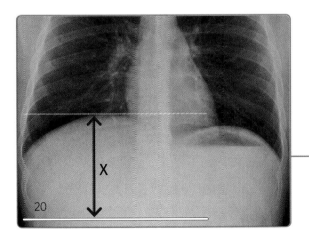

20

STEP 4
Measure from this point vertically, to the horizontal line – Distance X (Fig. 18).

STEP 5
On the PA x-ray, identify the top of the right hemidiaphragm (Fig. 19).

STEP 6
The inferior border of the right lung will be Distance X, from the top of the right hemidiaphragm (Fig. 20).

STEP 7
Confirm by following the lower lung vascular markings, or by direct visualization of the inferior lung margin.

STEP 8
Do the same with the left lung.

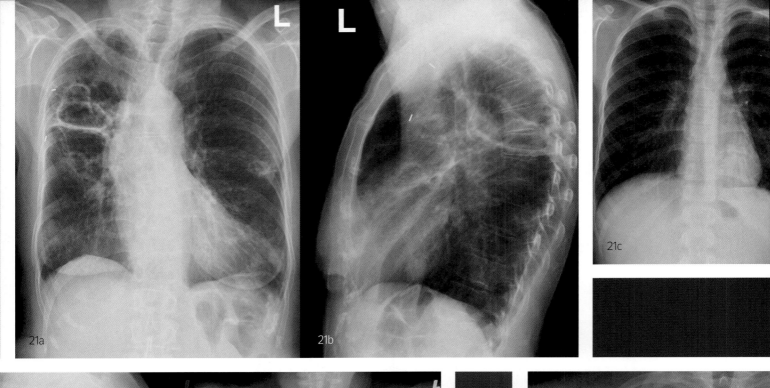

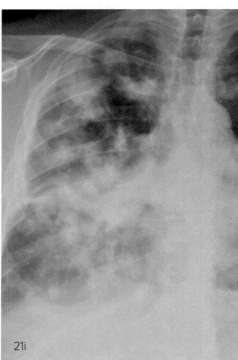

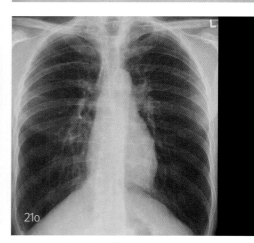

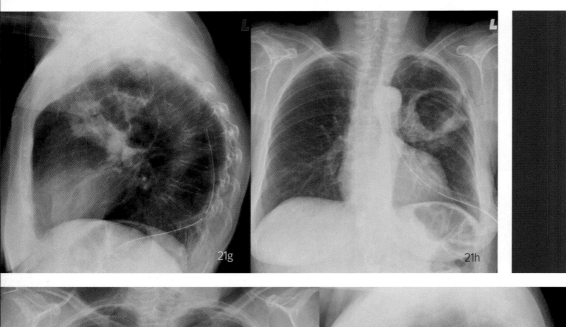

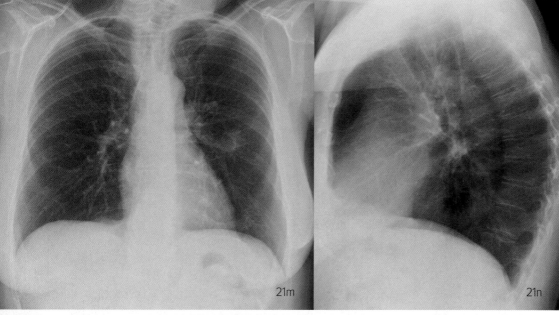

PATHOLOGY OF THE LUNGS & AIRSPACES

Example images of diseases and conditions that affect the lungs and airspaces.

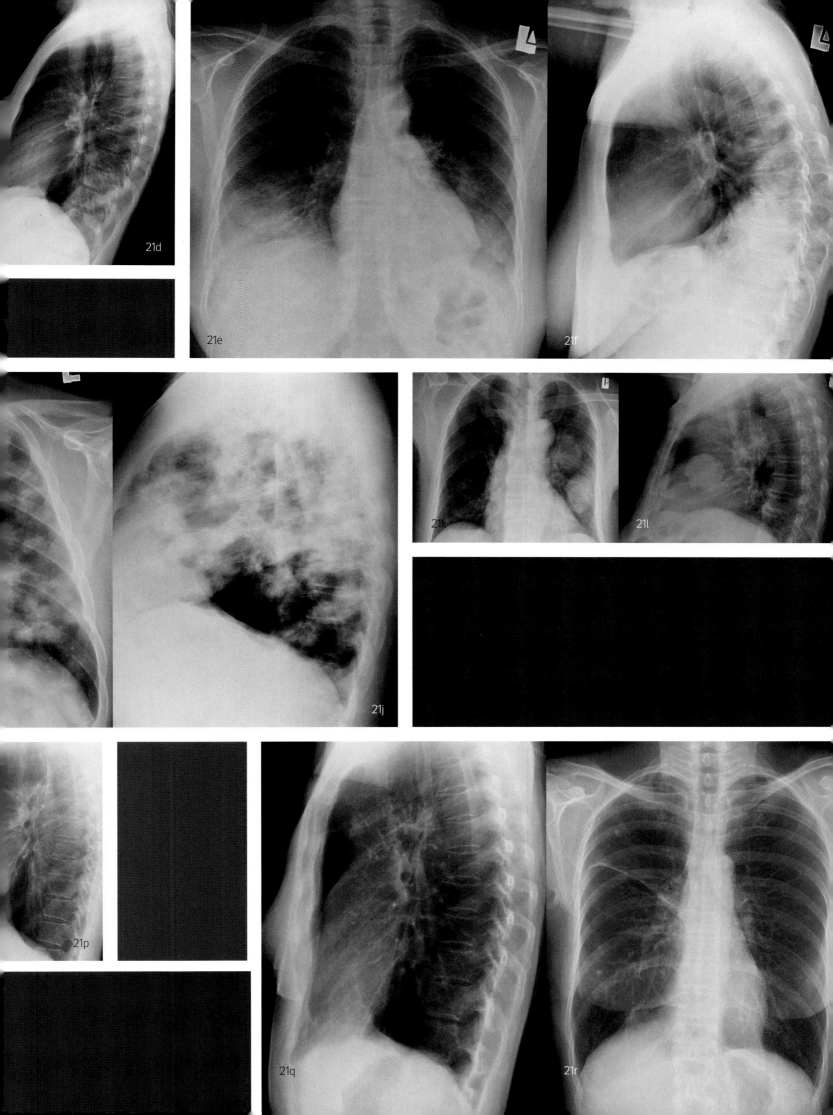

THE ABNORMAL LUNGS & AIRSPACES

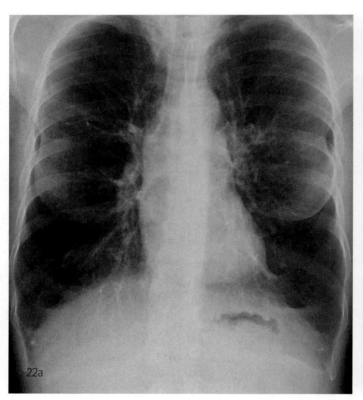

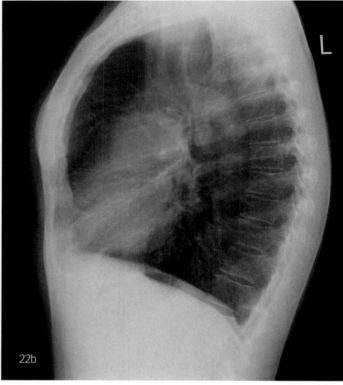

The Radiological Appearance of the Lungs and Airspaces Will Be Abnormal When

1. The grayscale of the lungs is too black or too white.

1a. Pathology that affects the lungs and shifts the grayscale to 'Too Black'

There are various pathologies involving the lungs that can cause the lungs to appear too black on an x-ray. The area of too black can: be focal or diffuse; be circumscribed by a thin or thick border; be solitary or multiple; be unilateral or bilateral; exist predominantly in one or a few lung segments or lobes.

Figure 22. COPD. Pathology can cause the grayscale of the lungs to appear too black. a, PA chest x-ray from a patient with COPD, b, lateral chest x-ray from the same patient.

Figure 23. Hyperinflated lungs. Pathology can cause the grayscale of the lungs to appear too black. a, PA chest x-ray from a patient with a previous pneumonectomy of the right lung causing hyperinflation of the right lung, b, lateral chest x-ray from the same patient.

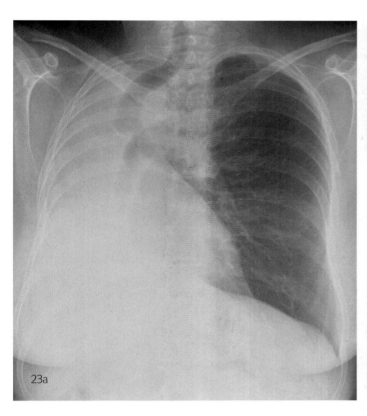

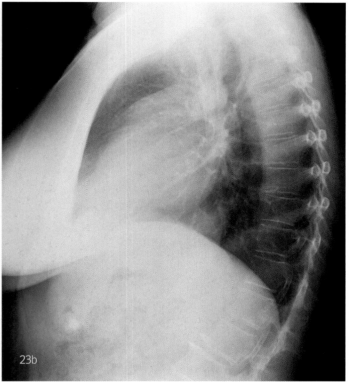

The abnormality of the grayscale of the lungs may be described as diffusely too black as seen when the lungs are hyperinflated (9). This can occur acutely during an asthma attack, or exist chronically in patients with chronic obstructive pulmonary disease (COPD) (Fig. 22a,b).

The diffuse pattern of too black may also be unilateral. A lung, or part of a lung, can hyperinflate in compensation for volume loss in another part of that lung (e.g., lobar atelectasis, lobectomy), or even to compensate for volume loss in the contralateral lung (e.g., pneumonectomy) (Fig. 23a,b). Hyperinflation related to emphysema may also be unilateral, or be predominant in a single, or few, lobes.

Did you catch the example on pages 458–459?
Fig. 21o,p – COPD

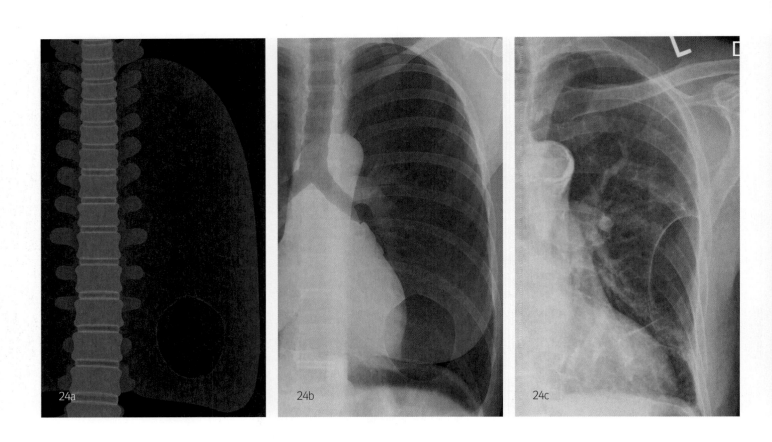

24a 24b 24c

The area of too black may be focal, and may be outlined by a thin line (e.g., pulmonary cyst , bleb or bullae) (Figs. 24a,b,c,d and 25a,b,c).

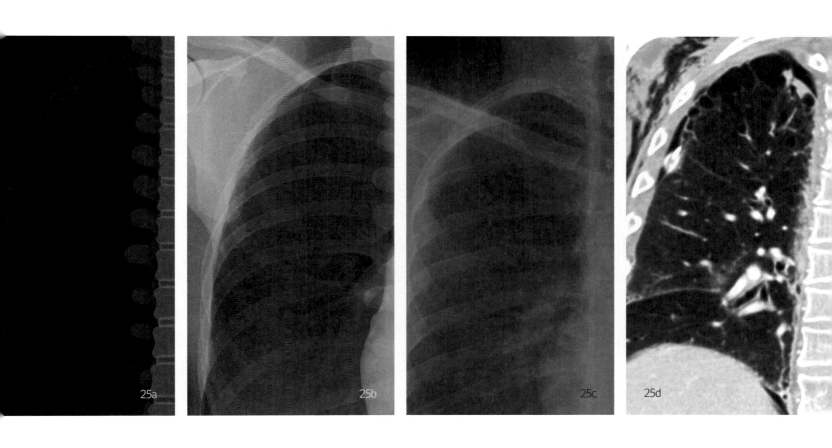

25a 25b 25c 25d

Figure 24. Pulmonary cyst. a, artistic representation of a pulmonary cyst, b, artistic representation of a pulmonary cyst with all thoracic structures, c, PA chest x-ray from a patient with a pulmonary cyst.

Figure 25. Pulmonary bleb. a, artistic representation of a pulmonary bleb, b, artistic representation of a pulmonary bleb with all thoracic structures, c, PA chest x-ray from a patient with a pulmonary bleb, d, CT scan from a patient with a bullae in apex of right lung.

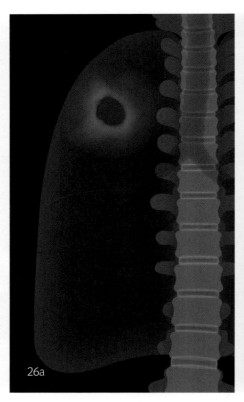
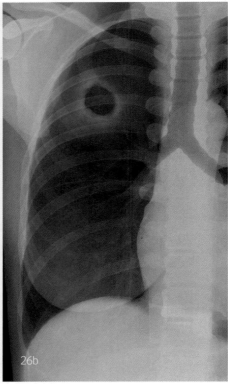
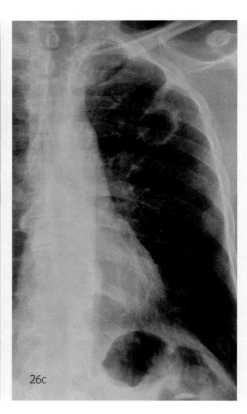

Alternatively, the area of too black may be bound by a thick irregular line (e.g., lung cavity) (Fig. 26a,b,c). The abnormality may be solitary or multiple (e.g., septic emboli) (Fig. 27).

When the lungs look too black, but are normal

Remembering that grayscale depends on the sum of the radiation absorption events (RAEs), the more soft tissue structures that the x-ray beam travels through, the whiter the image will appear. A lung with less soft tissues overlying it will look blacker on the x-ray. This is commonly seen in women who have had a mastectomy: the side with the removed breast will appear blacker than the other side (Fig. 28).

Similarly, the congenital absence (e.g., Polands Syndrome), or surgical removal, of ribs or muscles will cause the affected side to appear blacker. In these clinical cases,

Figure 26. Pulmonary cavity. a, artistic representation of a pulmonary cavity, b, artistic representation of a pulmonary cavity with all thoracic structures, c, PA chest x-ray from a patient with a pulmonary cavity.

Figure 27. Septic emboli. Pathology can cause the grayscale of the lungs to appear too black. as seen in this PA chest x-ray from a patient with septic emboli.

Figure 28. Mastectomy. Pathology can cause the grayscale of the lungs to appear too black as seen in this PA chest x-ray from a patient with a previous mastectomy.

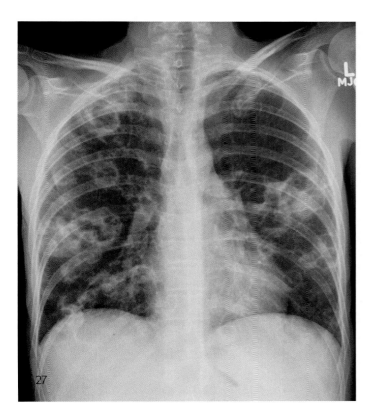

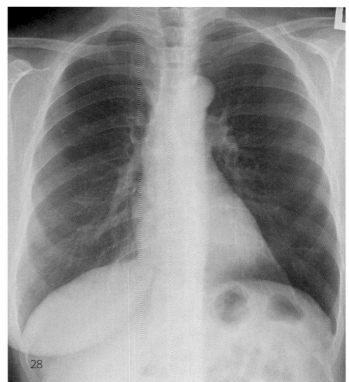

a thorough understanding of past surgical history is important prior to interpretation of the x-ray.

Did you catch the examples on pages 458–459?
Figs. 21a,b and 21g,h – Abscess (cavity)

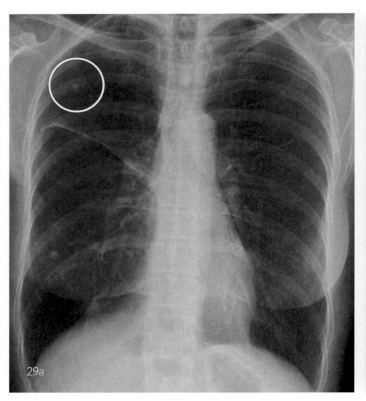

> When the lungs are too white, they can obscure or blend into other anatomical structures that lie adjacent to the lung pathology, causing the appearance of the silhouette sign (Pg. 484).

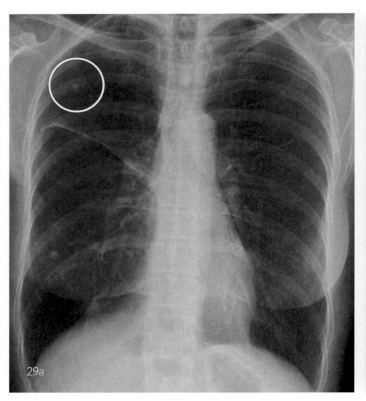

29a

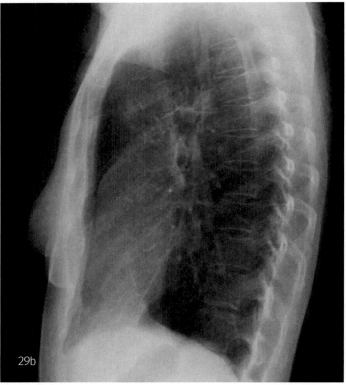

29b

1b. Pathology that affects the lungs and shifts the grayscale to 'Too White'

Pathologies involving the lungs are responsible for a variety of too white patterns. The too white area may: be focal, patchy or diffuse; segmental, lobar, exhibit predominance in the perihilar or peripheral regions or involve the entire lung; be unilateral or bilateral.

Describing the whiteness

Once you have determined that an abnormality exists that is causing the grayscale of the lung to be too white, it is important to describe the whiteness further.

The area of too white may be inhomogeneous, and contain areas that are even whiter. These very white areas are usually calcifications that remain as sequelae of granulomatous

Figure 29. Calcification. Pathology can cause the grayscale of the lungs to appear too white. a, PA chest x-ray from a patient with calcified granulomas, b, lateral chest x-ray from the same patient.

Figure 30. Barium in the lungs. Pathology can cause the grayscale of the lungs to appear too white. a, PA chest x-ray from a patient who inhaled barium, b, lateral chest x-ray from the same patient.

Sometimes the whiteness seen on the PA x-ray is difficult to explain. When this is the case, look at the lateral x-ray to see if the cause of this whiteness relates to pleural disease, or to a collapsed lobe (Ch. 18, Pg. 686).

!

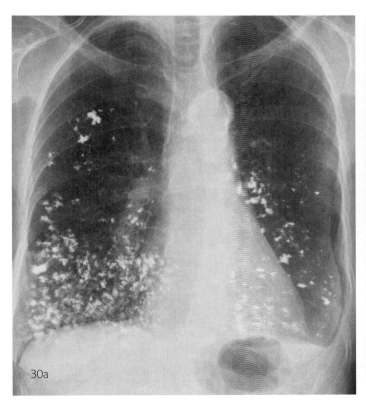

30a

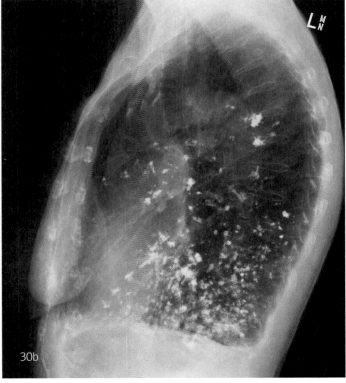

30b

disease within the lungs (Fig. 29a,b). The lungs will also be too white in patients who have aspirated barium during a radiological upper GI examination (Fig. 30a,b).

Did you catch the example on pages 458–459?
Fig. 21q,r – Calcified granulomas

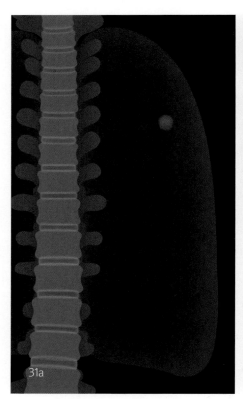

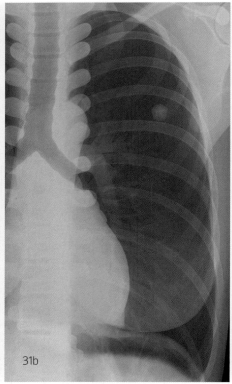

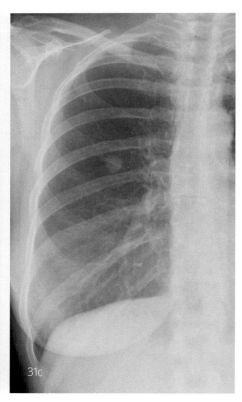

31a

31b

31c

The too white area may be homogeneous and well-circumscribed. Or the focal area may have an irregular spiculated border (as can be seen with some primary lung cancers).

If this area is less than 3 cm, it is called a solitary pulmonary nodule (Fig. 31a,b,c). If this area is greater than 3 cm, it is called a pulmonary mass (Fig. 32a,b,c) (12).

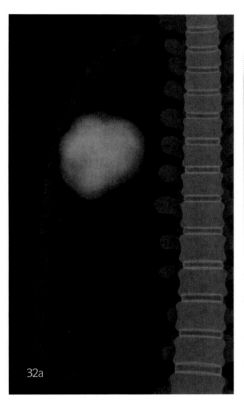

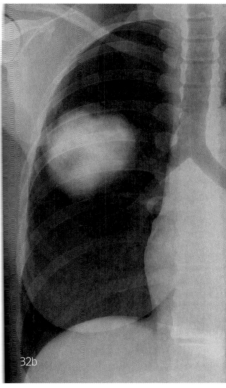

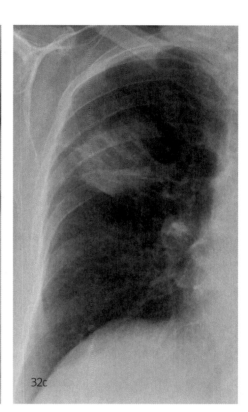

32a

32b

32c

Figure 31. Solitary pulmonary nodule (SPN). a, artistic representation of an SPN, b, artistic representation of an SPN with all thoracic structures, c, PA chest x-ray from a patient with an SPN in the right lung.

Figure 32. Pulmonary mass. a, artistic representation of a pulmonary mass, b, artistic representation of a pulmonary mass with all thoracic structures, c, PA chest x-ray from a patient with a pulmonary mass in the right lung.

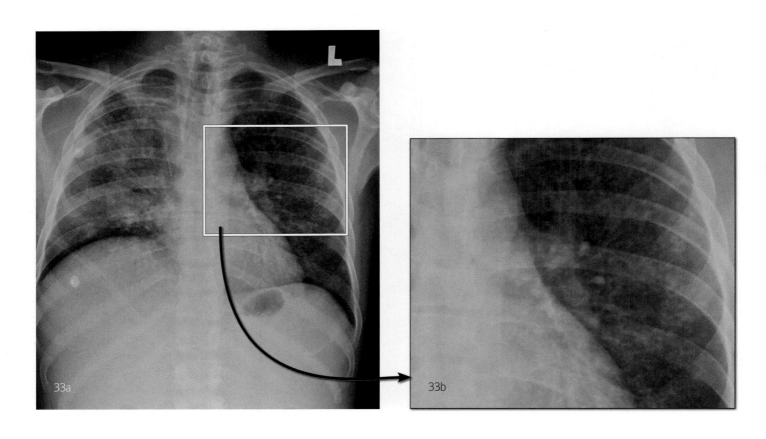

33a

33b

Acinar nodules

Lung nodules are usually associated with interstitial disease; however, nodules can also occur in air space disease. The classic acinar nodule has poorly defined margins, but is discrete enough to be identified as a distinct abnormality. It usually measures 4 to 10 mm in diameter, and may contain internal areas of too black, such as air bronchiolograms or air alveolograms (Fig. 33a,b)(12).

When the lungs look too white, but are normal

The normal lung parenchyma can look too white when the patient has taken a poor inspiration during the examination, or when the x-ray is intentionally taken in expiration. The lungs containing less air appear small and too white (Fig. 34).

The lungs can also look too white (and yet not diseased) when a large amount of soft tissue overlays the lungs, as seen in morbidly obese patients, or women with large breasts. The additional radiological density from breast implants (Fig. 35) will also make regions of the lungs look too white.

If the lungs appear too white and one of these causes is suspected, verification of the cause can be obtained by looking at the lateral x-ray.

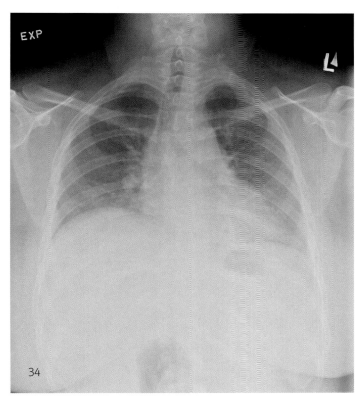

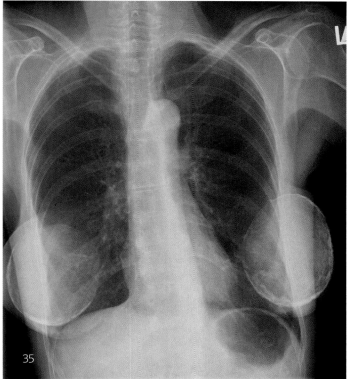

Figure 33. Acinar nodules. Pathology can cause the grayscale of the lungs to appear too white. a, PA chest x-ray form a patient with multiple acinar nodules, b, magnification from the same PA chest x-ray cropped to highlight the nodules in the left lung.

Figure 34. Poor inspiration. The grayscale of the lungs can appear too white even when normal as in this PA chest x-ray due to the patient taking a poor inspiration.

Figure 35. Breast implants. The grayscale of the lungs can appear too white even when normal, as in this PA chest x-ray from a patient with breast implants. The breast implants cause the grayscale of the lungs beneath them to appear too white.

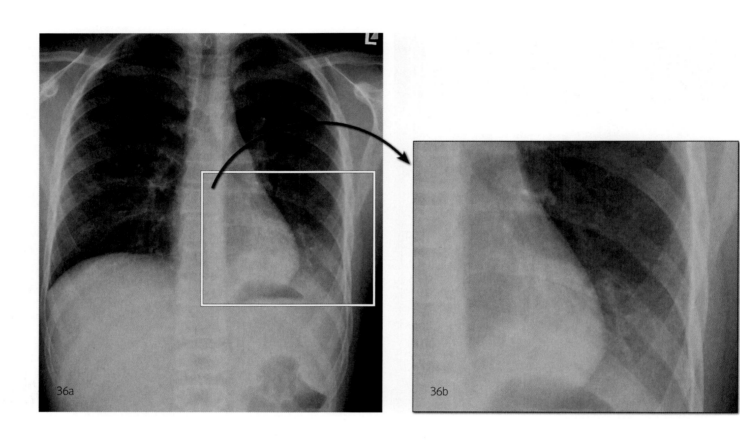

36a

36b

1c. When the lungs are too white AND too black

The focal area may be inhomogeneous, in that part of it is black and part of it is white.

A too white area may contain black branching areas within it – the air bronchogram sign (Fig. 36a,b), and the hallmark of airspace disease (Pg. 484). The air bronchograms will be caused when the airspaces are full of pus, blood, water or tumor (13).

Another example of this pattern of too white AND too black, is an air-fluid level associated with an infected bulla, or a lung abscess (Fig. 37a,b,c).

Figure 36. Air bronchogram sign. Pathology can cause the grayscale of the lungs to appear too white AND too black as in this PA chest x-ray from a patient with pneumonia. a, PA chest x-ray showing air bronchograms, b, magnification of the same PA chest x-ray cropped to highlight the air bronchograms.

Figure 37. Lung abscess. a, artistic representation of a lung abscess, b, artistic representation of a lung abscess with all thoracic structures, c, PA chest x-ray from a patient with a lung abscess in the left lung.

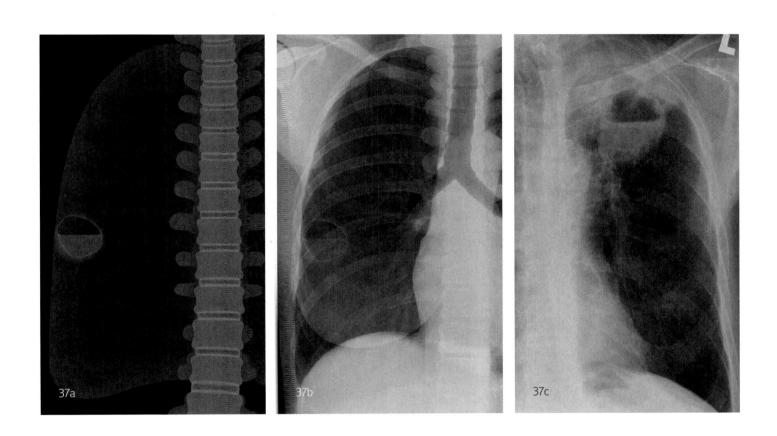

37a

37b

37c

Did you catch the examples on pages 458–459?
Figs. 21c,d and 21e,f – Air bronchograms

RADIOLOGY OF LUNG CANCER

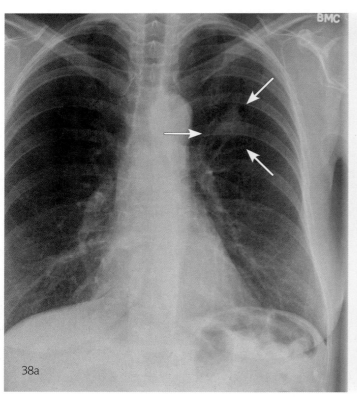

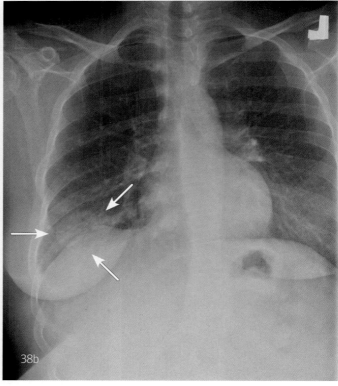

Chest x-rays still play an important role in identifying lung cancer. Unfortunately, we are not very good at identifying early cancers – experienced radiologists can miss up to 25% of small lung nodules! However, radiologists do much better identifying larger lesions.

When present, the appearance of a lung nodule (< 3 cm, **Pg. 468**) (Fig. 38a) or mass (> 3 cm, **Pg. 469**) (Fig. 38b) has to be further characterized. Is it calcified? Does it have large vessels coming in and out of it? Has it been seen on previous x-rays? What is the margin of the lesion like? Spiculated? Has it grown? Is it cavitating? Is there an associated effusion, chest wall involvement, or adenopathy? All of these features may help to establish whether or not the nodule or mass is a malignancy, and help in cancer staging (14).

Did you catch the examples on pages 458–459?
Figs. 21i,j and 21k.l – Metastases
Fig. 21m,n – Mass

Figure 38. Lung mass. a, PA chest x-ray from a patient with an ill-defined small lung mass in the left lung, b, PA chest x-ray from a patient with a large ill-definded lung mass in the right lung (arrows).

How is lung cancer staged?

Using the TNM classification that considers tumor size (T), nodal involvement (N), and secondary spread, metastasis (M) (15).

CHARACTERISTIC	SPECIFIC OBSERVATION	MEANING
Size	Greater than 2 cm	Suspect malignancy
	Less than 4 mm	Benign
Interval growth	Stable over 2 years	Benign
Shape (margin)	Spiculated	Suspect malignancy
Calcification	Diffuse, central, popcorn or laminated calcification	Benign
Other associated features	Effusion	Suspect malignancy
	Chest wall involvement	Suspect malignancy
	Adenopathy	Suspect malignancy

Table 12.3
Characteristics of an Opacity on a Chest X-ray and Their Meaning

RADIOLOGY OF EMPHYSEMA

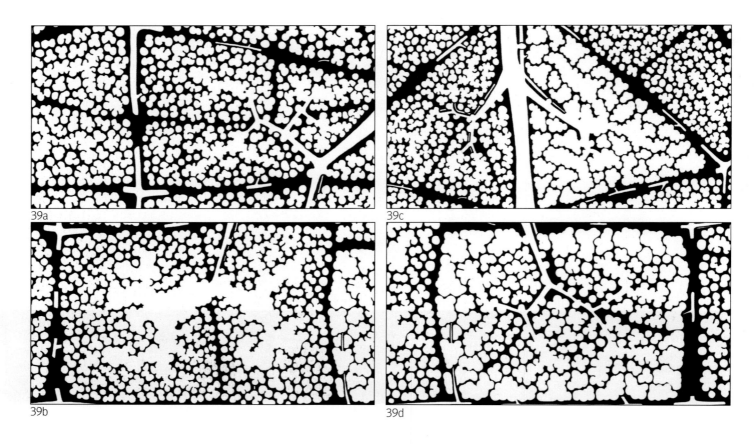

39a

39c

39b

39d

AMSER Emphysema is defined as abnormal, permanent enlargement of the air spaces distal to the terminal bronchioles. This is accompanied by the destruction of alveolar walls, without associated fibrosis. On a chest x-ray, the enlarged air spaces will make the lungs appear too black and hyperinflated.

Pulmonary emphysema is usually classified into three types: centrilobular (centriacinar), panlobular (panacinar), and paraseptal (Fig. 39b,c,d) (16,17).

Centrilobular emphysema is the most common form of emphysema, and involves the centriacinar airspace. Centrilobular emphysema usually involves the upper lobes and the superior segments of the lower lobes (Figs. 39b and 40).

Figure 39. Types of Emphysema. Illustration of the three types of emphysema, a, normal airspaces, b, centrilobular emphysema, c, panlobular emphysema, d, paraseptal emphysema.

Figure 40. Centrilobular emphysema. a, PA chest x-ray from a patient with centrilobular emphysema.

Figure 41. Panlobular emphysema. PA chest x-ray from a patient with panlobular emphysema.

476

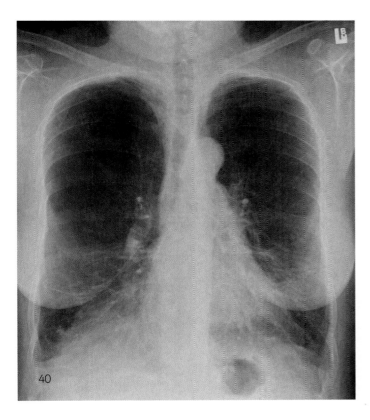

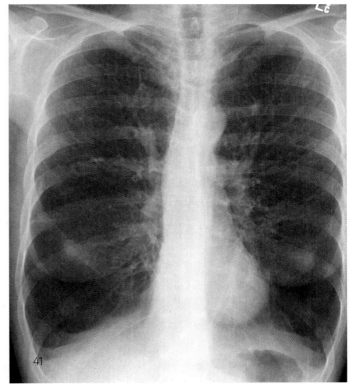

Panacinar emphysema involves the entire length of the secondary lobule, and may be caused by alpha 1-antitrypsin deficiency. This form of emphysema involves predominantly the lower lobes (Figs. 39c and 41).

Paraseptal emphysema is also called distal emphysema, and characteristically involves the periphery of the acini (Fig. 39d). This form of emphysema is usually very limited in extent and is associated with areas of pulmonary fibrosis, most often in the posterior aspect of the upper lobes. Paraseptal emphysema can be seen in combination with other forms of emphysema.

RADIOLOGY OF PNEUMONIA

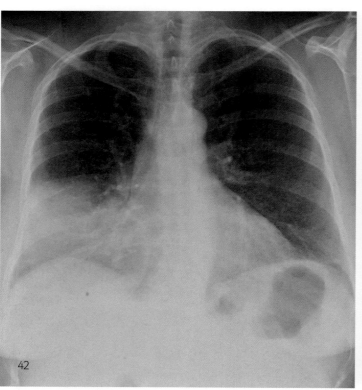

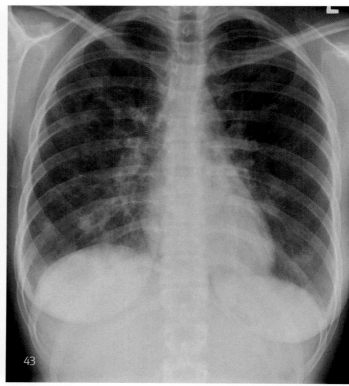

AMSER Pneumonia is an infection of the lower respiratory tract and remains one of the leading causes of death. Pneumonia can be caused by bacterial, viral, fungal and/or parasitic agents (18,19,20).

The infection is acquired through the airways and is confined to the lung parenchyma. Three main radiological patterns of pneumonia can develop: lobar or focal nonsegmental pneumonia, multifocal bronchopneumonia, focal or diffuse interstitial pneumonia (21,22).

Lobar, or focal, nonsegmental pneumonia is usually caused by *Streptococcus pneumoniae*. On an x-ray, the nonsegmental pneumonia is usually homogeneously white, with air bronchograms (Fig. 42). The opacity usually starts in the periphery of one lobe. Lobar pneumonias caused by *Klebsiella pneumoniae* and *Proteus* and

Figure 42. Lobar pneumonia. PA chest x-ray from a patient with lobar pneumonia.

Figure 43. Bronchopneumonia. PA chest x-ray from a patient with bronchopneumonia.

Figure 44. Interstitial pneumonia. PA chest x-ray from a patient with interstitial pneumonia.

Figure 45. Tuberculosis pneumonia. PA chest x-ray from a patient with a left upper lobe cavity secondary to tuberculosis.

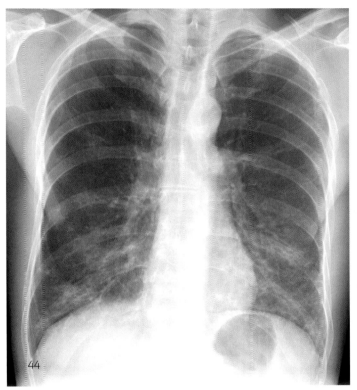

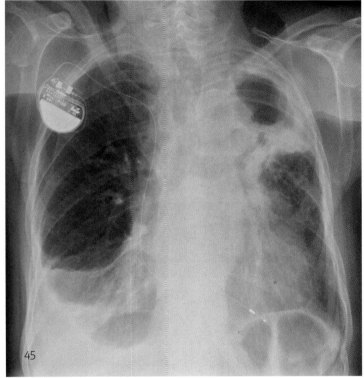

Morganella can initially appear the same as Streptococcal pneumonia, but can lead to abscess formation.

In bronchopneumonia the infection is centered on the larger airways with patchy lung involvement resulting in a patchy opacity pattern on x-rays (Fig. 43). There are usually no air bronchograms. Bronchopneumonias can be caused by *Staphylococcus aureus*, *Streptococcus pyogenes*, *Pseudomonas aeruginosa*, *Haemophilus influenzae*, and anaerobic bacteria. This type of pneumonia is sometimes called lobular (section of a lobe) pneumonia.

Radiologically, interstitial pneumonias can start as a fine reticular pattern, but in the later stages of infection can present as patchy, ill-defined multifocal opacities (Fig. 44). This pattern of infection is usually caused by infectious

agents such as *Haemophilus influenzae*, *Mycoplasma* or *Pneumocystis carinii*.

AMSER

Tuberculosis (TB) can cause pneumonia, but the radiological appearance of TB will vary depending on whether the infection is active or chronic.

In active pulmonary TB, air space disease usually occurs in the upper lungs (Fig. 45). There may be associated adenopathy within the mediastinum or hilum. Cavities can form within the consolidated lung.

The appearance of chronic inactive TB can vary from solitary calcified granulomas, to extensive bronchiectasis, scarring, and volume loss.

SUMMARY OF RADIOLOGICAL CHANGES
TO THE LUNGS & AIRSPACES

RADIOLOGICAL CHANGES		ASSOCIATED FINDINGS, DISEASES AND CONDITIONS
Grayscale changed	Too black	• Pulmonary cyst • Lung cavity • Septic emboli • Emphysema • Bilateral hyperinflation (asthma attack) • Unilateral hyperinflation (due to: lobar atelectasis, lobectomy, pneumonectomy)
	Too white	• Pneumonia • Solitary pulmonary nodule (SPN) • Pulmonary mass • Metastatic disease • Acinar nodules • Septic emboli • Calcifications due to granulomatous disease • Barium in the lungs (barium aspiration during upper GI exam) • Tuberculosis
	Too white AND too black	• Infected bulla • Lung abscess • Septic emboli

Table 12.4
Summary of Radiological Changes to the Lungs & Airspaces

Common Areas in Which Lung Pathology is Missed (Fig. 46a,b)

1. Below the upper edge of the diaphragms – obscured by abdominal organs (Fig. 47a,b)
2. Retrocardiac region – obscured by heart (Fig. 48a,b)
3. Apices - obscured by ribs and clavicles (Fig. 49a,b)
4. On the lateral, overlying the spine – obscured by vertebral bodies (Fig. 50a,b)

!

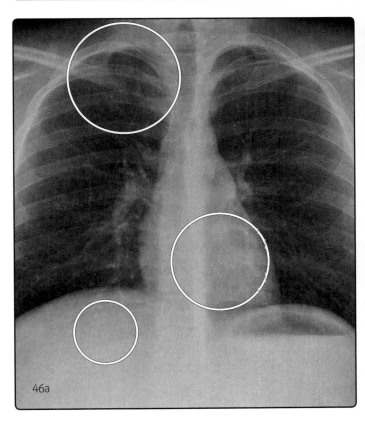

46a

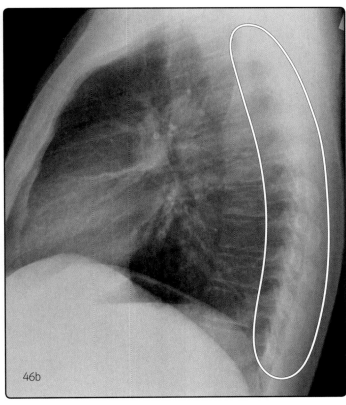

46b

Figure 46. Areas on a chest x-ray where lung pathology is commonly missed. a, PA chest x-ray with the three areas highlighted, b, lateral chest x-ray with the fourth region highlighted.

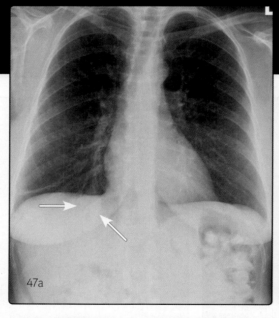

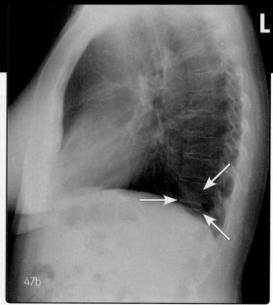

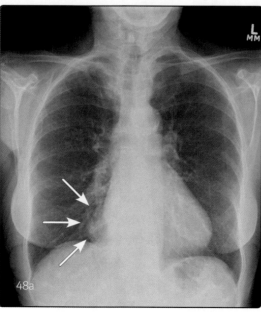

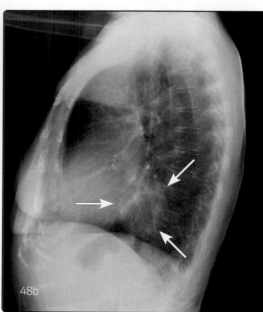

Figure 47. Pathology hidden below diaphragms. a, PA chest x-ray from a patient with an SPN (arrows) below the diaphragms, b, lateral chest x-ray from the same patient.

Figure 48. Pathology hidden behind heart. a. PA chest x-ray from a patient with a right lower lobe mass (arrows) hidden behind the heart, b. lateral chest x-ray from the same patient.

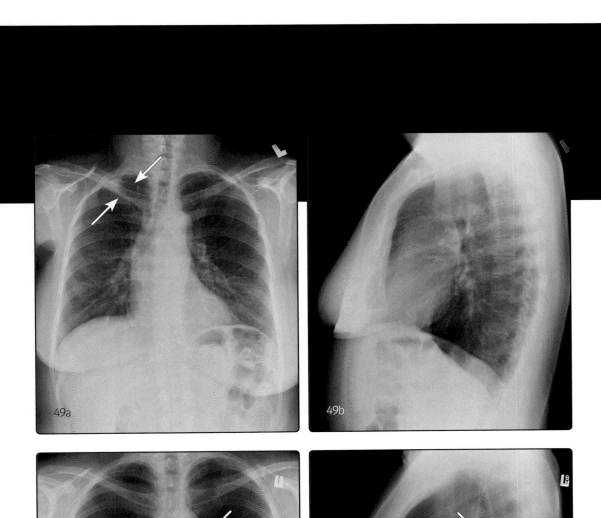

49a 49b

50a 50b

Figure 49. Pathology hidden in apices of lungs. a, PA chest x-ray from a patient with a right apical mass hidden in the apex of the right lung (arrows), b, lateral chest x-ray from the same patient.

Figure 50. Pathology hidden behind spine. a. PA chest x-ray from a patient with mass in left lower lobe (arrows), hidden by the spine, superiorly and medially, b, lateral chest x-ray from the same patient.

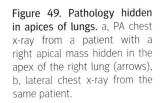

RADIOLOGICAL SIGNS
RELATED TO THE LUNGS & AIRSPACES

Air Bronchogram Sign (20)

AMSER   Normally, the peripheral bronchi are not visible on the chest x-ray because the walls of these bronchi are not thick enough to create an interface. The blackness of the air within the bronchi blends with the blackness of the air in the alveoli. However, if the alveoli are opacified, and the bronchi remain patent and full of air, the bronchi will become visible on the x-ray. The visualization of black branching bronchi within an opacified white lung is called an air bronchogram (if it involves the bronchi) (Fig. 51a,b,c), an air bronchiologram (if it involves the smaller bronchi and bronchioles), and an air alveologram (if it involves the alveoli).

An air bronchogram is indicative of airspace disease. Air bronchograms can be seen with pneumonia, pulmonary contusion and bleeding, pulmonary edema and bronchoalveolar cell carcinoma and lymphoma. The presence of an air bronchogram helps localize pathology to the respiratory zone of the lungs.

If the bronchi also become filled with fluid, cells or blood, the opacity will still be visible, but the black rectangles will disappear. In this case, there is no air bronchogram sign and the differential diagnosis will include a broader range of pathologies, including lung tumor.

The Silhouette Sign

AMSER   The silhouette sign occurs whenever two structures of similar radiological density are touching each other (Ch. 17, Pg. 654). When this occurs on x-ray, the two will appear as one structure (i.e., the interface between them is lost).

Spine Sign

AMSER   On the lateral x-ray, the posterior lungs will become blacker from superior to inferior. This normal gradient in grayscale is due to the fact that the lungs are wider and contain more air inferiorly. For this same reason, on the lateral x-ray, the thoracic vertebrae will look blacker more inferiorly. When pathology (e.g., tumor) is present, this gradient is lost - this is called the spine sign (Fig. 52a,b,c).

Figure 51. Air bronchogram sign. a, artistic representation of an the air bronchogram sign, b, artistic representation of an the air bronchogram sign with all thoracic structures, c, PA chest x-ray from a patient with left lower lobe pneumonia highlighting the air bronchogram sign.

Figure 52. Spine sign. a, artistic representation of an the spine sign, b, artistic representation of an the spine sign with all thoracic structures, c, PA chest x-ray from a patient with a posterior mediastinal tumor highlighting the spine sign.

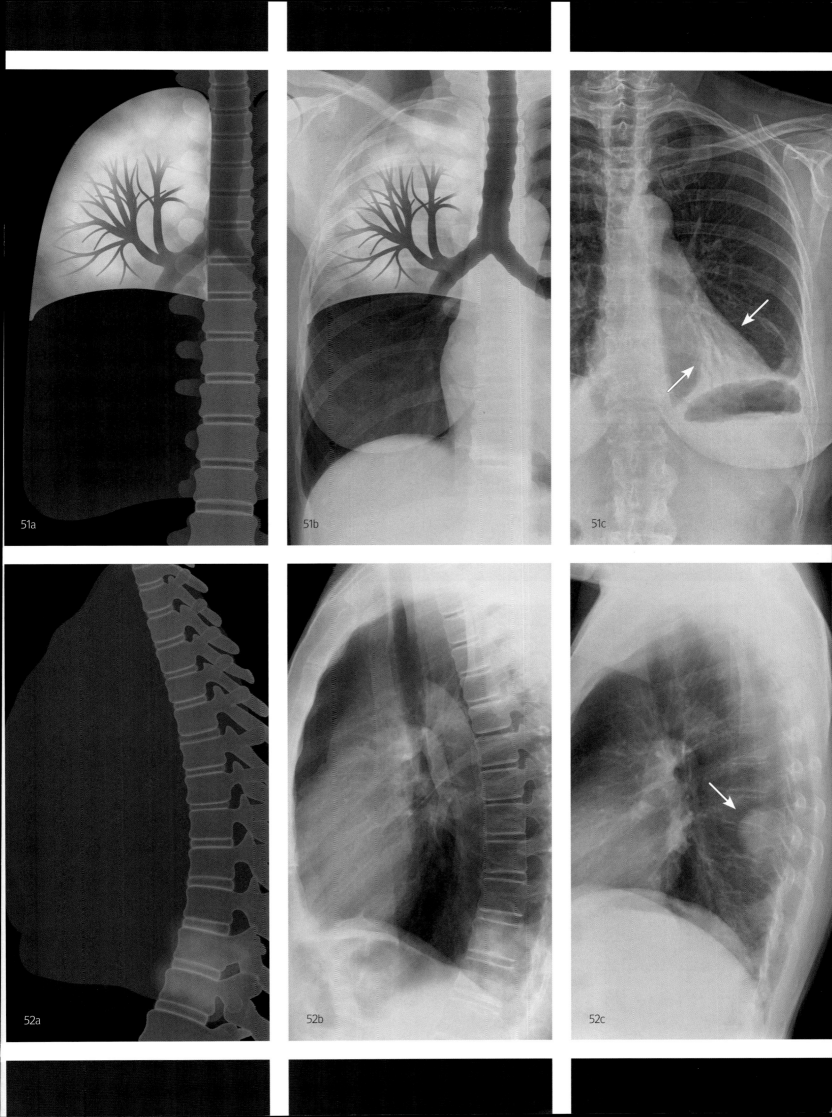

51a

51b

51c

52a

52b

52c

Visual Search of the Lungs

PA Chest X-ray

1. Start at the right apex (1).

2. Follow the lateral outline of the lung inferiorly to the right costophrenic angle (2).

3. Follow the inferior outline of the lung medially to the mediastinum (3).

4. Follow the medial outline of lung to the apex (4).

Complete the visual search by checking for any density changes across the thorax from top to bottom.

Follow the same instructions on the left.

VS

Lateral Chest X-ray

1. Start at the apex anteriorly (1).

2. Follow the outline of the lungs inferiorly to the diaphragm (2).

3. Follow the outline of the lungs posteriorly to the costovertebral angles (3).

4. Follow the posterior outline of lungs superiorly to the thoracic inlet (4).

Complete the visual search by checking for any density changes across the thorax from top to bottom.

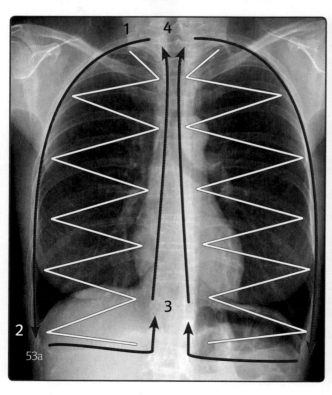

53a

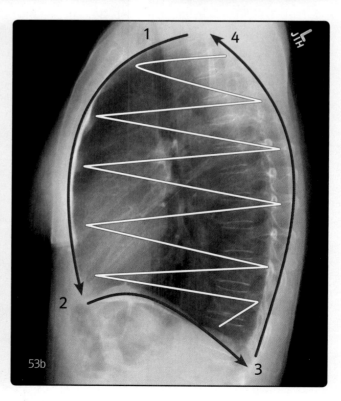

53b

Lung Radiological Analysis Checklist

GRAYSCALE

1   Is the grayscale of the lungs altered?

If **YES**, then describe.
Too white/too black/too white AND too black.
Right/left/bilateral.

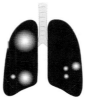

If **TOO WHITE**, then describe opacity.
Focal/diffuse.
Multiple/solitary.
Homogeneous/inhomogeneous.

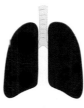

If **TOO BLACK**, then describe hyperlucency.
Focal/diffuse.
Multiple/solitary.
Pathological/mastectomy/surgery.
Homogeneous/inhomogeneous.

2   Is the normal branching of blood vessels obscured?

If **YES**, then describe.
Right/left/bilateral.

SIZE

3   Is the size of the lungs altered? (Does the blackness of the lungs extend all the way to the ribs?)

If **NO**, then describe.
Right/left/bilateral.
Increased/decreased.

OTHER

4   Are there any radiological signs related to the lungs?

If **YES**, then describe.
Air bronchogram.
Silhouette.
Spine.

5   Is there any evidence of previous surgery to the lungs?

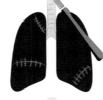

If **YES**, then describe.
Type of surgery and location.
Compare to previous CXR.

6   Are there any lines or tubes in the lungs?

If **YES**, then describe.
Give location of each relative to the carina, SVC and/or diaphragms.

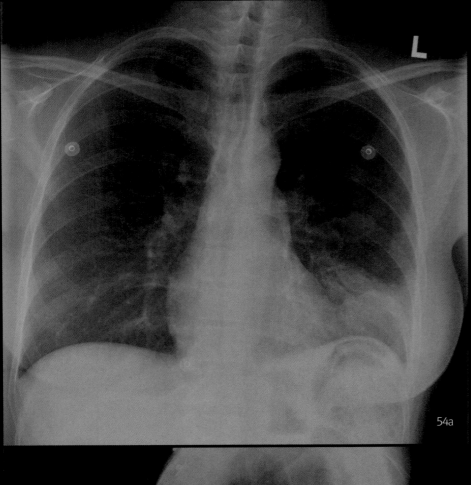

54a

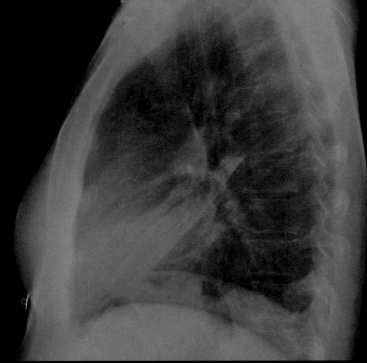

How would you describe your findings?

54b

You are the intern on call at a rural hospital. Your pager goes off when a 69-year-old female patient presents to the emergency department with a two-week history of flu-like symptoms, productive cough and fever. After a thorough history and examination, you suspect that she has a community-acquired pneumonia and proceed to investigate with lab work and a chest x-ray (Fig. 54a,b). You call the consultant on call and proceed to describe the x-ray findings.

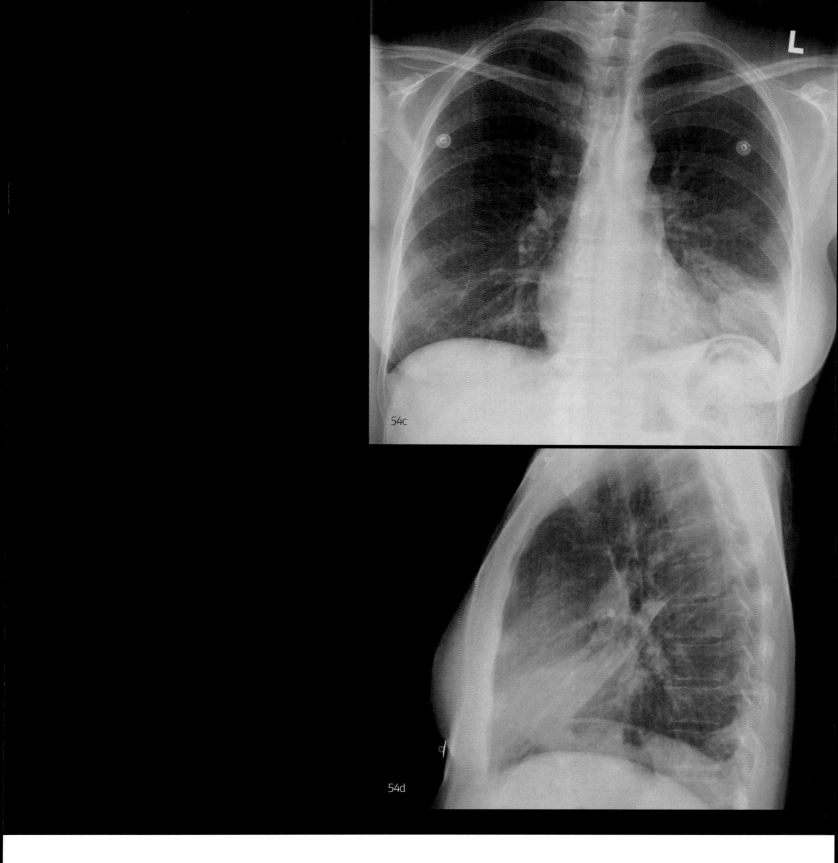

54c

54d

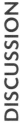

After reading this chapter, you should have an appreciation of the kind of pathology that can affect the lungs and airspaces. The most common of these are viral and bacterial infections of the lung parenchyma. Figures 54c and 54d show airspace consolidation within the right lung base. There are clear air bronchograms (Fig. 54c). Airspace consolidation can be caused by blood, pus, water and sometimes tumor in the airspaces. Compare the PA and lateral x-rays to see if you can localize the pathology to the affected lobe and segments.

Based on the findings, the diagnosis is lobar pneumonia (lingula, LUL).

DISCUSSION

References

1. Lewis, P.J., Shaffer, K., & Donovan, A. (Eds.). (2012). AMSER National Medical Student Curriculum in Radiology. http://aur.org/Secondary-Alliances.aspx?id=141.

2. Lewis, P.J., & Shaffer, K. (2005). Developing a national medical student curriculum in radiology. *Am. Coll. Radiol., 2*(1):8–11.

3. Ugalde, P., Camargo, J.J., & Deslaurieurs, J. (2007). Lobes, fissures and bronchopulmonary segments. *Thorac. Surg. Clin., 17*:587–599.

4. Nealy, W.C., Connolly, S.R., & Dalton, B.L. (1993). Naming the bronchopulmonary segments and the development of pulmonary surgery. *Ann. Thorac. Surg., 55*:184–188.

5. Jardin, M., & Remy, J. (1986). Segmental bronchovascular anatomy of the lower lobes: CT analysis. *AJR Am. J. Roentgenol., 147*(3):457–468.

6. Reid, L. (1958). The secondary lobule in the adult human lung, with special reference to its appearance in bronchograms. *Thorax, 13*(2):110–115.

7. Webb, W.R. (2006). Thin-section CT of the secondary pulmonary lobule: anatomy and the image—the 2004 Fleischner lecture. *Radiology, 239*(2):322–338.

8. Frija, J., de Kerviler, E., & Zagdanski, A.M. (1997). Radiologic anatomy of the inferior lung margins as demonstrated on computed radiography with enhancement of low frequencies. *Surg. Radiol. Anat. SRA., 19*(4):257–263.

9. Gibson, G.J. (1996). Pulmonary hyperinflation: a clinical overview. *Eur. Respir. J., 9*:2640–2649.

10. Fleischner, F.G. (1948). The visible bronchial tree; a roentgen sign in pneumonic and other pulmonary consolidations. *Radiology, 50*(2):184–189.

11. Tuddenham, W.J. (1984). Glossary of Terms for Thoracic Radiology: recommendations of the Nomenclature Committee of the Fleischner Society. *AJR Am. J. Roentengol., 143*: 509–517.

12. Itoh, H., Tokunaga, S., Todo, G., et al. (1978). Radiologicpathologic correlation of small lung nodules with special reference to peribronchial nodules. *AJR Am. J. Roentgenol., 130*:223–231.

13. Albert, R.H., & Russell, J.J. (2009). Evaluation of the solitary pulmonary nodule. *Am. Fam. Phys., 80*(8):827–831.

14. UyBico, S.J., Wu, C.C., Suh, R.D., et al. (2010). Lung cancer staging essentials: The new TNM staging system and potential imaging pitfalls. *RadioGraphics, 30*:1163–1181.

15. Takahashi, M., Fukuoka, J., Nitta, N., et al. (2008). Imaging of pulmonary emphysema: a pictorial review. *Int. J. Chron.Obstruct. Pulmon. Dis., 3*(2):193–204.

16. Goldin, J.G. (2009). Imaging the lungs in patients with pulmonary emphysema. *J. Thorac. Imaging, 24*(3):163–170.

17. Das, D., & Howlett, D.C. (2009). Chest x-ray manifestations of pneumonia. *Surgery (Oxford), 27*(10):453–455.

18. Franquet, T. (2001). Imaging of pneumonia: trends and algorithms. *Eur. Resp. J., 1*:196–208.

19. Ashizawa, K. (2009). Imaging of Pulmonary Furgal Infection. *Nippon Ishinkin Gakkai Zasshi, 50*:27–32.

20. Gefter, W.B. (1992). The spectrum of pulmonary aspergillosis. *J. Thorac. Imag., 7*:56–74.

21. Ramos, G., Orduña, A., & García-Yuste, M. (2001). Hydatid cyst of the lung: diagnosis and treatment. *World J. Surg., 25*(1):46–57.

22. Ganong, W. F. (2012) *Ganong's Review of Medical Physiology*, 24th ed. New York, NY: McGraw-Hill Professional.

CHAPTER 13
The INTERSTITIUM

importance

The interstitium is the scaffolding of the lung, and is involved in many chronic lung disorders. Patients with diseases of the interstitium usually present with non-specific clinical symptoms. An abnormal chest x-ray can often be the first clue to the presence of interstitial lung pathology. Identifying an abnormal interstitial pattern on an x-ray is essential for the early diagnosis and treatment of interstitial disease.

objectives

Skills

You will identify

- the different patterns of lung pathology (nodular, linear and reticular) on the PA and lateral chest x-rays.

- interstitial abnormalities based on location.

You will provide

- a pertinent differential diagnosis for the different lung patterns (nodular, linear and reticular).

Knowledge

You will review and understand

- the normal anatomy of the lung interstitium.

- common, important pathology of the lung interstitium.

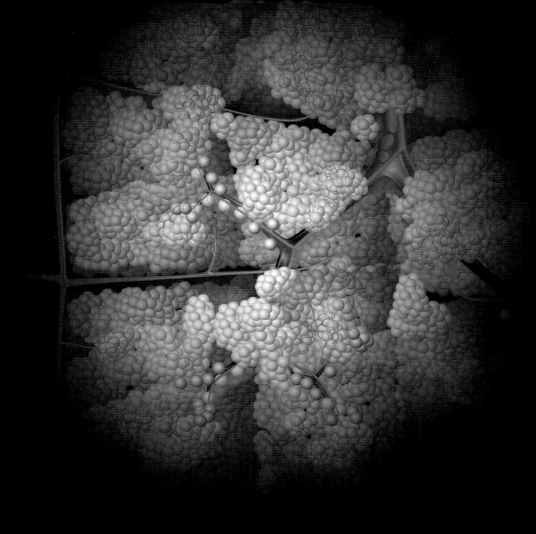

associated resources

This chapter maps to the following AMSER curriculum content (1,2).

1) Interstitial abnormalities
   Interstitial edema
   Extensive fibrosis (e.g., honeycombing, cystic fibrosis)

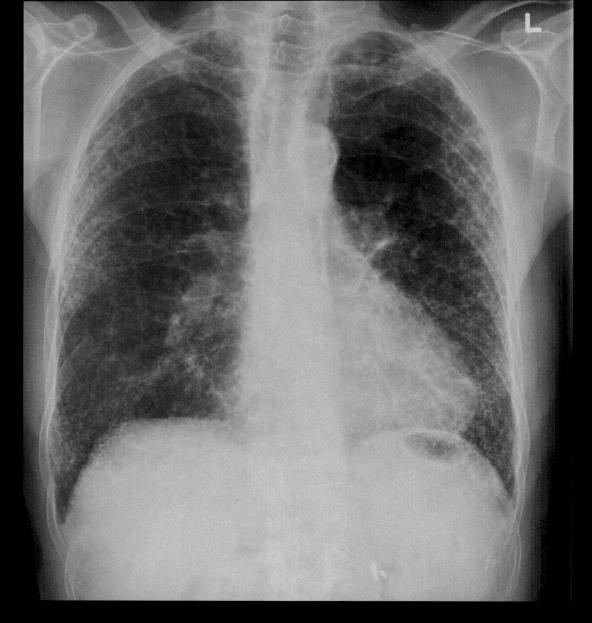

1a

An 80-year-old male is admitted to hospital with a 20-year history of dry cough, wheezing and a worsening of shortness of breath. He worked in construction for 55 years before retiring, and he claims he was exposed to asbestos on a daily basis. You suspect he may have pathology affecting the interstitium of his lungs. You order chest x-rays (Fig. 1a,b).

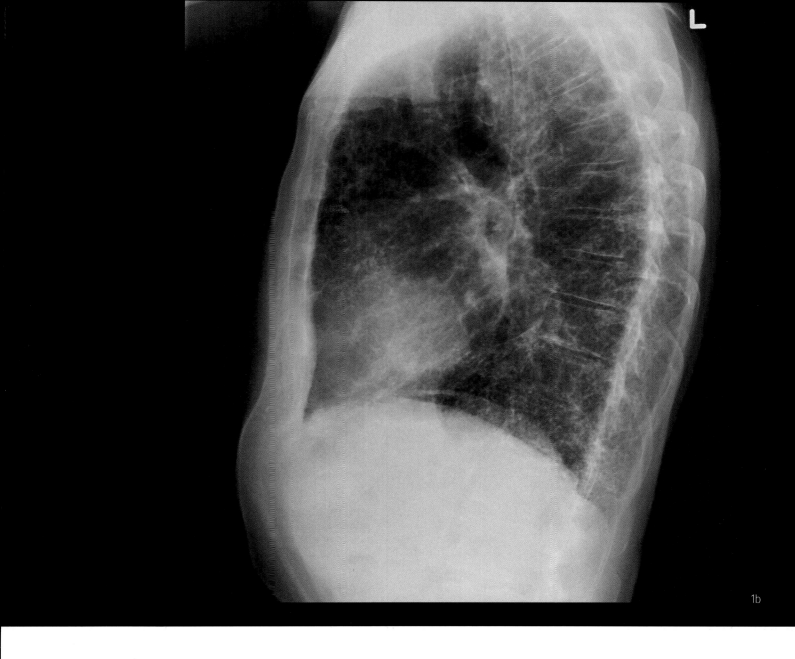

1b

How would you
describe your findings?

THE LUNG INTERSTITIUM

The word interstitium comes from the Latin *inter* and *sistere*, and means "whatever is placed between".

The interstitium of the lungs is the connective tissue scaffolding that holds the structure of the airspaces together. It is a network of fibers that extends from the central airways and vessels to the periphery of the lungs.

Components of the Interstitium

The lung interstitium can be divided into three different components (Fig. 2a,b):

1. Bronchovascular Interstitium – the interstitium that lies adjacent to the proximal vessels and airways.

2. Septal Interstitium – the interstitial fibers that connect the central bronchovascular interstitium with the peripheral interlobular septae.

3. Interlobular Septae – the part of the interstitium that defines the borders of the secondary lobules. The interlobular septal interstitium fibers are an extension of the subpleural fibers that invaginate into the lungs.

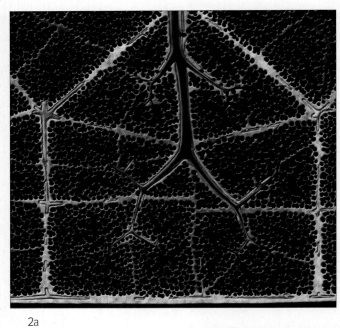

2a

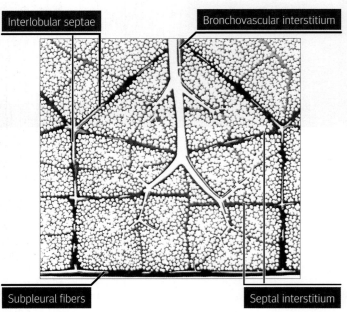

Interlobular septae

Bronchovascular interstitium

Subpleural fibers

Septal interstitium

2b

Figure 2. The components of the interstitium. a, artistic representation of the interstitial components of the secondary lobule of the lung as it would appear on high resolution computed tomography (HRCT), b, the interstitial components of the secondary lung lobule, labeled.

Radiological Shape and Grayscale of the Interstitium

The normal interstitium is not visible on chest x-rays for several reasons. Centrally, the fibers lie adjacent to the vessels and airways and, therefore, will not be seen as separate structures on the x-ray. Peripherally, the interstitium is so fine that it does not have enough radiodensity to be seen on the x-ray.

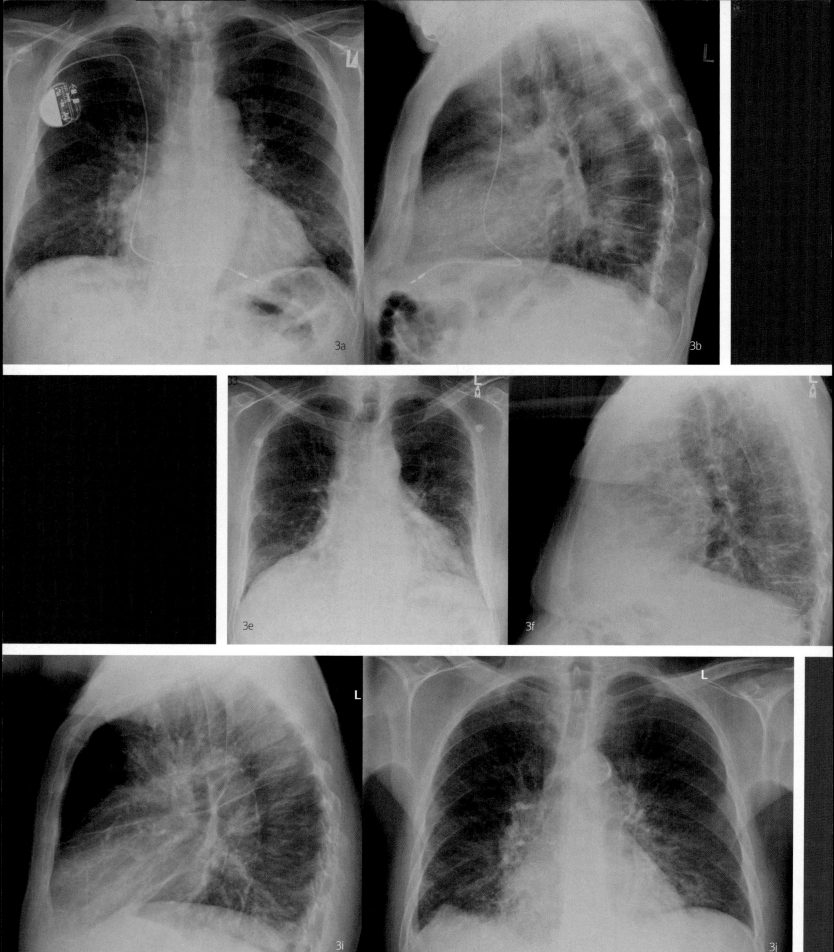

PATHOLOGY of the INTERSTITIUM

Example images of diseases and conditions that affect the interstitium.

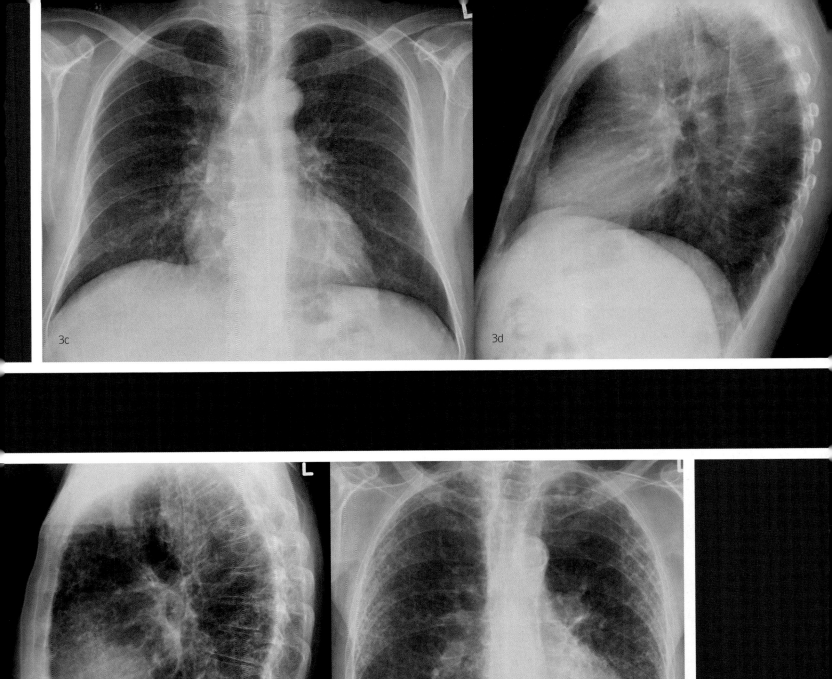

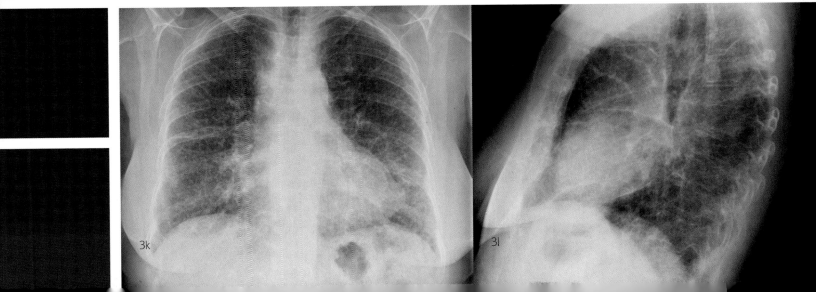

3c

3d

3g

3h

3k

3l

THE ABNORMAL INTERSTITIUM

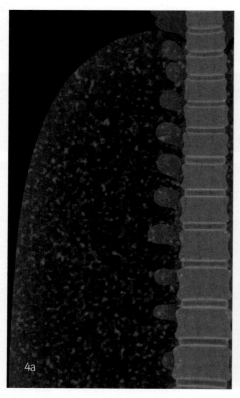 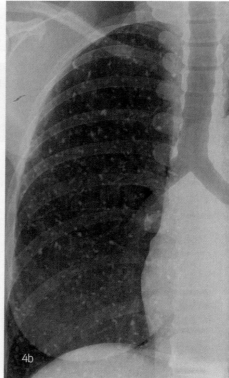 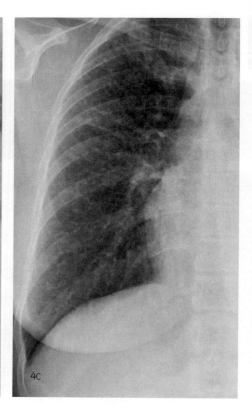

The Radiological Appearance of the Interstitium Will Be Abnormal When

1. the grayscale of the intersitium is too white.

1. Pathology that alters the interstitium and shifts the grayscale to 'Too White'

Pathology that affects the interstitium causes a shift in the normal grayscale to too white. Based on the pattern that is created by the areas of 'too white', abnormalities involving the interstitium can be further classified as:

i) predominantly nodular.

ii) predominantly reticular.

iii) predominantly linear, or.

iv) a mixed reticulonodular pattern.

Figure 4. Nodular pattern. a, artistic representation of a nodular pattern, b, artistic representation of a nodular pattern with all thoracic structures, c, PA chest x-ray from a patient with interstitial lung disease showing a nodular pattern.

Figure 5. Miliary pattern. a, artistic representation of a miliary pattern, b, artistic representation of a miliary pattern with all thoracic structures, c, PA chest x-ray from a patient with tuberculosis showing a typical miliary pattern.

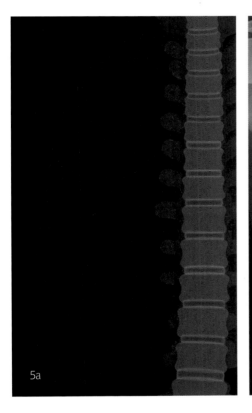 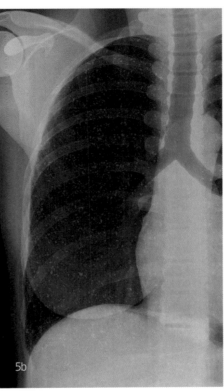 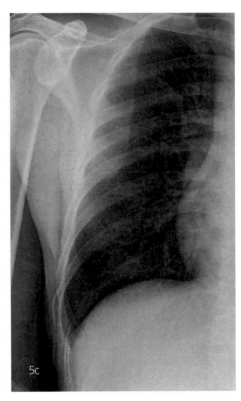

5a   5b   5c

I) Too many nodules

A nodular pattern as defined by the Fleisnner society is characterized by the presence of innumerable, small, rounded opacities that are discrete and range in diameter from 2 to 10 mm. The nodules are widespread in distribution and are without marginal spiculation (4). The nodules may, or may not, be calcified. Calcification usually implies chronicity.

Interstitial nodules differ from alveolar nodules radiologically in that they are homogeneous, very distinct, with clear, well-circumscribed borders, and they vary in size (Fig. 4a,b,c).

When there are multiple, less than 3 mm nodules in the lungs, this is described as a miliary pattern, or the micronodular pattern (Fig. 5a,b,c).

Did you catch the example on pages 498–499?
Fig. 3c,d – A miliary pattern in a patient with tuberculosis.

INTERSTITIUM Chapter 13 SECTION II

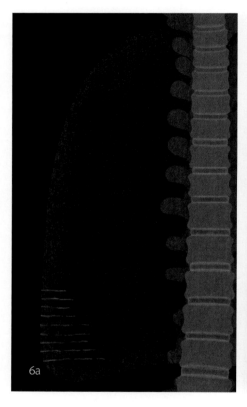

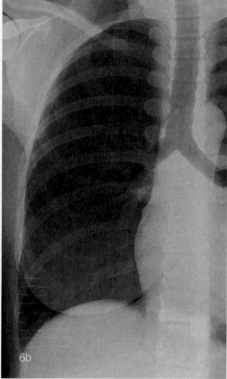

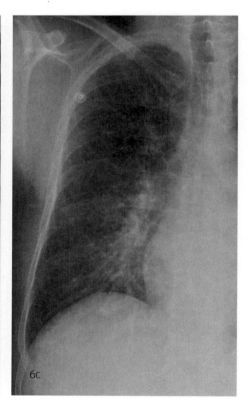

6a

6b

6c

II) Too many lines

The interstitial linear pattern is the result of thickening in, or around, the bronchovascular interstitium, the septal interstitium, or the interlobular septae (5).

Kerley B lines are an example of a linear pattern, representing a disease process involving the peripheral interlobular septae. The interlobular septae are an extension of subpleural fibers and start at the visceral pleura. Kerley B lines, therefore, extend all the way to the pleura (Fig. 6a,b,c).

Kerley A lines (Fig. 7a,b,c) are also a specific type of reticular pattern caused by the involvement of the septal interstitium. They connect the central bronchovascular interstitium with the peripheral interlobular septae. Kerley A lines are longer and usually thicker in caliber than Kerley B lines.

Figure 6. Kerley B lines. a, artistic representation of Kerley B lines, b, artistic representation of Kerley B lines with all thoracic structures, c, PA chest x-ray from a patient with congestive heart failure showing typical Kerley B lines.

Figure 7. Kerley A lines. a, PA chest x-ray from a patient with heart failure showing typical Kerley A lines, b, magnification of the same x-ray, Kerley A lines indicated (arrows).

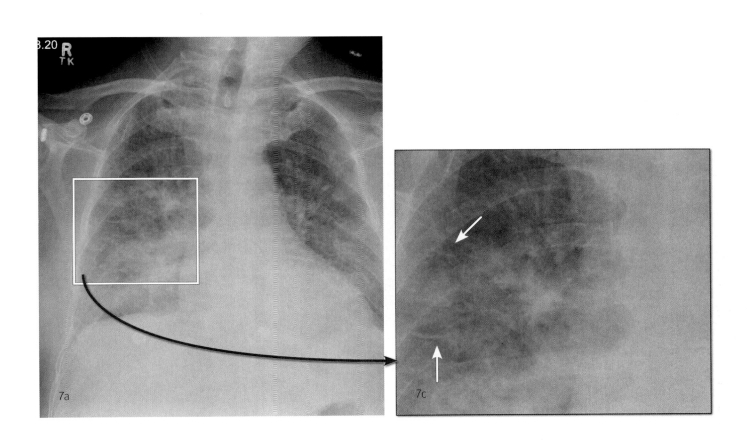

7a

7c

Did you catch the examples on pages 498–499?
Fig. 3a,b – Kerley B lines in a patient with heart failure.
Fig. 3k,l – An interstitial pattern in a patient with pulmonary interstitial lung disease.

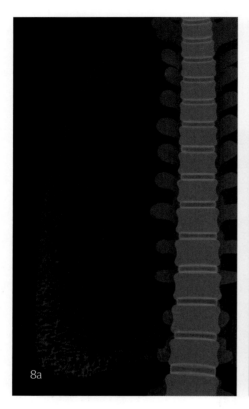
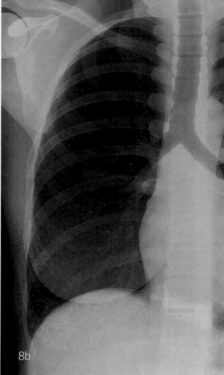
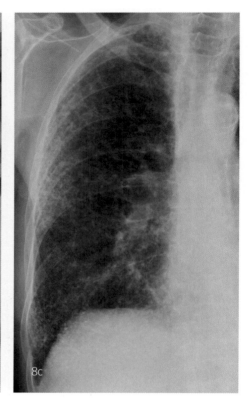

8a

8b

8c

III) The reticular pattern and too many circles

The reticular pattern is defined as a collection of innumerable, small, linear opacities, that together, produce an appearance resembling a net or web (Fig. 8a,b,c)(4).

A honeycomb pattern is a specific reticular pattern in which the web formed by the linear opacities resembles a true honeycomb. On an x-ray and CT scan, the pattern appears as a number of closely approximated ring shadows representing air spaces 5 to 10 mm in diameter, with walls 2 to 3 mm in thickness (Fig. 9a,b).

IV) The reticulonodular pattern

The reticulonodular pattern is defined as a collection of innumerable small, linear and micronodular opacities

Figure 8. Reticular pattern. a, artistic representation of a reticular pattern, b, artistic representation of reticular pattern with all thoracic structures, c, PA chest x-ray from a patient with interstitial lung disease showing a typical reticular pattern.

Figure 9. Honeycomb pattern. a, artistic representation of honeycomb pattern, b, axial CT scan showing the honeycomb pattern within the lung bases.

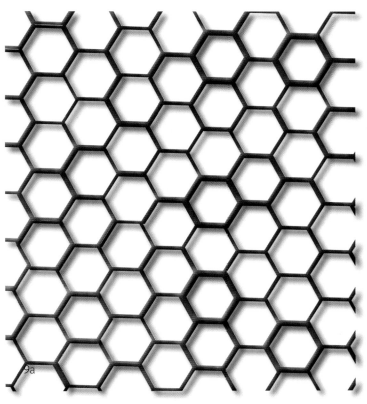

9a

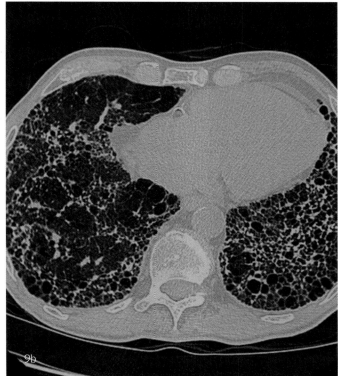

9b

that, together, produce an appearance resembling a net with small, superimposed nodules.

The differential diagnosis of disease processes that have both small nodules and reticulations is long. You can try to narrow down the differential diagnosis by determining which of the two patterns dominates. In most cases, a high resolution computed tomography (CT) scan is necessary to help establish a diagnosis.

Did you catch the example on pages 498–499?
Fig. 3g,h – A reticulonodular pattern in a patient with usual interstitial pneumonia.

How to identify interstitial nodules or lines on the chest x-ray

Since the blood vessels can have a linear appearance, the first step in identifying an abnormal reticular pattern is to be able to distinguish the normal vessels from pathology.

Normal blood vessels get smaller more peripherally, and will branch.

Abnormal reticulations will not usually change in size peripherally, and will not branch.

On a normal chest x-ray, there are very few vascular markings in the peripheral third of the lungs and in the retrosternal airspace. Therefore, with less blood vessel markings to confuse you, these areas provide an ideal backdrop to identify interstitial nodules and lines.

STEP 1
Confirm that the patient is midline and not rotated (Ch. 1, Pg. 32).

STEP 2
Start with the PA x-ray, and scan the periphery of lungs from inferior to superior (Fig. 10).

STEP 3
On the lateral, scan the retrosternal airspace from inferior to superior (Fig. 11).

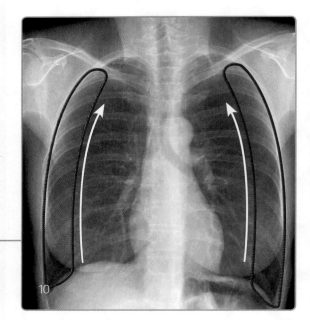

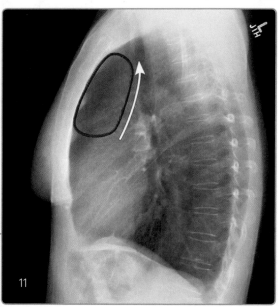

Blood vessels, when seen end-on on an x-ray, can also look like nodules and can be mistaken for interstitial pathology. Look for nodules in the periphery where vessels are not normally seen.

!

	PREDOMINANTLY NODULAR	PREDOMINANTLY RETICULAR	PREDOMINANTLY LINEAR	MIXED RETICULONODULAR
Key features	• Small round discrete opacities • 2 to 10 mm	• Small linear opacities • Net or web-like	• Thickening in or around the bronchovascular bundle, the perivenous bundles or the interlobular septae	• Small, linear micronodular opacities • Net-like with small superimposed nodules

Table 13.1
Summary of the Radiological Features of Interstitial Pathology – Patterns of Interstitial Disease

AUTHOR RECOMMENDATION
Confused about reticular and linear? Is there a difference? Many authors use linear and reticular synonymously. In our discussion, we define the two separately.

DIFFERENTIAL DIAGNOSES FOR INTERSTITIAL PATHOLOGY

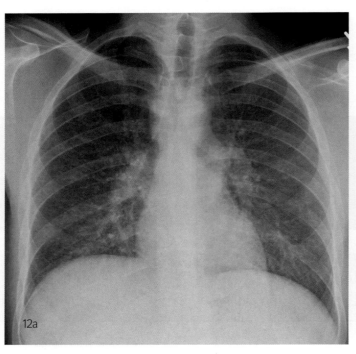

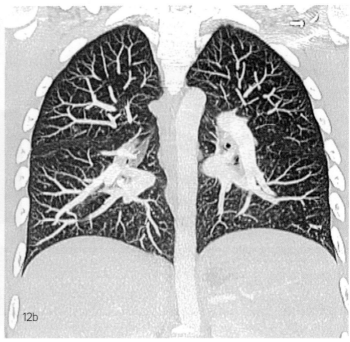

Differential Diagnosis for a Predominantly Small Nodular Interstitial Pattern

Common causes

Small nodules (Fig. 12a,b) can be caused by infectious disease processes, such as tuberculosis, or by non-infectious processes, such as metastases or silicosis. For this reason, it is appropriate to have a differential diagnosis based on whether the patient is febrile or afebrile.

If febrile, the differential diagnosis would include tuberculosis and histoplasmosis.

If afebrile, the differential diagnosis would also start with infectious causes, such as tuberculosis and histoplasmosis. However, you would then also include the following:

- Neoplastic causes – such as metastases from the thyroid gland.

- Occupational exposure – such as silicosis.
- Unknown etiology – such as sarcoidosis.

Rare causes

If all of the above are ruled out, then consider other rare disease processes that can cause interstitial nodules, such as: fungal infections, viral infections, and Histiocytosis X.

Figure 12. Small lung nodules. a, PA chest x-ray from a patient with miliary TB highlighting the presence of small lung nodules, b, CT scan from the same patient. Small nodules are present throughout both lungs.

Figure 13. Linear pattern. a, PA chest x-ray from a patient with heart failure highlighting a typical linear pattern, b, lateral chest x-ray from the same patient.

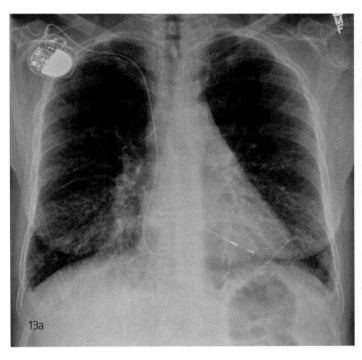

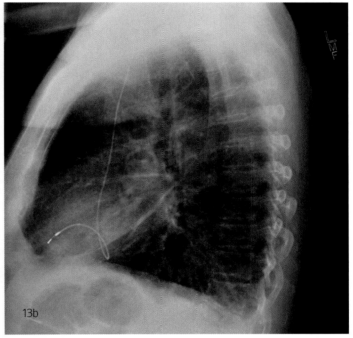

Differential Diagnosis for a Predominantly Linear Interstitial Pattern

Common causes

The differential diagnosis for a predominantly linear pattern (Fig. 13a,b) is formed on the basis of whether the patient is acutely ill or if the changes are chronic.

If acutely ill, the differential diagnosis must exclude cardiac causes, especially interstitial pulmonary edema. Other x-ray findings in cases of pulmonary edema are outlined in Chapter XX, page XX.

If the reticular changes are chronic, we again start with cardiac causes such as:

- Chronic congestive heart failure;
- Mitral valve stenosis;
- Left atrial myxoma.

Then the differential diagnosis would also include:

- Neoplastic causes – such as lymphangitic carcinomatosis.
- Occupational exposure – such as asbestosis.
- Unknown etiology – such as usual interstitial pneumonia, desquamative interstitial pneumonia (DIP), lymphocytic interstitial pneumonia (LIP), collagen vascular disease (e.g., rheumatoid arthritis, scleroderma), and systemic sclerosis.)

Rare causes

If all of the above are ruled out, then consider other rare disease processes that can cause an interstitial linear pattern such as: neurofibromatosis and tuberous sclerosis.

Did you catch the example on pages 498–499?
Fig. 3i,j – Pulmonary edema

INTERSTITIUM **Chapter 13** SECTION II

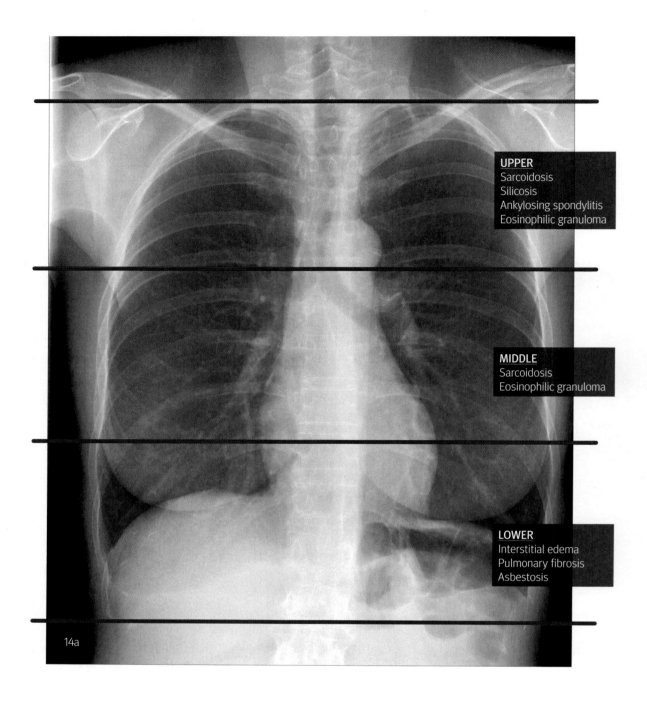

UPPER
Sarcoidosis
Silicosis
Ankylosing spondylitis
Eosinophilic granuloma

MIDDLE
Sarcoidosis
Eosinophilic granuloma

LOWER
Interstitial edema
Pulmonary fibrosis
Asbestosis

14a

Description of
Interstitial Changes by Location

In order to narrow the differential diagnosis of the interstitial lung processes, attempts have been made to describe the interstitial changes based on their predominate location: upper lobe, middle lobe or lower lobe; central or peripheral (Fig. 14a,b)(6).

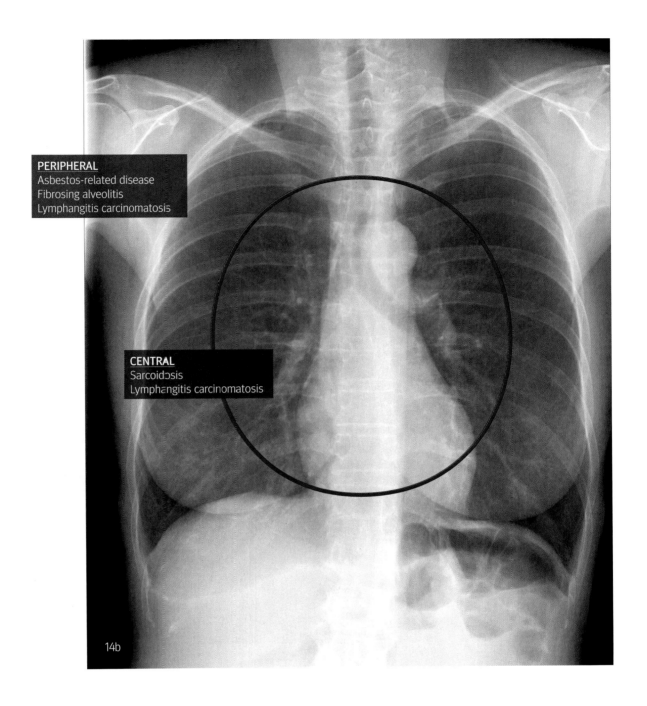

PERIPHERAL
Asbestos-related disease
Fibrosing alveolitis
Lymphangitis carcinomatosis

CENTRAL
Sarcoidosis
Lymphangitis carcinomatosis

14b

Figure 14. Localization of interstitial disease. a, upper, middle and lower lung fields, b, peripheral and central lung fields.

CHRONIC INTERSTITIAL LUNG DISEASE

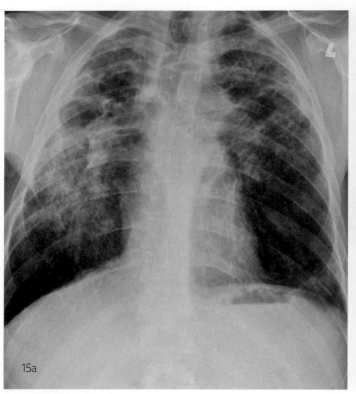

15a

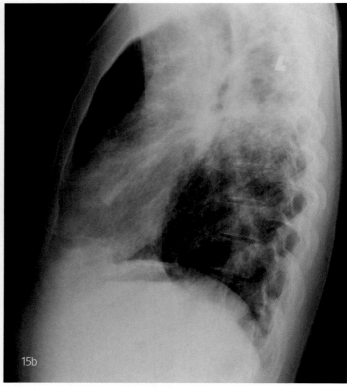

15b

Chronic interstitial lung processes can lead to progressive fibrosis within the lungs. The lung volumes are decreased and there is distortion of the lung architecture (Fig 15a,b). If the changes are predominantly in the upper lobe, the fibrosis can lead to elevation of both hila; if predominantly in the lower lobe, the hila can be retracted inferiorly. A honeycomb pattern can be present. Although the course of the interstitial lung disease can be better quantified with high resolution CT, the progression of the disease can be identified on a standard chest x-ray by carefully comparing the current x-rays with all previous available chest examinations.

Figure 15. Fibrosis in chronic interstitial lung disease. a, PA chest x-ray from a patient with chronic interstitial lung disease, b, lateral chest x-ray from the same patient.

Figure 16. Pulmonary fibrosis. a, PA chest x-ray from a patient with long standing pulmonary fibrosis, b, lateral chest x-ray from the same patient.

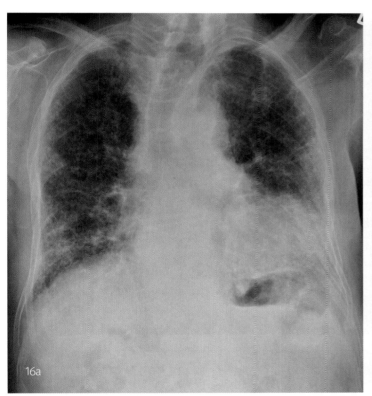

16a

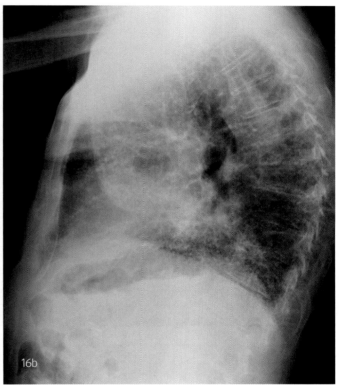

16b

Ordinary pulmonary fibrosis
(different from interstitial fibrosis)

Scarring of the lung that occurs as the result of healing processes will be seen as distinct linear, randomly-distributed, opacities on x-ray (Fig. 16a,b).

Did you catch the example on pages 498–499?
Fig. 3e,f – Idiopathic pulmonary fibrosis

Visual Search of the Interstitium

***Same as for lung (Ch. 12, Pg.486), but pay special attention to the inferior lateral portions of both lungs on the PA and the retrosternal air space on the lateral. ***

PA Chest X-ray

1. Start at the right apex (1).

2. Follow the lateral outline of the lung inferiorly to the right costophrenic angle (2).

3. Follow the inferior outline of the lung medially to the mediastinum (3).

4. Follow the medial outline of the lung to the apex (4).

Complete the visual search by checking for any density changes across the thorax from top to bottom.

Follow the same instructions on the left.

Lateral Chest X-ray

1. Start at the top anteriorly (1).

2. Follow the outline of the lungs inferiorly to the diaphragm (2).

3. Follow the outline of the lungs posteriorly to the costovertebral angles (3).

4. Follow the posterior outline of lungs superiorly to the thoracic inlet (4).

Complete the visual search by checking for any density changes across the thorax from top to bottom.

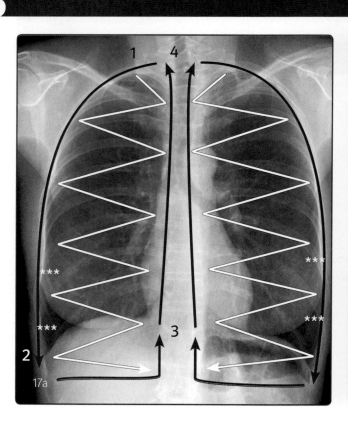

17a

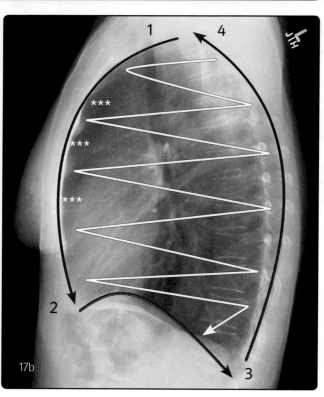

17b

514

Interstitium Radiological Analysis Checklist

GRAYSCALE

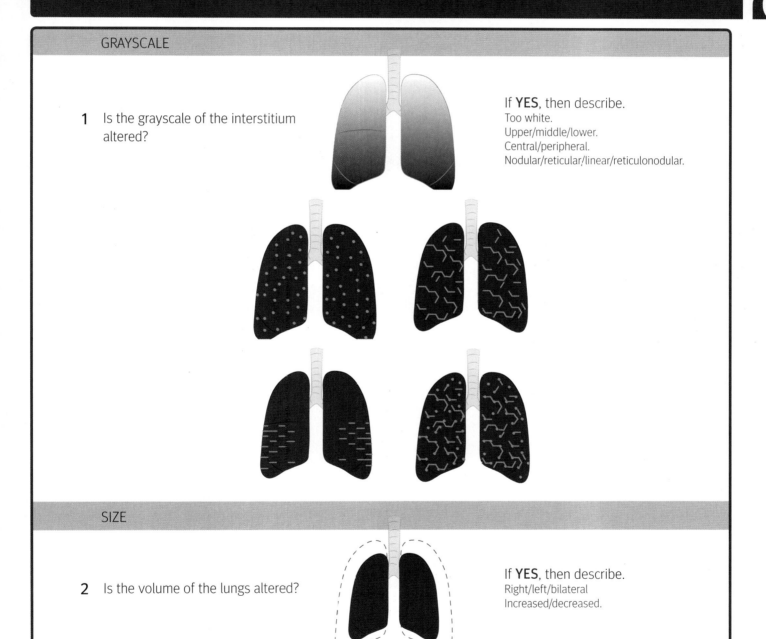

1 Is the grayscale of the interstitium altered?

If **YES**, then describe.
Too white.
Upper/middle/lower.
Central/peripheral.
Nodular/reticular/linear/reticulonodular.

SIZE

2 Is the volume of the lungs altered?

If **YES**, then describe.
Right/left/bilateral
Increased/decreased.

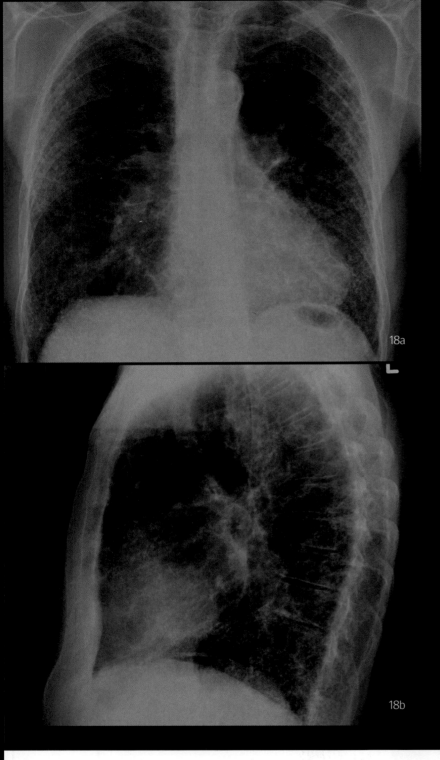

18a

18b

How would you describe your findings?

CASE STUDY

An 80-year-old male is admitted to hospital with a 20-year history of dry cough, wheezing, and a worsening of shortness of breath. He worked in construction for 55 years before retiring, and he claims he was exposed to asbestos on a daily basis. You suspect he may have pathology affecting the interstitium of his lungs. You order chest x-rays (Fig. 18a,b).

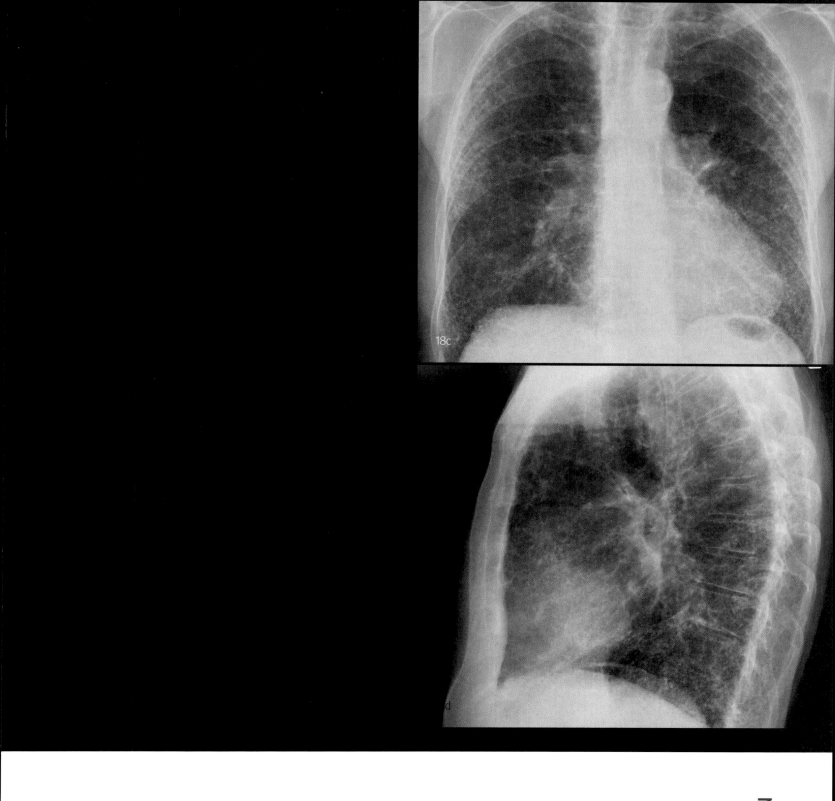
18c

Interstitial lung findings can be difficult to identify on a chest x-ray. In this case, a predominantly reticular interstitial pattern is evident (Fig. 18c,d). The additional lines are most evident in the periphery of both lungs where normally the lungs are void of any markings.

Based on the findings, the diagnosis is idiopathic pulmonary fibrosis.

References

1. Lewis, P.J., Shaffer, K., & Donovan, A. (Eds.). (2012). AMSER National Medical Student Curriculum in Radiology. http://aur.org/Secondary-Alliances.aspx?id=141.

2. Lewis, P.J., & Shaffer, K. (2005). Developing a national medical student curriculum in radiology. *Am. Coll. Radiol., 2*(1):8–11.

3. Webb, W.R., Müller, N.L., & Naidich, D.P. (2008). *High-resolution CT of the Lung,* 4th ed. Philadelphia, PA: Lippincott Williams & Wilkin.

4. Tuddenham, W.J. (1984). Glossary of Terms for Thoracic Radiology: recommendations of the Nomenclature Committee of the Fleischner Society. *AJR Am. J. Roentengol., 143*: 509–517.

5. Kerley, P. (1993). Radiology in heart disease. *Br. Med. J., 2*:594–597.

6. Ryu, J.H., Olson, E.J., Midthun, D.E., & Swensen, S.J. (2002). Diagnostic approach to the patient with diffuse lung disease. *Mayo Clinic Proc., 77*(11):1221–1227.

CHAPTER 14
The CHEST WALL
& DIAPHRAGMS
(the peripheral zone)

importance

The lungs and heart are protected within the body by the bony thorax, by the ribs, diaphragms and spine. However, on a chest x-ray, these structures overlap with the lungs and mediastinum, and can make chest x-ray interpretation difficult.

If you do not understand the radiological anatomy of the chest wall and diaphragms, you can erroneously interpret normal structures as abnormal, or abnormal structures as normal.

objectives

Skills

You will develop

- a systematic approach to evaluating the chest wall and diaphragms.

You will identify

- the normal anatomy of the chest wall, including ribs, sternum, scapulae, breasts and thoracic vertebrae on the PA and lateral chest x-rays.

- the breast and nipple shadows (as well as changes related to a previous mastectomy) on the PA and lateral chest x-rays.

- both hemidiaphragms on the PA and lateral chest x-rays.

- the common pathology of the chest wall (including collapsed vertebrae, pectus deformity of the chest, rib fracture and rib destruction) on the PA and lateral chest x-rays.

Knowledge

You will review and understand

- the normal anatomy of the chest wall.

- the radiological anatomy of the chest wall.

- what constitutes an abnormal chest wall and diaphragms.

- the pathological conditions affecting the chest wall and diaphragms.

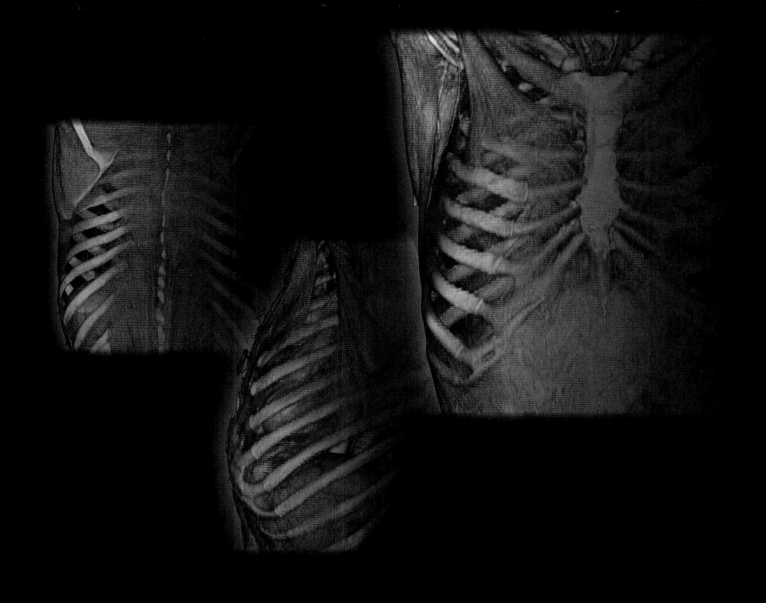

associated resources

This chapter maps to the following AMSER curriculum content (1,2).

1) Normal radiological anatomy
    Diaphragms
    Bone and soft tissues:
        Thoracic spine
        Scapulae
        Clavicles
        Sternum
        Ribs

2) Common normal variants
    Cervical ribs

3) Pathological conditions affecting the chest wall and diaphragms
    Rib fracture (musculoskeletal radiology)
    Diaphragmatic rupture

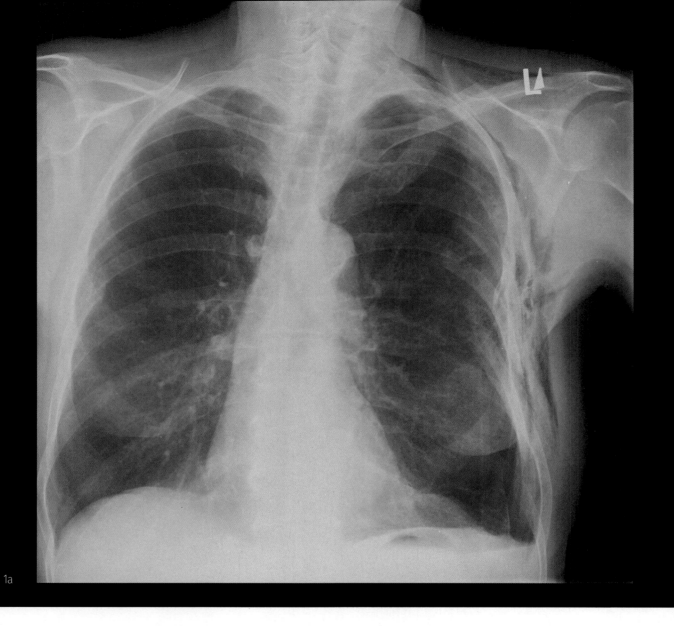

1a

A 65-year-old female presents to the emergency department after having fallen down a flight of stairs. She complains of chest pain that is worse with breathing and movement. Her rib cage is tender and she winces when palpated. You are worried that she may have fractured her ribs and you order a chest x-ray examination (Fig. 1a,b). The emergency department consultant asks you to describe the x-ray findings.

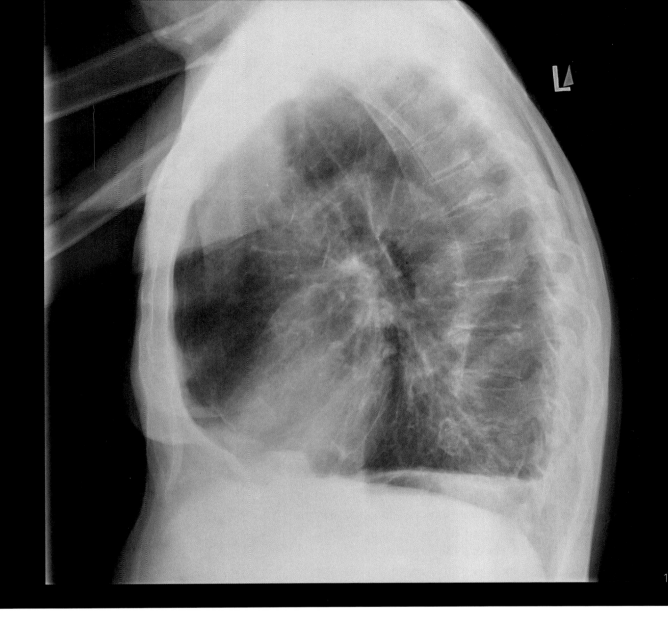

1b

How would you
describe your findings?

THE CHEST WALL
& DIAPHRAGMS

The chest wall and diaphragms define the boundary of the thoracic (or chest) cavity (Fig. 2a,b). The chest wall is an airtight, expandable, cone-shaped cage, comprised of bones, fat and muscle. The bony structures – primarily the ribs, the sternum and the vertebrae – are collectively called the thoracic cage, and protect the lung, heart and other internal structures of the thorax. The muscular structures of the chest wall (including the diaphragms) are important for the mechanics of breathing, aiding in the ventilatory process of the lung.

The Bony Thorax

The chest wall is made up of anterior, posterior and lateral aspects (Fig. 3a,b,c).

The anterior (ventral) wall of the bony thorax is shorter than the posterior wall. It extends from the suprasternal notch superiorly to the xiphoid process inferiorly. The anterior chest wall is formed by the sternum and the anterior portions of the ribs. The posterior chest wall is formed by the 12 thoracic vertebrae, their transverse

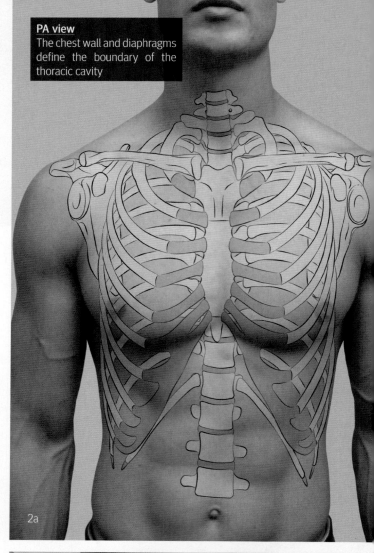

PA view
The chest wall and diaphragms define the boundary of the thoracic cavity

2a

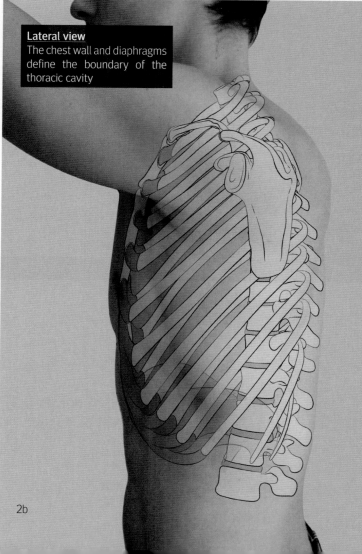

Lateral view
The chest wall and diaphragms define the boundary of the thoracic cavity

2b

Figure 2. Surface anatomy localization of the bony thorax. a, frontal perspective, b, lateral perspective.

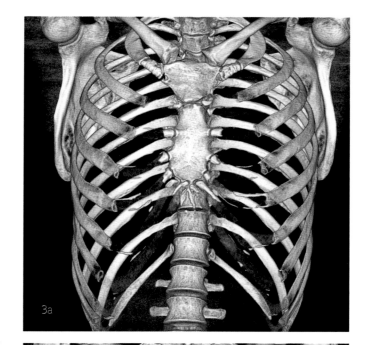

processes, and the 12 posterior aspects of the ribs. The lateral aspects of the chest wall consist of the upper 10 ribs, which slope obliquely downward from their posterior attachment sites.

The superior aperture of the bony thorax (also called either the thoracic inlet or the thoracic outlet), is a downwardly-slanted, 5-10 cm, kidney-shaped opening, bounded by the first ribs and respective costal cartilage laterally, the manubrium anteriorly, and the body of the first thoracic vertebra posteriorly (3).

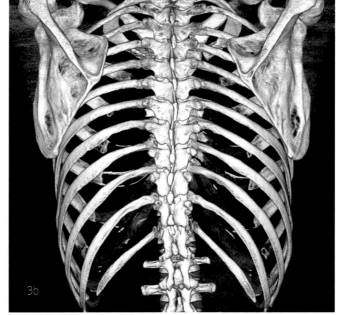

The inferior aperture of the bony thorax is bounded by the 12th vertebra and 12th rib posteriorly, the cartilage of the 7th to 10th ribs laterally, and the xiphisternal joint anteriorly. It is much wider than the superior aperture, and is enclosed by the diaphragm.

The costal margin refers to the inferior margin of the lowest rib and the costal cartilage.

The upper ventral portion of the thoracic cage is covered by the clavicles. Laterally, it is covered by the shoulder girdles and vessels; dorsally, it is covered in part by the scapulae.

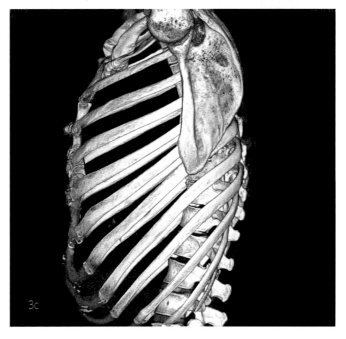

Figure 3. The bony thorax. 3D volume rendering (from CT data) of the thorax, a, frontal perspective, b, posterior perspective, c, lateral perspective.

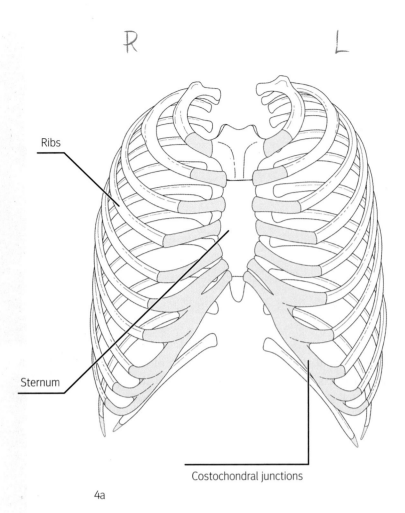

Ribs

Sternum

Costochondral junctions

4a

The Ribs

Each normal individual has 12 pairs of ribs making up the rib cage (Fig. 4a,b)(4). The ribs are numbered with respect to their attachment on the vertebrae. The 1st to 7th ribs are referred to as true ribs, due to their direct articulation with the sternum via the costochondral junctions. The 8th through 10th ribs are referred to as false ribs because they articulate with the costal cartilage of the 7th rib. The 11th and 12th ribs are called floating ribs, as they do not articulate with the sternum or costal cartilage anteriorly.

NORMAL VARIANT
Additional cervical or lumbar ribs may be found as normal variants.

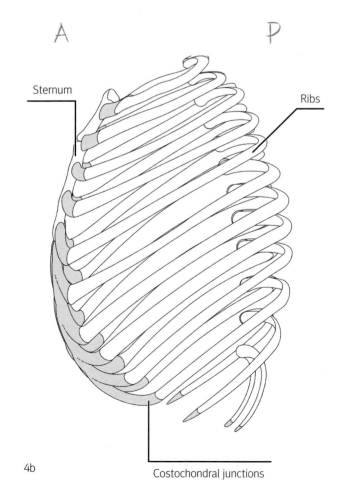

Sternum

Ribs

Costochondral junctions

4b

Figure 4. Anatomy of the ribs. Illustrations of the ribs, a, frontal perspective, b, lateral perspective.

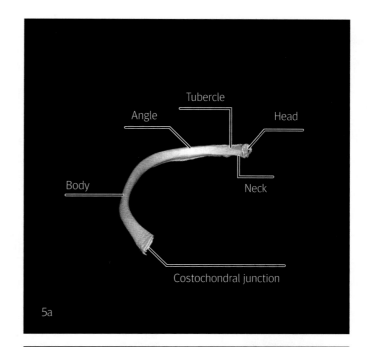

5a

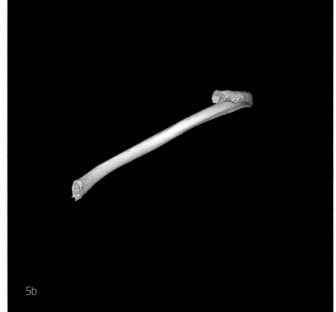

5b

Each rib is composed of a head, neck, tubercle and body (Fig. 5a,b,c) The head of the rib articulates with the facets of two adjacent vertebral bodies. The tubercle articulates with the transverse process. The neck is located between the head and tubercle. The body of the rib is the longest part of the rib, which articulates with the costal cartilage anteriorly. The most posterior part of the body of the rib is referred to as the angle of the rib. Each of the 12 ribs has a linear groove which courses along the length of its inferior aspect. This costal groove carries the intercostal nerves and vessels.

Figure 5. A rib. 3D volume rendering from CT data of a rib, a, frontal perspective, b, lateral perspective, c, horizontal perspective.

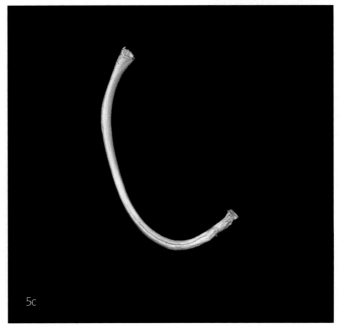

5c

Radiological Shape and Grayscale of the Ribs

The ribs are examples of cancellous bones. Each rib is comprised of an external cortical region and an internal medullary portion. The cortical portion is visible on x-rays as a thin, less than 1 mm, white line that clearly defines the outer borders of the ribs (Fig. 6a,b,c). The superior border of each rib is clear and easy to identify. Because of the natural irregularity of the inferior border of the ribs, the inferior border may be less distinct. On the PA x-ray, the ribs will have a ribbon shape. The posterior part runs horizontally, and gradually curves inferiorly and anteriorly. The exceptions are the 11th and 12th ribs — these are short ribs and usually only course horizontally.

On the lateral x-ray, the ribs will look like ribbons running from posterior superior to anterior inferior (Fig. 7a,b,c).

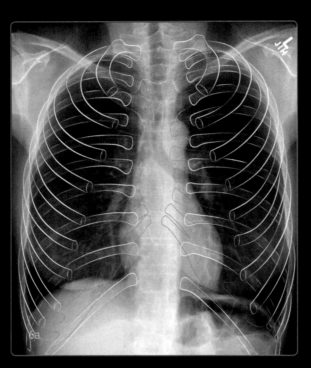

6a

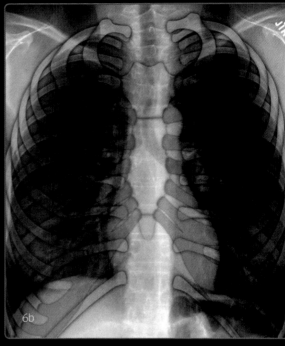

6b

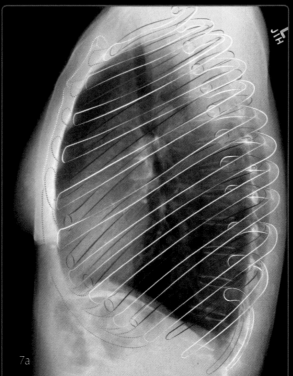

7a

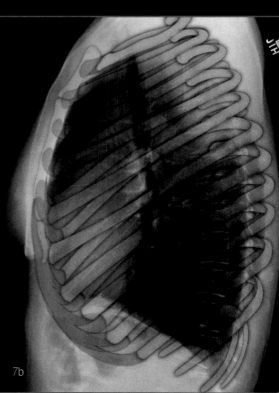

7b

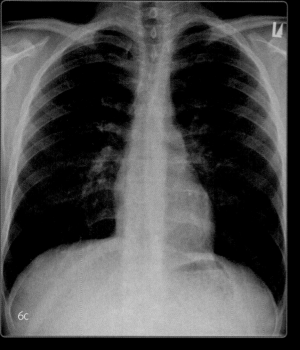

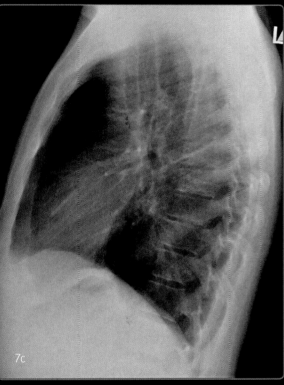

Figure 6. Radiological anatomy of the ribs from the frontal perspective. a, PA chest x-ray with the ribs outlined, b, PA chest x-ray with a grayscale illustration of the ribs overlay, c, PA chest x-ray cropped to highlight the ribs.

Figure 7. Radiological anatomy of the ribs from the lateral perspective. a, lateral chest x-ray with the ribs outlined, b, lateral chest x-ray with a grayscale illustration of the ribs overlay, c, lateral chest x-ray cropped to highlight the ribs.

Cartilaginous portions of the ribs anterior to the costochondral junction can also calcify (Fig. 9a,b). This calcification can appear in the form of lines and dots and can mimic lung pathology.

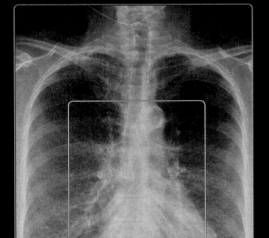

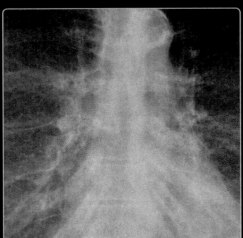

The posterior and lateral parts of the ribs are easily identified on the chest x-ray. The anterior part of the ribs has a cartilage matrix and is usually not visible on x-rays. In some cases, calcification can be present at the junction of the bony and cartilaginous portions. These costochondral calcifications are easily identified on x-rays (Fig. 8a,b). The x-ray appearance of the costochondral calcifications appears to be gender specific; in males they have a convex shape and in females a concave shape.

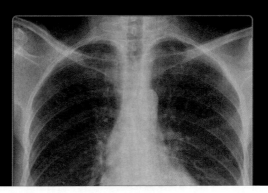

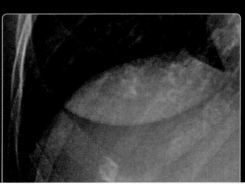

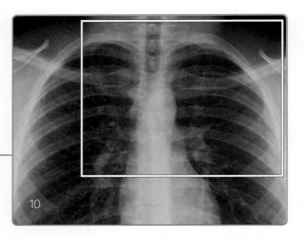

10

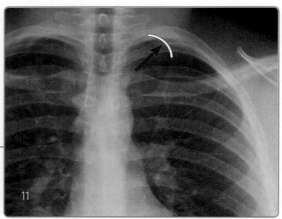

11

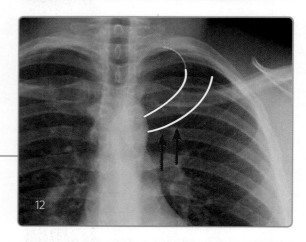

12

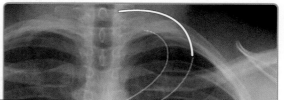

How to count the ribs on the PA x-ray

Learning to count the ribs is important for accurately localizing pathology in the thorax.

STEP 1
Confirm that the patient is midline and not rotated (Ch. 1, Pg. 32).

STEP 2
Focus your visual attention on the thoracic inlet on the right or left side – in this example we focus on the left side (Fig. 10).

STEP 3
Identify the superior edge of the 1st rib at the apex of the left lung (Fig. 11).

STEP 4
Follow this superior edge anteriorly. Identify the inferior edge of this 1st rib (Fig. 12).

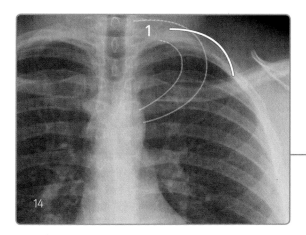

14

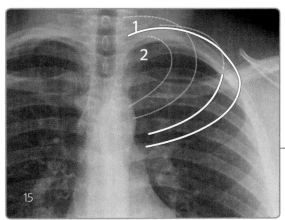

15

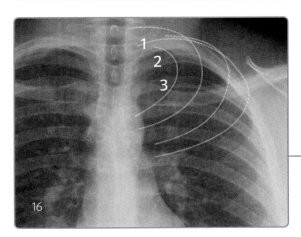

16

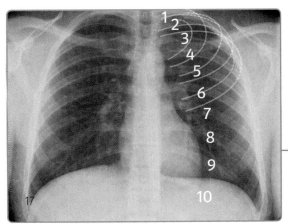

17

STEP 6
You can now identify the superior edge of the 2nd rib with confidence (Fig. 14).

STEP 7
Follow this rib forward as you did with the 1st rib. Find the lower edge of the 2nd rib, anteriorly, and follow it back (Fig. 15).

STEP 8
Then find the 3rd rib (Fig. 16).

STEP 9
Do this for all remaining ribs. As you move inferiorly, it will become easier to identify both the superior and inferior edge of each rib, without needing to follow the ribs anteriorly and then posteriorly (Fig. 17).

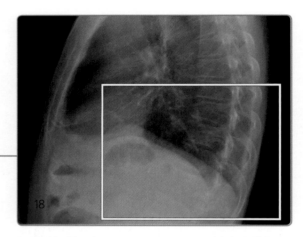

How to differentiate the right and left ribs on the lateral x-ray

Differentiating the right and left ribs on the lateral x-ray helps to localize the origin of pathology in the pleura and lungs.

STEP 1
Focus your vision on the posterior inferior aspect of the thorax (Fig. 18).

STEP 2
Identify two sets of ribs posteriorly and inferiorly (Fig. 19).

STEP 3
The larger of the two sets of ribs are the magnified right ribs (Fig. 20)(5).

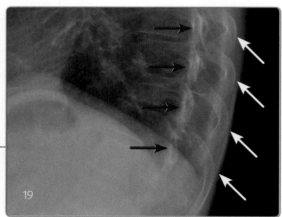

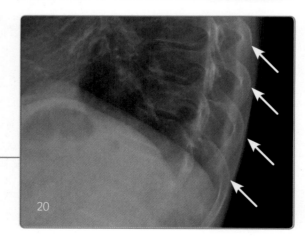

534

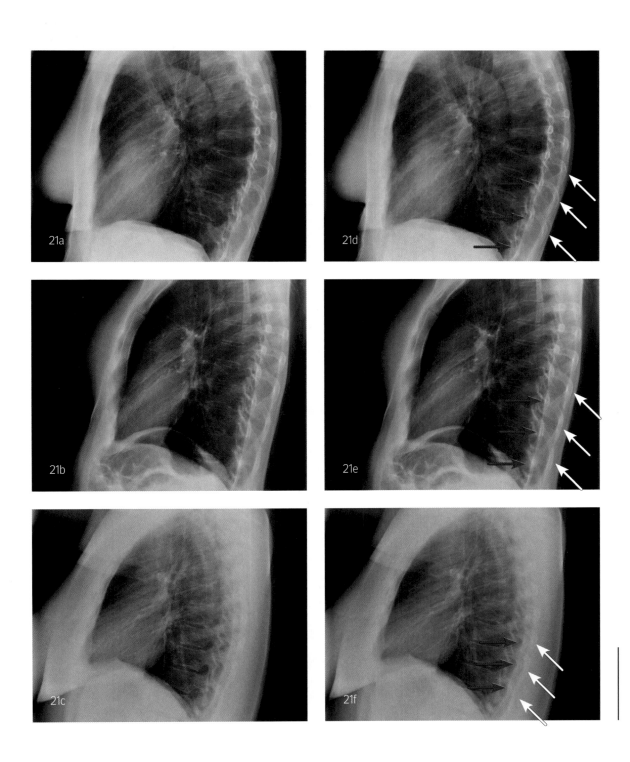

Figure 21. Differentiating right and left ribs. a-c, example lateral chest x-rays cropped to highlight the ribs, d-f, corresponding lateral x-ray annotated.

21a

21b

21c

21d

21e

21f

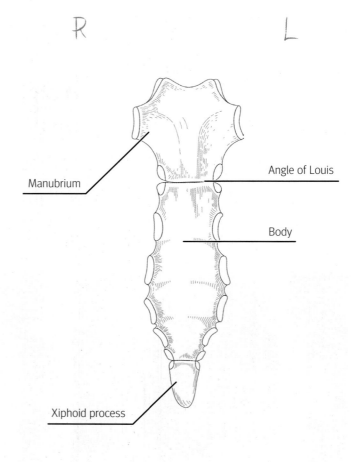

R   L

Manubrium

Angle of Louis

Body

Xiphoid process

22a

The Sternum

The sternum is divided into the manubrium, the body and
the xiphoid process (Figs. 22a,b,c,d). The word *sternum* is
derived from Latin and means "shield". The first seven pairs
of ribs articulate directly with the sternum, out of which
the 1st rib articulates with the manubrium, and the 2nd to
7th ribs articulate with the body of the sternum. The ribs
articulate anteriorly with the sternum via costochondral
cartilage. The sternal angle (angle of Louis) is an important
surface and radiological landmark (Pg. 540). This angle
lies at the level of the fourth thoracic vertebrae (T4). The
sternum also articulates with the clavicles (collar bones).

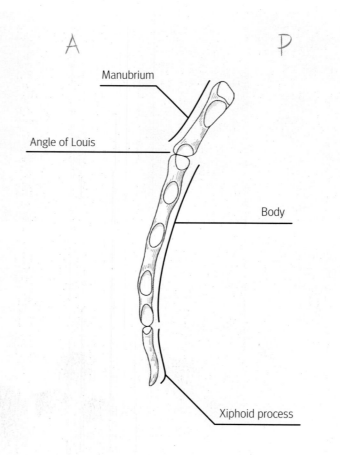

A   P

Manubrium

Angle of Louis

Body

Xiphoid process

22b

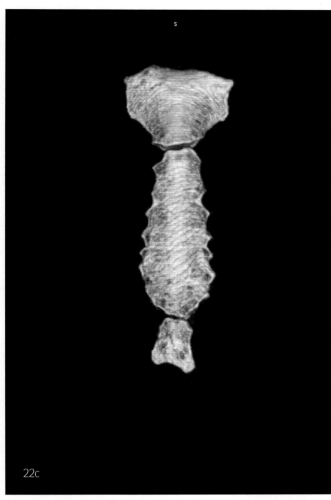

22c

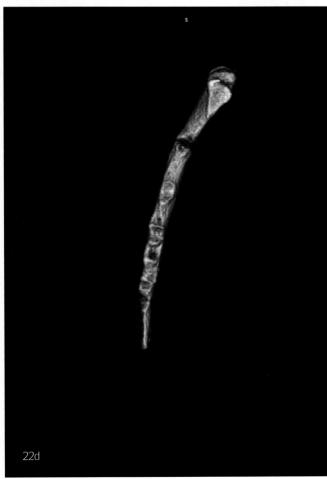

22d

Figure 22. Anatomy of the sternum.
a, Illustration of the sternum from the frontal perspective, b, illustration of the sternum from the lateral perspective. c, 3D volume rendering (from CT data) of the sternum from the frontal perspective, d, 3D volume rendering (from CT data) of the sternum from the lateral perspective.

537

Radiological Shape and Grayscale of the Sternum

The cortical outline of the sternum is difficult to clearly visualize on the PA x-ray because of overlap with the mediastinum (Fig. 23a,b,c)(6). The superior border of the sternum, at the sternal notch, is visible between the medial border of both clavicles (Fig. 23c).

The anterior and posterior cortical outlines of the sternum are visible on the lateral x-ray (Fig. 24a,b,c)(6). A normal break is present in the upper third of the sternum. This represents the junction between the body and the manubrium, and is called the angle of Louis (Fig. 24c).

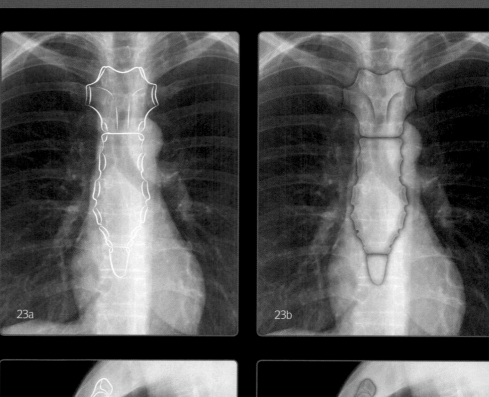

23a

23b

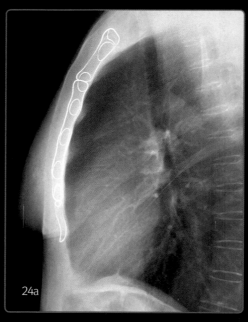

24a

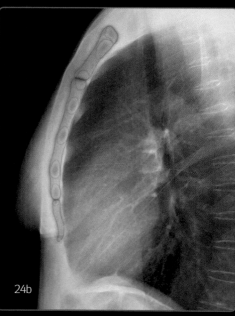

24b

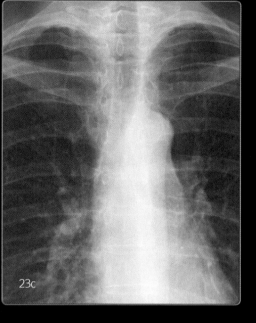

23c

Figure 23. Radiological anatomy of the sternum from the frontal perspective. a, PA chest x-ray with the sternum outlined, b, PA chest x-ray with a grayscale illustration of the sternum overlay, c, PA chest x-ray cropped to highlight the sternum. Notice that on the PA x-ray, the sternum is not well visualized.

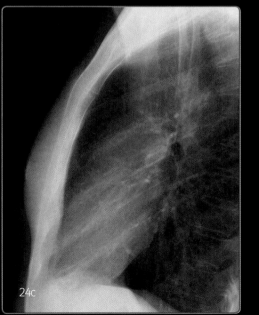

24c

Figure 24. Radiological anatomy of the sternum from the lateral perspective. a, lateral chest x-ray with the sternum outlined, b, lateral chest x-ray with a grayscale illustration of the sternum overlay, c, lateral chest x-ray cropped to highlight the sternum.

How to identify the sternum and the angle of Louis on the lateral x-ray

The angle of Louis is a useful landmark within the thorax for delineating the border of the superior and inferior mediastinum. Knowing how to identify the sternum and the angle of Louis on the lateral x-ray is essential for mediastinal classification.

STEP 1
Focus your vision on the anterior part of the thorax, where the lungs and heart touch the anterior chest wall (Fig. 25).

STEP 2
Identify the anterior and posterior cortical outlines of the sternum. The cortex of the sternum produces two thin, white cortical lines (Fig. 26).

STEP 3
The angle of Louis is found where the manubrium and body of the sternum join together (Fig. 27).

?

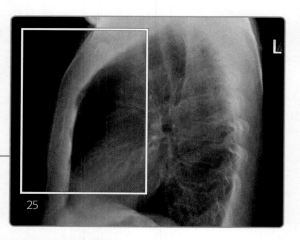

25

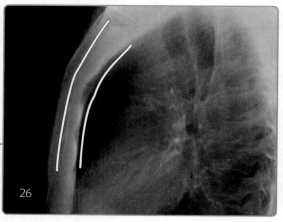

26

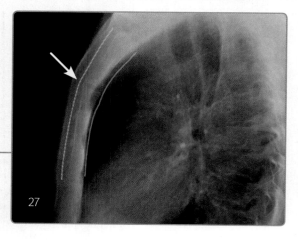

27

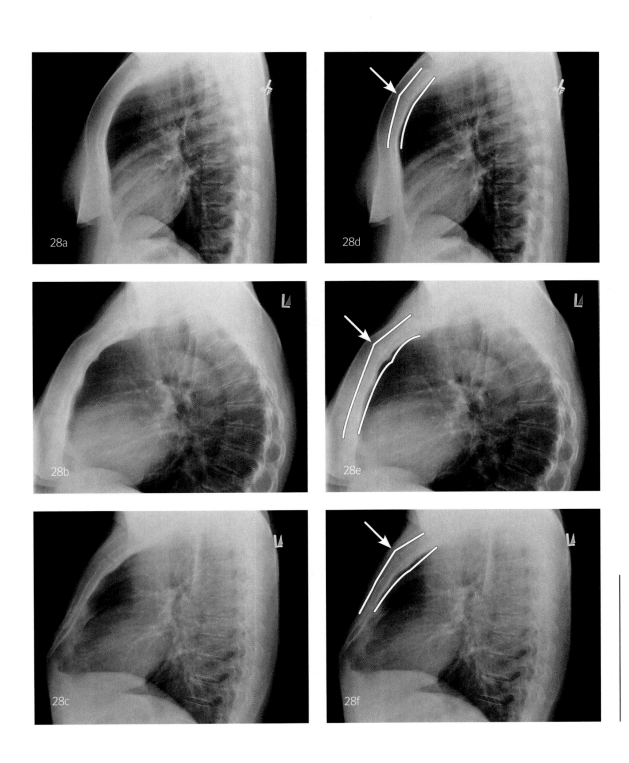

Figure 28. Identifying the sternum and angle of Louis on the lateral chest x-ray. a-c, example lateral chest x-rays cropped to highlight the sternum, d-f, corresponding lateral chest x-rays annotated to show the position of the sternum and the Angle of Louis.

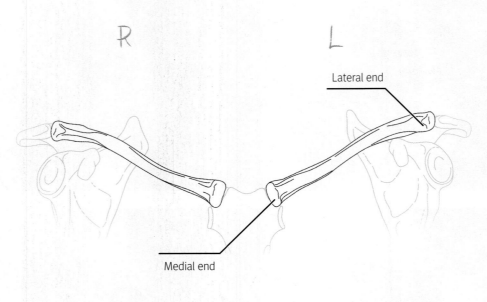

29a

The Clavicles

The clavicle is a long, thin bone that connects the thorax with the upper extremity. The clavicle can be divided into a shaft and two ends – medial and lateral (Fig. 29a,b). It articulates medially with the manubrium sterni, and laterally with the scapula.

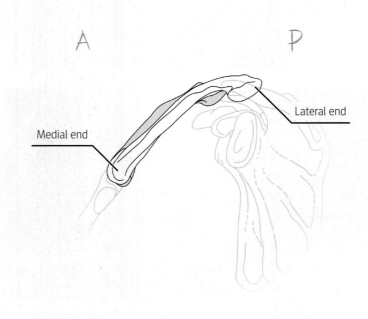

Figure 29. Anatomy of the clavicles.
Illustrations of the clavicles, a, frontal perspective, b, lateral perspective.

29b

Radiological Shape and Grayscale of the Clavicles

The cortical outline of the clavicle can be clearly seen on PA chest x-rays, oriented horizontally, overlying the lung apices (Fig. 30a,b,c). Because of their location, they can make the identification of a small pneumothorax, or a small apical mass, difficult.

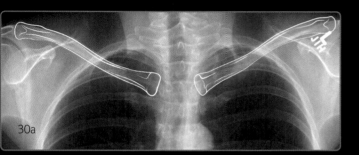

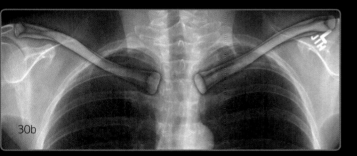

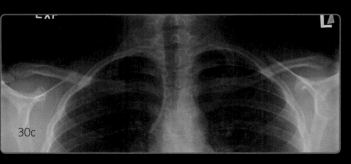

Figure 30. Radiological anatomy of the clavicles from the frontal perspective. a, PA chest x-ray with the clavicles outlined, b, PA chest x-ray with a grayscale illustration of the clavicles overlay, c, PA chest x-ray cropped to highlight the clavicles.

R   L

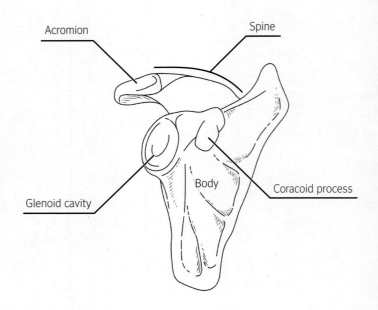

Acromion

Spine

Glenoid cavity

Body

Coracoid process

31a

The Scapulae

The word *scapula* is derived from Latin and means "a spade". The scapulae are triangular-shaped, flat bones that articulate with the clavicles and the humeral heads (Fig. 31a,b,c,d,e). Each scapula is comprised of a body, scapular spine, acromion, glenoid cavity, and coracoid process. The body of the scapula has lateral and medial borders.

A   P

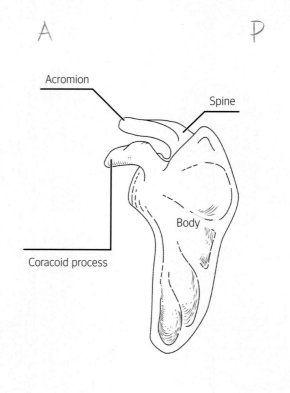

Acromion

Spine

Body

Coracoid process

31b

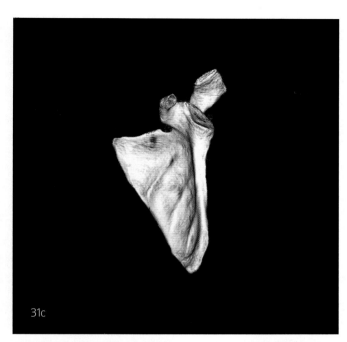

31c

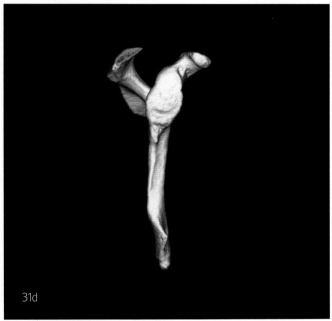

31d

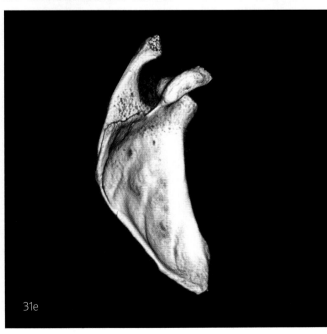

31e

Figure 31. Anatomy of the scapulae.
a, Illustration of the right scapula from
the frontal perspective, b, illustration of
the right scapula from the medial-lateral
perspective, c, 3D volume rendering
(from CT data) of the left scapula from
the frontal perspective, d, 3D volume
rendering (from CT data) of the left
scapula from the lateral perspective, e, 3D
volume rendering (from CT data) of the
left scapula from the medial perspective.

Radiological Shape and Grayscale of the Scapulae

The cortex of the scapulae will produce a thin, white line on an x-ray.

On a properly performed PA chest x-ray, the scapulae should be positioned such that the cortical line corresponding to the medial border of the scapulae bodies do not overlay the thoracic cavity (Fig. 32a,b,c).

On the lateral x-ray, the scapulae will normally be seen overlying the posterior superior part of the thorax (Fig. 33a,b,c).

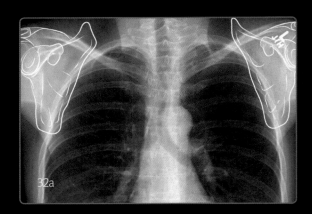

32a

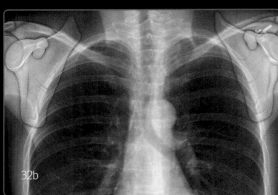

32b

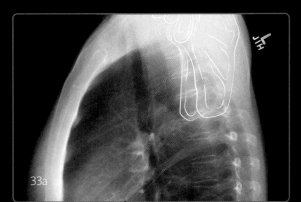

33a

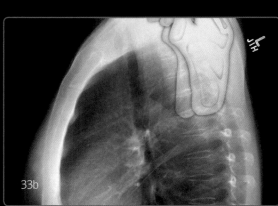

33b

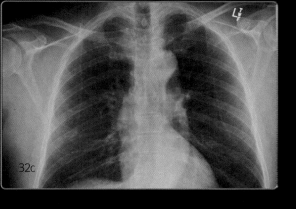

32c

Figure 32. Radiological anatomy of the scapulae from the frontal perspective. a, PA chest x-ray with the scapulae outlined, b, PA chest x-ray with a grayscale illustration of the scapulae overlay, c, PA chest x-ray cropped to highlight the scapulae.

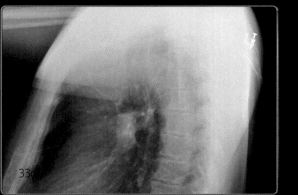

33c

Figure 33. Radiological anatomy of the scapulae from the lateral perspective. a, lateral chest x-ray with the scapulae outlined, b, lateral chest x-ray with a grayscale illustration of the scapulae overlay, c, lateral chest x-ray cropped to highlight the scapulae.

If the positioning of the patient is not optimal, the medial borders of the scapulae will overlay the thoracic cavity and may mimic the visceral pleura seen with a pneumothorax (Fig. 34). It is, therefore, very important to distinguish the scapulae with certainty on the PA x-ray.

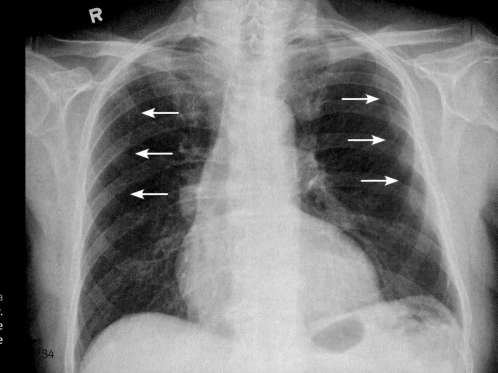

Figure 34. Scapulae can mimic a pneumothorax on the PA chest x-ray. **PA chest x-ray highlighting the scapulae (arrows). Note how they can be mistaken for a pneumothorax.**

In addition, given their position and orientation, the two vertical lines that indicate the medial aspects of the scapulae can be mistaken for the borders of the trachea on the lateral x-ray (Fig. 35).

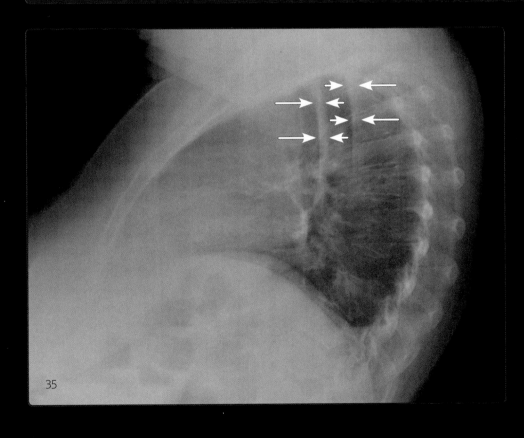

35

Figure 35. Scapulae can mimic the trachea on the lateral x-ray. **Lateral chest x-ray with the scapulae highlighted (arrows). Note how they can be mistaken for the trachea.**

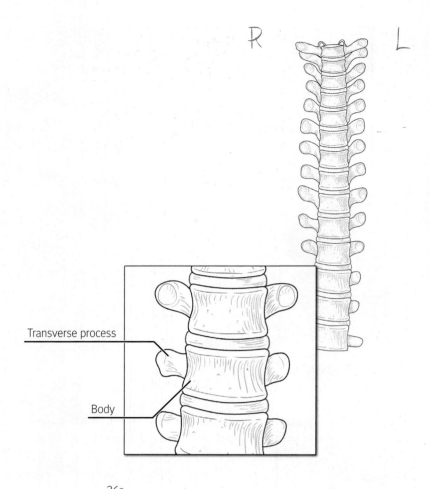

Transverse process

Body

36a

The Thoracic Spine

In the normal person, 12 thoracic vertebrae are present – each with a body, pedicles, laminae and a spinous process (Fig. 36a,b,c,d,e).

The vertebral bodies measure approximately 15 to 27 mm in height, with the dimensions gradually increasing from superior to inferior (7). Each of the vertebrae is separated from the next vertebra by a disc.

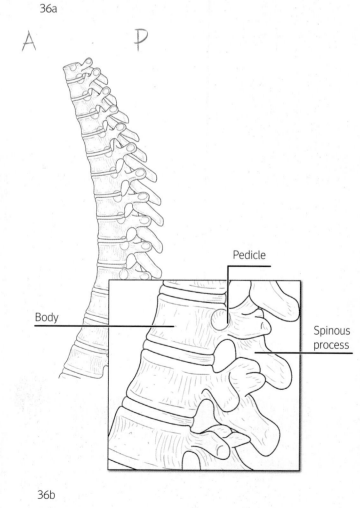

Pedicle

Body

Spinous process

36b

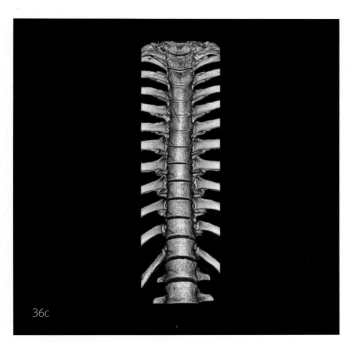

36c

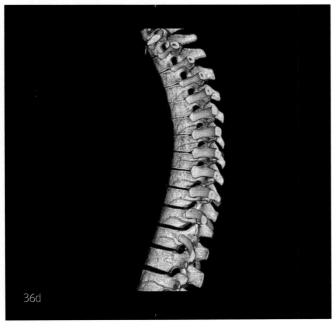

36d

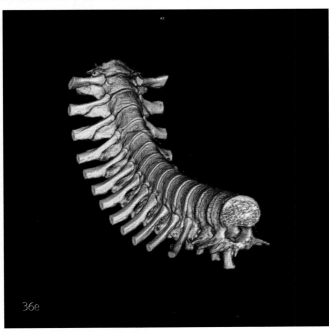

36e

Figure 36. Anatomy of the thoracic spine. a, Illustration of the thoracic spine from the frontal perspective, b, illustration of the thoracic spine from the lateral perspective, c, 3D volume rendering (from CT data) of the thoracic spine from the frontal perspective, d, 3D volume rendering (from CT data) of the thoracic spine from the lateral perspective, e, 3D volume rendering (from CT data) of the thoracic spine as seen end-on.

Radiological Shape and Grayscale of the Spine

On the PA x-ray, the vertebral bodies line up in a straight, vertical column (Fig. 37a,b,c). The cortical outline of the vertebrae is seen as a white rectangle, and the pedicles are seen as white ovals.

On the lateral x-ray, the vertebral bodies also appear as white rectangles stacked one on another; however, the vertebral alignment forms a smooth kyphotic curve (Fig. 38a,b,c). The thoracic spinous processes are difficult to identify because of their overlap with the ribs. The discs are comprised of cartilaginous tissue and are not visualized on x-rays; they appear as dark spaces between the vertebral bodies.

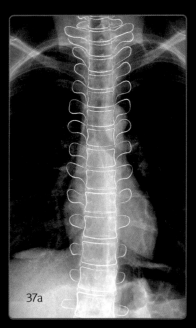

37a

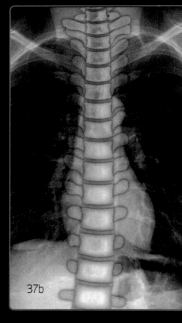

37b

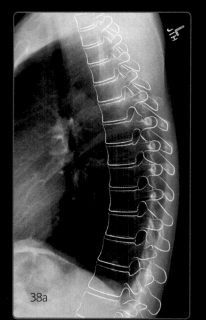

38a

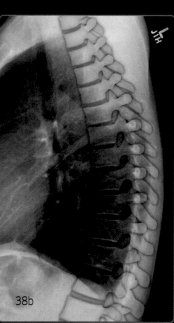

38b

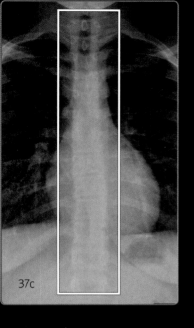

Figure 37. Radiological anatomy of the thoracic spine from the frontal perspective. a, PA chest x-ray with the thoracic spine outlined, b, PA chest x-ray with a grayscale illustration of the thoracic spine overlay, c, PA chest x-ray cropped to highlight the thoracic spine.

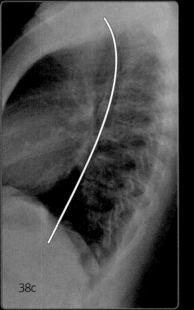

Figure 38. Radiological anatomy of the thoracic spine from the lateral perspective. a, lateral chest x-ray with the thoracic spine outlined, b, lateral chest x-ray with a grayscale illustration of the thoracic spine overlay, c, lateral chest x-ray cropped to highlight the thoracic spine.

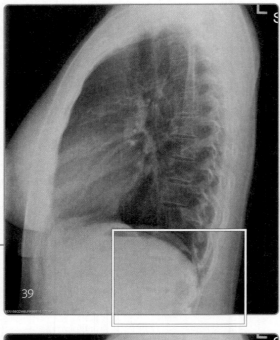

How to count the vertebral bodies on the lateral x-ray

Learning to count the vertebral bodies is important to accurately label vertebral body pathology, such as fractures.

STEP 1
Focus on the vertebral bodies, posteriorly and inferiorly (Fig. 39).

STEP 2
Identify the lowest rib, and follow this rib to its articulation with the corresponding vertebral body. This is the twelfth thoracic vertebra – T12 (Fig. 40).

STEP 3
Count the vertebral bodies starting with T12 (Fig. 41).

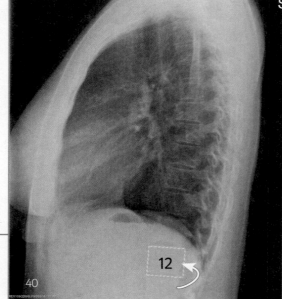

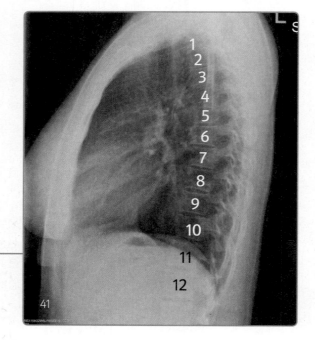

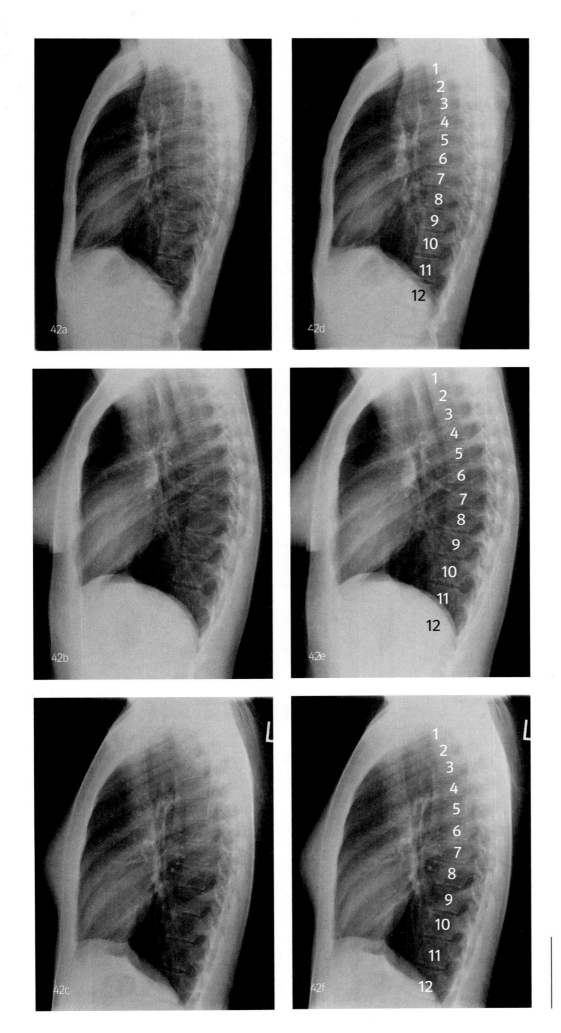

Figure 42. Counting the vertebrae on the lateral chest x-ray. a-c, example lateral chest x-rays to highlight the vertebrae, d-f, corresponding lateral chest x-rays annotated to show the correct numbering of the vertebrae.

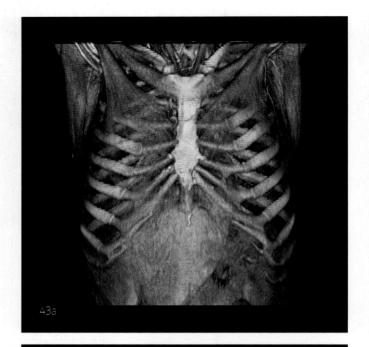

The Muscles, Skin and Subcutaneous Tissues

The most external part of the thorax is comprised of muscles, subcutaneous tissue, and skin (Fig. 43a,b,c). Abnormalities of these structures can alter the appearance of the other anatomical structures on a chest x-ray.

The Breasts

The breasts are positioned over the pectoralis major muscle, and usually extend from the level of the 2nd rib to the level of the 6th rib anteriorly. The superior lateral quadrant of the breast extends diagonally upwards towards the axillae and is known as the axillary tail of Spence. A thin layer of mammary tissue extends from the clavicle above to the 7th or 8th ribs below, and from the midline to the edge of the latissimus dorsi posteriorly.

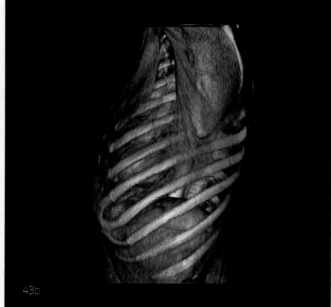

The breasts are modified sudoriferous (sweat) glands, present in both sexes. Each breast has one nipple surrounded by the areola. The breast is composed of glandular tissue (mammary glands), connective tissue (collagen and elastin), adipose tissue (fat), and Cooper's ligaments.

Breasts vary in both size and shape, and in their content of fibrous, glandular and adipose tissue, which influences their appearance on the radiological examinations.

Figure 43. Anatomy of the external thorax. 3D volume rendering (from CT data) of the muscles comprising the external thorax, a, frontal perspective, b, lateral perspective, c, posterior perspective.

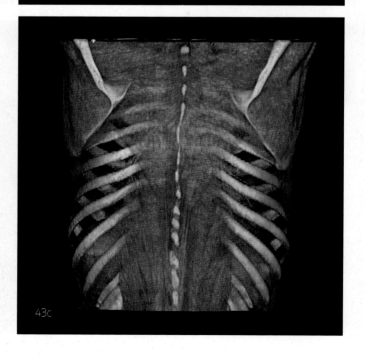

Radiological Shape and Grayscale
of the Muscles, Skin and Subcutaneous Tissues (I)

The major muscle visible on the x-ray is the pectoralis major. When visible, this muscle gives an increased opacity over the upper lateral aspect of the hemithorax (Fig. 44).

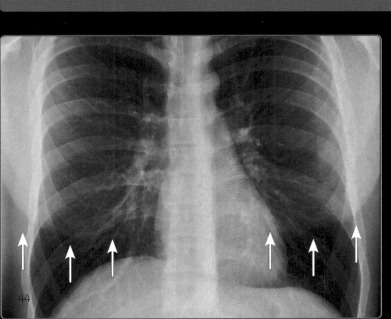

Figure 44. Radiological anatomy of the pectoralis muscle.
PA chest x-ray highlighting the pectoralis muscle.

44

Radiological Shape and Grayscale
of the Muscles, Skin and Subcutaneous Tissues (II)

The skin and adipose tissues will form the most lateral edges of the chest x-ray (Fig. 45). Just superior to the clavicles, the soft tissues form a skin/air interface, visible on the PA chest x-ray as a distinct edge called the companion shadow (Fig. 46)(8).

Figure 45. Radiological appearance of the skin and adipose tissue. **PA chest x-ray highlighting the skin and adipose tissue forming the lateral edges of the chest x-ray (arrows).**

Figure 46. The companion shadow. **PA chest x-ray cropped to highlight the companion shadow (arrows).**

Figure 47. Excess adipose on the chest x-ray. **Excess adipose tissue increases scatter radiation and decreases image quality. a, PA chest x-ray with excess adipose tissue, b, lateral chest x-ray from the same patient. Note how gray and blurry the x-ray appears.**

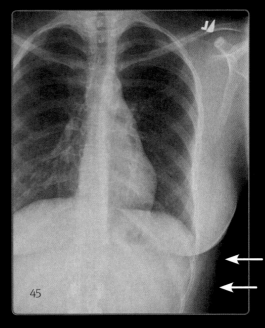

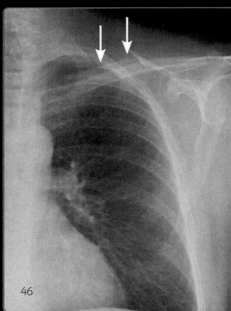

Adipose tissue can increase scatter radiation on the x-ray, and decrease image quality. The more adipose tissue, the more gray the x-ray will look (Fig. 47a,b).

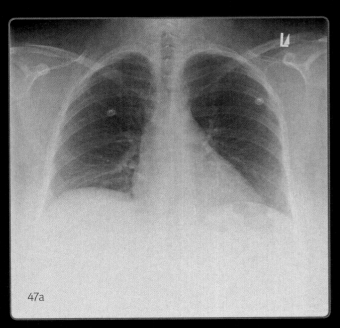

47a

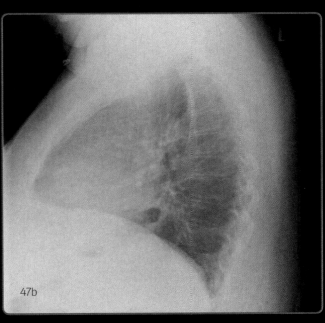

47b

Radiological Shape and Grayscale of the Breasts & Nipples

On the PA chest x-ray, in women, the breasts appear as oval-shaped opacities, overlying the inferior hemithorax, bilaterally (Fig. 48a,b,c). There is tremendous variation in shape and size of the breasts, even from side to side. Depending on the size of the breasts, they can overlay a significant part of the hemithorax or can overlap the upper abdomen, without obscuring the lungs. The inferior border of each breast is clearly seen because the breast interfaces with air; the superior border of each breast is not defined.

On the lateral chest x-ray, the breasts can easily be identified anteriorly. Because of this anterior location, the breasts do not overlap with the intrathoracic structures on the lateral chest x-ray.

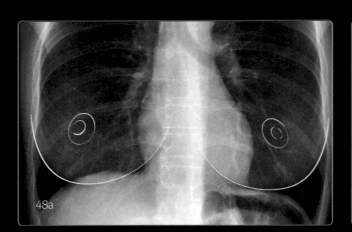

48a

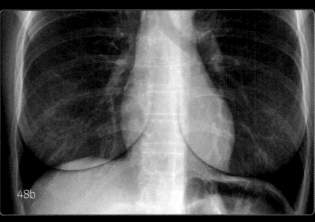

48b

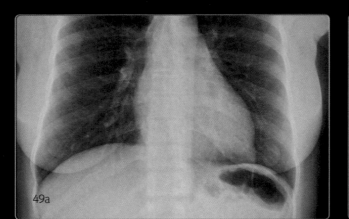

49a

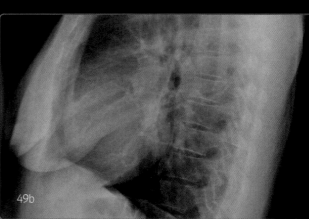

49b

Nipples also vary in size and shape. Because of the shape of the nipples, they interface with air, and frequently are seen as distinct round opacities. Nipple opacities can be seen in women and men, and can mimic lung nodules (Fig. 49a,b). The nipple opacities can be differentiated from nodules by identifying the nipples on the lateral x-ray, or by repeating the chest x-rays with nipple markers (Fig. 49c).

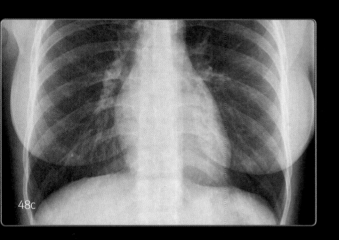

Figure 48. Radiological anatomy of the breasts from the frontal perspective. a, PA chest x-ray with the breasts outlined, b, PA chest x-ray with a grayscale illustration of the breasts overlay, c, PA chest x-ray cropped to highlight the breasts.

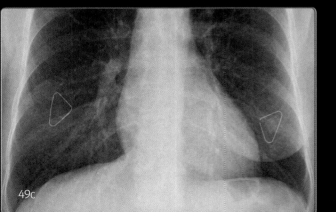

Figure 49. Radiological anatomy of the nipples. a, PA chest x-ray highlighting the nipples, b, lateral chest x-ray highlighting the nipples, c, PA chest x-ray with nipple markers (arrows).

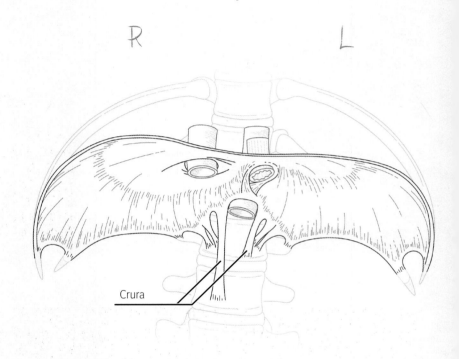

50a

The Diaphragms

The diaphragms are large muscles that lie under the lungs, and separate the thoracic cavity from the abdominal cavity (Fig. 50a,b)(9,10). Anteriorly, the diaphragms attach to the sternum, and to the lower six ribs and their cartilage. Posteriorly, the diaphragms have two crura. The crura attach to the first through third (L1 to L3) lumbar vertebral bodies on the right, and the first and second (L1 and L2) lumbar vertebral bodies on the left.

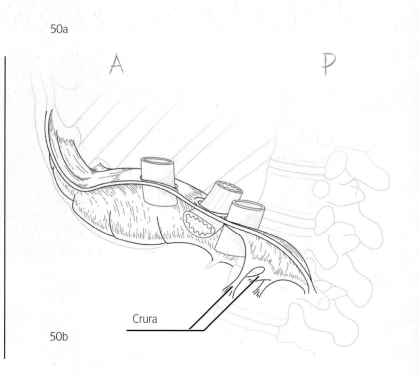

50b

Figure 50. Anatomy of the diaphragms. Illustration of the diaphragms, a, frontal perspective, b, lateral perspective.

Position of Diaphragms in the Normal Population on the PA X-ray [11]

Right hemidiaphragm higher – 94.2%
Left hemidiaphragm higher – 1.4%
Both hemidiaphragms the same – 4.4%

Diaphragm eventration refers to focal elevation of a diaphragm that is non-paralytic, and is associated with focal muscular aplasia, and thinning. The abdominal structures bulge into the thorax at this focal area of diaphragmatic muscle weakness (Fig. 51a,b) (12).

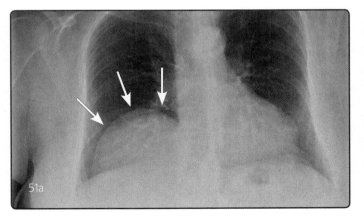

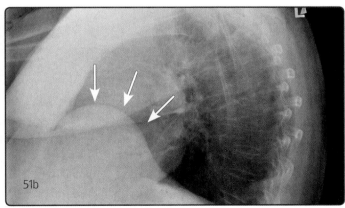

Figure 51. Diaphragm eventration. a, PA chest x-ray from a patient with diaphragm eventration, b, lateral chest x-ray from the same patient.

Radiological Shape and Grayscale of the Diaphragms

The diaphragms are not thick enough to be seen as separate structures. The location of the diaphragms on the PA and lateral x-rays is inferred by the position of the lungs, because the inferior border of the lungs lie on the diaphragms (Figs. 52a,b,c, and 53a,b,c).The right hemidiaphragm is usually higher than the left.

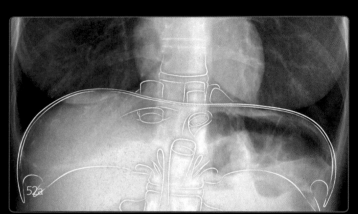

52a

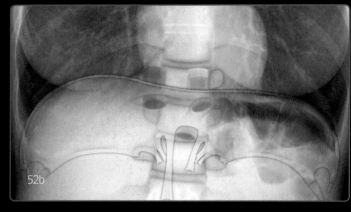

52b

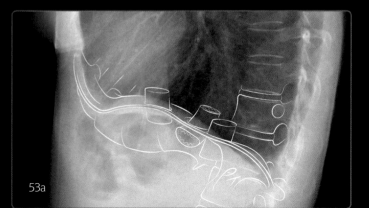

53a

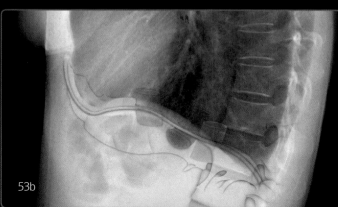

53b

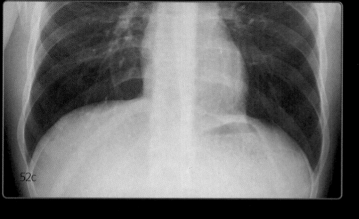

Figure 52. Radiological anatomy of the diaphragms from the frontal perspective. a, PA chest x-ray with the diaphragms outlined, b, PA chest x-ray with a grayscale illustration of the diaphragms overlay, c, PA chest x-ray cropped to highlight the diaphragms.

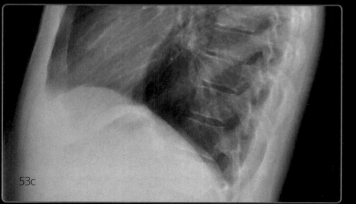

Figure 53. Radiological anatomy of the diaphragms from the lateral perspective. a, lateral chest x-ray with the diaphragms outlined, b, lateral chest x-ray with a grayscale illustration of the diaphragms overlay, c, lateral chest x-ray cropped to highlight the diaphragms.

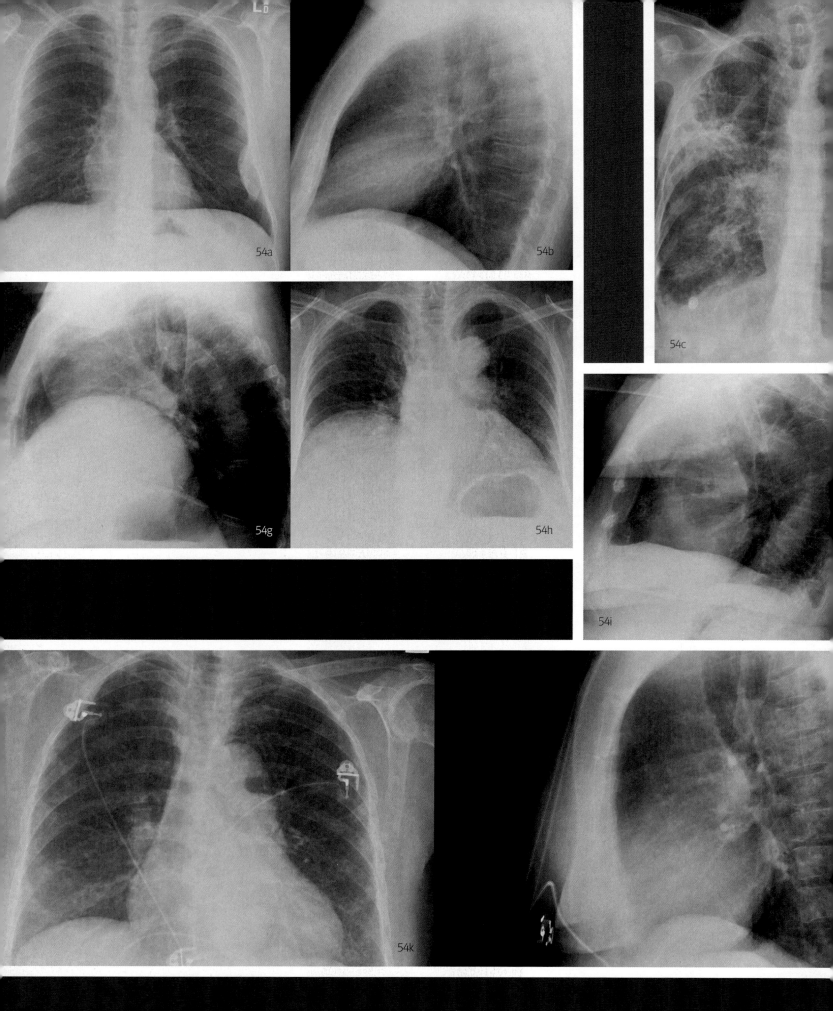

PATHOLOGY of the CHEST WALL & DIAPHRAGMS

Example images of diseases and conditions that affect the chest wall and diaphragms.

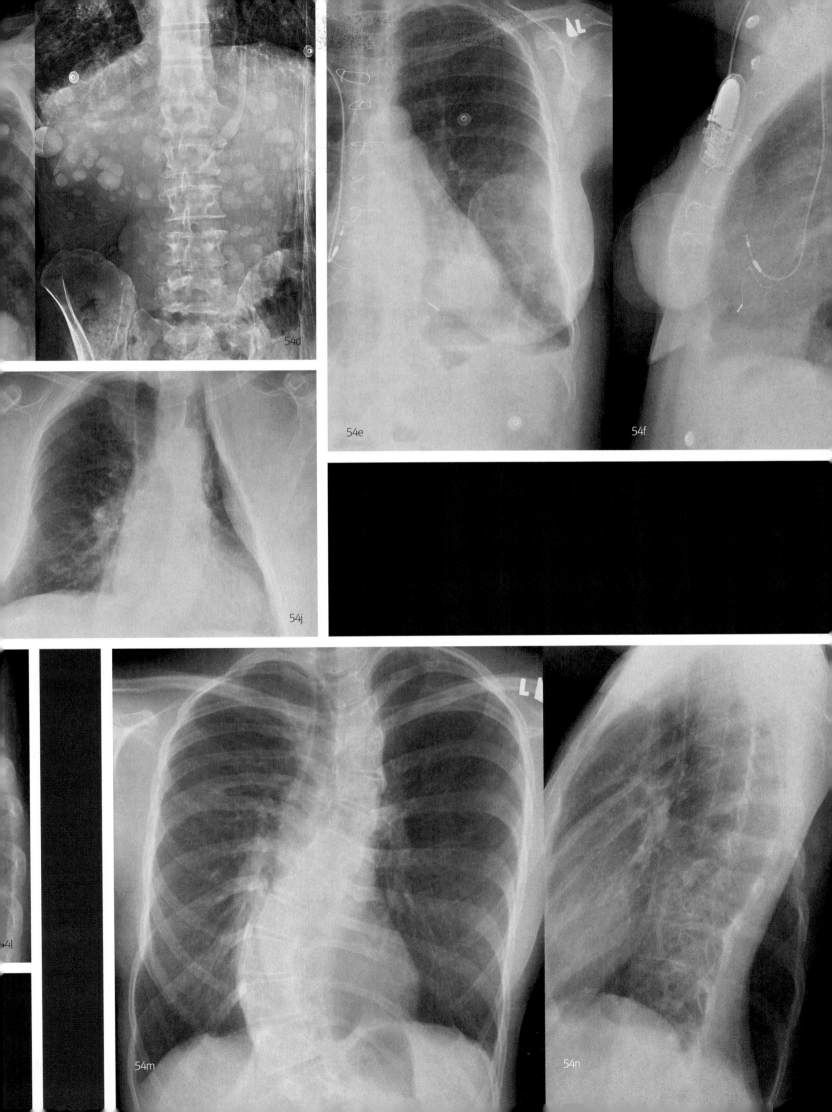

54d

54e

54f

54j

54l

54m

54n

THE ABNORMAL
CHEST WALL & DIAPHRAGMS

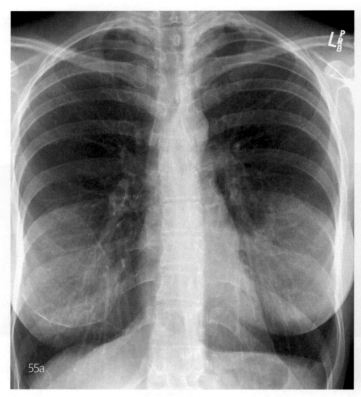 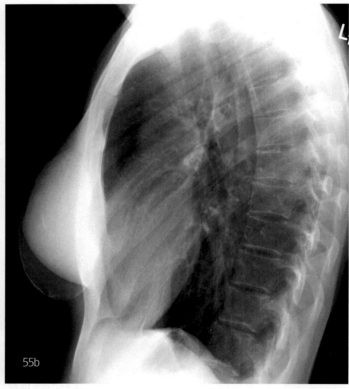

55a   55b

The Radiological Appearance of the Chest Wall and Diaphragms Will Be Abnormal When

1. The grayscale of the chest wall, diaphragms, or both, is too white or too black (Fig. 55a,b).

2. The size of the chest wall, diaphragms, or both, is enlarged or reduced.

3. The position of the chest wall, diaphragms, or both, is shifted.

4. The shape of the chest wall, diaphragms, or both, is distorted (Fig. 56a,b).

5. Special Case: Abnormal congenital development.

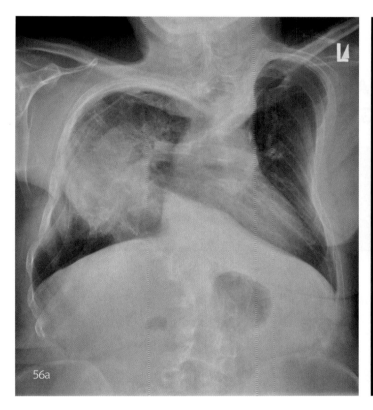

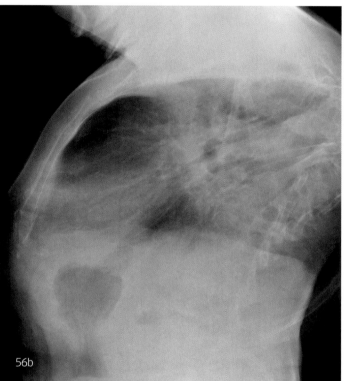

Figure 55. Breast implants. Breast implants can cause the grayscale of the chest wall to appear too white. a, PA chest x-ray from a patient with breast implants, b, lateral chest x-ray from the same patient.

Figure 56. Scoliosis. Scoliosis can cause the chest wall to change in shape. a, PA chest x-ray from a patient with scoliosis, b, lateral chest x-ray from the same patient.

SUMMARY OF RADIOLOGICAL CHANGES
TO THE CHEST WALL & DIAPHRAGMS

RADIOLOGICAL CHANGES TO THE....		...RIBS	...STERNUM	...CLAVICLES
1. Change in grayscale	Too white	• Fracture healing (Fig. 54a,b) • Metastasis (Fig. 54k,l)	• Fracture healing • Metastasis (Fig. 54k,l)	• Fracture healing • Metastasis (Fig. 54k,l)
	Too black	• Bone destruction • Acute fracture	• Bone destruction • Acute fracture	• Bone destruction • Acute fracture
2. Change in size	Increase	• Bone expansion secondary to tumor • Old healed fracture	• Bone expansion secondary to tumor • Old healed fracture	• Bone expansion secondary to tumor • Old healed fracture
	Decrease	• Surgery (Fig. 54i,j) • Neurofibromatosis	• Surgery • Neurofibromatosis	
3. Change in position		• Pectus excavatum • Pectus carinatum	• Pectus excavatum • Pectus carinatum	• Dislocated acromioclavicular or sternoclavicular joint
4. Change in shape		• Previous trauma • Surgery	• Previous trauma • Surgery	• Previous trauma • Surgery
5. Special cases: Abnormal congenital development		• Congenitally fused • Supernumary ribs		

Table 14.1.
Summary of Radiological Changes to the Chest Wall & Diaphragms

...SCAPULAE	...SPINE	...SKIN, SUBCUTANEOUS TISSUES & MUSCLES	...BREASTS	...DIAPHRAGMS
		• Skin moles • Neurofibroma (Fig. 54c,d) • Calcifications		
• Fracture healing • Metastasis (Fig. 54k,l)	• Fracture healing • Metastasis (Fig. 54k,l)	*** ARTIFACTS: skin piercing ***	• Breast implants (Fig. 54e,f) • Calcified implants	• Diaphragmatic hernias if does not contain air
• Bone destruction • Acute fracture	• Bone destruction • Acute fracture	• Surgical emphysema	• Mastectomy • Abscess	• Diaphragmatic hernias if contain air
• Bone expansion secondary to tumor • Old healed fracture	• Bone expansion secondary to tumor • Old healed fracture		• Partial mastectomy • Developmental asymmetry	• Post-traumatic rupture
	• Bone collapse due to fracture			
• Winged scapulae	• Scoliosis (Fig. 54m,n) • Rotoscoliosis			• Elevated secondary to diaphragmatic paralysis (Fig. 54g,h)
• Previous trauma • Surgery	• Previous trauma • Surgery	• Previous trauma • Surgery	• Previous trauma • Surgery	• Flattening with lung hyperinflation
		• Poland syndrome (absent pectoralis major muscle)		• Bochdalek hernia • Morgagni hernia

What is not a part of the normal chest wall and may be present on the chest x-rays? (Fig. 57a,b,c,d)

1.   ECG leads
2.   Central venous catheters
3.   Pacemakers
4.   Ventilation tubes and extensions in ICU patients
5.   Hair bands and clips
6.   Buttons and clips of clothing
7.   Jewellery
8.   Coins and currency in pockets

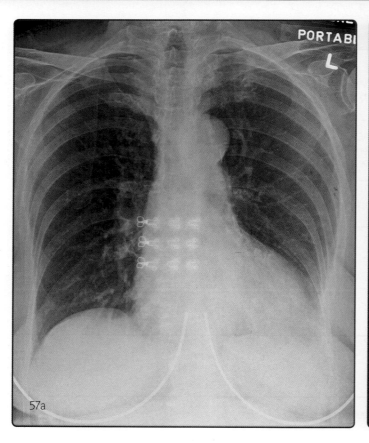

57a

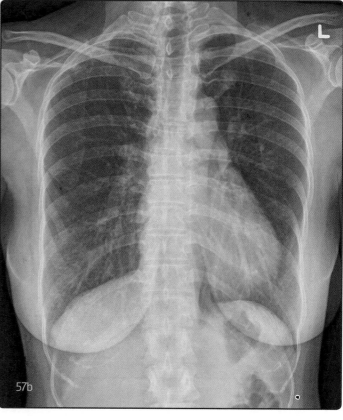

57b

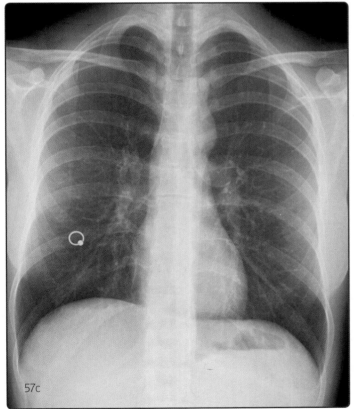

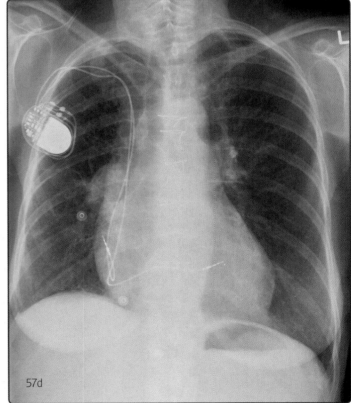

Figure 57. Other items on a chest x-ray. Many items that are not part of the normal chest wall may also be seen on a chest x-ray. a, PA chest x-ray with clips (internal) and wire from clothing (external), b, PA chest x-ray from a patient with clothing artifact, c, PA chest x-ray from a patient with a nipple ring, d, PA chest x-ray from a patient with a pacemaker.

THE PERIPHERY OF THE CHEST X-RAY

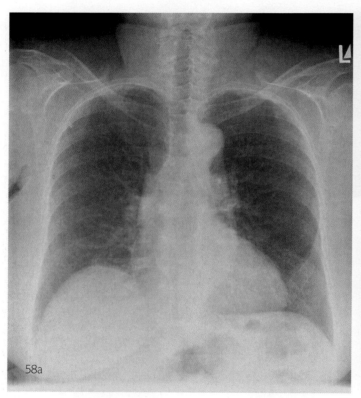

58a

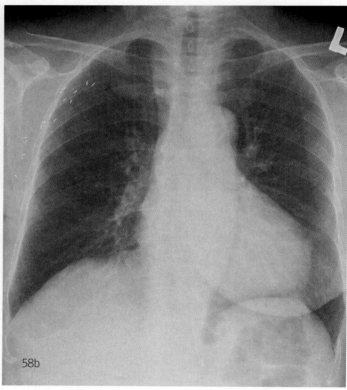

58b

In addition to information about the thorax, the chest x-ray examination can also provide valuable information about other anatomical areas outside of the thoracic cavity, including:

- Axillary region and shoulders.
- Lower neck.
- Upper abdomen.

Axillary Region

Without prior history, the presence of surgical clips (unilateral or bilateral) in the axillary region (Fig. 58a,b), especially in women, may be an indicator of previous breast surgery, and axillary dissection. The presence of a breast shadow does not preclude previous surgery, as a breast-sparing lumpectomy may have been performed. Prominent soft tissue densities in the axillary regions may be caused by adenopathy.

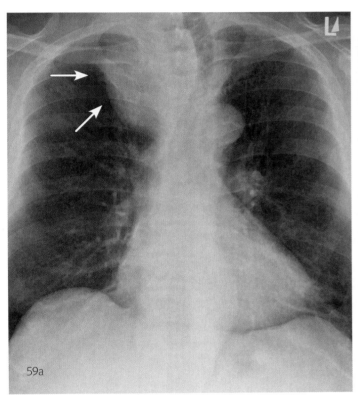

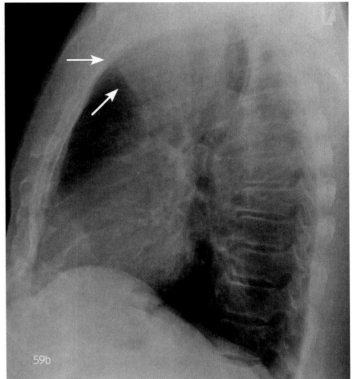

Lower Neck and Thoracic Outlet

The fascia of the lower neck extends into the upper mediastinum, and provides a path for the spread of disease from the neck into the thorax (13).

The key to identifying neck pathology is identifying airway narrowing or displacement. In thin patients, soft-tissue changes in the neck can also be seen as soft-tissue asymmetry and a change in grayscale.

Thyroid enlargement is a common abnormality in the neck region that can extend into the thorax (Fig. 59a,b).

The differential diagnosis of disease processes in the neck extending into the thorax includes the following.

- Tumor
- Aadenopathy
- Infection,
- Hematoma.

Figure 58. Surgical clips. a, PA chest x-ray from a patient with surgical clips visible in the right axilla, b, PA chest x-ray from a second patient with surgical clips visible in the right axilla.

Figure 59. Enlarged thyroid. Thyroid (arrows) displaces the trachea. a, PA chest x-ray from a patient with an enlarged thyroid, b, lateral chest x-ray from the same patient showing the enlarged thyroid (arrows) displacing the trachea.

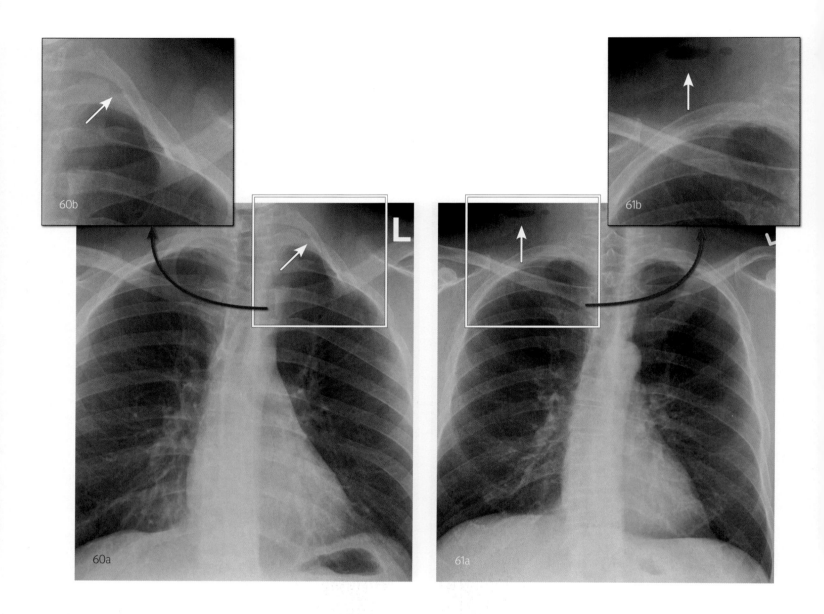

Thoracic outlet syndrome

AMSER A common variant of development is the presence of cervical ribs, either unilaterally or bilaterally (Fig. 60a,b). Cervical ribs can cause thoracic outlet syndrome, by compressing on the brachial plexus and the subclavian vessels.

Abnormal collections of air and calcifications can occur and be seen in the neck. Air in the neck region may indicate an infection (Fig. 61a,b), or the superior extension of mediastinal air (pneumomediastinum) (Fig. 62). Calcifications may indicate significant peripheral vascular disease, or be an indicator of a systemic calcium metabolism disorder.

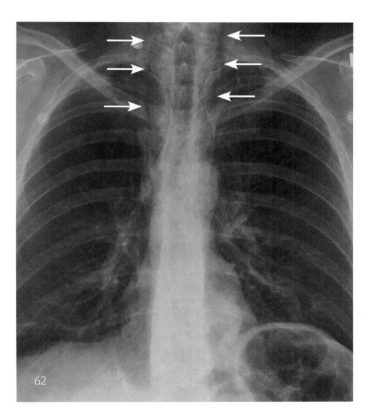

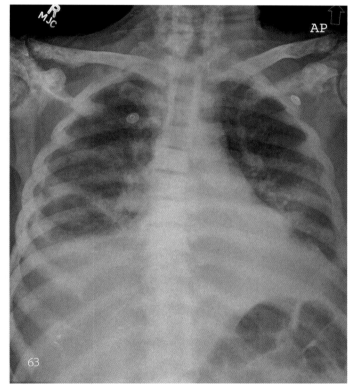

Shoulders

Any disease process that involves the bones or joints can involve the shoulders. Joint or bony destruction may be an indicator of infection or metastatic disease (Fig. 63). Clavicle and shoulder joint erosions can occur with rheumatoid arthritis.

Figure 60. Cervical ribs. A common normal variant in development is the presence of extra, cervical ribs. PA chest x-ray from a patient with a left cervical rib (arrow).

Figure 61. Neck abscess. Air in the neck may indicate an infection. PA chest x-ray from a patient with an abscess (arrow) in the right neck.

Figure 62. Air in the neck. The air of a pneumomediastinum can extend superiorly into the neck. PA chest x-ray from a patient with a pneumomediastinum extending into the neck region (arrows).

Figure 63. Metastatic disease. Widespread bone destruction into the shoulders may be an indicator of infection or metastatic disease. PA chest x-ray highlighting widespread bone destruction from a patient with prostatic cancer.

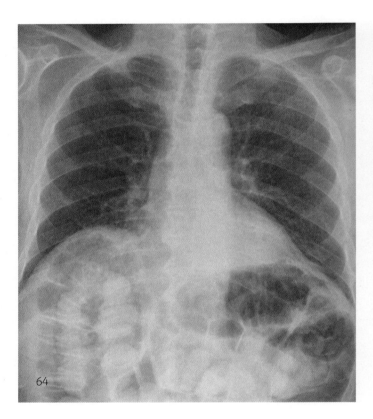

64

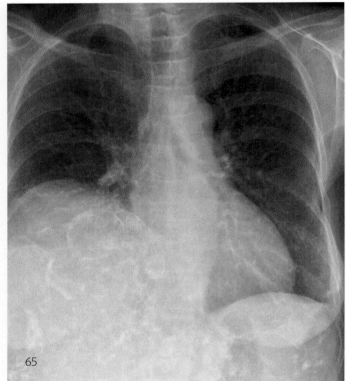

65

Upper Abdomen

Intra-abdominal pathology can occasionally be seen on chest x-rays (12). This can include:

- Bowel dilatation related to bowel obstruction (Fig. 64).
- Bowel wall thickening related to colitis.
- Liver or spleen enlargement.
- Calcifications in the right upper quadrant from calcified gallstones, calcified liver and kidney cysts (Fig. 65).
- Renal calculi on adrenal calcifications.
- Calcifications in the midline from chronic pancreatitis.
- Calcification in the left upper quadrant from renal calculi, left adrenal calcification, specific granulomas, pancreatic tail calcifications.
- Abnormal intramural gas from emphysemous cholecystitis, emphysemous pyelonephritis, ischemic bowel, liver, renal, or pancreatic abscess.
- Free air related to viscous perforation (Fig. 66a,b).

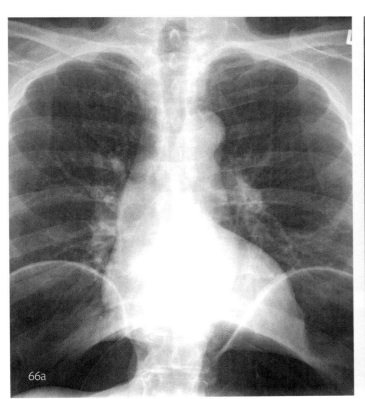

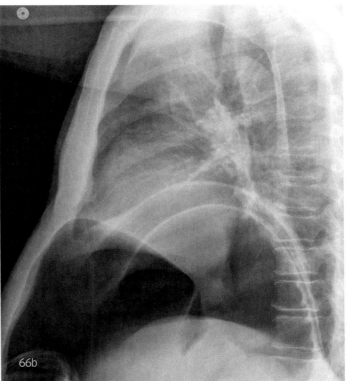

Figure 64. **Bowel obstruction.** PA chest x-ray from a patient with a bowel obstruction, showing distended bowel loops.

Figure 65. **Calcifications.** PA chest x-ray from a patient with extensive intra-abdominal calcifications. Numerous calcified liver and kidney cysts in a patient with long-standing renal failure.

Figure 66. **Free intra-abdominal air.** a, PA chest x-ray from a patient with massive free intra-abdominal air, b, lateral chest x-ray from the same patient.

Visual Search of the Chest Wall & Diaphragms

PA Chest X-ray

1. Start at the right apex.

2. Follow the rib counting method to outline the superior and inferior cortex of each rib.

3. Complete the rib search by checking the opacity of each rib.

4. Check cortical outline and density of each scapula.

5. Check cortical outline and density of each clavicle.

6. Check the lateral edges of the spine through the heart.

7. Check the contour of both diaphragms.

VS

Lateral Chest X-ray

1. Check the cortical outline and opacity of the sternum.

2. Check the cortical outline and density of each vertebral body.

3. Check the cortical outline and density of each rib, posteriorly.

4. Check the contour of both diaphragms.

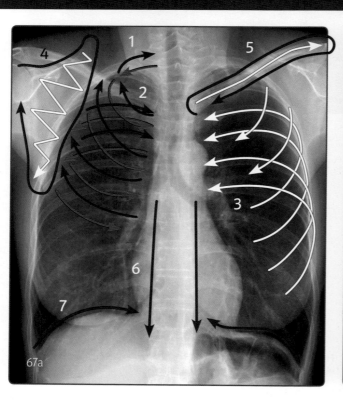

67a

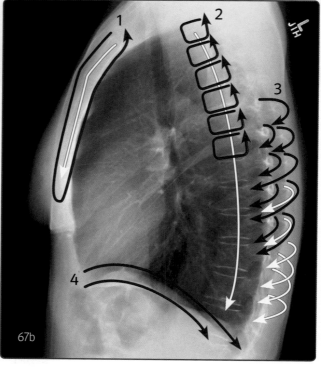

67b

Chest Wall & Diaphragms Radiological Analysis Checklist

To confidently state that the chest wall and diaphragms are normal all parts of the checklist should indicate a normal appearance.

BONY THORAX (Spine, ribs, clavicles, scapulae, sternum)

GRAYSCALE

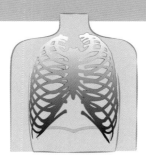

1   Is the grayscale of the bones altered?

If **YES**, then describe.
Too white/too black.
Bone density.
Cortical outline.
Fractures/bone destruction.

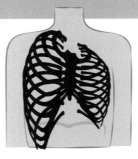

2   Are any abnormal opacities present?

If **YES**, then describe.
Give number and location.
Focal/diffuse.

POSITION

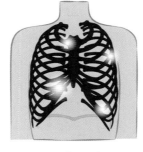

3   Is the position of the bony thorax (ribs, spine, clavicles, sternum, scapulae) altered?

If **YES**, then describe.
Right/left.
Anterior/posterior.
Elevated/depressed.

OTHER

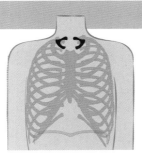

4   Are there any accessory ribs?

If **YES**, then describe.
Cervical/lumbar
Give number and position.

SOFT TISSUES

GRAYSCALE

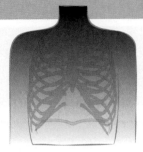

5 Is the grayscale of the soft tissues altered?

If **YES**, then describe.
Too white/too black.

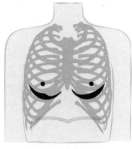

6 Are breast, pectoral folds and/or nipple shadows present?

If **YES**, then describe.
Right/left/bilateral.
If not sure, repeat CXR with nipple markers.

SIZE

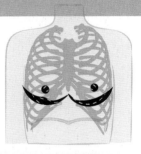

7 Is the size of the breasts altered?

If **YES**, then describe.
Right/left/bilateral
Increased/decreased.

DIAPHRAGMS

POSITION

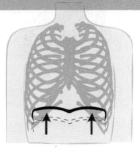

8 Is the position of the diaphragm(s) altered?

If **YES**, then describe.
Right/left/bilateral.
Elevated/depressed.

SHAPE

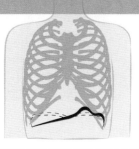

9 Is the shape of the diaphragm(s) altered?

If **YES**, then describe.
Right/left/bilateral.
Describe shape.

10 Is there a presence of bowel loops or stomach in the thoracic cavity?

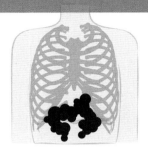

If **YES**, then describe.
Right/left.
Anterior/posterior.

11 Are there any external objects that are not part of the normal chest wall?

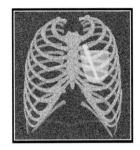

If **YES**, then describe.
ECG leads/buttons and clips on clothing/hair bands and clips/jewellery/coins and currency in pockets.

12 Is there any evidence of previous surgery to the chest wall or diaphragms?

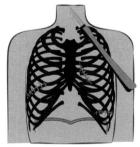

If **YES**, then describe.
Type of surgery and location.
Compare to previous CXR.

13 Are there any lines or tubes in the chest wall?

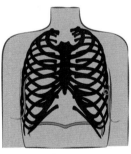

If **YES**, then describe.
Give location of each relative to the carina, SVC and/or diaphragms.

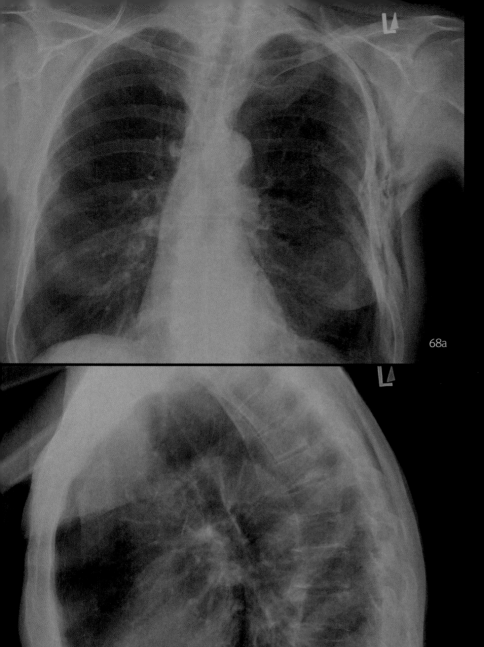

68a

68b

How would you
describe your
findings?

A 65-year-old female presents to the emergency department after having fallen down a flight of stairs. She complains of chest pain that is worse with breathing and movement. Her rib cage is tender and she winces when palpated. You are worried that she may have fractured her ribs and you order a chest x-ray examination (Fig. 68a,b). The emergency department consultant asks you to describe the x-ray findings.

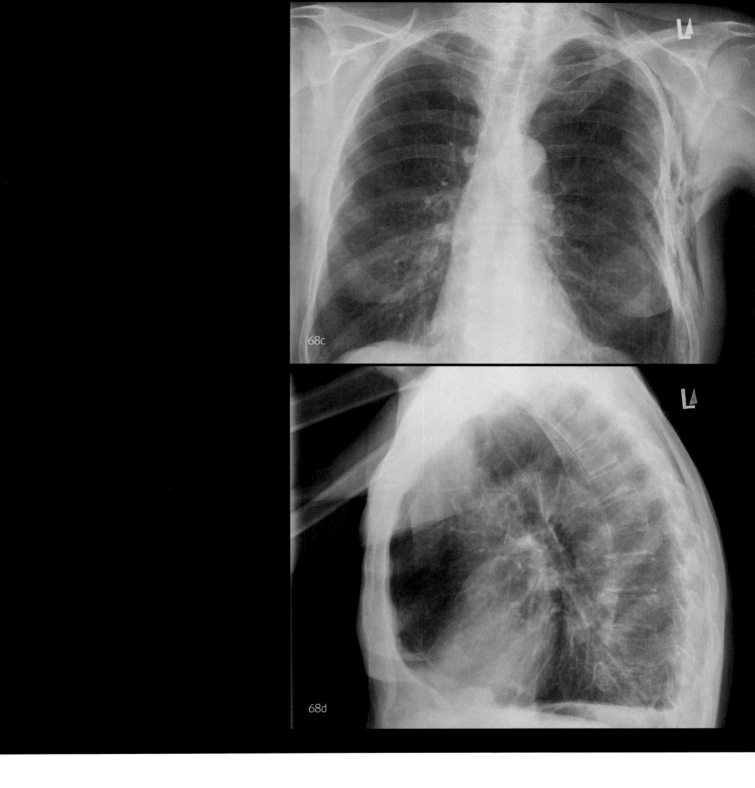

68c

68d

DISCUSSION

Possible pathology of the chest wall and diaphragms should always be included in your differential diagnosis when a patient presents with chest pain. Figures 68c and 68d show multiple left rib fractures and surgical emphysema. Make sure you examine each rib carefully so as not to miss comminuted fractures or hairline fractures.

Based on the findings, the diagnosis is post-traumatic rib fracture and surgical emphysema.

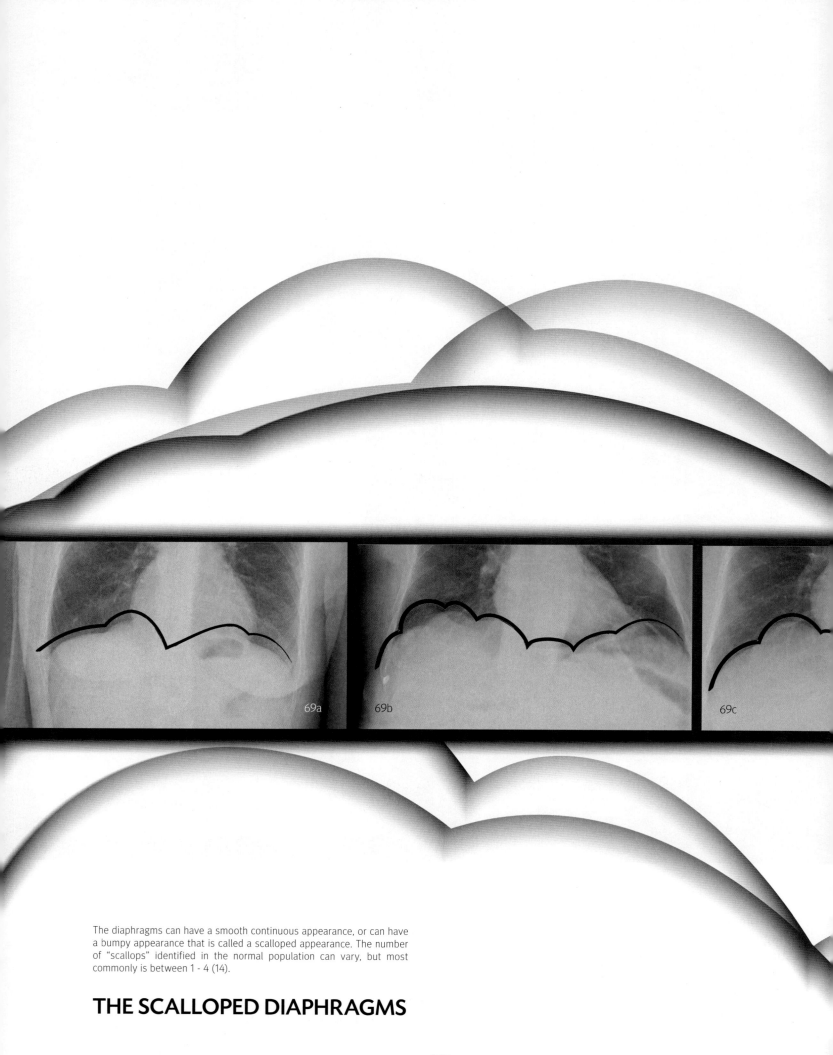

The diaphragms can have a smooth continuous appearance, or can have a bumpy appearance that is called a scalloped appearance. The number of "scallops" identified in the normal population can vary, but most commonly is between 1 - 4 (14).

THE SCALLOPED DIAPHRAGMS

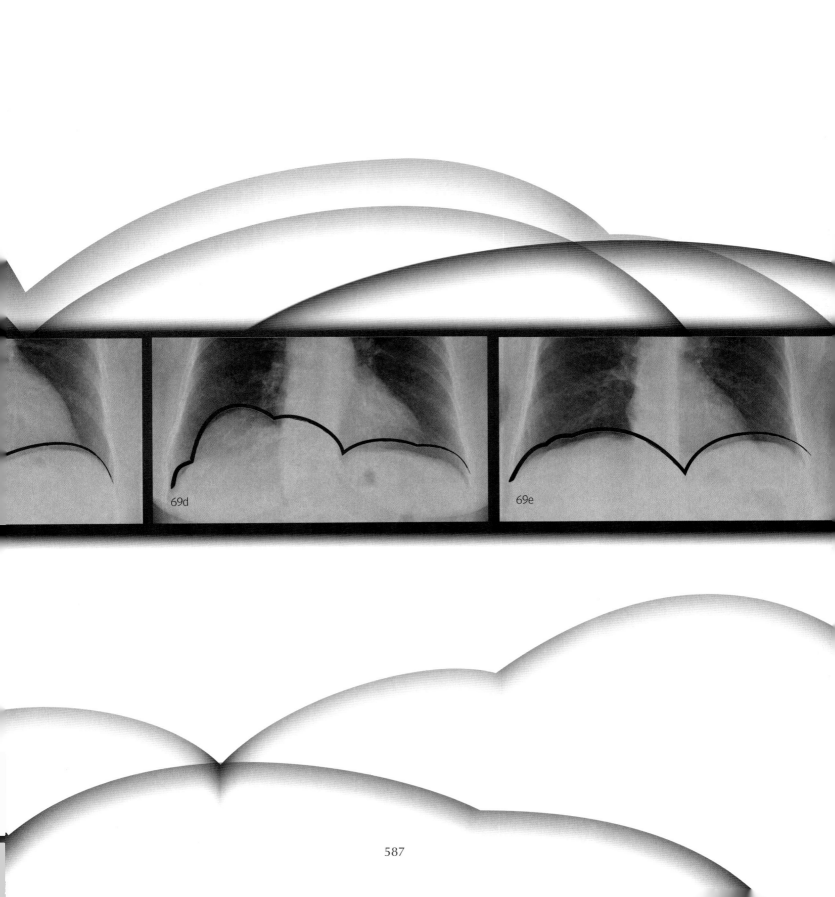

69d

69e

References

1. Lewis, P.J., Shaffer, K., & Donovan, A. (Eds.). (2012). AMSER National Medical Student Curriculum in Radiology. http://aur.org/Secondary-Alliances.aspx?id=141.

2. Lewis, P.J., & Shaffer, K. (2005). Developing a national medical student curriculum in radiology. *Am. Coll. Radiol., 2*(1):8–11.

3. Urschel, H.C. Jr. (2007). Anatomy of the thoracic outlet. *Thorac. Surg. Clin., 17*(4):511–520.

4. Kurihara, Y., Yakushiji, Y.K., Matsumoto, J., et al. (1999). The ribs: anatomic and radiologic considerations. *Radiographics, 19*(1):105–190.

5. Naidich, J.B., Naidich, T.P., Hyman, R.A., et al. (1979). The big rib sign: localization of basal pulmonary pathology in lateral projection utilizing differential magnification of the two hemithoraces. *Radiology, 131*:1–8.

6. Carrier, G., Fréchette, E., Ugalde, P., & Deslauriers, J. (2007). Correlative anatomy for the sternum and ribs, costovertebral angle, chest wall muscles and intercostal spaces, thoracic outlet. *Thorac. Surg. Clin., 17*(4):521–528.

7. Cilad, I., & Nissan, M. (1985). Sagittal evaluation of elemental geometrical dimensions of human vertebrae. *J. Anat., 143*:115–120.

8. Amory, H.I., & Sieber, P.E. (1953). The supraclavicular shadows in chest film interpretation. *Radiology, 61*(1):8–12.

9. Kleinman, P.K., & Raptopoulos, V. (1985). The anterior diaphragmatic attachments: and anatomic and radiologic study with clinical correlates. *Radiology, 155*:289–293.

10. Panicek, M., Benson, B., & Gottlieb, H. (1988). The diaphragm: Anatomic, pathologic, and radiologic considerations. *RadioGraphics, 8*(3):385–425.

11. Abiru, H., Ashizawa, K., Hashmi, R., & Hayashi, K. (2005). Normal radiographic anatomy of thoracic structures: analysis of 1000 chest radiographs in Japanese population. *Br. J. Radiol., 78*:398–404.

12. Sandstrom, C.K., & Stern, E.J. (2011). Diaphragmatic hernias: A spectrum of radiographic appearances. *Curr. Probr. Diagn. Rad., 40*(3):95–115.

13. Deslauriers, J. (2007). Anatomy of the neck and cervicothoracic junction. *Thorac. Surg. Clin., 17*(4):529–547.

14. Lennon, E.A., & Simon, G. (1965). The height of the diaphragm in the chest radiograph of normal adults. *Br. J. Radiol., 38*:937–943.

CHAPTER 15
CONSTRUCTING
the X-RAY IMAGE

importance

In the preceding chapters, you reviewed the radiological anatomy of the various anatomical structures within the thorax. It is important to understand the radiological anatomy of the individual structures, but also how all of these structures together form the x-ray image. This chapter provides a different perspective on the chest x-ray – it will enable you to get a deeper understanding of the radiological anatomy through the reconstruction of the chest x-ray from its various grayscale components.

In this chapter, the chest x-ray image is rebuilt, step-by-step, to form a complete picture.

objectives

Skills

You will identify

- key anatomical structures on the reconstructed PA and lateral chest x-rays.

Knowledge

You will review and understand

- the radiological anatomy of all of the structures within the thorax.
- the anatomical layout of the thorax by the reconstruction of the PA and lateral x-rays.

associated resources

This chapter maps to the following AMSER curriculum content (1,2).

1) Normal Anatomy: Chest x-ray (CXR) - PA and lateral

a) Lungs
   Trachea and carina
   Right and left main bronchi

b) Heart
   Aorta
   Pulmonary veins

c) Mediastinum
   Superior vena cava
   Subclavian vessels
   Azygos vein
   Carina
   Right and left main pulmonary arteries
   Azygo-esophageal stripe (line, or recess)
   Right paraspinal stripe (line)
   Left paraaortic stripe (line)

d) Bone and soft tissues
   Thoracic spine
   Scapulae
   Clavicles
   Diaphragms

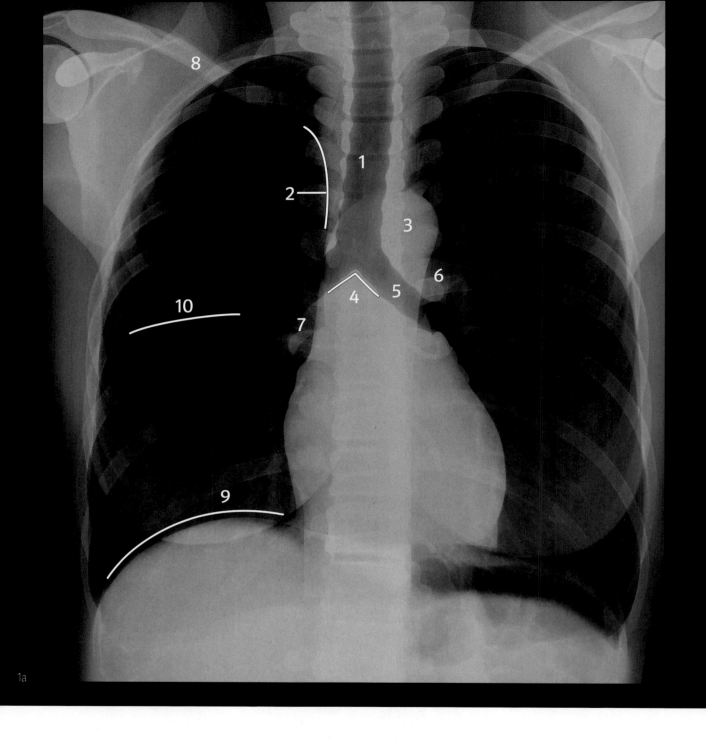

1a

CASE STUDY

The following PA and lateral chest x-rays (Fig. 1a,b) have been constructed in layers of important anatomical structures.

PA X-ray

Aortic arch	Left pulmonary artery
Carina	Right hemidiaphragm
Clavicle	Right pulmonary artery
Horizontal fissure	Superior vena cava
Left main stem bronchus	Trachea

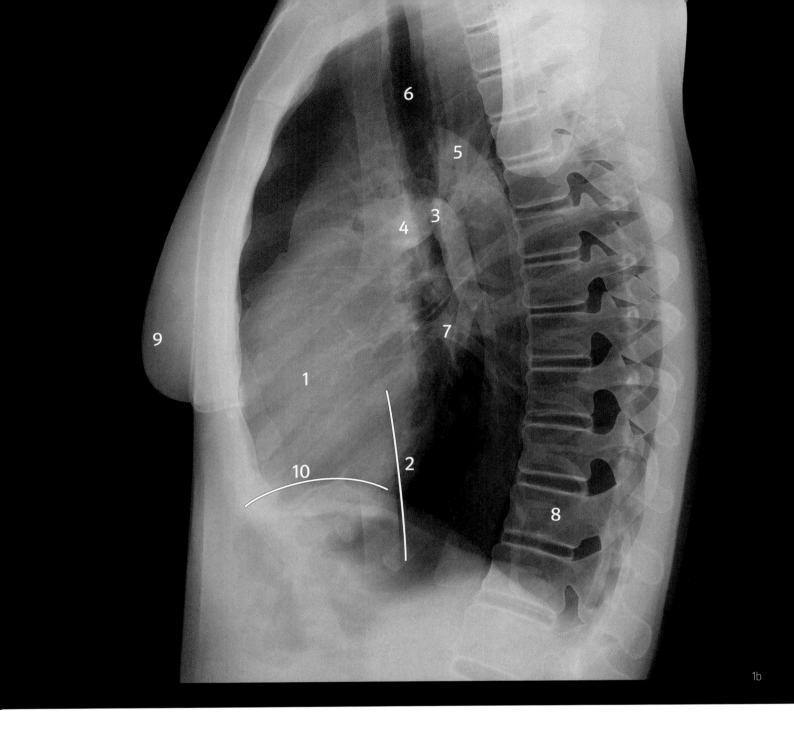

Lateral X-ray

Aortic arch
Breast
Diaphragm
Heart
Inferior vena cava

Left pulmonary artery
Pulmonary veins
Right pulmonary artery
Trachea
Vertebrae

Can you match
each number
to the anatomical
structure listed?

CONSTRUCTING
THE PA CHEST X-RAY

The PA chest x-ray will be reconstructed in the following steps.

We start the construction of the PA x-ray image with the grayscale of the lungs added to a black canvas (Fig. 2). If the x-ray beam does not encounter any anatomical structures before it hits the x-ray detectors, it will make the image look black. The canvas we start with is black and corresponds to the air on an x-ray that is seen outside of the body. The lungs are faintly outlined and will have some opacity because of the blood within the blood vessels of the lungs.

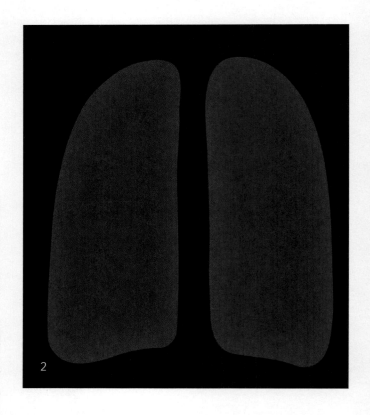

2

We now add the vertebrae. These are usually easy to identify because of their well-defined white outline (Fig. 3). In this illustration, the vertebral bodies can be clearly seen because we have not yet added overlying structures.

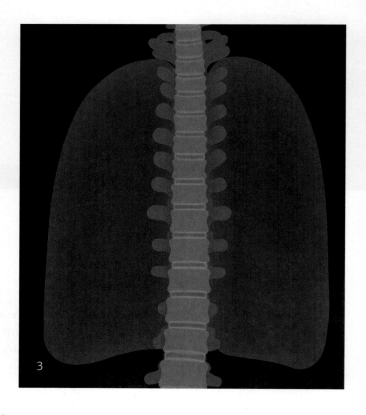

3

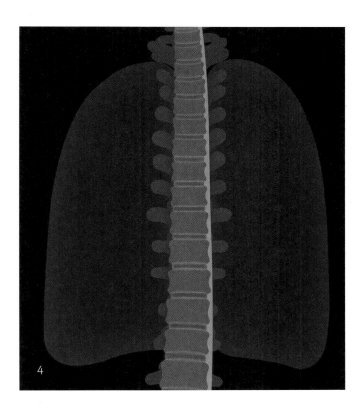

4

The soft tissues beside the vertebral column will appear as a white vertical stripe (Fig. 4), that is seen on most PA x-rays. This is referred to as the left paraspinal stripe (line).

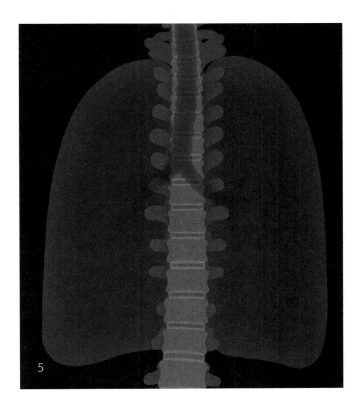

5

The trachea, radiologically, is a black rectangle that stops at the carina (the T4 level) (Fig. 5). The main stem bronchi also look like black rectangles.

AMSER

The soft tissues adjacent to the right border of the trachea form a thin, white, vertical stripe (Fig. 6) – the right paratracheal stripe (line).

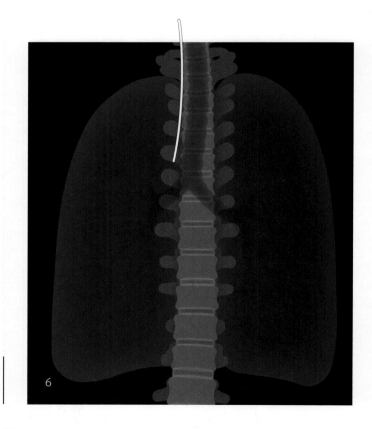

6

596

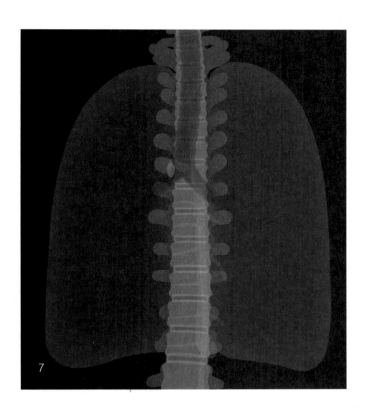

7

The esophagus and azygos vein course vertically and create a white, vertical stripe overlying the left side of the vertebral bodies (Fig. 7). The left-most edge of this stripe is called the azygo-esophageal stripe (line, or recess). The azygos vein, where it drains into the superior vena cava, can be identified as a white, oval structure, sitting on the right main stem bronchus.

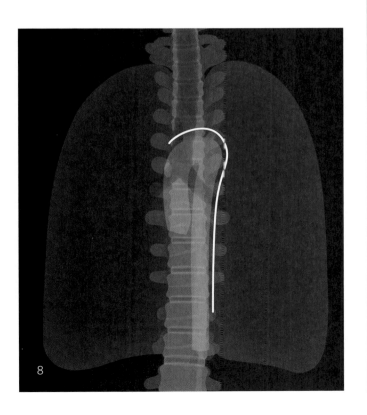

8

The aorta has a candy-cane shape, and lies in the mid-thorax (Fig. 8). On the PA chest x-ray, only the left, lateral wall of the vertical portion of the aorta is visible and this forms the left paraaortic line (stripe).

AMSER

The heart (Fig. 9) contributes a significant amount of whiteness to the mediastinum centrally and interiorly.

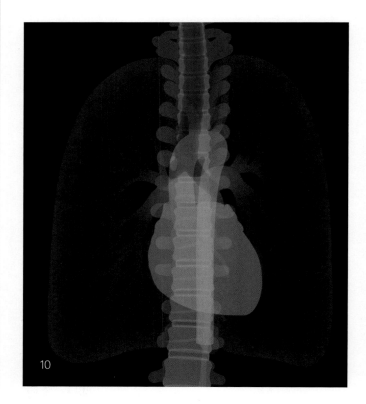

AMSER

The pulmonary arteries (Fig. 10) form an H-shaped structure centrally. The horizontal bar of the H lies centrally within the mediastinum. For simplification, the more peripheral arterial branches are not shown.

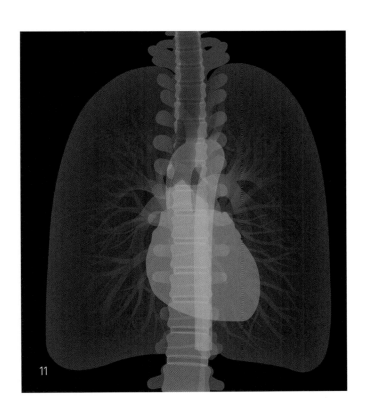

The superior pulmonary veins (Fig. 11) lie lateral to the arteries, but usually cannot be differentiated from them on an x-ray. The inferior pulmonary veins course horizontally, joining the superior pulmonary veins as they drain into the left atrium. For simplification, the more peripheral venous branches are not shown.

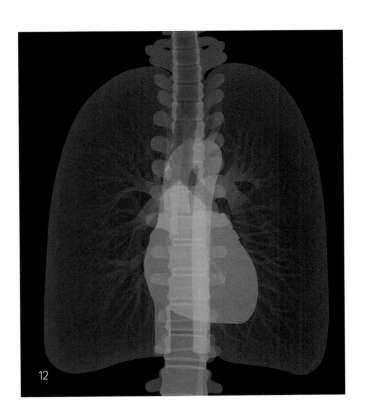

Above the aortic arch, the edges of the mediastinum (Fig. 12) are formed by the superior vena cava (SVC) on the right and the subclavian artery on the left. This is called the vascular pedicle.

Similar to the vertebral bodies, the posterior ribs have a distinct, white, cortical outline that makes them easy to identify (Fig. 13). The ribs outline the lateral edges of the lungs and pleura.

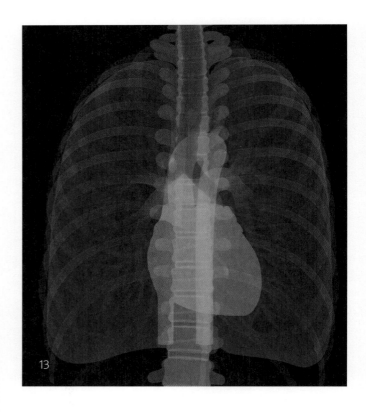

The diaphragms, scapulae and clavicles define the upper and lower borders of the thorax (Fig. 14).

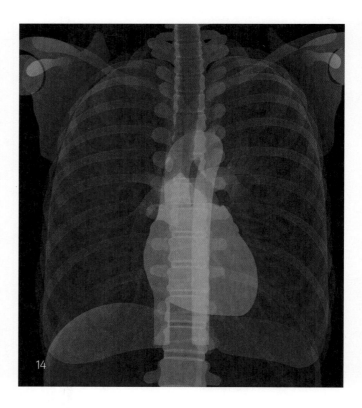

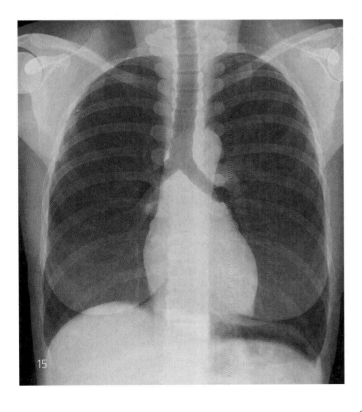

15

By adding the mediastinal fat and the soft tissues of the chest wall, the PA x-ray image is now completed (Fig. 15).

Compare the reconstructed PA chest x-ray with the real PA chest x-ray found on the front foldout cover.

CONSTRUCTING
THE LATERAL CHEST X-RAY

The lateral chest x-ray can be reconstructed in the following steps.

As with the PA chest x-ray, we start the construction of the lateral x-ray image with a black background canvas. We give the lungs the same grayscale as on the PA x-ray. The lungs are faintly outlined (Fig. 16).

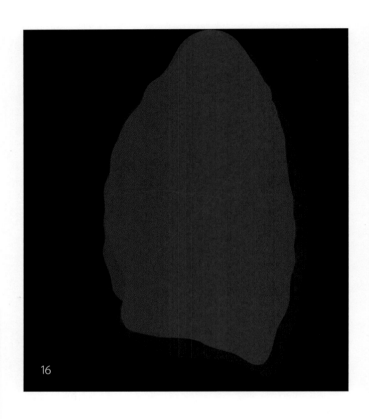

16

We now add the vertebrae. These are usually easy to identify because of their well-defined, white outline (Fig. 17). On a lateral x-ray, the vertebral bodies are easily identified posteriorly.

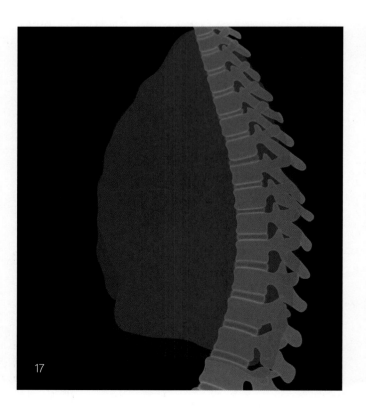

17

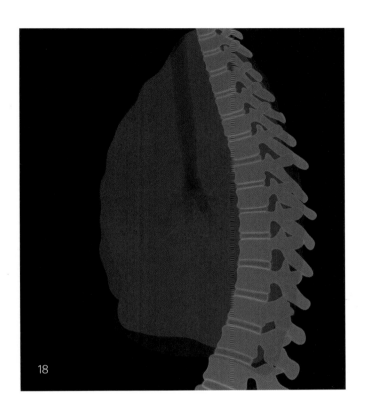

The trachea, radiologically, is a black rectangle that stops at the carina (Fig. 18). On the lateral chest x-ray, the main stem bronchi can sometimes be seen as black circles within the rectangle. The bronchus intermedius appears as the continuation of the trachea, inferiorly.

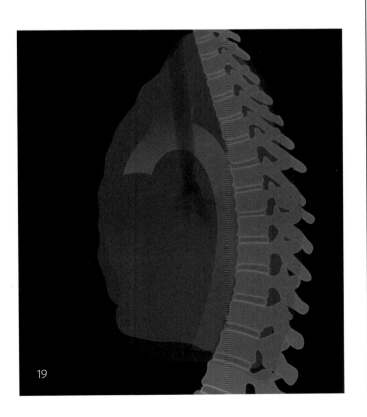

The aorta has a candy cane-shape in the mid-thorax (Fig. 19). The ascending aorta, aortic arch and parts of the descending aorta are visible on the lateral chest x-ray, identified posteriorly.

The heart (Fig. 20) contributes a significant amount of whiteness to the mediastinum anteriorly and inferiorly.

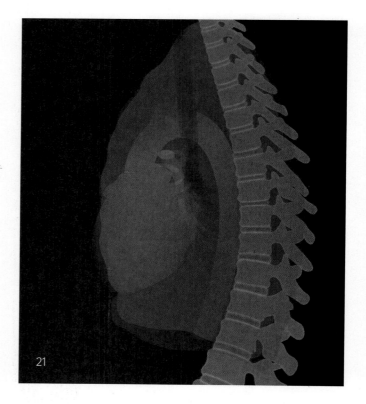

The right pulmonary artery (RPA)(Fig. 21) forms a white oval centrally and anterior to the trachea.

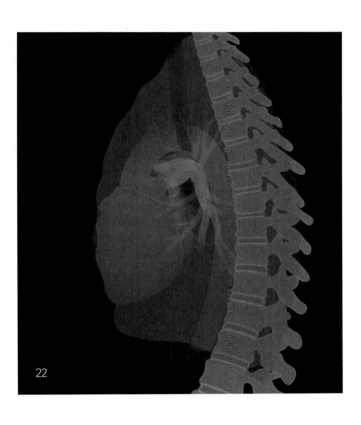

The left pulmonary artery (LPA)(Fig. 22) courses over the left main stem bronchus and forms an arch – "the little arch".

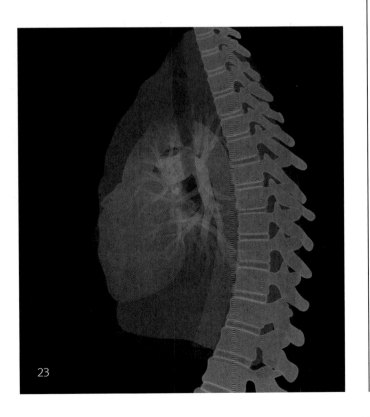

The superior pulmonary veins are difficult to differentiate from the arteries. The inferior pulmonary veins course horizontally and, similar to the superior pulmonary veins, drain into the left atrium (Fig. 23).

The ribs have a distinct, white, cortical outline that makes them easy to identify (Fig. 24).

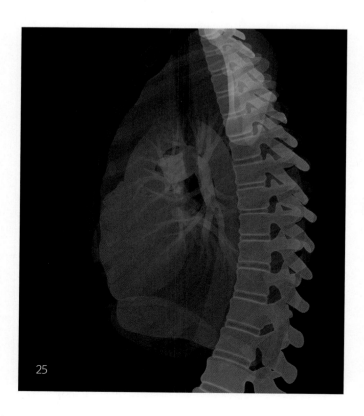

24

The diaphragms, scapulae and clavicles define the upper and lower borders of the thorax (Fig. 25).

25

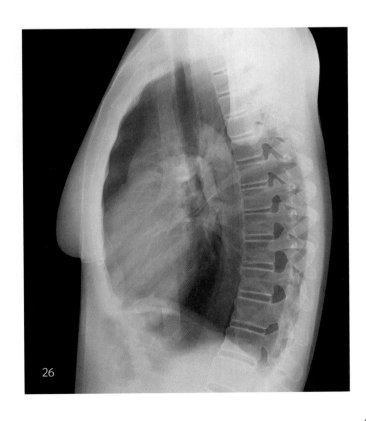

26

By adding the superior vessels (the carotid and brachiocephalic arteries), mediastinal fat and soft tissues of the chest wall, the lateral x-ray image is now completed (Fig. 26).

Compare the reconstructed lateral chest x-ray with the real lateral chest x-ray found on the back foldout cover.

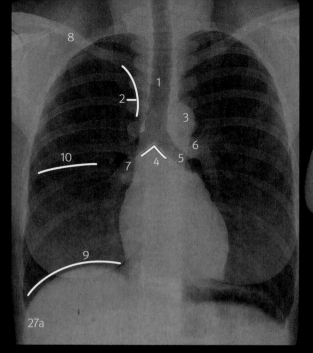

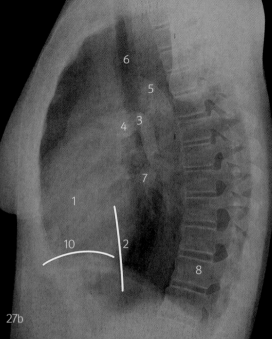

Can you match each number to the anatomical structure listed?

27a

27b

The following PA and lateral chest x-rays (Fig. 27 a,b), have been constructed in layers of important anatomical structures.

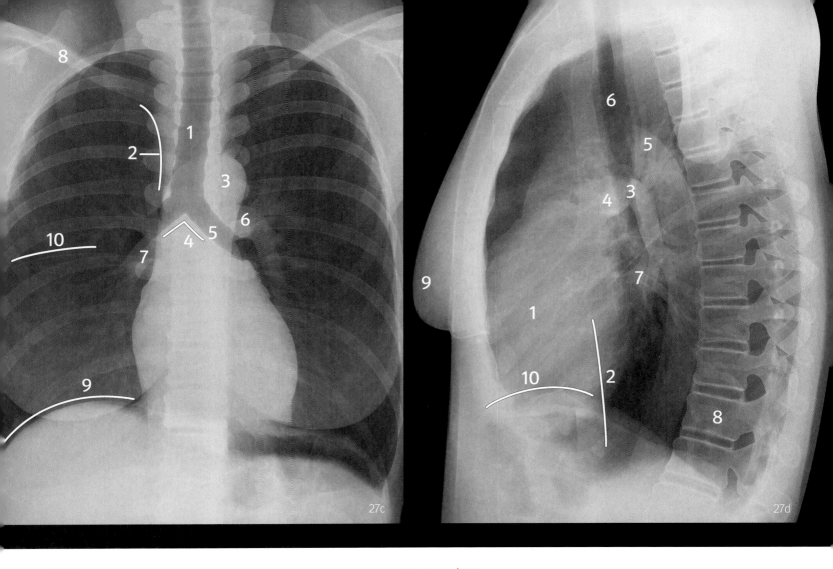

PA X-ray

1. Trachea
2. Superior vena cava
3. Aortic arch
4. Carina
5. Left main stem bronchus
6. Left pulmonary artery
7. Right pulmonary artery (descending branch)
8. Clavicle (right)
9. Right hemidiaphragm
10. Horizontal fissure in right lung

Lateral X-ray

1. Heart
2. Inferior vena cava
3. Left pulmonary artery
4. Right pulmonary artery
5. Aortic arch
6. Trachea
7. Pulmonary veins (inferior)
8. Vertebrae
9. Breast
10. Diaphragm (right hemidiaphragm)

DISCUSSION

References

1. Lewis, P.J., Shaffer, K., & Donovan, A. (Eds.). (2012). AMSER National Medical Student Curriculum in Radiology. http://aur.org/Secondary-Alliances.aspx?id=141.

2. Lewis, P.J., & Shaffer, K. (2005). Developing a national medical student curriculum in radiology. *Am. Coll. Radiol., 2*(1):8–11.

PUTT
TOGE

Having reviewed Sections I and II, you now have a good understanding of what the normal anatomical structures and pathology look like on a chest x-ray and are ready to put it all together.

Section III is divided into 8 Chapters. Section III starts with a chapter on how to interpret the chest x-ray; this is where you begin to put your new knowledge into practice. Now that you know what to look for, we'll help you do so in a systematic way to ensure the accurate identification of pathology.

Subsequent chapters show you how to apply this knowledge to more complex chest x-rays.

In this section you will learn further interpretive skills such as how to accurately localize pathology and how to use the digital technologies with the interpretive process.

Finally, you will learn when it is appropriate to order a chest x-ray.

CHAPTER 16
HOW TO INTERPRET
A CHEST X-RAY

importance

You have already been introduced to the concept of chest x-ray interpretation in Chapter 5. Chapters 7-14 covered normal radiological anatomy and the radiological appearance of chest pathology. Now that you have a clearer understanding of what can be seen on a chest x-ray, in this chapter you will learn how to put this knowledge together into a new skill – chest x-ray interpretation.

objectives

Skills

You will identify

- all of the important landmarks on a chest x-ray that are necessary for the interpretive process.

- the key features of a high quality x-ray and a poor quality x-ray.

Knowledge

You will review and understand

- the six phase process of chest x-ray interpretation.

- the latest technologies and systems that are used in modern radiology.

- how to set up an account and use a PACS system.

- how the PACS system can enhance x-ray interpretation and how this digital system differs from an analog system.

This chapter maps to the following AMSER curriculum content (1,2).

1) Chest x-ray interpretation.

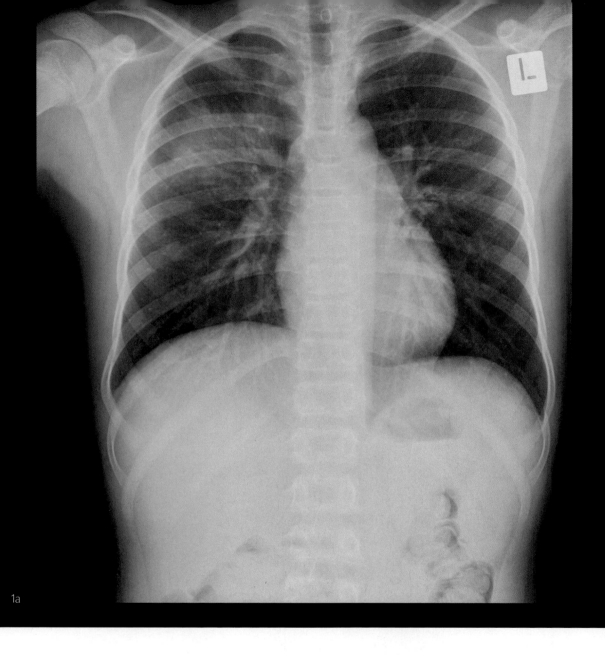

1a

You are working on-call overnight as an intern in the emergency department. At morning rounds you are asked to interpret the chest x-rays (Fig. 1a,b) of a patient you saw during the night. The patient is a 44-year-old non-immunocompromised male with a history of productive cough, fever and elevated white blood cell count (WBC).

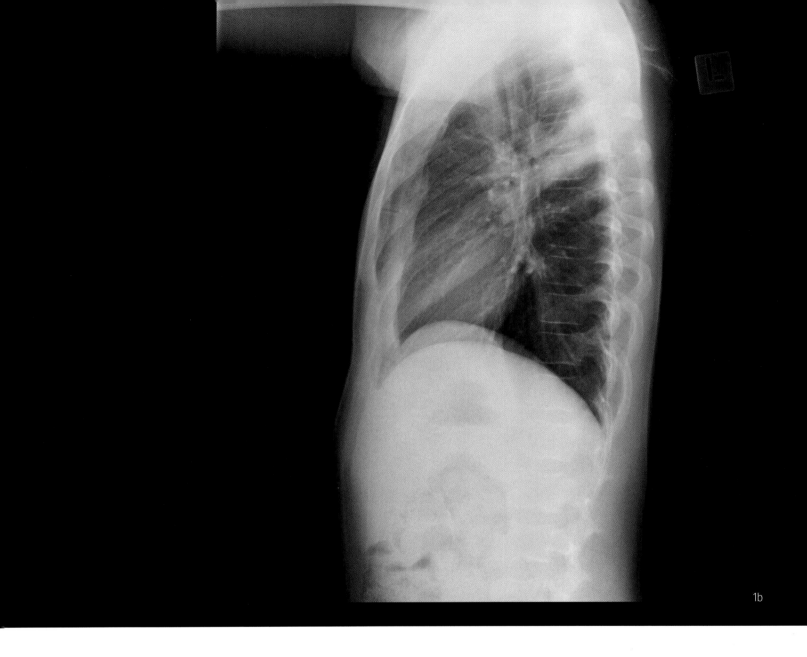

1b

How would you present
the PA and lateral
chest x-ray findings?

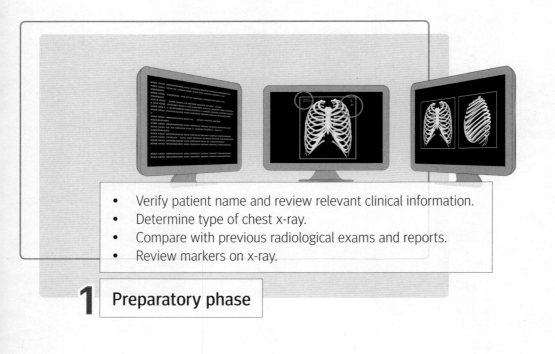

- Verify patient name and review relevant clinical information.
- Determine type of chest x-ray.
- Compare with previous radiological exams and reports.
- Review markers on x-ray.

1 Preparatory phase

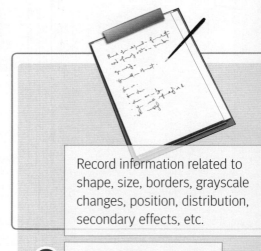

Record information related to shape, size, borders, grayscale changes, position, distribution, secondary effects, etc.

3 Descriptive phase

2 Visual identification phase

- Compare to normal.
- Scan x-ray using systematic approach.

2

INTERPRETATION OF THE CHEST X-RAY

Having reviewed the preceding chapters you are now ready to tackle the task of chest x-ray interpretation.

The interpretive process will follow 6 phases or steps as previously described (Chapter 5).

1. Preparatory phase
2. Visual identification phase
3. Descriptive phase
4. Summary phase
5. Differential diagnosis phase
6. Communication phase

Figure 2. Phases of x-ray interpretation. Diagram of the phases of interpretation. 1, preparatory phase, 2, visual identification phase, 3, descriptive phase, 4, summary phase, 5, differential diagnosis phase, 6, communication phase.

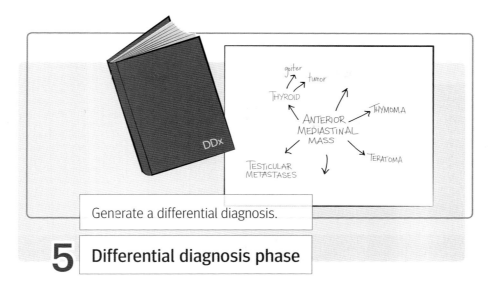

Generate a differential diagnosis.

5 **Differential diagnosis phase**

4 **Summary phase**

Generate a summary statement based on key findings.

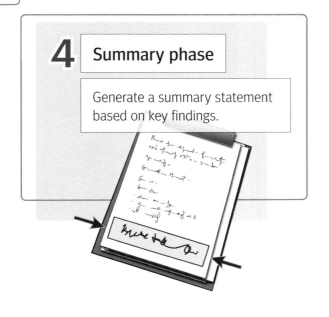

6 **Communication (action) phase**

Communicate the next steps (eg., treatment plan, further tests, etc.).

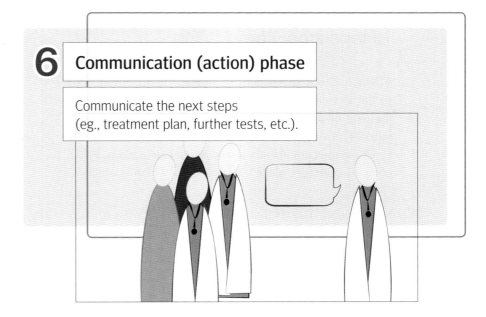

1. Preparatory Phase

ALWAYS check the patient demographics to ensure they fit the examination you are viewing. Make certain that the date of the examination is accurate and check for all relevant previous examinations (Fig. 3a,b). In PACS, it is easy to mix up the current with the previous examinations. When comparing images, make sure you know which is which.

Know your patient's history

- Has the patient had previous thoracic surgery?
- Are there known anatomical variations such as dextrocardia / situs inversus?
- Does the patient have a chest-wall deformity such as pectus excavatum or scoliosis?
- When you examined the patient clinically did you observe any physical findings that could influence the chest x-ray examination (e.g., a palpable thyroid)?

Review the technical aspects of the examination: Is it a good x-ray?

- Is the patient properly centered?
- Has the patient taken a good inspiration?
- Is the examination overexposed? Underexposed?
- Are there any artifacts preventing interpretation of the x-ray?

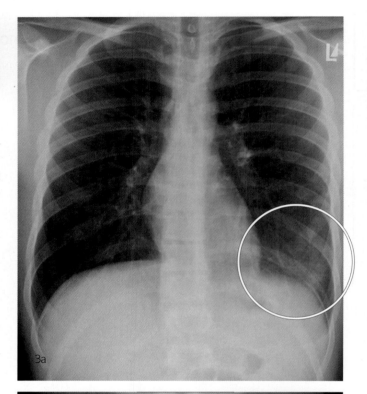

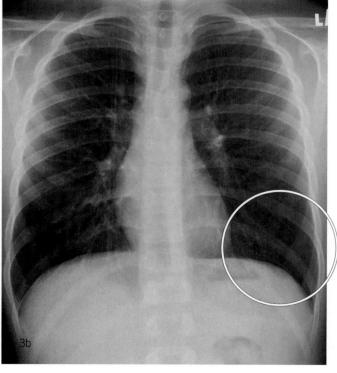

Figure 3. Compare with previous examinations. a, PA chest x-ray from a patient with an opacity in left lung base that is easily identified when compared to the previous normal examination in 3b, b, normal (previous) PA chest x-ray from the same patient.

Chest X-ray Quality Checklist

In order to make sure that the chest x-ray examination is of good quality, all parts of the checklist should indicate good quality.

rc

PATIENT POSITIONING

1 Is the patient position correct?
(rotation/centering)

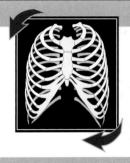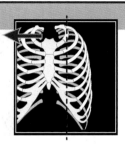

If **NO**, then describe.
Rotated left/right.
Shifted left/right.

INSPIRATION

2 Did the patient take a good inspiration?

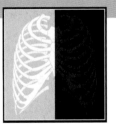

If **NO**, then describe.
Give number of posterior ribs visible.

EXPOSURE

3 Is the x-ray of adequate exposure?

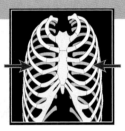

If **NO**, then describe.
Under-exposed/over-exposed.

ARTIFACTS & SHARPNESS

4 Is the x-ray free from external artifacts?
(Are artifacts obscuring part of the image?)

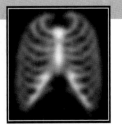

If **NO**, describe.
Hair/clothes/lines/jewellery.

5 Is the x-ray sharp?
(not blurry due to motion artifact)

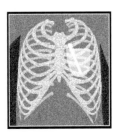

If **NO**, may need to
repeat chest x-ray.

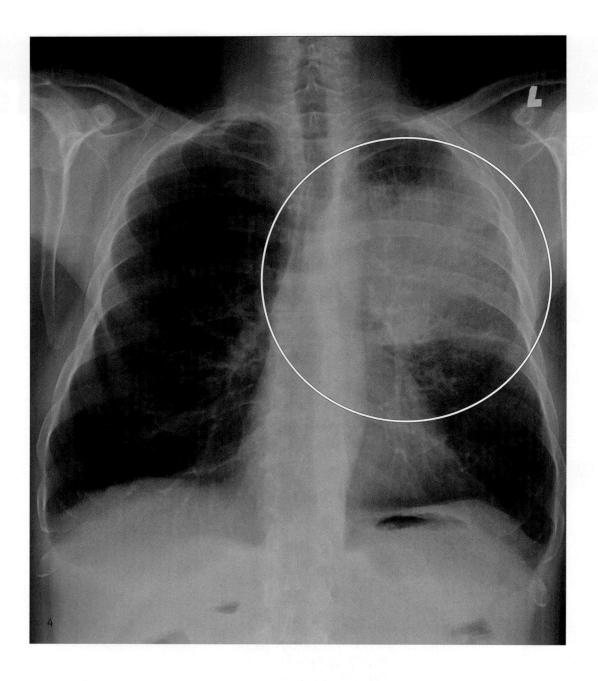

2. Visual Phase

Do you immediately see an abnormality? (Fig. 4)

If no ➡️ Continue with systematic visual search.

If yes ➡️ Is the abnormality too black or too white?
➡️ Continue with systematic visual search.

The systematic visual search will include the airways (trachea & bronchi), the heart, the mediastinum, the hilum, the pleura, the lungs and interstitium, and the chest walls and diaphragms.

Figure 4. Obvious abnormality. An example of a PA chest x-ray with an obvious abnormality in the left upper thorax.

Figure 5. Visual search - Part I. Typical PA and lateral chest x-rays with the paths of the visual searches illustrated. a,b, the trachea and bronchi, c,d, the heart and pericardium (cardiac zone), e,f, the mediastinum (mediastinal zone).

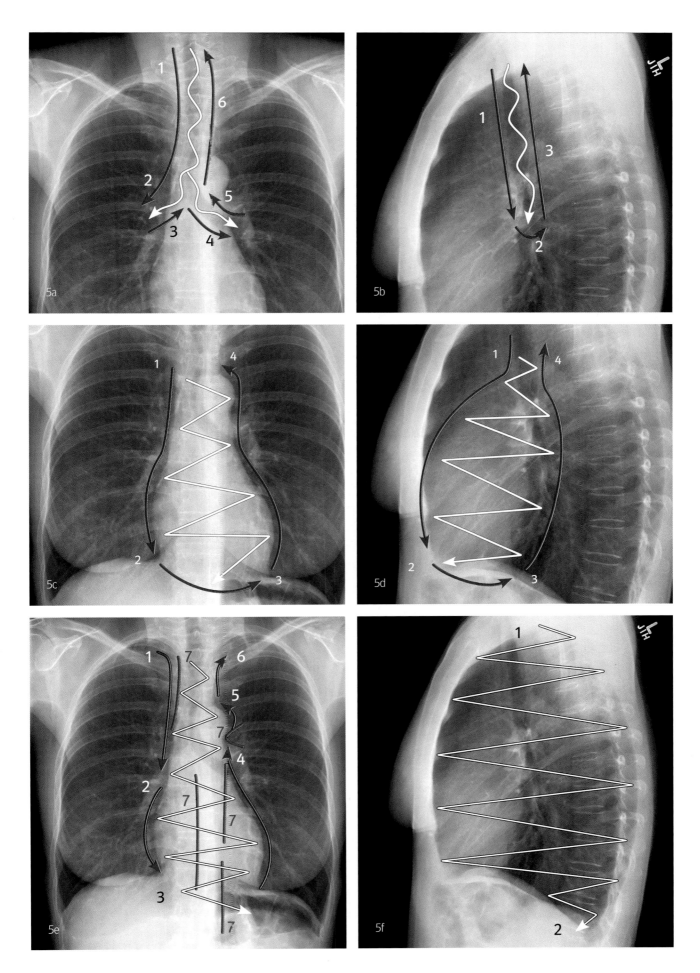

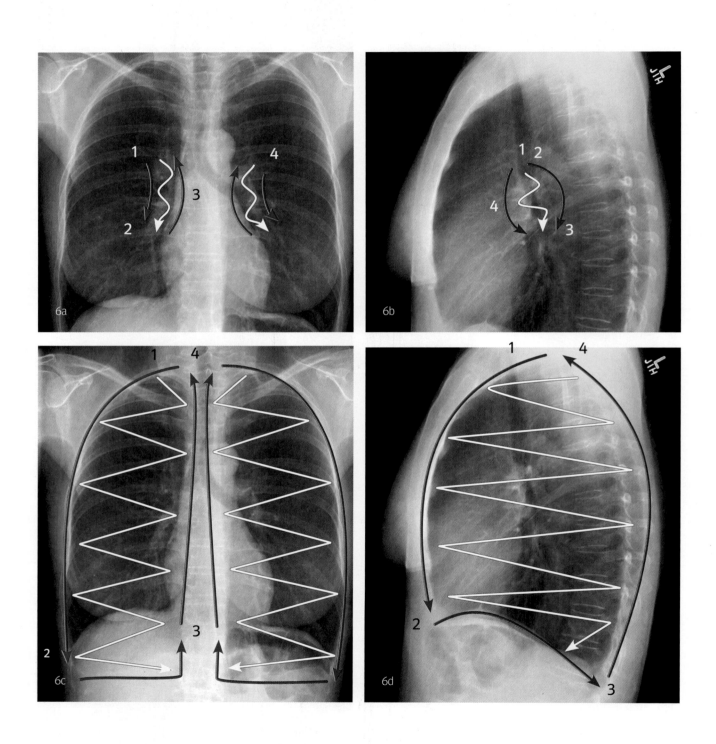

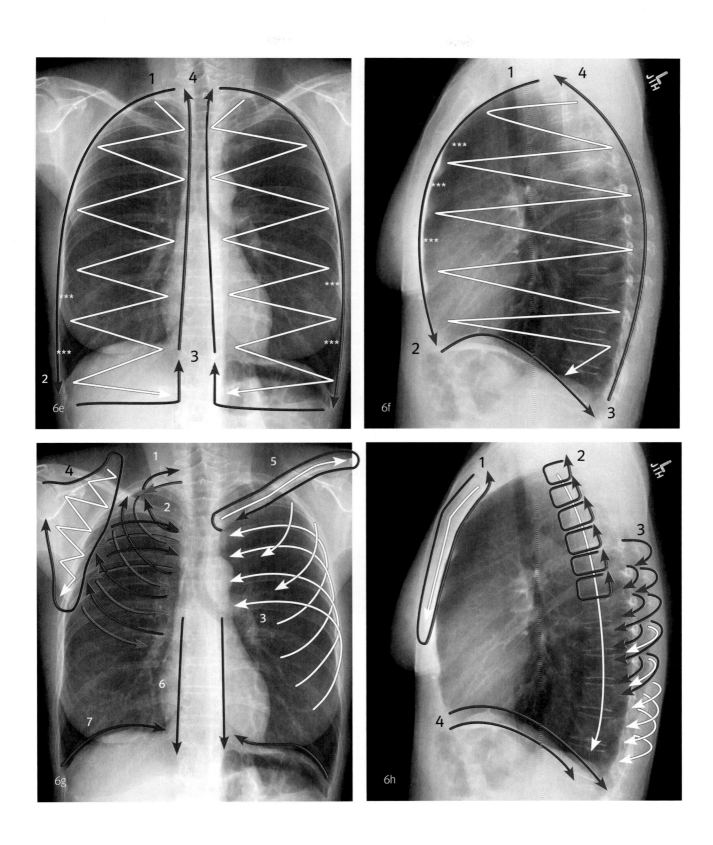

Figure 6. Visual search - PART II. Typical PA and lateral chest x-rays with the paths of the visual searches illustrated. a,b, the hilum (hilar zone), c,d, the pleura (pleural zone), e,f, the lungs and interstitium (lung zone), g,h, the chest wall and diaphragms (peripheral zone).

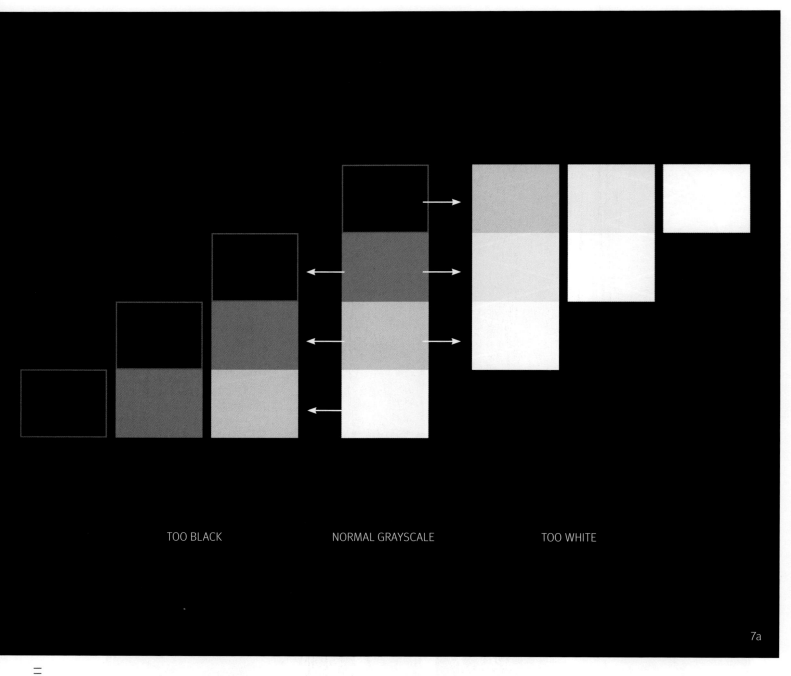

TOO BLACK   NORMAL GRAYSCALE   TOO WHITE

7a

3. Descriptive Phase

In the descriptive phase the positive and negative findings are established and named.

Most pathology can be described by how they change the grayscale (Ch. 3). The radiological findings will manifest as a shift in grayscale to too white or too black, a change in size of the structure, a shift of the grayscale shadow created by the structure, or a change in the shape of the structure's grayscale shadow (Fig. 7a,b,c,d).

How we describe the grayscale changes forms the basis for the following anatomy-specific checklists.

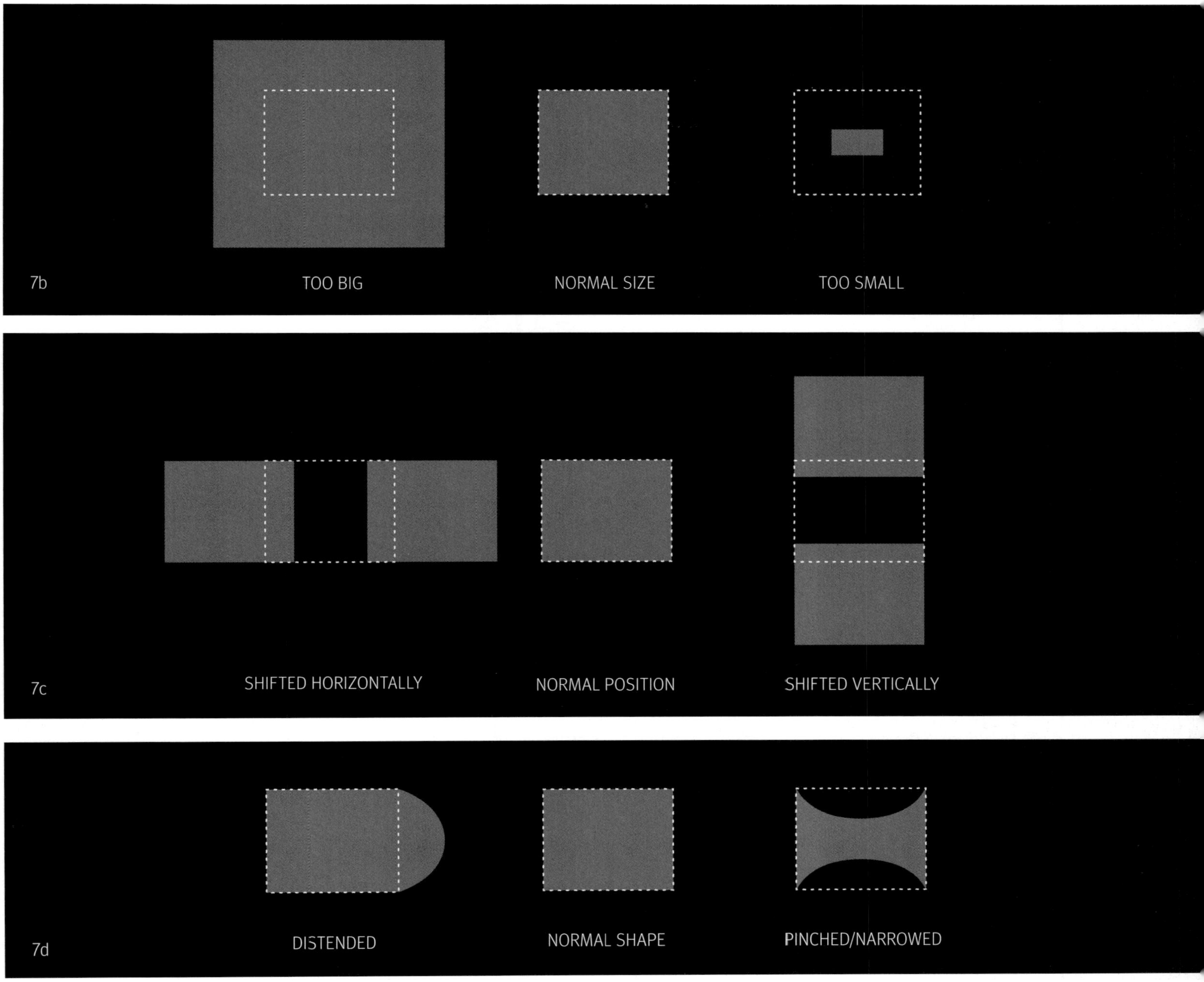

Figure 7. Changes to grayscale shadows due to pathology. a, pathology can cause the grayscale shift to "too white", or "too black", b, change in size, c, change in position, d, change in shape.

Trachea & Proximal Bronchi Radiological Analysis Checklist

To confidently state that the trachea and proximal bronchi are normal, all parts of the checklist should indicate a normal appearance.

GRAYSCALE

1   Is the grayscale of the trachea altered?

If **YES**, then describe.
Too white/too black.

POSITION

2   Is the trachea deviated?

If **YES**, then describe.
Right/left.
Anterior/posterior.

3   Is the carina angle greater than 90 degrees?

If **YES**, then describe.
Give angle measurement.

SHAPE

4   Is the shape of the trachea narrowed?

If **YES**, then describe.
Focal/diffuse.

5   Is there a visible mass deviating/ narrowing the trachea?

If **YES**, then describe.
Size/position.

OTHER

6   Are there any radiological signs related to the trachea?

If **YES**, then describe.
Air bronchogram.
Tram line.

7   Is there any evidence of previous surgery to the trachea and/or bronchi?

If **YES**, then describe.
Type of surgery and location.
Compare to previous CXR.

8   Are there any lines or tubes in the trachea?

If **YES**, then describe.
Give location of each relative to the carina.

Hilum Radiological Analysis Checklist

To confidently state that the hilum is normal all parts of the checklist should indicate a normal appearance.

GRAYSCALE

1 Is the grayscale of the hilum altered?

If **YES**, then describe.
Too white (too dense)
Right/left/bilateral.

SIZE

2 Is the size of the hilum altered?

If **YES**, then describe.
Too big/too small.
Right/left/bilateral.

POSITION

3 Is the position of the hilum shifted?

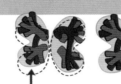

If **YES**, then describe.
Elevated/depressed.
Medial/lateral.
Anterior/posterior.
Right/left/bilateral.

SHAPE

4 Is the H-shape of the hila distorted on the PA x-ray?

If **YES**, then describe.
Lobulated/irregular.
Right/left/bilateral.

5 Are one or both of the arches distorted on the lateral x-ray?

If **YES**, then describe.
Aorta narrowed/distended.
LPA narrowed/distended.

OTHER

6 Is the AP window normal?

If **NO**, then describe.
Blurred/obscured.
Too big/too small.

7 Are there any radiological signs related to the hilum?

If **YES**, then describe.
Hilar convergence.
Hilar overlay.
H-sign.

8 Is there any evidence of previous surgery to the hilum?

If **YES**, then describe.
Type of surgery and location.
Compare to previous CXR.

Mediastinum Radiological Analysis Checklist

To confidently state that the mediastinum is normal, all parts of the checklist should indicate a normal appearance.

GRAYSCALE

1   Is the grayscale of the mediastinum altered?

If **YES**, then describe.
Too white/too black.
Pathology/lipomatosis.

SIZE

2   Is the size of the mediastinum altered?

If **YES**, then describe.
Too big.
Right/left.
Anterior/middle/posterior compartment.

SHAPE

3   Are the mediastinal contours abnormal?

If **YES**, then describe.
Right/left.
Distorted/missing/additional.

POSITION

4   Is the position of the mediastinum shifted?

If **YES**, then describe.
Right/left.
Anterior/posterior.

OTHER

5   Is the AP window normal?

If **NO**, then describe.
Blurred, obscured.
Too big/too small.

6   Are the lines and stripes normal?

If **NO**, then describe.
Too wide/irregular/missing.

7   Are there any radiological signs related to the mediastinum?

If **YES**, then describe.
123.
hilar overlay.
Iceberg.
Silhouette.

8   Is there any evidence of previous surgery to the mediastinum?

If **YES**, then describe.
Type of surgery and location.
Compare to previous CXR.

9   Are there any lines or tubes in the mediastinum?

If **YES**, then describe.
Give location of each relative to the carina and SVC.

Heart & Pericardium Radiological Analysis Checklist

To confidently state that the heart and pericardium are normal all parts of the checklist should indicate a normal appearance.

GRAYSCALE

1. Is the grayscale of the cardiopericardial silhouette altered?

If **YES**, then describe.
Too white/too black.

SIZE

2. Is the size of the cardiopericardial silhouette altered?

If **YES**, then describe.
Too big/too small.
Pathological/magnification effect/pectus excavatum.

POSITION

3. Is the position of the cardiopericardial silhouette shifted?

If **YES**, then describe.
Up/down.
Right/left.
Anterior/posterior.

SHAPE

4. Is the shape of the cardiopericardial silhouette distorted?

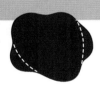

If **YES**, then describe.
Name specific contour.
Pathological/normal variant.

OTHER

5. Is there any evidence of previous surgery to the heart or pericardium?

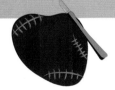

If **YES**, then describe.
Type of surgery and location.
Compare to previous CXR.

CONGESTIVE HEART FAILURE

6. Are there signs of vascular redistribution?

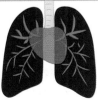

If **YES**, then describe.
Pulmonary venous hypertension/
pulmonary arterial hypertension /
shunt vascularity.

7. Are there signs of edema?

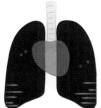

If **YES**, then describe.
Interstitial/alveolar.
Kerley A/Kerley B/cuffing.

Pleura Radiological Analysis Checklist

To confidently state that the pleura is normal, all parts of the checklist should indicate a normal appearance.

GRAYSCALE

1 Do the lungs extend all the way to the ribs?

    If **NO**, is the grayscale of the pleura altered?

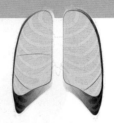

If **YES**, then describe.
Too white/too black/too white AND too black.
Right/left/bilateral.

SIZE

2 Is the size of the pleural space altered?

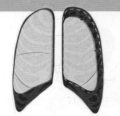
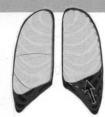

If **YES**, then describe.
Right/left/bilateral.
Give size of pneumothorax or pleural effusion.

POSITION

3 Are the fissures shifted?

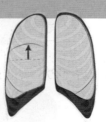

If **YES**, then describe.
Elevated/depressed.
Medial/lateral.

SHAPE

4 Is the shape of the lateral or posterior costophrenic angles altered?

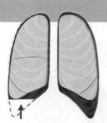
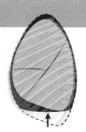

If **YES**, then describe.
Right/left/bilateral.
Blunted.

OTHER

5 Are there any radiological signs related to the pleura?

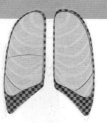

If **YES**, then describe.
Pseudotumor.
Deep sulcus.

Lung Radiological Analysis Checklist

To confidently state that the lungs are normal, all parts of the checklist should indicate a normal appearance.

rc

GRAYSCALE

1 Is the grayscale of the lungs altered?

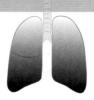

If **YES**, then describe.
Too white/too black/too white AND too black.
Right/left/bilateral.

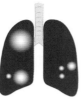

If **TOO WHITE**, then describe opacity.
Focal/diffuse.
Multiple/solitary.
Homogeneous/inhomogeneous.

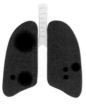

If **TOO BLACK**, then describe hyperlucency.
Focal/diffuse.
Multiple/solitary.
Pathological/mastectomy/surgery.
Homogeneous/inhomogeneous.

2 Is the normal branching of blood vessels obscured?

If **YES**, then describe.
Right/left/bilateral.

SIZE

3 Is the size of the lungs altered? (Does the blackness of the lungs extend all the way to the ribs?)

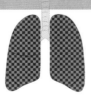

If **NO**, then describe.
Right/left/bilateral.
Increased/decreased.

OTHER

4 Are there any radiological signs related to the lungs?

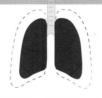

If **YES**, then describe.
Air bronchogram.
Silhouette.
Spine.

5 Is there any evidence of previous surgery to the lungs?

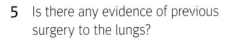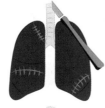

If **YES**, then describe.
Type of surgery and location.
Compare to previous CXR.

6 Are there any lines or tubes in the lungs?

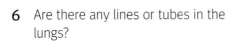

If **YES**, then describe.
Give location of each relative to the carina, SVC and/or diaphragms.

Interstitium Radiological Analysis Checklist

To confidently state that the interstitium is normal, all parts of the checklist should indicate a normal appearance.

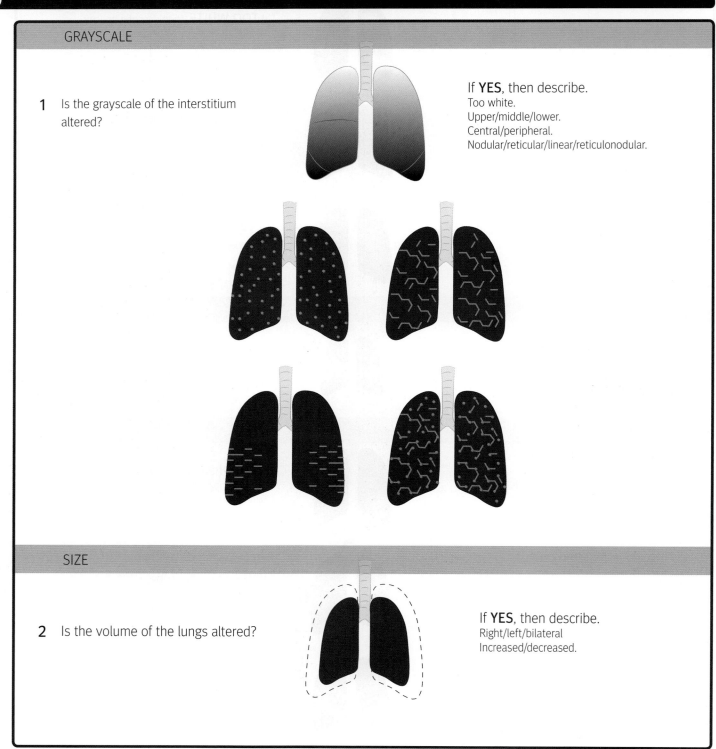

GRAYSCALE

1   Is the grayscale of the interstitium altered?

If **YES**, then describe.
Too white.
Upper/middle/lower.
Central/peripheral.
Nodular/reticular/linear/reticulonodular.

SIZE

2   Is the volume of the lungs altered?

If **YES**, then describe.
Right/left/bilateral
Increased/decreased.

Chest Wall & Diaphragms Radiological Analysis Checklist

To confidently state that the chest wall and diaphragms are normal all parts of the checklist should indicate a normal appearance.

BONY THORAX (Spine, ribs, clavicles, scapulae, sternum)

GRAYSCALE

1   Is the grayscale of the bones altered?

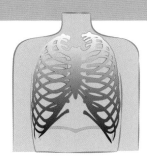

If **YES**, then describe.
Too white/too black.
Bone density.
Cortical outline.
Fractures/bone destruction.

2   Are any abnormal opacities present?

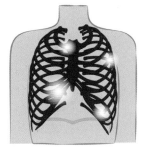

If **YES**, then describe.
Give number and location.
Focal/diffuse.

POSITION

3   Is the position of the bony thorax (ribs, spine, clavicles, sternum, scapulae) altered?

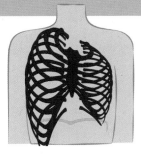

If **YES**, then describe.
Right/left.
Anterior/posterior.
Elevated/depressed.

OTHER

4   Are there any accessory ribs?

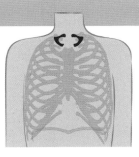

If **YES**, then describe.
Cervical/lumbar
Give number and position.

SOFT TISSUES

GRAYSCALE

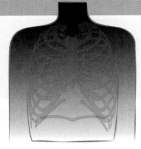

5 Is the grayscale of the soft tissues altered?

If **YES**, then describe.
Too white/too black.

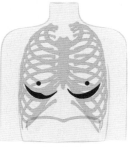

6 Are breast, pectoral folds and/or nipple shadows present?

If **YES**, then describe.
Right/left/bilateral.
If not sure, repeat CXR with nipple markers.

SIZE

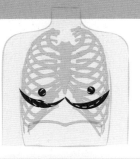

7 Is the size of the breasts altered?

If **YES**, then describe.
Right/left/bilateral
Increased/decreased.

DIAPHRAGMS

POSITION

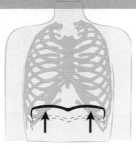

8 Is the position of the diaphragm(s) altered?

If **YES**, then describe.
Right/left/bilateral.
Elevated/depressed.

SHAPE

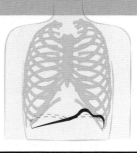

9 Is the shape of the diaphragm(s) altered?

If **YES**, then describe.
Right/left/bilateral.
Describe shape.

10 Is there a presence of bowel loops or stomach in the thoracic cavity?

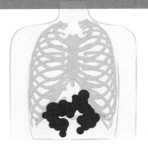

If **YES**, then describe.
Right/left.
Anterior/posterior.

11 Are there any external objects that are not part of the normal chest wall?

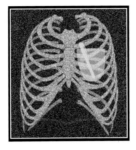

If **YES**, then describe.
ECG leads/buttons and clips on clothing/ hair bands and clips/jewellery/coins and currency in pockets.

12 Is there any evidence of previous surgery to the chest wall or diaphragms?

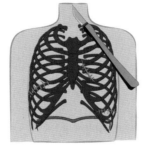

If **YES**, then describe.
Type of surgery and location.
Compare to previous CXR.

13 Are there any lines or tubes in the chest wall?

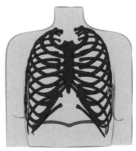

If **YES**, then describe.
Give location of each relative to the carina, SVC and/or diaphragms.

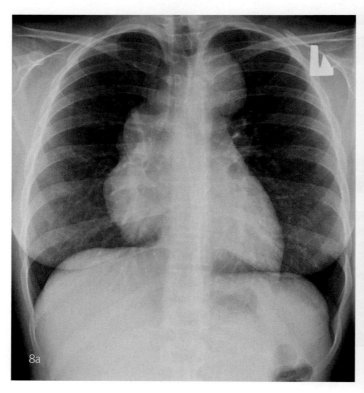

8a

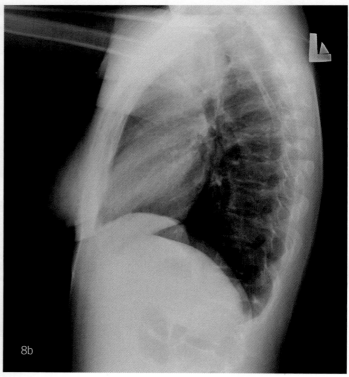

8b

4. Summary Phase

In the summary phase the radiological findings are grouped together into meaningful clusters, and summarized into brief phrases. These clusters describe the radiological pattern or sign from which the differential diagnosis list is created (Fig. 8a,b,c).

There may only be finding leading to a single component summary (e.g., anterior mediastinal tumour) or there may be multiple findings requiring a multi-component summary (e.g., anterior mediastinal tumour AND RUL pneumonia AND left pleural effusion).

The summary statement should include all relevant positive findings AND all relevant negative information.

5. Differential Diagnosis Phase

An initial radiological differential diagnosis is formulated based on the summary phase(s). Two or three of the most likely causes of the finding should be given (Fig. 8d). Any life-threatening causes should be considered first. The other causes listed should be listed in order based on how common they are. The differential diagnosis should also

be linked to the clinical findings and to previous imaging.

Air bronchograms in a patient with chest trauma will have a different significance to air bronchograms in a patient with cough, fever and a productive cough.

In the acute setting it is important to establish which of the findings are relevant and contributing to the patients clinical situation.

Establishing what is or is not relevant is easier if previous images are available. Previous x-rays and reports will give definite clues to what is chronic. This is extremely important because a radiological finding will have different significance in the acute versus the chronic setting.

In the visual phase, each of the abnormalities is identified. The descriptive phase is applied to each of the abnormalities; a summary is formulated for each of the findings.

At this point, two methods can be used to establish the differential diagnosis. One method (recommended) is to create a differential diagnosis for each finding separately and look for the common origin of the changes. The second method is to try and make a diagnosis based on pathology that can manifest with the identified findings. The risk with the second method is that two, three or even more unrelated pathologies can exist in the patient.

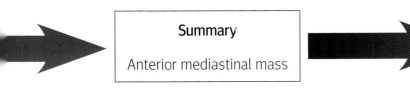

Summary

Anterior mediastinal mass

Differential diagnosis

Thymoma
Thyroid (goiter, tumor)
Teratoma
Testicular carcinoma metastases

8c   8d

Example Case

Summary

1. Left hilar mass.
2. Multiple lung nodules.

In this case, make a differential diagnosis for a left hilar mass and a second differential diagnosis for multiple lung nodules. At the very end put the two differential diagnoses together in the clinical context:

Clinical Context A: Smoker with weight loss.

Bronchogenic carcinoma with lung metastasis.

Clinical Context B: Smoker who has worked in gold mine with history of occupational lung disease.

May still be bronchogenic carcinoma with lung metastasis OR may be bronchogenic carcinoma with nodules secondary to silicosis.

6. Communication Phase (Action Phase) – now that you found it, what next?

The communication phase will vary depending on who is interpreting the x-rays.

The chest x-ray examination is ordered for specific clinical reasons – the radiological findings are part of the clinical diagnostic journey and should be treated as such.

- If it is an acute finding, then appropriate treatment should be started.
- If it is an unexpected acute finding, then immediate action should be taken.
- If you are uncertain of the findings, then seek immediate help from a radiologist.
- If the plain x-ray findings are not clear, additional tests may be required to narrow the differential diagnosis.

Figure 8. Differential diagnosis of an anterior mediastinal mass. a, PA chest x-ray from a patient with an anterior mediastinal mass, b, lateral chest x-ray from the same patient, c, summary, d, differential diagnosis.

Picture Archiving and Communication System (PACS) & Chest X-ray Interpretation

Picture Archiving and Communication System (PACS) has revolutionized access to radiological examinations and reports. PACS was introduced in the early 1990's as a computer system designed to provide aid in diagnostic image reading and data management. PACS is composed of image acquisition devices, network display devices, image servers and archives, and storage devices. PACS allows immediate access to images following completion of the examination, making early diagnosis and intervention possible. PACS are found in most larger radiology departments, and are gaining popularity in smaller community centers.

The PACS workstation (Fig. 9a)

Important findings such as a pneumothorax or malpositioned endotracheal tubes may be missed on low resolution monitors. Therefore, formal interpretation of chest x-rays is usually performed on high-resolution monitors. The minimal resolution requirement for chest x-ray interpretation is 2048 X 1536. In the Radiology Department the monitors are typically two 2K x 2K color or grayscale monitors. High-resolution monitors are also installed wherever primary interpretation of the x-rays occurs; for example, in the Emergency Department and Intensive Care Unit.

PACS provides a radiological clinical record for the patient in your institution: PACS has the radiological report attached to the examination, and may provide previous x-rays automatically for comparison. PACS allows multiple clinical staff to view the images simultaneously and give advice. Residents believe that PACS has positively affected their learning experience (3).

The viewing environment

The optimum viewing and interpretation environment has appropriate lighting and controlled noise (4). Ideally, the lighting should be indirect and subdued. Background noise should be at a minimum (this includes noise from other students, and physicians). If you are performing a primary interpretation make sure that the monitors are of adequate resolution to make a confident interpretation.

Setting up a PACS account and user preferences

It is usually hospital policy that each PACS user must have a personal login and password. These are required because of privacy concerns – with personal logins, the use of PACS can be monitored and audited by the hospital information department and by the privacy officer. A user login can usually be obtained through the diagnostic imaging department PACS coordinator after appropriate credentialing.

Your login and password information should be secure and saved in a safe place. Once you are logged in you are taking responsibility for the PACS usage. Each time you finish using the PACS workstation, log off.

The PACS coordinator can also help first time PACS users to setup personal preferences for image viewing. If you do not know which presets to select, do not worry, the PACS software has presets to start you on your interpretive journey the first time you login.

Using PACS to aid in interpretation

After you have successfully logged into PACS, you will need to do the following.

Identifying the patient

Patients can be identified in the PACS database by entering the patient name, the patient hospital identification number, or the radiology check-in number specific for the examination that was ordered.

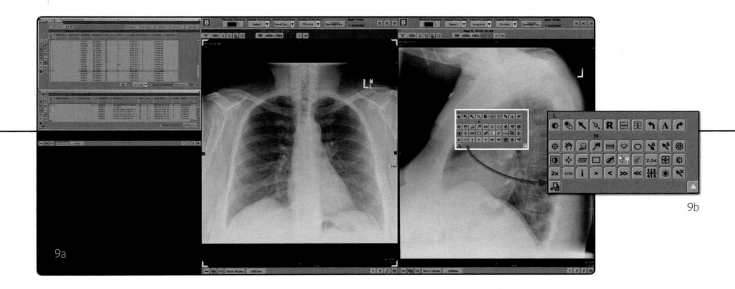

9a

9b

Identifying the relevant examination

Once you have identified the correct patient, PACS will list all of the examinations on that patient that are found in PACS. When you select the examination you wish to view, the chest x-ray images will show on the monitors. If you are on a two monitor viewing station two images will appear. If you are on a one monitor station only one image will appear.

Identifying relevant previous examination(s)

Depending on how the system is configured, the most recent relevant examination(s) should also appear. On a two monitor system the two examinations will appear side by side and are ready for comparison. On a one monitor system you will need to toggle between the two examinations.

On PACS there is usually a pull down menu option that will allow you to select which examination you choose to compare to the current examination. It is sometimes very valuable to review several previous examinations to identify subtle disease progression.

Setting the viewing screens

On a two monitor system, set up the examinations so that the two PA images are side by side. Do the same for the lateral images. Make sure that the image brightness is adequate.

Examining the images in detail

You are now ready to start the interpretive process as outlined in this book. Use the PACS tools to help you with the interpretation process.

Reviewing the examination reports

The radiology report attached to the examination is an important component to patient care. Use the report as a learning tool to verify the findings that you have made.

Viewing tools

PACS has various tools that allow for augmented image assessment (Fig. 9b). There are various PACS vendors, and each PACS system has some variability in functionality but most have similar viewing tools.

Some of the more commonly used tools on the PACS are the following:

Magnification

Usually two types: one being the magnifying glass that allows for focused magnification; the second is general magnification of the image.

Value: Allows focusing vision on certain structures.

Video invert

Changes grayscale so black becomes white and white becomes black.

Value: Highlights bones.

Window and level

This feature allows the user to control grayscale levels displayed on the monitor.

Value: Allows adjustment of image to highlight pathology.

Reset

After changing the window levels, you may want to revert back to the initial image appearance. There is usually a reset button that does just that. This is usually done automatically after you close the examination.

Figure 9. PACS. a, PACS three monitor system, b, PACS tools.

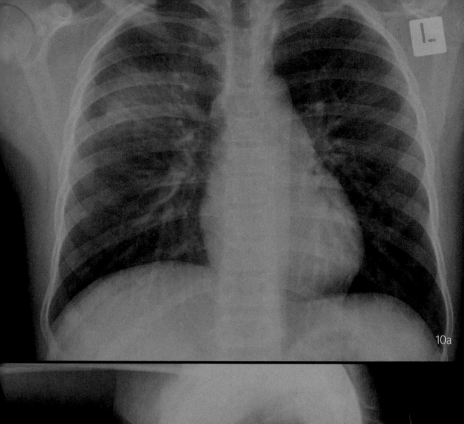

10a

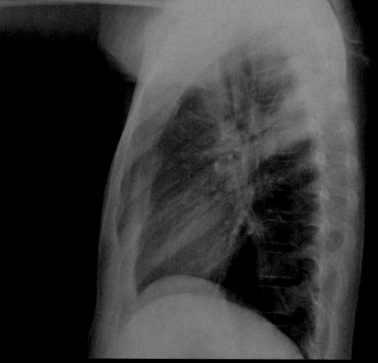

10b

How would you present the PA and lateral chest x-ray findings?

You are working on-call overnight as an intern in the emergency department. At morning rounds you are asked to interpret the chest x-rays (Fig. 10a,b) of a patient you saw during the night. The patient is a 44-year-old non-immunocompromised male with a history of productive cough, fever and elevated white blood cell count (WBC).

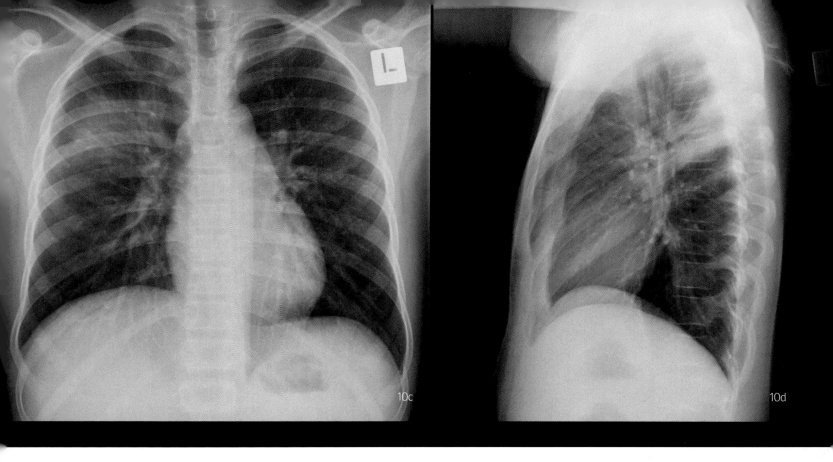

10c

10d

Presenting the Clinical Case at Rounds

"I am presented with PA and lateral chest x-rays (Fig. 10c,d) of a 44-year-old male patient with a history of productive cough, fever and elevated white blood cell count (WBC). A previous chest x-ray examination dated .... is available for comparison."
"The examination is of good technical quality."

Preparatory phase

"The examination is abnormal. On both images an area of too white is identified within the upper right hemithorax. The abnormality is localized to the right upper lobe. Air bronchograms are identified consistent with airspace disease. There is no associated calcification or cavitation. The remaining lung fields are clear. There is normal pulmonary vasculature."
"The pleural, mediastinal, hilar and chest wall regions are normal. No cardiac abnormalities."

Visual and descriptive phase

"In summary, there is evidence of airspace disease in the RUL of the lung."

Summary phase

"The differential diagnosis of air space disease includes: fluid within the airspaces, infection, and hemorrhage, or less commonly, tumor. Because of the patient's clinical symptoms the most likely diagnosis is RUL pneumonia."

Differential diagnosis phase

"Repeat chest x-ray examination only if no clinical improvement following appropriate antibiotic treatment."

Communication phase

DISCUSSION

643

References

1. Lewis, P.J., Shaffer, K., & Donovan, A. (Eds.). (2012). AMSER National Medical Student Curriculum in Radiology. http://aur.org/Secondary-Alliances.aspx?id=141.

2. Lewis, P.J., & Shaffer, K. (2005). Developing a national medical student curriculum in radiology. *Am. Coll. Radiol.* 2(1):8–11.

3. Mullins, M.E., Mehta, A., Patel, H., et al. (2001). Impact of PACS on the education of radiology residents. *Acad. Radiol.* 8:67–73

4. Krupinski, E.A. (2006). Technology and perception in the 21st-century reading room. *J. Am. Coll. Radiol. JACR.* 3(6):433–440.

CHAPTER 17
LOCALIZATION of DISEASE in the THORAX

importance

In the previous chapters, you learned how to discriminate normal and abnormal structures on the chest x-ray. Now we will look at how to localize the abnormal findings within the thorax. The accurate localization of pathology is an important step in establishing a differential diagnosis and for communicating your findings to the patient and other members of the healthcare team. This chapter will teach you several useful methods to correctly localize pathology within the thorax on a chest x-ray, particularly within the lungs.

objectives

Skills

You will identify

- the landmarks used in the grid method.
- the lobes (and segments) of the lungs, using the grid method.

You will localize

- normal and abnormal findings within the thorax, both within the lungs and other structures, on the PA and lateral chest x-rays.

Knowledge

You will review and understand

- the three localization methods and how to apply these to both the PA and lateral chest x-rays.

- the important radiological signs that can help with the localization of pathology.

associated resources

This chapter maps to the following AMSER curriculum content (1,2).

1) Lungs
   Right upper lobe (RUL)
   Right lower lobe (RLL)
   Right middle lobe (RML)
   Left upper lobe (LUL)
   Left lower lobe (LLL)

2) Minor and major fissures

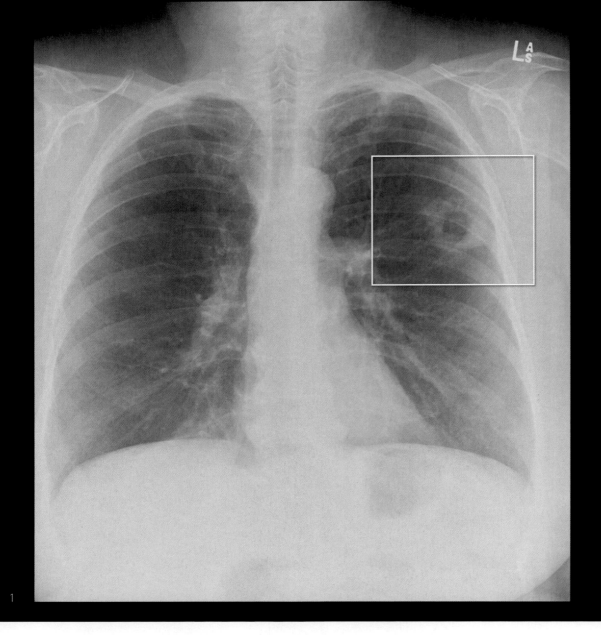

1

CASE STUDY

This PA chest x-ray shows a lesion in the left hemithorax (Fig. 1).

How would you determine the exact anatomical origin of the lesion?

List the potential anatomical locations from which this lesion could be originating.

LOCALIZATION OF DISEASE IN THE THORAX

Two of the key ingredients to successful interpretation of the chest x-ray examination are the discrimination between normal and abnormal, and the correct localization of the identified abnormality. The process of localizing pathology can be difficult on a chest x-ray because of the overlap of anatomical structures (discussed in Chapter 2).

Figure 2 illustrates a chest lesion that appears within the mid-right thorax on the PA x-ray. What are the possible locations of the lesion from the PA x-ray alone? As you have already learned, an x-ray is all-inclusive in that it includes overlapping information from all structures along the PA axis. Therefore, the lesion could lie anywhere from the front of the thorax to the back. The potential structures to consider for localization are: the anterior chest wall, the anterior pleura, the mediastinum, the hilum, the lung, the posterior pleura, the posterior chest wall and artifacts.

So how do we establish the location of the lesion?

Three methods to facilitate the localization of thoracic pathology are described in this chapter. These three methods are all based on the process of elimination, and include: the possibility method, the characterization method, and the grid method.

1. The Possibility Method

The first method is called the possibility method. In our illustrative case (Fig. 2a), we have already established that from the PA x-ray alone, the possibilities include the anterior chest wall, anterior pleura, lung, posterior pleura, and posterior chest wall, as well as artifacts outside of the patient. The lateral chest wall, lateral pleura, mediastinum, hila and diaphragms can be eliminated. To further narrow down the possibilities, the lateral chest x-ray is required.

If on the lateral chest x-ray (Fig. 2b) the opacity lies centrally, then the anterior chest wall, the anterior pleura,

the posterior pleura and the posterior chest wall can be eliminated. Therefore the opacity, through the process of elimination, lies within the lung.

In a second illustrative case, the lesion on the PA x-ray (Fig. 3a) lies in the mid-right hemithorax, but more medially. In this case, the possibilities from the PA x-ray include the anterior chest wall, the anterior pleura, the mediastinum, the right hilum, the lung, the posterior pleura, and the posterior chest wall, as well as artifacts outside of the patient.

If on the lateral chest x-ray (Fig. 3b) the opacity lies anteriorly – and can clearly be seen as separate from the anterior chest wall and anterior pleura – then the anterior chest wall, anterior pleura, right hilum, posterior pleura and posterior chest wall can be eliminated. Therefore, the opacity, through the process of elimination, lies either within the anterior mediastinum or within the lung.

Summary of the possibility method:

- Establish the possible locations from the PA x-ray.
- Narrow down the possibilities from the lateral x-ray.

On many chest x-rays, the localization process is completed with this method. However, if after using this method the localization is still uncertain, proceed to the next method.

Figure 2. The possibility method - Case 1. a, PA chest x-ray with a spherical lesion overlying the right hemithorax. From the PA x-ray alone we can conclude the lesion lies in the right hemithorax, but we do not know how far anterior or posterior the lesion lies. b, lateral chest x-ray with a spherical lesion overlying the mid thorax. Using the lateral x-ray, we can see that the lesion lies centrally, and we can eliminate the anterior and posterior compartments of the thorax. Together with the PA x-ray, we can determine the lesion lies within the right lung

Figure 3. The possibility method - Case 2. a, PA chest x-ray with a spherical lesion overlying the right hemithorax, medially. From the PA x-ray alone we can only conclude that it lies in the right hemithorax. b, lateral chest x-ray with a spherical lesion overlying the anterior thorax. Using the lateral x-ray we can see that the lesion lies anteriorly, yet posterior to the chest wall, and we can eliminate the most anterior and the posterior structures of the thorax. Together with the PA x-ray, we can determine that the lesion lies within the right anterior mediastinum or anterior right lung.

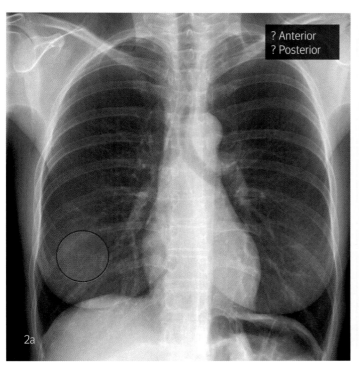

? Anterior
? Posterior

2a

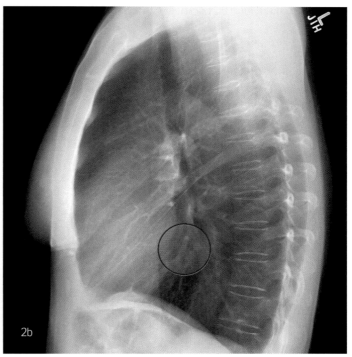

2b

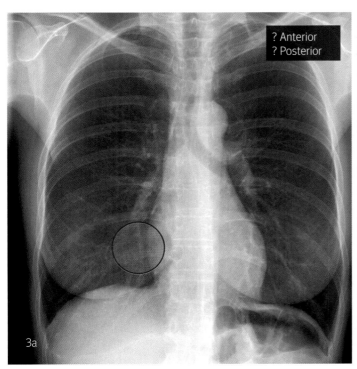

? Anterior
? Posterior

3a

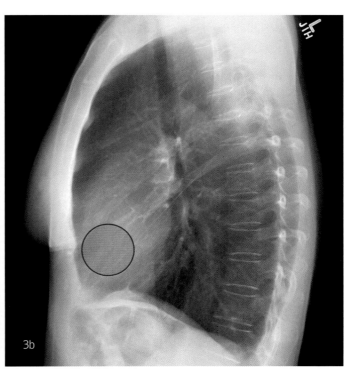

3b

2. The Characterization Method

Once we have narrowed down the localization using the possibility method, you can pinpoint the pathology further, based on the appearance of the abnormality. This is called the characterization method.

The characteristics of lesions that aid in their localization are summarized below. For information on the imaging characteristics of pathology that involve specific anatomical structures, see the associated chapter in Section II.

If the lesion is associated with bone destruction, the lung and pleura can be eliminated, and the lesion localized to the chest wall (Ch. 14).

If the lesion has a border that is not clearly outlined, then the lesion probably originates from the pleura or chest wall (Ch. 11, Ch.14) (3,4).

If there is a clean outline of the lesion, and all of the borders are visible, the lesion probably originates from the lung (Ch. 12).

The effect the lesion has on neighboring structures (i.e., mass effect) can also give a clue to the origin of the lesion. For example, a mass deviating the trachea probably originated from the mediastinum (Fig. 4a,b).

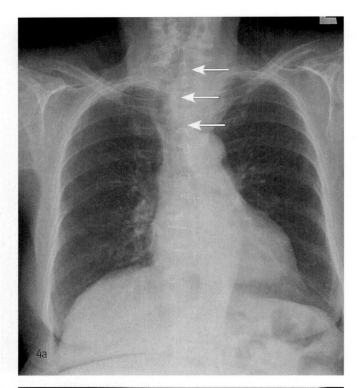

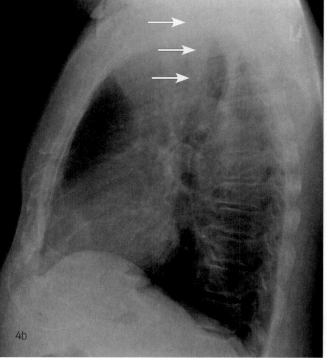

Figure 4. The characterization method. The effect the lesion has on other structures, or the mass effect, is part of the characterization method that can be used to localize a lesion. a, PA chest x-ray with a deviated trachea (arrows) due to a mass in the mediastinum, b, lateral chest x-ray in which the trachea (arrows) is displaced posteriorly by an anterior mediastinal mass.

If the lung pathology extends to a fissure, a straight edge will be visible. The position of the opacity relative to the fissure can be used for localization (Fig. 5a,b).

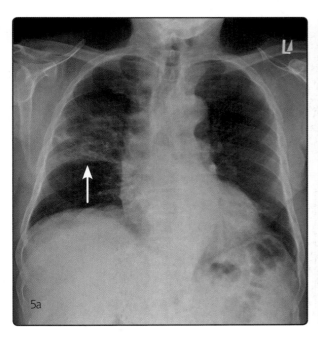
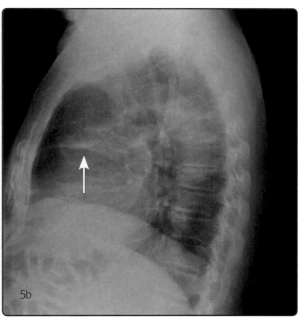

5a

5b

Figure 5. Localization of lung pathology using the fissures. The position of an opacity relative to a fissure can be used to localize lung pathology. a, PA chest x-ray with consolidation of the right lung that abuts the horizontal fissure (arrow) and forms a straight edge, b, lateral chest x-ray from the same patient, showing a similar pattern (arrow).

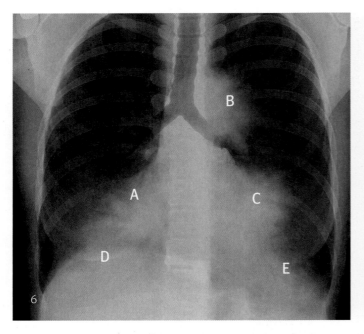

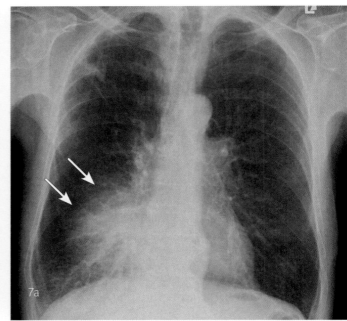

STRUCTURE OBLITERATED	LOCATION OF LUNG PATHOLOGY
(A) Right heart border	Anterior segment RUL or RML
(B) Left border or aortic knob	Apicoposterior segment of LUL
(C) Left heart border	Lingula of LUL
(D) Right hemidiaphragm	RLL
(E) Left hemidiaphragm	LLL

Table 17.1
Using the Silhouette Sign to Localize Pathology to the Lung Lobes and Segments

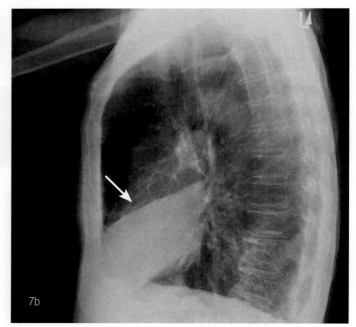

The silhouette sign will appear when an intrathoracic lesion touches a border of an adjacent anatomical structure, and the normally clearly defined border is obliterated (Fig. 6).

When the lesion is within a lung segment or lobe, the silhouette sign helps localize to that segment or lobe (Fig. 7a,b).

Large lesions that occupy a significant portion of the thorax present a specific challenge in localization. In these cases, find the epicenter of the abnormality – the location of the epicenter will usually define the origin of the abnormality (Fig. 8a,b,c,d).

Figure 6. The silhouette sign is used to localize pathology. The silhouette sign can be used to localize pathology to the lobes of the lungs. PA chest x-ray highlighting the five potential structures that, if obliterated, could signify lung pathology as listed in Table 17.1.

Figure 7. The silhouette sign. a, PA chest x-ray with a mass in the right middle lobe (arrows) that is abutting and obscuring the right heart border, b, lateral chest x-ray from the same patient; right middle lobe involvement is confirmed (arrow).

654

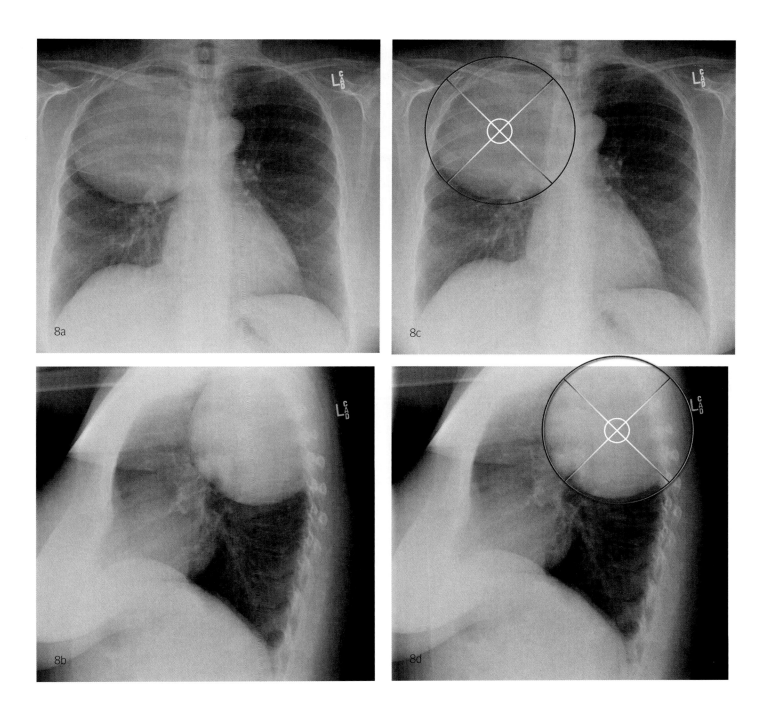

3. Grid Method

The third method for localization, called the grid method, is a modification of the possibility method. In this method, you use grid lines to localize pathology.

In the following section, the use of this method, as applied to localizing pathology within the lobes of the lungs, is described in detail. The localization of pathology within components of the mediastinum is described in Chapter 9. The localization of pathology to the hilar zone is described in Chapter 8.

Figure 8. Large lesions pose a challenge for localizing pathology. If you localize the epicenter of the abnormality, you will usually be correct in naming that as the anatomical zone of origin. a, PA chest x-ray with a large mass in the right upper hemithorax, b, lateral chest x-ray from the same patient, with a large mass in the upper hemithorax posteriorly, c, PA chest x-ray with the location of the epicenter highlighted; the epicenter of the mass overlies the right lung, d, lateral chest x-ray with the epicenter highlighted; the mass overlies the lungs.

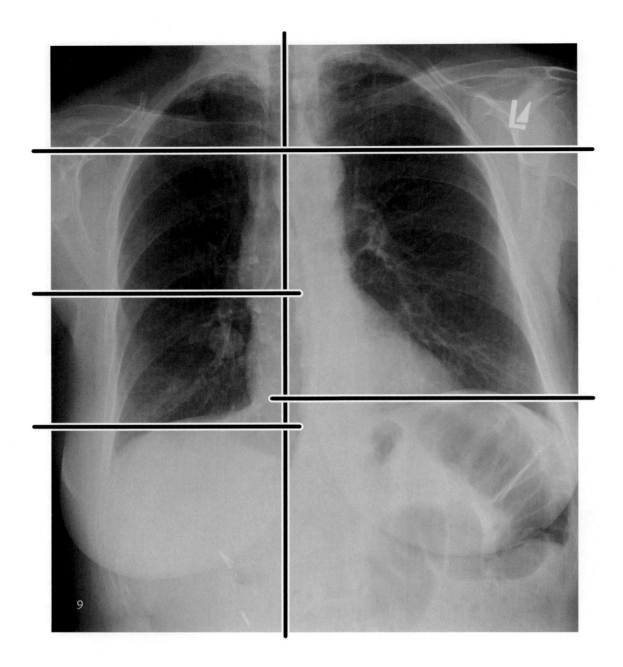

9

LOCALIZING DISEASE TO THE LOBES OF THE LUNGS - THE GRID METHOD

AMSER Pathology can occur in any of the lobes of the lungs. In the right lung, pathology may exist in the right upper lobe (RUL), right middle lobe (RML) or right lower lobe (RLL). In the left lung, there are only two possibilities: the left upper lobe (LUL) or left lower lobe (LLL).

Pathology can be localized to specific lobes of the lungs using the grid method (Fig. 9) and the process of elimination. A series of horizontal and vertical lines are superimposed on the x-ray x-rays to divide the lungs into regions that roughly correspond to the lobes of the lungs.

We first use the PA x-ray to start the localization process – eliminating those lobes in which the pathology cannot exist. Then we use the lateral x-ray to confirm and/or further localize the pathology – by continuing to eliminate non-possibilities until only one lobe remains.

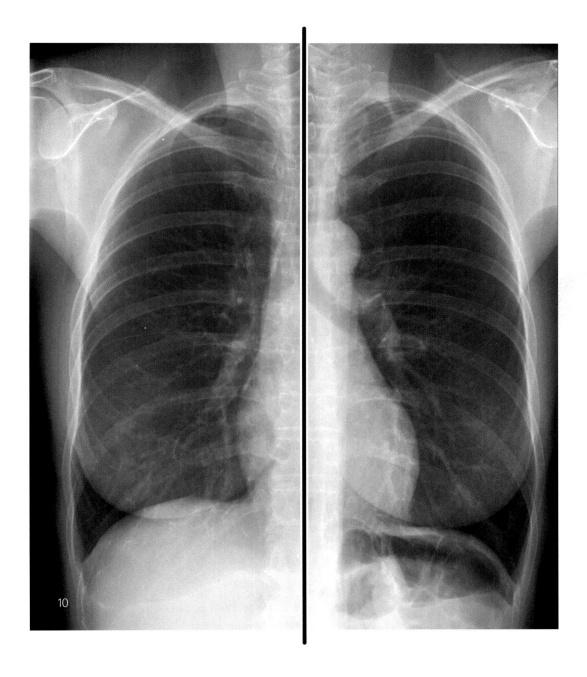

Grid Lines on the PA X-ray

Vertical grid line

On the PA chest x-ray, there is one vertical grid line that runs in the center of the PA x-ray, in the craniocaudal direction, vertically, parallel to the long axis of the spine (Fig. 10).

Figure 9. The grid method. In the grid method a series of defined lines are used to localize a lesion. PA chest x-ray with all of the grid lines used in the grid method.

Figure 10. The vertical grid line on the PA chest x-ray. On the PA chest x-ray one vertical grid line is used; it is drawn in the midline. PA chest x-ray highlighting the position of the vertical grid line.

Horizontal grid lines

On the PA x-ray, each lung has a different number of horizontal grid lines reflecting their unique anatomy (Fig. 13a,b).

The right lung

AMSER In the right lung, there are three horizontal grid lines (Fig. 11a) – the three lines are positioned to align with the anatomy of the fissures.

The most superior of the three lines (upper horizontal grid line) is drawn at the level of the top of the aortic arch (A). This line corresponds to the superior tip of the oblique fissure, and defines the border between the posterior superior aspect of the RLL below and the RUL above.

The second line (middle horizontal grid line), lies at the level of the horizontal fissure (B). The middle horizontal grid line overlies the horizontal fissure on the PA x-ray, and defines the border between the RUL above and the RML below.

The third and lowest horizontal line (lower horizontal grid line), lies at the level of the top of the right hemidiaphragm (C). This line corresponds to the inferior tip of the oblique fissure. The oblique fissure is not visible on the PA chest x-ray, but we know that, anatomically, the inferior anterior limit of the oblique fissure lies approximately at the level of the top of the diaphragms. The lower horizontal grid line defines the border between the RML above and the RLL below.

The left lung

AMSER On the left, there are only two horizontal grid lines. As on the right, the most superior of the two lines (upper horizontal grid line) lies at the level of the top of the aortic arch (D). However, on the left, there is only one fissure (the oblique fissure – there is no minor fissure) and therefore, only one additional grid line is necessary to localize pathology (Fig. 11b).

The second horizontal line lies at the level of the top of the left hemidiaphragm (lower horizontal grid line) and corresponds to the inferior tip of the oblique fissure (E).

Figure 11. The horizontal grid lines on the PA chest x-ray. There are 5 horizontal grid lines on the PA chest x-ray, three on the right lung, and two on the left. a, right side of the PA chest x-ray highlighting the position of the right lung horizontal grid lines, b, left side of the PA chest x-ray highlighting the position of the left lung horizontal grid lines.

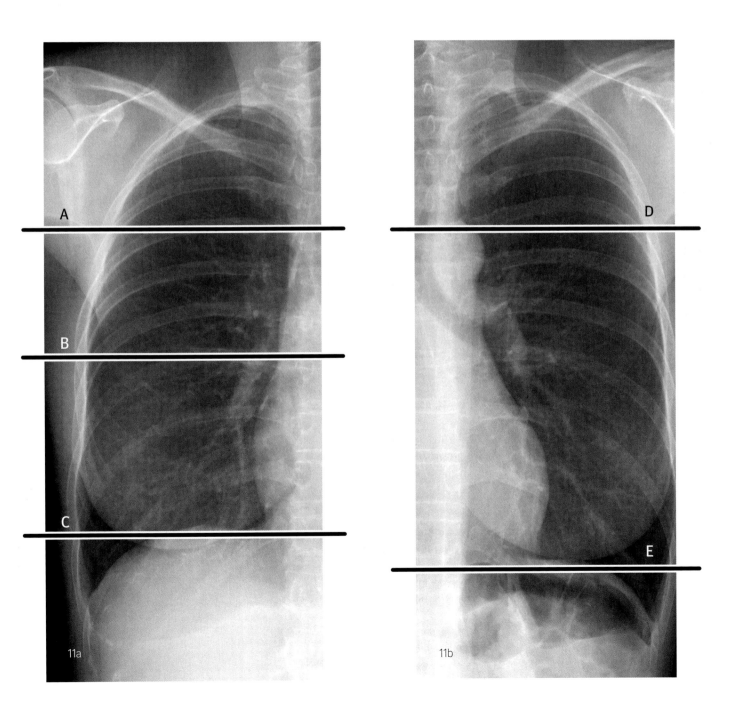

11a

11b

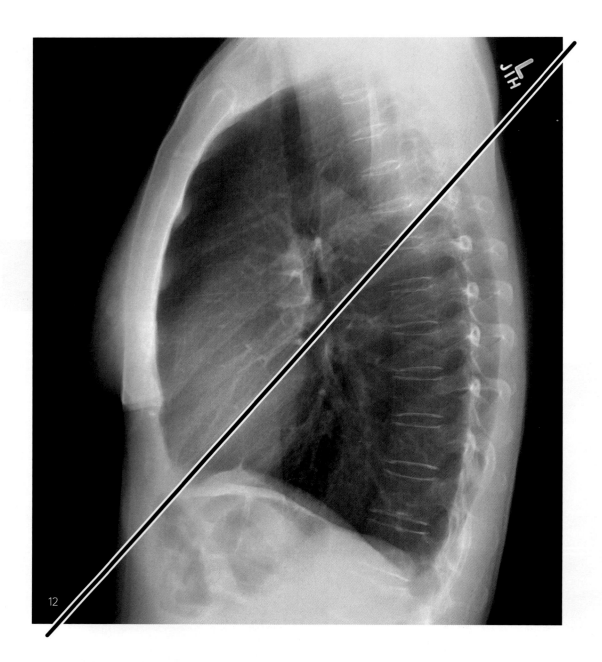

12

AMSER   Grid Lines on the Lateral X-ray:

Oblique grid line

On the lateral x-ray the "vertical" grid line runs in an oblique orientation, corresponding to the oblique fissures – the oblique grid line (Fig. 12). The right and left oblique fissures course almost identically, on the lateral chest x-ray and therefore, this grid line runs along the course of both left and right oblique fissures. The oblique grid line defines the border between lobes on both the left and the right lungs.

Within the right lung, the oblique grid line defines the border between the RUL and the RML anteriorly and the RLL posteriorly.

On the left lung the oblique grid line defines the border between the LUL anteriorly, and the LLL posteriorly.

Figure 12. The Oblique grid line on the lateral chest x-ray. On the lateral chest x-ray one oblique grid line is used. Lateral chest x-ray highlighting the position of the oblique grid line.

Figure 13. The horizontal grid line on the lateral chest x-ray. On the lateral chest x-ray one horizontal grid line is used, and is only relevant for localizing pathology in the right lung. Lateral chest x-ray highlighting the position of the oblique grid line and horizontal grid line.

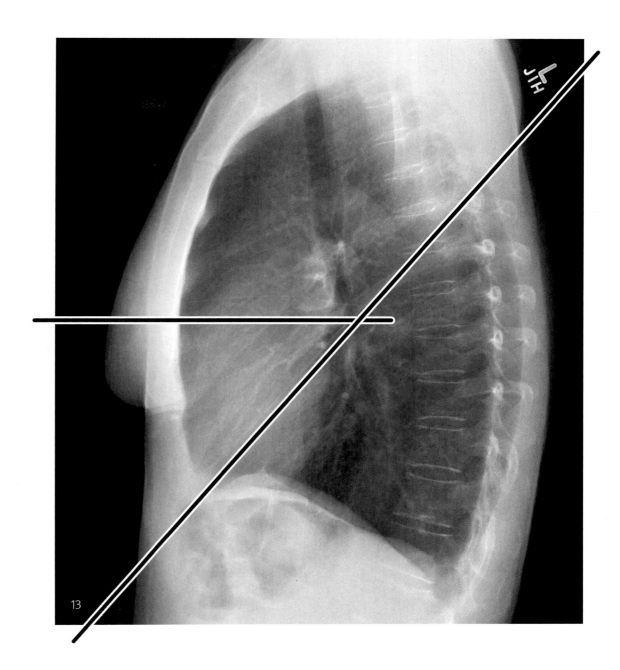

13

Lateral horizontal grid line

On the lateral x-ray, there is only one useful horizontal grid line used to define the lobes. This horizontal grid line is positioned at the level of the horizontal fissure on the right lung (lateral horizontal grid line) (Fig. 13). This line defines the border between the RML below and the RUL above. Note that the horizontal grid line on the lateral x-ray is short and terminates posteriorly at the oblique fissure (oblique grid line). This grid line is only relevant for localizing pathology to the right lung.

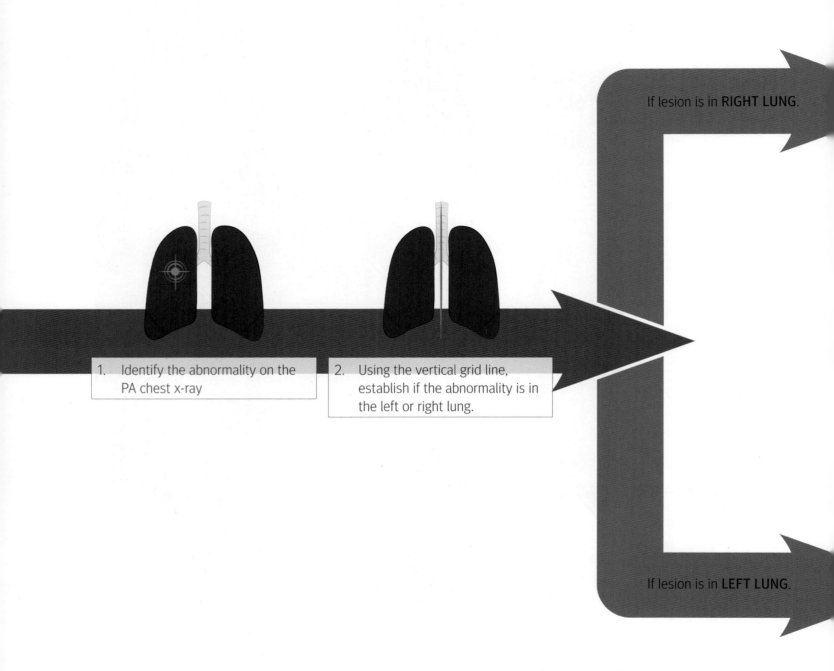

1. Identify the abnormality on the PA chest x-ray

2. Using the vertical grid line, establish if the abnormality is in the left or right lung.

If lesion is in **RIGHT LUNG**.

If lesion is in **LEFT LUNG**.

How to use the grid method to localize pathology in the lungs

When you first identify pathology on the PA x-ray, localize it to the left or the right lung. Then, using the horizontal grid lines on the PA x-ray, determine in which lobes the pathology may reside, and eliminate the lobes in which the pathology cannot exist. When the location of the abnormality is pinpointed as far as possible using the PA x-ray, the lateral x-ray is then used to make the final determination or confirmation.

?

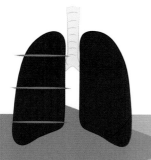
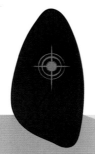
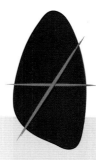

3. Using the horizontal grid lines, establish if the abnormality is:
- In the apical region (apex), above the upper horizontal grid line,
- Above the minor fissure (middle horizontal grid line),
- Between the minor fissure and diaphragm,
- Below the diaphragm (lower horizontal grid line).

If in the **APEX, STOP**.
The lesion is in the **RUL**.

If **BELOW THE DIAPHRAGM, STOP**. The lesion is in the **RLL**.

4. If the abnormality is below the apex and above the diaphragm, identify the abnormality on the lateral chest x-ray.

5. Using the lateral chest x-ray and the oblique grid line, establish if the abnormality is:
- In front of the oblique fissure,
- Behind the oblique fissure.

If the lesion is in **FRONT OF THE OBLIQUE FISSURE**, it is in the **RML**.

If the lesion is **BEHIND THE OBLIQUE FISSURE**, it is in the **RLL**.

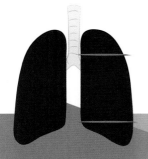
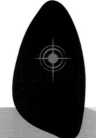
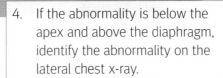
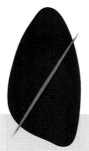

3. Using the horizontal grid lines, establish if the abnormality is:
- In the apical region (apex), above the upper horizontal grid line,
- Above the diaphragm and below the upper horizontal grid line,
- Below the diaphragm (lower horizontal grid line).

If the lesion is **ABOVE THE UPPER GRID LINE, STOP**.
It is in the **LUL**.

If the lesion is **BELOW THE DIAPHRAGM, STOP**.
It is in the **LLL**.

4. If the abnormality is below the apex and above the diaphragm, identify the abnormality on the lateral chest x-ray.

5. Using the lateral chest x-ray and the oblique grid line, establish if the abnormality is:
- In front of the oblique fissure,
- Behind the oblique fissure.

If the lesion is in **FRONT OF THE OBLIQUE FISSURE**, it is in the **LUL**.

If the lesion is **BEHIND THE OBLIQUE FISSURE**, it is in the **LLL**.

USING THE GRID METHOD TO LOCALIZE PATHOLOGY IN THE LUNGS

The following section presents some example scenarios of lung pathology localized to the right and left lungs.

AMSER Pathology in the right lung

If, on the PA x-ray, the pathology is noted to be to the right of the vertical grid line, the left lung can, therefore, be eliminated and the pathology is located at some position in the right lung. The horizontal grid lines are used to further localize the abnormality.

Scenario 1: If the lesion lies above the level of the aortic arch (upper horizontal grid line) (Fig. 14), the RLL and RML can be eliminated and the lesion localized to the RUL, even without the lateral x-ray. The lateral x-ray is used to confirm the localization.

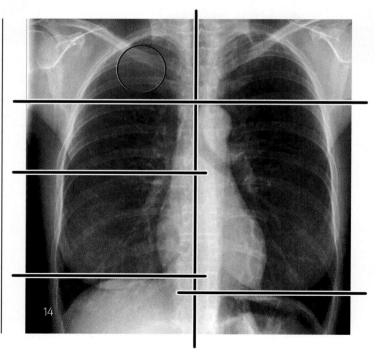

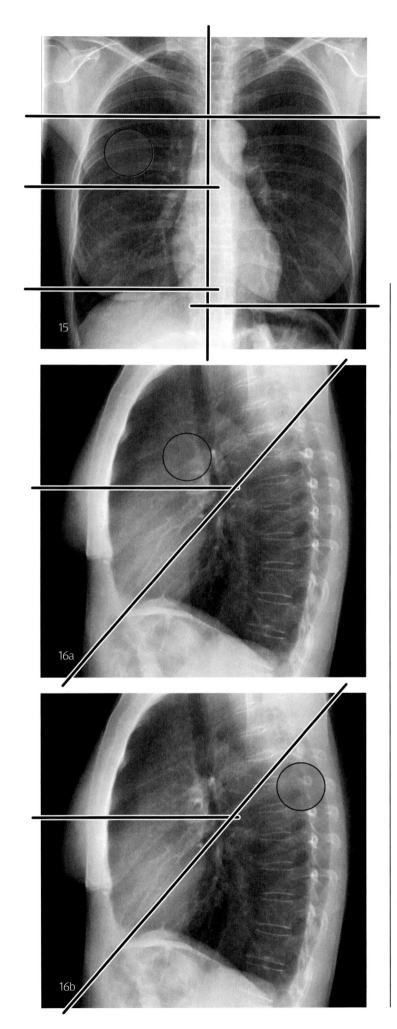

Scenario 2: If the lesion is identified within the right lung, above the minor fissure (middle horizontal grid line), but below the upper horizontal line, then the RML can be eliminated (Fig. 15). Two possibilities remain; RUL and RLL.

If, on the lateral x-ray, the lesion lies anterior to the oblique fissure (right oblique grid line) (Fig. 16a), the RLL can be eliminated and the lesion is localized to the RUL.

If, on the lateral x-ray, the lesion lies posterior to the oblique fissure (oblique grid line) (Fig. 16b), the RUL can be eliminated and the lesion localized to the RLL.

Scenario 3: If the lesion is identified within the right lung, below the minor fissure (middle horizontal grid line) and above the right hemidiaphragm (lower horizontal grid line) (Fig. 17), the RUL can be eliminated. Two possibilities remain; the RML and RLL.

If, on the lateral x-ray, the lesion lies anterior to the oblique fissure (oblique grid line) (Fig. 18a), the RLL can be eliminated and the lesion localized to the RML.

If, on the lateral x-ray, the lesion lies posterior to the oblique fissure (oblique grid line) (Fig. 18b), the RML can be eliminated and the lesion localized to the RLL.

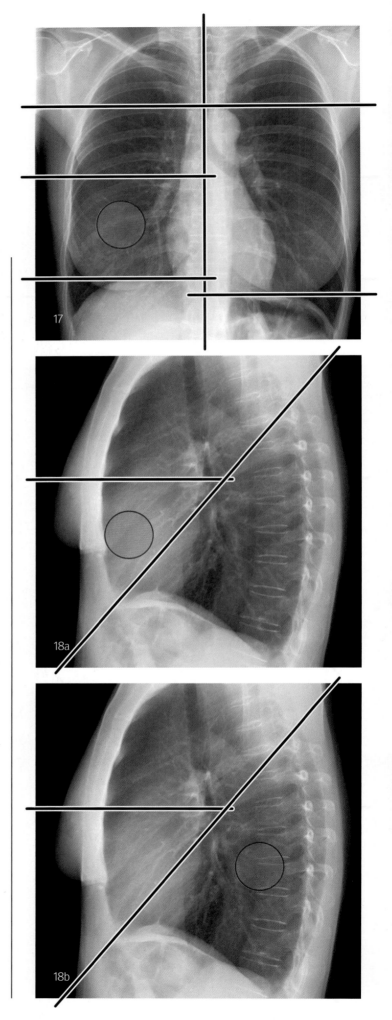

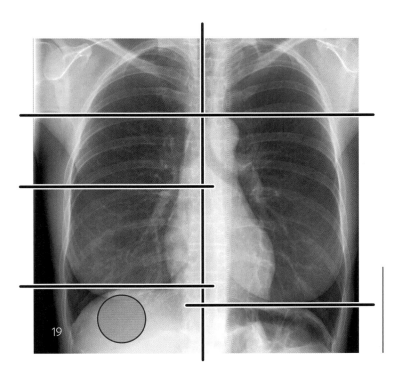

Scenario 4: If the lesion lies below the level of the top of the right hemi diaphragm (lower horizontal grid line) (Fig. 19), the RUL and RML can be eliminated and the lesion localized to the RLL, even without the lateral x-ray. The lateral x-ray is used to confirm the localization.

AMSER Pathology in left lung

If, on the PA x-ray, the pathology is noted to be to the left of the vertical grid line, the right lung can be eliminated and the pathology is located at some position in the left lung. The horizontal grid lines are used to further localize the abnormality.

Scenario 1: If, on the PA x-ray, the lesion lies above the upper horizontal grid line, the lesion can only lie within the LUL (Fig. 20). The lateral x-ray is used to confirm the localization.

Scenario 2: If, on the PA x-ray the lesion lies below the lower horizontal grid line, the LUL can be eliminated and the lesion localized to the LLL (Fig. 21). The lateral x-ray is used to confirm the localization.

Scenario 3: If, on the PA x-ray, the lesion lies below the upper horizontal grid line and above the lower horizontal grid line (Fig. 22), the lesion can lie within either the LLL or the LUL. Neither lobe is eliminated. The lateral x-ray is necessary for localization.

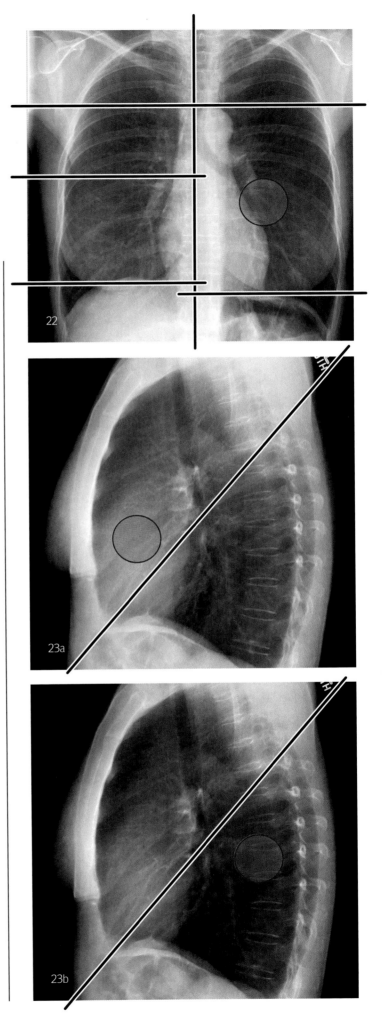

If, on the lateral x-ray, the lesion lies anterior to the oblique fissure (left oblique grid line) (Fig. 23a), the LLL can be eliminated and the lesion localized to the LUL.

If, however, on the lateral x-ray, the lesion lies posterior to the oblique fissure (left oblique grid line) (Fig. 23b), the LUL can be eliminated and the lesion localized to the LLL.

669

Using the Possibilities Method to Localize Disease to the Lung Segments

After accurately localizing pathology to a lung lobe, it is then possible to localize the pathology to individual segments. The two lungs differ in total number of segments, as they do with number of lobes. There are ten lung segments on the right and eight lung segments on the left. For more information on lung segments, review the discussion in Chapter 12, Page 446.

The lungs are not geometrical structures and, as such, there are variations in size of the segments (6).

The following, therefore, only serves as a general guide to localization to individual segments.

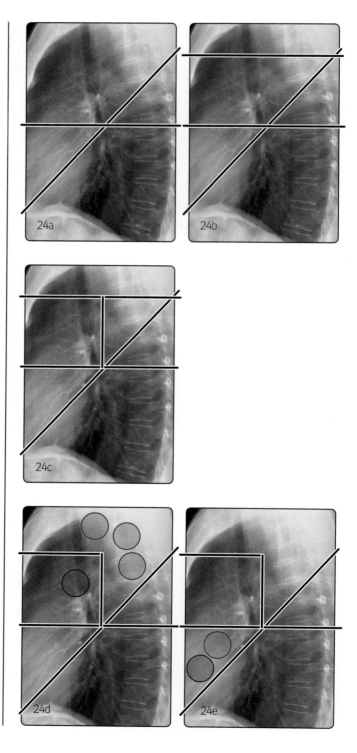

If the lesion lies within the LUL, then there are four possibilities.

1. Apicoposterior segment.
2. Anterior segment.
3. Superior lingular segment.
4. Inferior lingular segment.

The LUL can be divided by two horizontal lines and a vertical line. The first horizontal line (lower left horizontal line) corresponds to the horizontal line used on the lateral x-ray for localizing pathology in the right lung. This line defines the border between the lingular segments (below this line) and the remaining segments of the LUL (Fig. 24a).

A second horizontal line (upper left horizontal line) is drawn, extending anteriorly from the superior posterior end of the oblique fissure (Fig. 24b).

A vertical line is also drawn from the posterior end of the lower left horizontal line, superiorly to the upper left horizontal line (Fig. 24c).

If the lesion lies above the upper left horizontal line and/or posterior to the vertical line, it will be localized to the apicoposterior segment (Fig. 24d; pink circles). If the lesion lies inferior to the upper left horizontal line and above the lower left horizontal line, then the apicoposterior and lingular segments can be eliminated. The lesion can only lie in the anterior segment (Fig. 24d; purple circle).

Below the left lower horizontal line lies the lingula. If the lesion lies in the superior aspect of the lingula, it will lie within the superior lingular segment (Fig. 24e; pink circle). If the lesion lies inferiorly, then it must be in the inferior lingular segment (Fig. 24e; purple circle).

If the lesion lies within the LLL, then there are four possibilities.

1. Apical segment.
2. Posterior basal segment.
3. Anteromedial basal segment.
4. Lateral basal segment.

The LLL is divided by a horizontal line (as in the right lung) that lies at the level of the minor fissure, but extends posteriorly (Fig. 25a). A lesion above this line lies in the apical segment of the LLL (Fig. 25b).

The localization to the basal segment (below the horizontal line) of the LLL is also similar to the right, except that the anterior and medial segments are usually fused.

Divide the LLL below the horizontal line into thirds, using two equidistant vertical lines (Fig. 26a). If the lesion lies in the posterior third, it will be localized to the posterior basal (Fig. 26b; p nk circle). If it lies in the anterior third then it will be localized to the anteromedial basal segment (Fig. 26b; purple circle). This segment overlaps the middle third. If the lesion lies within the middle third, then it must lie in the lateral basal segment, as the anterior and medial segments are fused (Fig. 26b; blue circle).

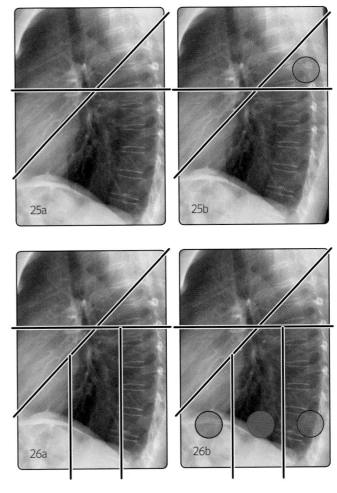

25a

25b

26a

26b

671

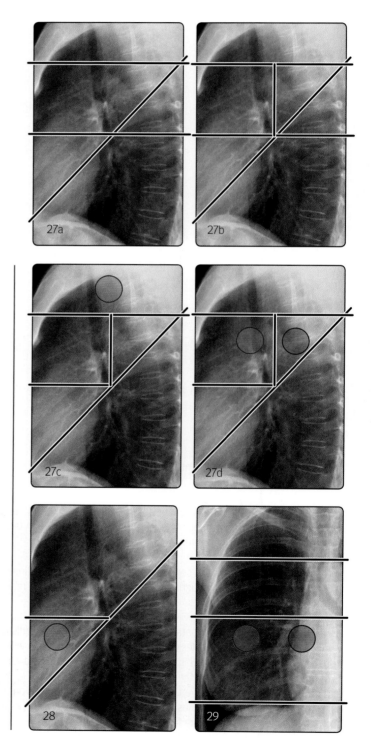

If the lesion lies within the RUL, then there are three possibilities.

1. Apical segment.
2. Anterior segment.
3. Posterior segment.

On a lateral chest x-ray, the RUL lies anterior to the oblique fissure. Find the posterior end of the oblique fissure. Draw a horizontal line extending anteriorly from this point (Fig. 27a).

Starting at the midpoint of this first line, draw a second line perpendicular to this first line through the remaining portion of the RUL inferiorly (Fig. 27b).

If the lesion lies superior to this line, then the anterior and posterior segments can be eliminated. The lesion can only lie in the apical segment (Fig. 27c). If the lesion lies inferior to the horizontal line, the apical segment can be eliminated. The lesion will lie within the anterior or posterior RUL segment, depending on whether it is anterior or posterior to the vertical line, respectively (Fig. 27d).

If the lesion lies within the RML (Fig. 28), then there are two possibilities.

1. Medial segment.
2. Lateral segment.

Look on the PA x-ray. If the lesion lies close to the heart, it can be localized to the medial segment (Fig. 29; purple circle). If it lies laterally, then it can be localized to the lateral segment (Fig. 29; pink circle).

If the lesion lies within the RLL, then there are five possibilities.

1. Apical.
2. Medial basal.
3. Anterior basal.
4. Lateral basal.
5. Posterior basal.

We can draw a horizontal line through the RLL at the level of the minor fissure (Fig. 30a).

If the lesion lies above this line, then the lesion lies in the apical segment (Fig. 30b).

If the lesion lies below this line, then there are four possibilities.

1. Medial basal.
2. Anterior basal.
3. Lateral basal.
4. Posterior basal.

On the lateral x-ray, divide the RLL with two equidistant vertical lines (Fig. 31a).

If the lesion lies within the anterior third, then it must lie within the anterior basal segment (Fig. 31b; pink circle). If it lies within the posterior third, then it must lie within the posterior basal segment (Fig. 31b; purple circle).

If the lesion lies within the middle third (Fig. 31c), then there are two possibilities

1. Medial basal.
2. Lateral basal.

The PA x-ray is needed to establish which of these two segments the lesion lies within (Fig. 32). If the lesion lies medially, then the lateral basal segment can be eliminated. The only possible segment is the medial basal. If the lesion lies laterally, then the medial basal is eliminated. The lesion can only lie within the lateral basal segment.

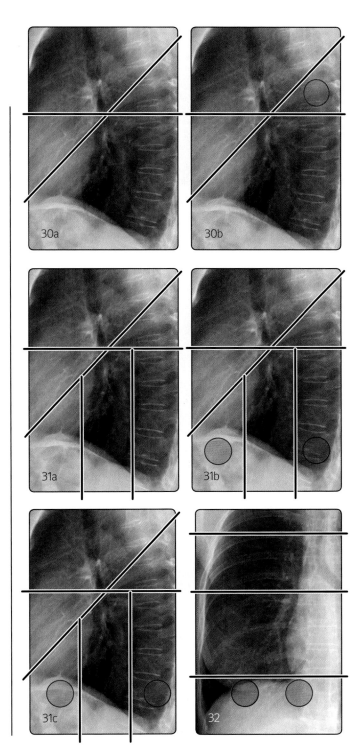

673

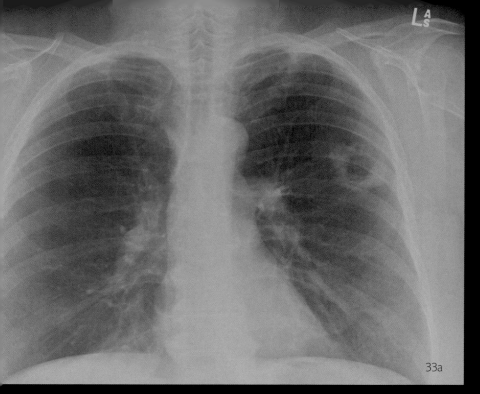

33a

List the potential anatomical locations from which this lesion could be originating.

How would you determine the exact anatomical origin of the lesion?

This PA chest x-ray shows a lesion in the left hemithorax (Fig. 33a).

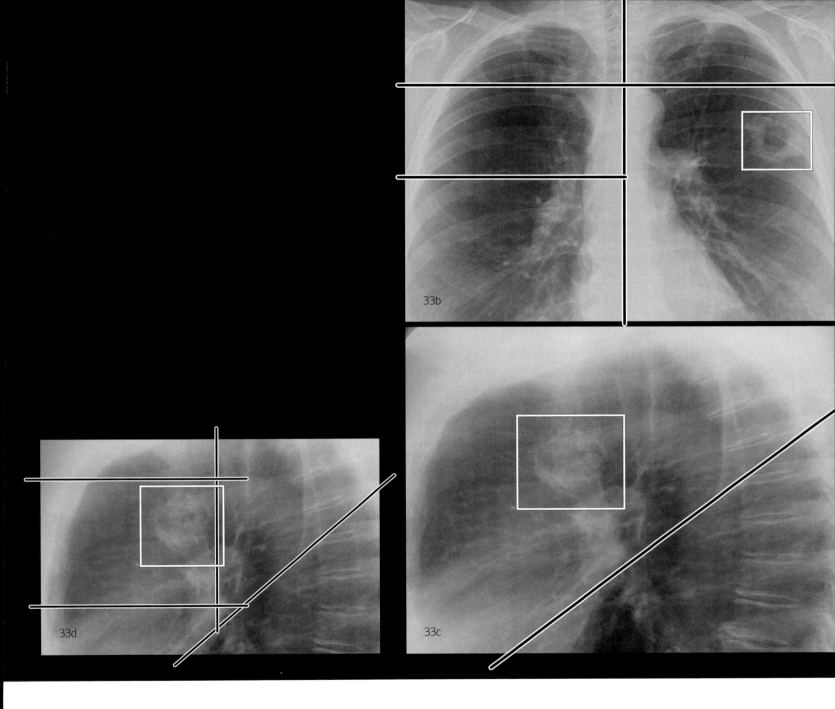

33b

33c

33d

The white opacity seen on the PA x-ray cannot be definitively localized on the PA x-ray; the lateral x-ray is needed.

Using the grid/possibility method of localization, we add the grid lines to this x-ray (Fig. 33b). Based on the position of the lesion relative to the grid lines, the lesion can lie within either the LUL or the LLL. Then, by using the lateral x-ray and adding the grid lines (Fig. 33c), we can now eliminate the LLL. Therefore, we can localize the opacity to the LUL.

By adding the grid lines applicable to the LUL (Fig. 33d), the lingular and the apicoposterior segments can be eliminated. The opacity is localized to the anterior segment of the LUL.

References

1. Lewis, P.J., Shaffer, K., & Donovan, A. (Eds.). (2012). AMSER National Medical Student Curriculum in Radiology. http://aur.org/Secondary-Alliances.aspx?id=141.

2. Lewis, P.J., & Shaffer, K. (2005). Developing a national medical student curriculum in radiology. *Am. Coll. Radiol. 2*(1):8–11.

3. Volk, M., Strotzer, M., & Feuerbach, S. (2000). Case of the month. Intrapulmonary or extrapulmonary? *Br. J. Radiol., 73*(868):451–452.

4. Ellis, R. (1977). Incomplete border sign of extrapleural masses. *JAMA, 237*(25):2748.

5. Felson, B., & Felson, H. (1950). Localization of intrathoracic lesions by means of the postero-anterior roentgenogram; the silhouette sign. *Radiology, 55*(3):363–374.

6. Ugalde, P., deCamargo, J., & Deslauriers, J. (2007). Lobes, fissures, and bronchopulmonary segments. *Thorac. Surg. Clin., 17*(4):587–599.

CHAPTER 18
ATELECTASIS &
LOBAR COLLAPSE

importance

Atelectasis is a frequently encountered abnormality on chest x-rays. Since the presence of collapse may indicate serious underlying pathology, confident recognition of collapse on an x-ray is an essential skill.

objectives

Skills

You will identify

- specific radiological features of lobar collapse on the PA and lateral chest x-rays.

- the location of the collapse on the PA and lateral chest x-rays.

You will be able to

- create a differential diagnosis for lobar collapse and for volume loss within a lung.

Knowledge

You will review and understand

- the definition and the classification of lobar collapse.

- the common etiologies and pathophysiology of lobar collapse.

- the clinical features of lobar collapse.

- why and how pathology changes the radiological appearance of the lungs when collapse has occurred.

associated resources

This chapter maps to the following AMSER curriculum content (1,2).

1) Radiological identification of lobar collapse

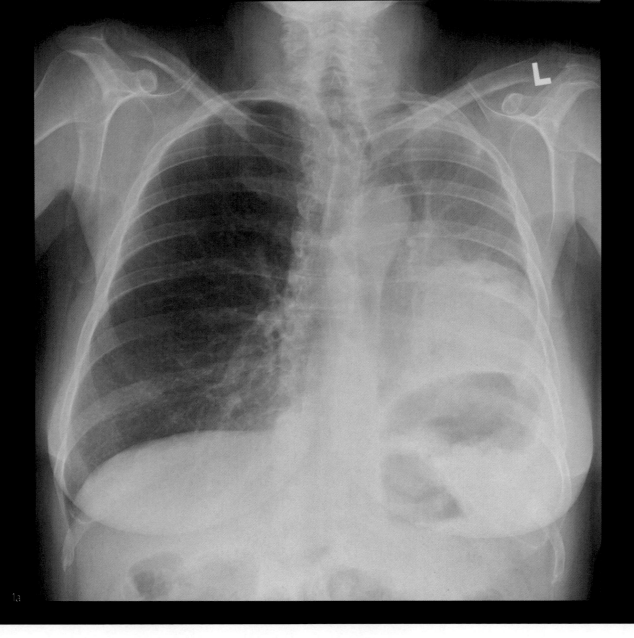

1a

You are the surgical intern on call overnight and you are called to see a 66-year-old female who is one-day post-laparoscopic cholecystectomy. She has a low-grade fever and has become mildly tachypnoeic. You suspect that she may have an infection, or atelectasis. You request a chest x-ray (Fig. 1a,b), and are asked to report your findings to the consultant.

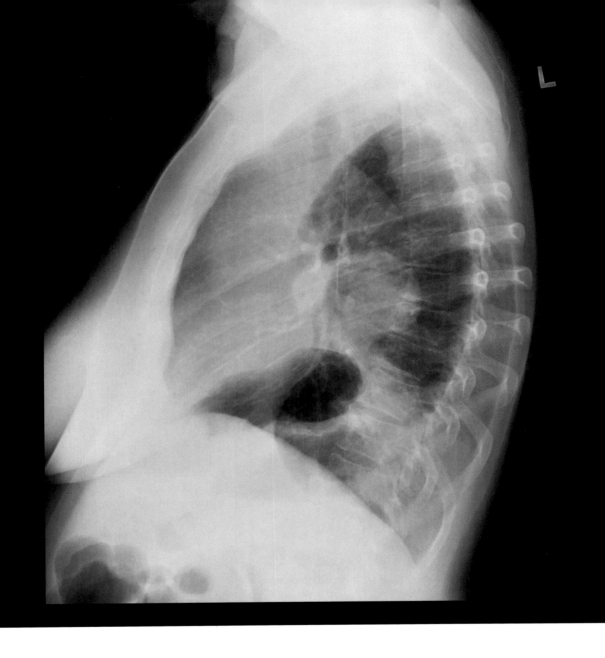

1b

What do you tell
the consultant?

ATELECTASIS

Atelectasis is a term that is derived from the Greek words *a*, *tekos*, and *ectasisis*, meaning "without complete expansion" (3). The Fleishner Society describes atelectasis as reduced inflation of all, or part of, the lung (4). Generally, 'collapse' is used interchangeably with atelectasis, but usually represents a more severe form of atelectasis. In this chapter, 'collapse' is used to describe atelectasis involving the lobes of the lungs.

Causes of Atelectasis

There are five mechanisms of atelectasis.

1. Postobstructive atelectasis.
2. Compressive atelectasis.
3. Cicatricial or rounded atelectasis.
4. Adhesive atelectasis.
5. Passive atelectasis.

1. Postobstructive atelectasis

The most frequent cause of atelectasis is obstruction. The main obstructive causes include: mucous plugging, foreign body aspiration, and the presence of a tumor. The atelectasis occurs as the result of reabsorption of air, distal to the obstruction.

Obstruction within the lung can occur at any level of the large or small bronchi (Fig. 2a,b). The complete obstruction of a lobar bronchus will lead to lobar collapse, whereas the complete obstruction of a segmental bronchus will lead to segmental atelectasis.

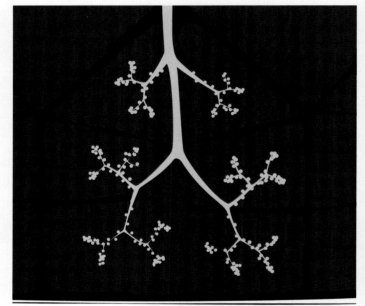

2a

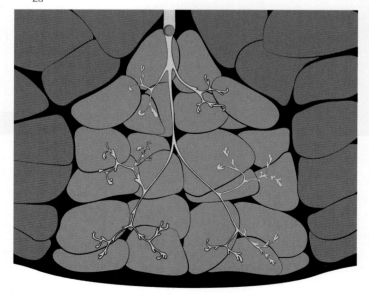

2b

2. Compressive atelectasis

Compressive atelectasis occurs when a space-occupying process, existing within the thorax, compresses the lung parenchyma and forces air out of the alveoli (Fig. 3)(5).

3. Cicatricial or rounded atelectasis

Cicatrization atelectasis results from parenchymal scarring (Fig. 4). The volume loss can occur because the scarring is either directly obstructing the bronchi, or is involving the parenchyma and preventing expansion. A granulomatous disease, such as chronic tuberculosis or sarcoidosis, commonly causes this type of atelectasis.

One type of cicatricial atelectasis is rounded atelectasis, also called folded-lung syndrome or Blesovsky syndrome (6,7). This occurs when the lung folds, or curls, into a ball as a result of fibrous bands and adhesions to the visceral pleura. This form of atelectasis is commonly found in asbestos workers.

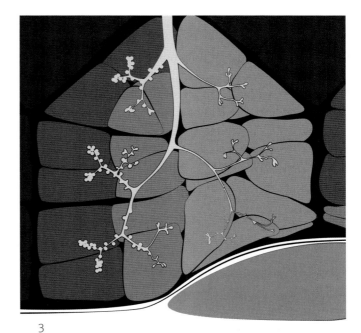
3

Figure 2. Postobstructive atelectasis. The most common cause of atelectasis is obstruction of the airways. Schematic representation of the mechanism of obstructive atelectasis. a, normal secondary lobule structure, b, changes due to postobstructive atelectasis.

Figure 3. Compressive atelectasis. Compressive atelectasis is due to the compression of the alveoli from an external source. Illustration of the changes due to compressive atelectasis.

Figure 4. Cicatricial (rounded) atelectasis. Cicatricial atelectasis is caused by parenchymal scarring. Illustration of the changes due to atelectasis secondary to scarring.

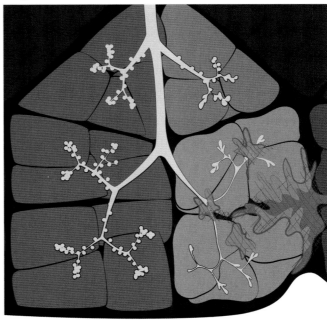
4

4. Adhesive atelectasis

Adhesive atelectasis results from a surfactant deficiency. Surfactant lowers the surface tension of the alveoli and therefore, plays an important role in preventing the alveoli from collapsing. The loss of surfactant production, or the inactivation of surfactant, leads to atelectasis. This is seen in acute respiratory distress syndrome (ARDS)(Fig. 5) and similar disorders.

5. Passive atelectasis

Passive atelectasis occurs when there is a loss of contact between the parietal and visceral pleurae. This occurs with pleural effusions or with a pneumothorax. Air or fluid within the pleural space causes a loss of negative pressure and therefore, there is nothing to maintain the expansion of the lungs to the limits of the chest wall. The elastic properties of the lungs are preserved and therefore, the lungs relax, or recoil, which results in the loss of volume. A pleural effusion will cause more atelectasis in the lower lung zones, whereas the upper lobes are more typically affected by a pneumothorax (Fig. 6).

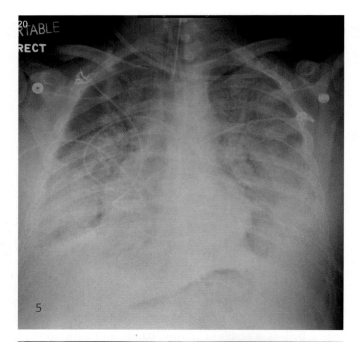

Figure 5. Adhesive atelectasis. Adhesive atelectasis occurs when there is a surfactant deficiency, as is seen in ARDS. PA chest x-ray from a patient with ARDS.

Figure 6. Passive atelectasis. Passive atelectasis occurs when there is a loss of contact between the pleural layers. PA chest x-ray of a pneumothorax causing passive atelectasis (arrows).

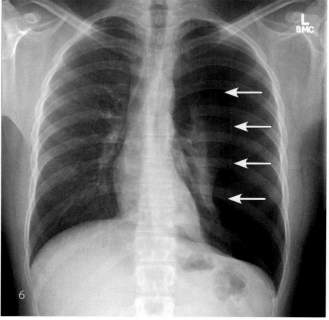

Clinical Risk Factors for Atelectasis

Collapse frequently occurs in the post-operative patient – especially those who have had thoracic and upper abdominal surgery – due to hypoventilation (i.e., shallow breathing) in response to pain. Furthermore, surgical manipulation and anesthesia can disrupt the normal production of surfactant and interfere with the proper functioning of the diaphragm. Both of these complications can then lead to atelectasis that is usually basilar or segmental in distribution.

Atelectasis may also occur following direct blunt injury to the chest. This is due to hypoventilation, because of pain secondary to rib or sternal fractures. Atelectasis can also result from a traumatic pneumothorax or hemothorax.

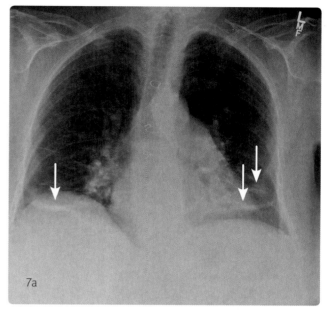

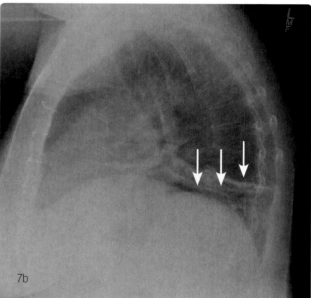

Subsegmental Atelectasis

Hypoventilation leads to subsegmental atelectasis – an atelectasis that has a linear or disc shape, with multiple separate areas of involvement. The atelectasis will appear as white bands, usually abutting the pleura, and is seen more frequently within the lung bases (Fig. 7a,b). These bands can vary from a few millimeters to one centimeter in thickness. Subsegmental atelectasis is used synonymously with the terms plate, plate-like or discoid atelectasis (8).

Figure 7. Subsegmental atelectasis. Subsegmental atelectasis is caused by hypoventilation, and is seen most frequently at the lung bases. a, PA chest x-ray with subsegmental atelectasis in both lower lobes (arrows), b, lateral chest x-ray showing subsegmental atelectasis in both lower lobes (arrows).

RADIOLOGICAL APPEARANCE OF ATELECTASIS

The lungs are normally full of air. When atelectasis occurs, the air in the involved lung (or part of) gets resorbed, and that region of lung parenchyma becomes visible as an opacity on the x-ray. The size and radiological appearance of the lung opacity will depend on the location and the amount of lung involved. Atelectasis can involve: the entire lung, the lobes (lobar atelectasis), the lung segments (segmental atelectasis), or parts of a segment (subsegmental atelectasis).

At the same time, the remainder of the ipsilateral lung – and even the contralateral lung – may over-inflate as if to fill the void created by the atelectasis, causing a shift in the fissures. In fact, the hallmark, and only direct sign of atelectasis, is the shift of the fissures. The direction of the fissure shift characterizes which lobe of the lung is involved. Shift of the fissures usually requires significant volume loss.

Radiological Signs/Features of Lobar Collapse

The radiological signs/features of lobar collapse can be divided into direct and indirect (9).

Direct sign of collapse

- The hallmark, and only direct sign, of collapse is the shift of the fissures (Fig. 8a,b).

Indirect signs of collapse

- Increased lung opacity (Fig. 9a).
- Compensatory hyperinflation of the surrounding lung (Fig. 9b).
- Obscured cardiac, mediastinal, or diaphragmatic borders (Fig. 9c).
- Crowding of pulmonary vessels (Fig. 9d).
- Elevated diaphragm (Fig. 9e).
- Hilar displacement (Fig. 9f).
- Crowding of the ribs (Fig. 9g).

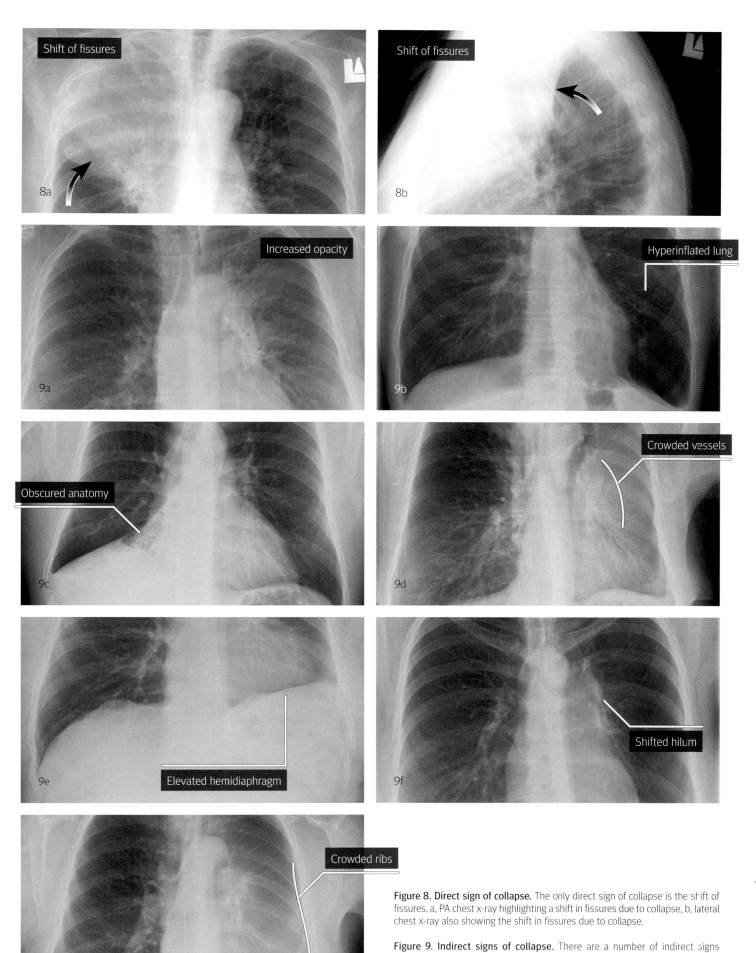

Figure 8. Direct sign of collapse. The only direct sign of collapse is the shift of fissures. a, PA chest x-ray highlighting a shift in fissures due to collapse, b, lateral chest x-ray also showing the shift in fissures due to collapse.

Figure 9. Indirect signs of collapse. There are a number of indirect signs that can be used to identify collapse, as shown in these PA chest x-rays. a, increased lung opacity, b, compensatory hyperinflation, c, obscured anatomy, d, crowding of pulmonary vessels, e, elevated diaphragms, f, hilar displacement, g, crowding of the ribs.

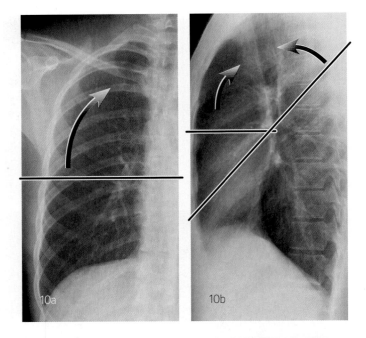

10a

10b

Right upper lobe collapse

In right upper lobe (RUL) collapse, the direction of collapse is superior, medial, and anterior (Figs. 10a,b & 12-17).

On the PA x-ray (Fig. 11a), there is an area that is too white in the upper zone of the right lung. The minor fissure shifts superiorly and medially, the trachea can be deviated to the right, and the ribs over the area can be closer together than normal. In addition, the mediastinum may look widened. The right hilum will look smaller and will be elevated. The right hemidiaphragm may be elevated.

On the lateral chest x-ray (Fig. 11b), there is also an area that is too white in the upper zone of the right lung, the superior part of the oblique fissure above the hilum shifts anteriorly and superiorly, and the minor fissure shifts superiorly.

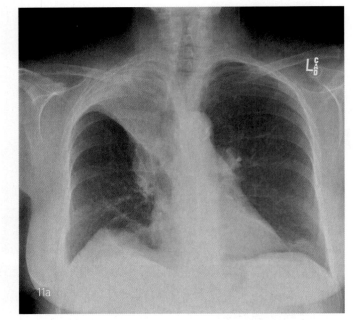

11a

Figure 10. Direction of fissure shift in right upper lobe (RUL) collapse. a, PA chest x-ray highlighting direction of RUL collapse (arrow), b, lateral chest x-ray highlighting direction of RUL collapse (arrows).

Figure 11. Right upper lobe (RUL) collapse. a, PA chest x-ray showing grayscale change in the superior aspect of the right hemithorax related to RUL collapse, b, lateral chest x-ray showing grayscale change the superior aspect of the right hemithorax related to RUL collapse.

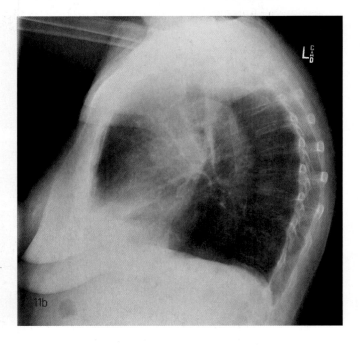

11b

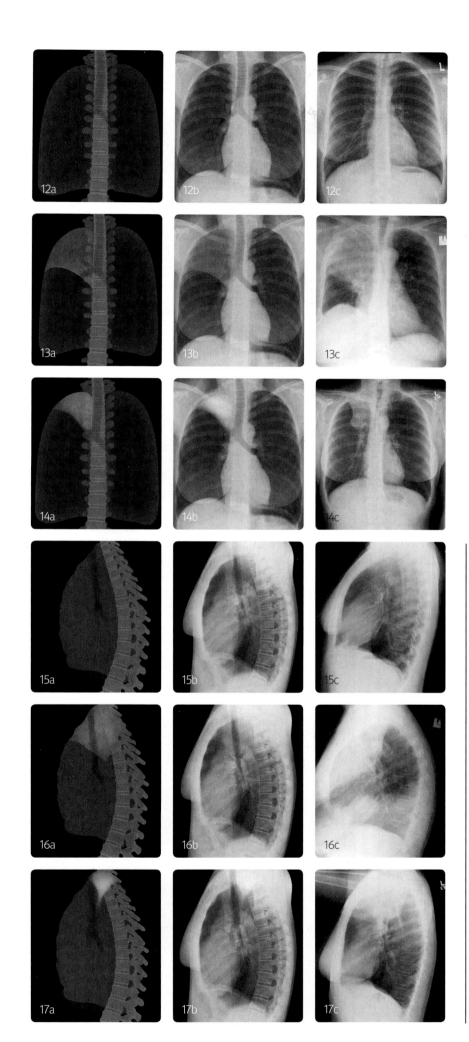

Figure 12. Right upper lobe (RUL) collapse series - normal, frontal view. a, artistic representation of normal lungs, b, artistic representation of normal lungs with all thoracic structures, c, PA chest x-ray showing normal lung grayscale.

Figure 13. Right upper lobe (RUL) collapse series - partial collapse, frontal view. a, artistic representation of partial RUL collapse, b, artistic representation of partial RUL collapse with all thoracic structures, c, PA chest x-ray showing change in grayscale due to partial RUL collapse.

Figure 14. Right upper lobe (RUL) collapse series - advanced collapse, frontal view. a, artistic representation of advanced RUL collapse, b, artistic representation of advanced RUL collapse with all thoracic structures, c, PA chest x-ray showing change in grayscale due to advanced RUL collapse.

Figure 15. Right upper lobe (RUL) collapse series - normal, lateral view. a, artistic representation of normal lungs, b, artistic representation of normal lungs with all thoracic structures, c, lateral chest x-ray showing normal lung grayscale.

Figure 16. Right upper lobe (RUL) collapse series - partial collapse, lateral view. a, artistic representation of partial RUL collapse, b, artistic representation of partial RUL collapse with all thoracic structures, c, lateral chest x-ray showing change in grayscale due to partial RUL collapse.

Figure 17. Right upper lobe (RUL) collapse series - advanced collapse, lateral view. a, artistic representation of advanced RUL collapse, b, artistic representation of advanced RUL collapse with all thoracic structures, c, lateral chest x-ray showing change in grayscale due to advanced RUL collapse.

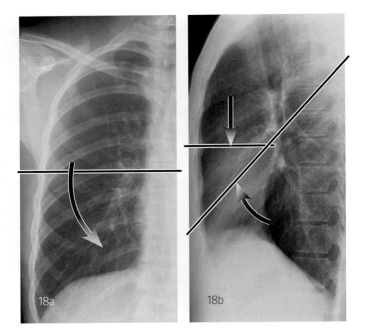

Right middle lobe collapse

AMSER In right middle lobe (RML) collapse, the direction of collapse is inferior and medial (Fig. 18a,b).

RML collapse can be very difficult to spot on the PA x-ray because the changes caused by the collapse may be subtle. This subtlety is a result of the direction of the x-ray beam relative to the collapse and the relatively small size of the RML. RML collapse is much more obvious on the lateral x-ray (the area of collapse will be quite white), because the position of the collapse relative to the direction of the x-ray beam is oriented to facilitate its visibility.

When RML collapse is evident on a PA x-ray (Fig. 19a), the upper part of the lower zone may look 'too white', which can interfere with the clarity of the right heart border (silhouette sign, Ch. 17, Pg. 654), the right diaphragm may be slightly raised, and usually, the minor fissure shifts inferiorly and medially. The right heart border may be obscured, especially with medial segment collapse.

On the lateral chest x-ray (Fig. 19b), there is a triangular-shaped area of too white (a triangular opacity), with its apex at the hilum and its base spanning between the diaphragm and sternum. On the lateral x-ray, the minor fissure shifts inferiorly, and the anterior inferior part of the oblique fissure shifts superiorly.

Figure 18. Direction of fissure shift in right middle lobe (RML) collapse. a, PA chest x-ray highlighting direction of RML collapse (arrow), b, lateral chest x-ray highlighting direction of RML collapse (arrows).

Figure 19. Right middle lobe (RML) collapse. a, PA chest x-ray showing subtle grayscale change in the inferior aspect of the right hemithorax related to RML collapse, b, lateral chest x-ray showing more prominent grayscale change in the inferior aspect of the right hemithorax related to RML collapse.

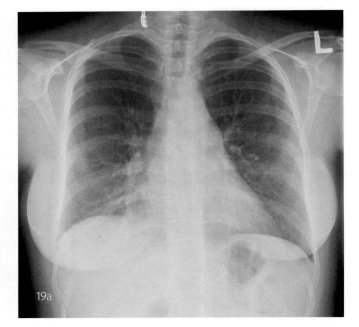

19a

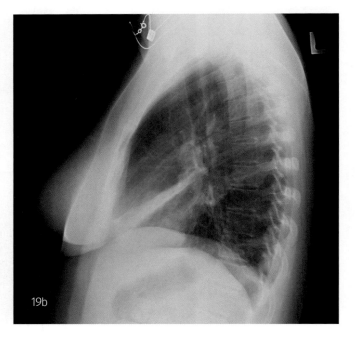

19b

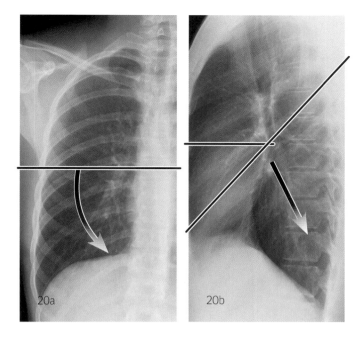

Right lower lobe collapse

In right lower lobe (RLL) collapse, the direction of collapse is inferior and posterior (Fig. 20a,b).

On the PA x-ray (Fig. 21a), RLL collapse usually causes a too white area above the diaphragm that obscures the right border of the heart (silhouette sign). The minor fissure will shift inferiorly and posteriorly. The right hilum will look smaller and will be depressed. The right hemidiaphragm may be elevated. The right main stem bronchus will be pulled into a more vertical position.

On the lateral x-ray (Fig. 21b), there is usually a triangular area near the posterior part of the lung field that looks too white, and the oblique fissure shifts inferiorly and posteriorly.

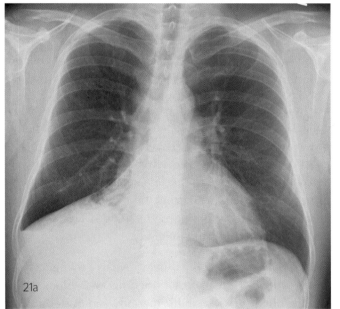

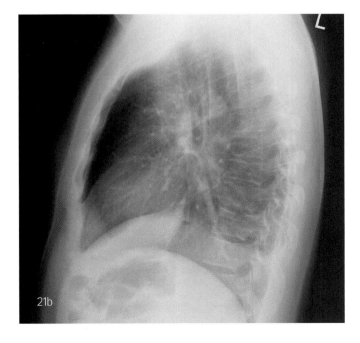

Figure 20. Direction of fissure shift in right lower lobe (RLL) collapse. a, PA chest x-ray highlighting direction of RLL collapse (arrow), b, lateral chest x-ray highlighting direction of RLL collapse (arrow).

Figure 21. Right lower lobe (RLL) collapse. a, PA chest x-ray showing subtle grayscale change in the inferior aspect of the right hemithorax related to RLL collapse, b, lateral chest x-ray showing subtle grayscale change in the inferior aspect of the right hemithorax related to RLL collapse.

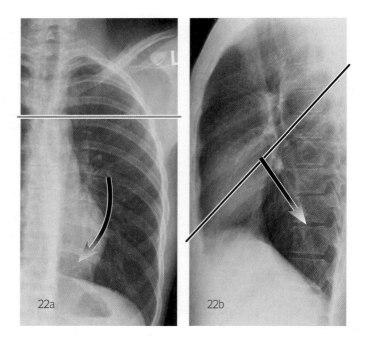
22a 22b

Left lower lobe collapse

AMSER In left lower lobe (LLL) collapse, the direction of collapse is posterior, inferior and medial (Figs. 22a,b & 24-29).

LLL collapse can be very easy to oversee because, when collapsed, the LLL is positioned behind the heart. An area of too white can be spotted behind the heart on the PA chest x-ray (Fig. 23a). The left hilum will look smaller and will be depressed. The left hemidiaphragm may be elevated. The left main stem bronchus will be pulled into a more vertical position. The oblique fissure will be displaced posteriorly and inferiorly.

The lateral x-ray (Fig. 23b), usually reveals a triangular area that is too white at the posterior corner of the lung fields, and the oblique fissure shifts inferiorly and posteriorly.

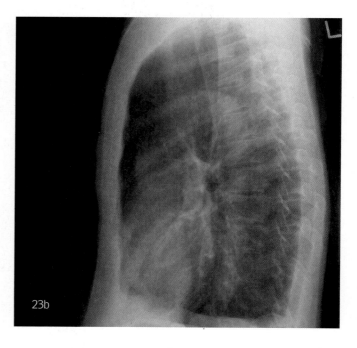
23a
23b

Figure 22. Direction of fissure shift in left lower lobe (LLL) collapse. a, PA chest x-ray highlighting direction of LLL collapse (arrow), b, lateral chest x-ray highlighting direction of LLL collapse (arrow).

Figure 23. Left lower lobe (LLL) collapse. a, PA chest x-ray showing subtle grayscale change in the inferior aspect of the left hemithorax related to LLL collapse, b, lateral chest x-ray showing subtle grayscale change in the inferior aspect of the left hemithorax related to LLL collapse.

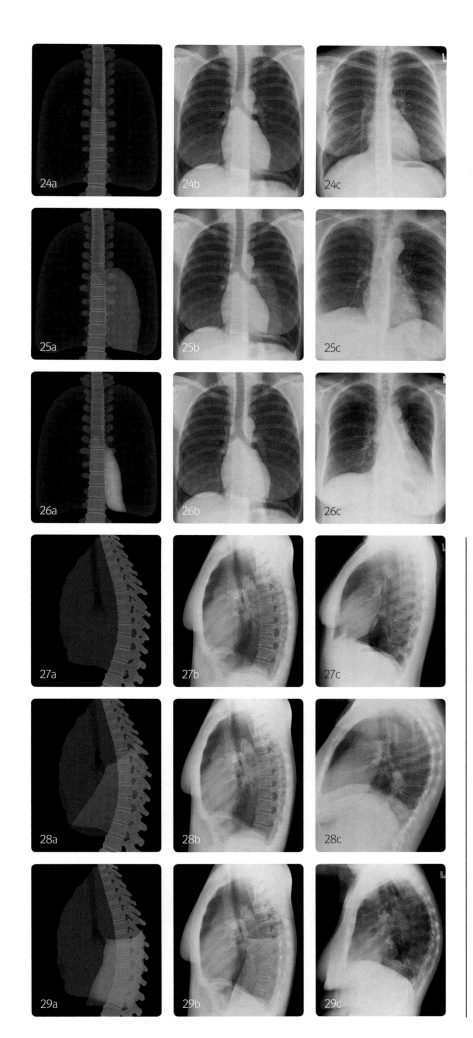

Partial collapse of the LLL is a frequent feature of post-operative PA chest x-rays.

Figure 24. Left lower lobe (LLL) collapse series - normal, frontal view. a, artistic representation of normal lungs, b, artistic representation of normal lungs with all thoracic structures, c, PA chest x-ray showing normal lung grayscale.

Figure 25. Left lower lobe (LLL) collapse series - partial collapse, frontal view. a, artistic representation of partial LLL collapse, b, artistic representation of partial LLL collapse with all thoracic structures, c, PA chest x-ray showing change in grayscale due to partial LLL collapse.

Figure 26. Left lower lobe (LLL) collapse series - advanced collapse, frontal view. a, artistic representation of advanced LLL collapse, b, artistic representation of advanced LLL collapse with all thoracic structures, c, PA chest x-ray showing change in grayscale due to advanced LLL collapse.

Figure 27. Left lower lobe (LLL) collapse series - normal, lateral view. a, artistic representation of normal lungs, b, artistic representation of normal lungs with all thoracic structures, c, lateral chest x-ray showing normal lung grayscale.

Figure 28. Left lower lobe (LLL) collapse series - partial collapse, lateral view. a, artistic representation of partial LLL collapse, b, artistic representation of partial LLL collapse with all thoracic structures, c, lateral chest x-ray showing change in grayscale due to partial LLL collapse.

Figure 29. Left lower lobe (LLL) collapse series - advanced collapse, lateral view. a, artistic representation of advanced LLL collapse, b, artistic representation of advanced LLL collapse with all thoracic structures, c, lateral chest x-ray showing change in grayscale due to advanced LLL collapse.

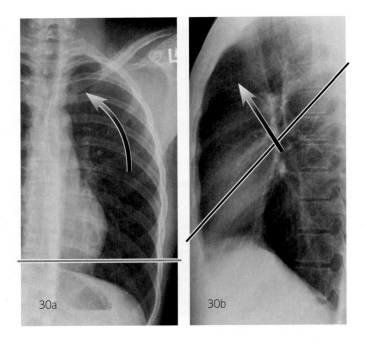

30a 30b

Left upper lobe collapse

In left upper lobe (LUL) collapse, the direction of collapse is superior, anterior and medial (Fig. 30a,b).

When the LUL collapses, the entire left lung field may look slightly too white. This does not indicate a complete left lung collapse. It is because the LUL lies in front of (and encompasses the whole of) the left lower lobe (LLL) anatomically and, therefore, there is no easy manner by which to distinguish whether the opacity lies in the LUL or entire left lung on the PA x-ray. In LUL collapse, the major fissure shifts upwards and medially on the PA x-ray (Fig. 31a). The remaining LLL will hyperinflate, causing the blood vessels in the LLL to look more separate (splayed) than normal.

On the lateral x-ray (Fig. 31b), the oblique fissure shifts anteriorly, and an area that looks too white can sometimes be seen at the top of the lung fields.

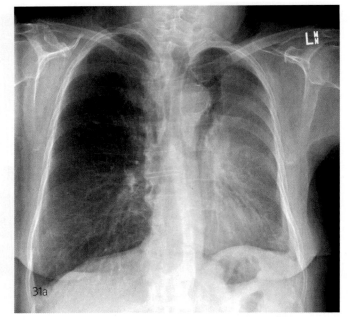

31a

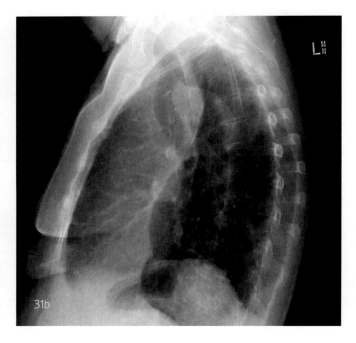

31b

Figure 30. Direction of fissure shift in left upper lobe (LUL) collapse. a, PA chest x-ray highlighting direction of LUL collapse (arrow), b, lateral chest x-ray highlighting direction of LUL collapse (arrow).

Figure 31. Left upper lobe (LUL) collapse. a, PA chest x-ray showing subtle grayscale change in the superior aspect of the left hemithorax related to LUL collapse, b, lateral chest x-ray showing subtle grayscale change in the superior aspect of the left hemithorax related to LUL collapse.

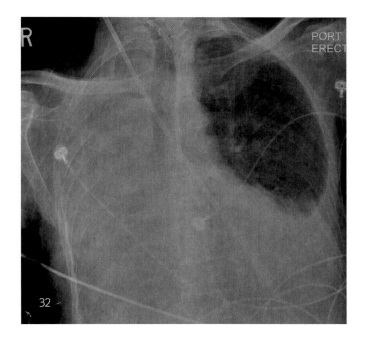

Collapse of the entire lung

Occasionally, with a central obstructing lesion, the entire lung can collapse. The radiological appearance is one of total opacification of the affected hemithorax (Fig. 32). This is sometimes called a whiteout. The volume loss causes deviation of the trachea and a shift of the mediastinum to the affected side. The opposite lung will hyperinflate and may herniate across the midline.

The main differential diagnoses for complete opacification of a hemithorax are massive pleural effusion, or a previous pneumonectomy.

An effusion (Fig. 33a,b), will produce midline shift in the opposite direction. However, collapse and effusion often coexist – in this case there may be minimal shift.

Previous pneumonectomy may be identified by signs of the previous surgery, such as visible sutures or clips, or by a rib abnormality.

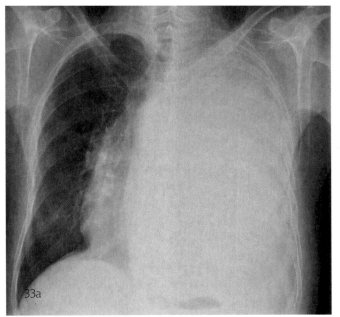

AMSER

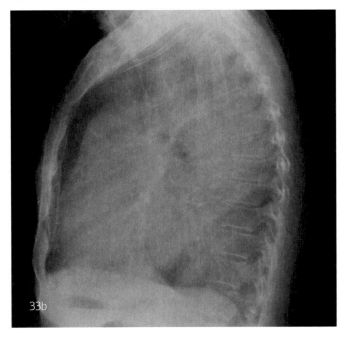

Figure 32. Collapse of the entire right lung. PA x-ray showing collapse of the entire right lung. Note the direction of shift of the trachea towards the collapsed lung.

Figure 33. Collapse of the entire left lung. a, PA x-ray showing collapse of the entire left lung caused by a massive left pleural effusion. Note the direction of shift of the trachea away from the collapsed lung, b, lateral chest x-ray – diffuse whiteness through almost the entire chest.

RADIOLOGICAL SIGNS ASSOCIATED WITH COLLAPSE

Upper Triangle Sign

In RLL collapse, a triangular opacity can be visible in the upper right hemithorax, medially. This is caused by the partial shift of the superior mediastinal structures to the right, secondary to the lower lobe collapse (Fig. 34)(10).

Golden S Sign

The minor fissure in RUL collapse is usually convex superiorly. In certain cases, it may appear concave, because of an underlying mass lesion. This is called the Golden S Sign (Fig. 35)(11,12).

Tenting Sign

Tenting of the diaphragmatic pleura (tenting or juxtaphrenic peak sign) is another helpful sign of RUL atelectasis (Fig. 35)(13).

Luftsichel Sign

In LUL collapse, the LUL shifts anteriorly and superiorly. Occasionally, a hyperexpanded superior segment of the LLL is positioned between the atelectatic upper lobe and the aortic arch. This gives the appearance of a crescent to the aerated lung and is referred to as the luftsichel sign (Fig. 36a,b)(14).

Top of the Aortic Knob Sign

The top of the aortic knob sign is seen on the PA x-ray when the left lower lobe collapses, and the superior mediastinum shifts and obliterates the aortic arch (a special example of the silhouette sign).

Figure 34. Upper triangle sign. PA chest x-ray from a patient with right lower lobe (RLL) collapse, with the upper triangle sign highlighted.

Figure 35. Golden S sign & tenting sign. PA chest x-ray from a patient with right upper lobe collapse, with the golden S and tenting signs evident.

Figure 36. Luftsichel sign. a, AP chest x-ray from a patient with left upper lobe (LUL) collapse with the luftsichel sign evident. b, lateral chest x-ray from the same patient.

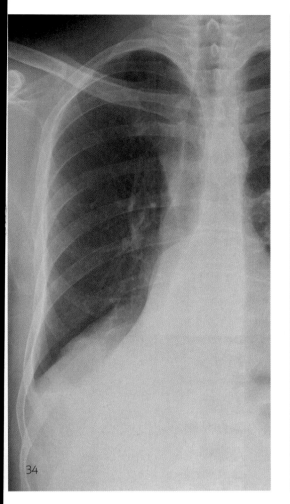

34

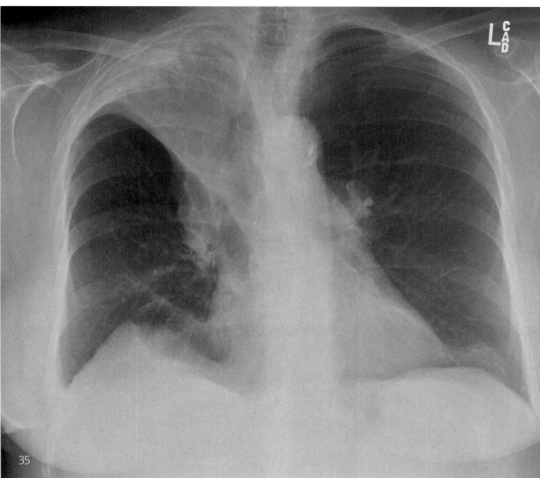

35

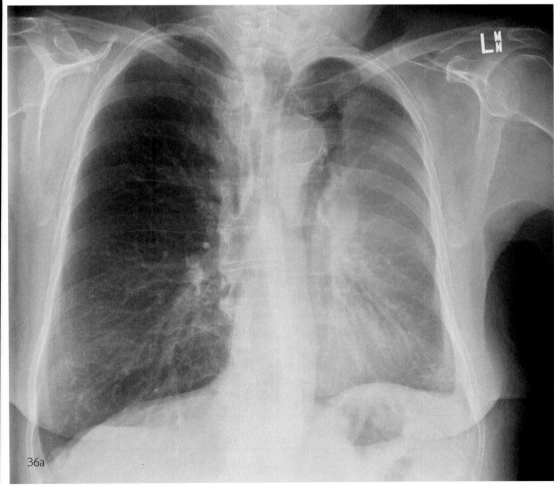

36a

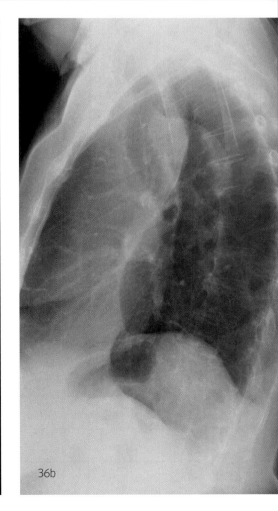

36b

Collapse and the Supine Chest X-ray

When evaluating the acutely ill ICU patient, you will not have the luxury of a lateral x-ray. The presence of atelectasis in these patients is important to recognize and treat ... BUT ... the appearance of collapse on a supine film may differ from the PA film. Therefore, the characteristics of atelectasis specific to the supine x-ray are important to recognize. These characteristics are discussed in detail in Chapter 19 (Pg. 722).

DIFFERENTIAL DIAGNOSIS OF ATELECTASIS

Although atelectasis is readily detectable on an x-ray, other pathologies that may similar radiologically must be excluded.

DIFFERENTIAL DIAGNOSIS	CLUE
Asbestosis	Clinical history of asbestos exposure; look for pleural plaques and calcifications.
Pneumonia	Clinical history; look for air bronchograms.
Pulmonary embolism	Clinical history.
Pulmonary fibrosis	Clinical history; look for previous chest x-rays.
Lung cancer	Clinical history – always suspect if collapse is present!!

Table 18.1
Clues for the Differential Diagnosis of Atelectasis

Atelectasis Radiological Analysis Checklist

This checklist is to be used if you suspect lobar collapse. The direction of the fissure shift characterizes which lobe of the lung is collapsed (15,16,17,18,19).

1 Is the position of the fissures shifted?

If **NO**, then lobar collapse can be excluded. **STOP**.

If **YES**, then describe for PA and lateral view.
Minor/oblique fissure (right/left).
Superior/inferior..
Medial/lateral.
Anterior/posterior.

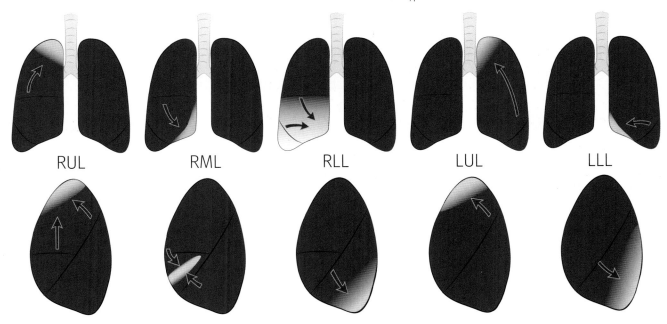

RUL RML RLL LUL LLL

DIRECTION OF COLLAPSE		DIRECTION OF FISSURE SHIFT ON THE PA X-RAY		DIRECTION OF FISSURE SHIFT ON THE LATERAL X-RAY	
		Minor	Oblique	Minor	Oblique
RUL	Superior, medial, and anterior	Superior and medial		Superior	Superior and anterior (superior portion only)
RML	Inferior and medial	Inferior and medial		Inferior	Superior (anterior inferior portion only)
RLL	Inferior and posterior	Inferior and medial	Inferior and medial		Inferior and posterior
LUL	Superior, anterior, and medial		Superior and medial		Anterior
LLL	Posterior, inferior, and medial		Inferior and medial		Inferior and posterior

Table 18.2
The Direction of Shift of the Fissures in Lobar Collapse

Confirming lobar collapse

The following characteristics are used to confirm your suspicion of lobar collapse (15,16,17,18,19).
If any of these are present, they confirm lobar collapse. If none are present, this does not exclude lobar collapse.

GRAYSCALE OF COLLAPSED LUNG

1   Is the grayscale of the collapsed
lobe increased?

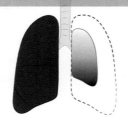

If **YES**, then confirms collapse.
Describe.
Slightly white/very white.

HYPERINFLATION

2   Is there hyperinflation of the
surrounding lung?

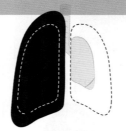

If **YES**, then confirms collapse.
Describe.
Right/left.
Partial/full.

HILAR SHIFT

3   Is the hilar position shifted in the
direction of the lobar collapse?

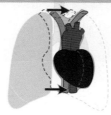

If **YES**, then confirms collapse.
Describe.
Elevated/depressed
Right/left.
Anterior/posterior.

MEDIASTINAL SHIFT

4   Is the mediastinum shifted in the
direction of the lobar collapse?

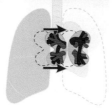

If **YES**, then confirms collapse.
Describe.
Right/left.

ELEVATED DIAPHRAGM

5   Is the ipsilateral diaphragm
elevated?

If **YES**, then confirms collapse.
Describe.
Right/left..

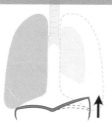

ATELECTASIS **Chapter 18** SECTION III

RIB CROWDING

6 Is there ipsilateral rib crowding?

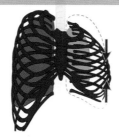

If **YES**, then confirms collapse.
Describe.
Right/left.
Upper/lower.

VESSEL CROWDING

7 Is there crowding of the pulmonary vessels?

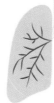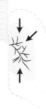

If **YES**, then confirms collapse.
Describe.
Right/left.
Upper/lower.

OBSCURED BORDERS

8 Are any of the cardiac, mediastinal or diaphragmatic borders obscured?

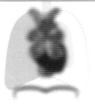

If **YES**, then confirms collapse.
Describe.
Right/left.
Heart/aorta.

SIGNS

9 Are any radiological signs of collapse present?

If **YES**, then confirms collapse.
Describe.
Upper triangle.
Golden S.
Tenting.
Luftsichel.
Top of aortic knob.

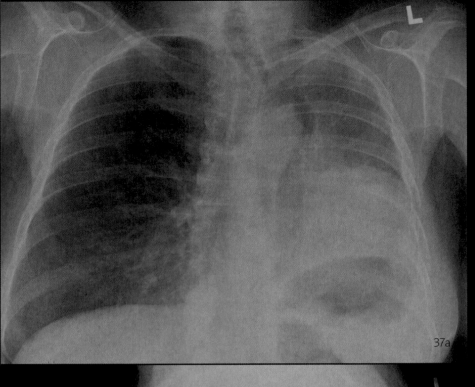

37a

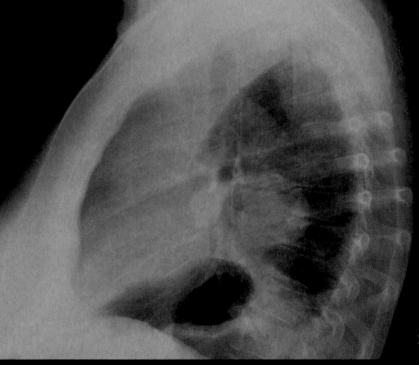

37b

What do you tell the
consultant?

You are the surgical intern on call overnight and you are called to see a 66-year-old female who is one-day post-laparoscopic cholecystectomy. She has a low-grade fever and has become mildly tachypnoeic. You suspect that she may have an infection, or atelectasis. You request a chest x-ray (Fig. 37a,b), and are asked to report your findings to the consultant.

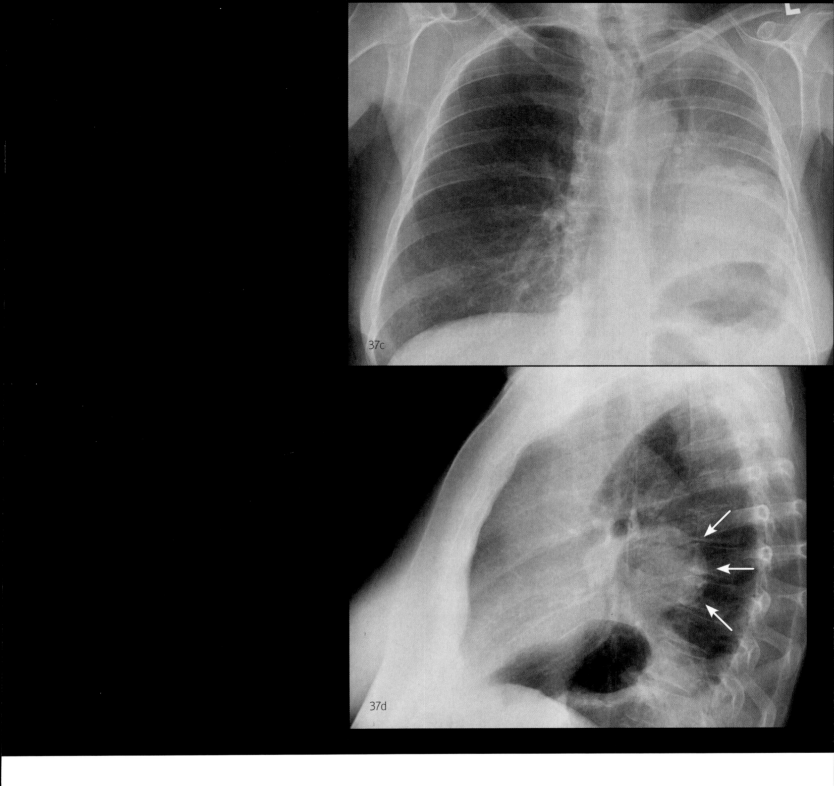

37c

37d

Direct and indirect findings are consistent with a left upper lobe collapse. The lateral image (Fig. 37d) also shows a mass centrally (arrows). Lung cancer is suspected and further follow up required.

Based on these findings, the diagnosis is left upper lobe collapse caused by a lung tumor.

References

1. Lewis, P.J., Shaffer, K., & Donovan, A. (Eds.). (2012). AMSER National Medical Student Curriculum in Radiology. http://aur.org/Secondary-Alliances.aspx?id=141.

2. Lewis, P.J., & Shaffer, K. (2005). Developing a national medical student curriculum in radiology. *Am. Coll. Radiol.* 2(1):8–11.

3. Haubrich, W.S. (2003). *Medical Meanings: A Glossary of Word Origins*, 2nd ed. Philadelphia, PA: ACP Press.

4. Tuddenham, W. (1984). Glossary of terms for thoracic radiology: recommendations of the Nomenclature Committee of the Fleischner Society. *AJR Am. J. Roentgenol.,143*:509–517.

5. Woodring, J.H. (1988). Determining the cause of pulmonary atelectasis: a comparison of plain radiography and CT. *AJR Am. J. Roentgenol.,150*(4):757–763.

6. Blesovsky, A. (1996). The folded lung. *Br. J. Dis. Chest, 60*(1):19–22.

7. McHugh, K., & Blaquiere, R.M. (1989). CT features of rounded atelectasis. *AJR Am. J. Roentgenol., 153*(2):257–260.

8. Westcott, J.L., & Cole, S. (1985). Plate atelectasis. *Radiology, 155*(1):1–9.

9. Lubert, M., & Krause, G.R. (1951). Patterns of lobar collapse as observed radiographically. *Radiology, 56*(2):165–182.

10. Kattan, K.R., Felson, B., Holder, L.E., & Eyler, W.R. (1975). Superior mediastinal shift in right-lower-lobe collapse: the "upper triangle sign". *Radiology, 116*(02):305–309.

11. Gupta, P. (2004). The Golden S sign. *Radiology, 233*(3):790–791.

12. Lemyze, M., Grunderbeeck, N.V., Gasan, G., & Thevenin, D. (2011). Golden s sign. *Am. J. Respir. Crit. Care Med., 183*(1):131.

13. Kattan, K.R., Eyler, W.R., & Felson, B. (1980). The juxtaphrenic peak in upper lobe collapse. *Semin. Roentgenol., 15*(2):187–193.

14. Blankenbaker, D.G. (1998). The luftsichel sign. *Radiology, 208*(2):319–320.

15. Proto, A.V., & Tocino, I. (1980). Radiographic manifestations of lobar collapse. *Semin. Roentgenol., 15*(2):117–173.

16. Proto, A.V. (1996). Lobar collapse: basic concepts. *Eur. J. Radiol., 23*(1):9–22.

17. Woodring, J.H., & Reed, J.C. (1996). Radiographic manifestations of lobar atelectasis. *J. Thorac. Imaging, 11*(2):109–144.

18. Ashizawa, K., Hayashi, K., Aso, N., & Minami, K. (2001). Lobar atelectasis: diagnostic pitfalls on chest radiography. *Br. J. Radiol., 74*(877):89–97.

19. Mintzer, R.A., Sakowicz, B.A., & Blonder, J.A. (1988). Lobar collapse. Usual and unusual forms. *Chest, 94*(3):615–620.

CHAPTER 19

The PORTABLE (AP) CHEST X-RAY: The critically ill patient

importance

Critically ill patients that require a chest x-ray need special consideration. The examination is performed at the bedside using portable x-ray equipment. For technical reasons portable examinations are performed with the patient in the anterior-posterior (AP) position rather than in the conventional posterior-anterior (PA) orientation.

This chapter explores the differences between the AP and the PA view. Although technically challenging, if you apply the same principles that were presented for the PA view to the AP view, you will minimize your chances of missing any pathology, and maximize your ability to make appropriate clinical decisions concerning very sick patients.

objectives

Skills

You will identify

- a portable (AP) chest x-ray.

- the key differences between AP and PA chest x-rays.

- the key features and pathologies that commonly characterize a portable (AP) chest x-ray (e.g., ARDS, atelectasis, pneumothorax, pneumomediastinum, and pleural effusions).

Knowledge

You will review and understand.

- the indications and technical considerations for a portable chest x-ray.

- the problems that are specific to the intensive care unit patient that may require routine daily x-ray examinations.

- the common pitfalls in portable chest x-ray interpretation.

associated resources

This chapter maps to the following AMSER curriculum content (1,2).

1) Atelectasis

2) Pleural abnormalities

3) Cardiac abnormalities

4) Interstitial abnormalities

5) Emergency "don't miss" findings
Supine pneumothorax (deep sulcus sign)
Pulmonary edema (interstitial and alveolar)
Pneumomediastinum
Aortic rupture (supine chest x-ray)

6) Limitations of Modalities
Posterior-Anterior (PA) versus Anterior-Posterior (AP)
Supine x-rays

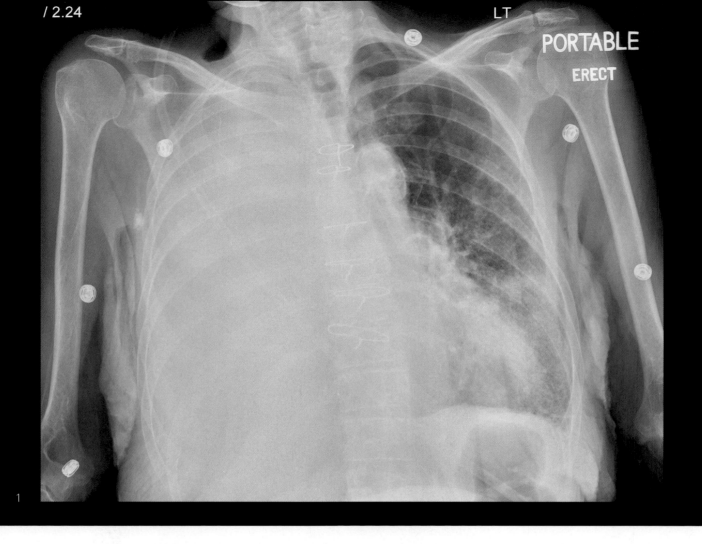

1

LT

PORTABLE

ERECT

CASE STUDY

You are working in the intensive care unit. Your non-ventilated patient on I.V. heparin developed acute shortness of breath and a drop in hemoglobin. You cannot hear any breath sounds on the right. You order a portable chest x-ray (Fig. 1).

What are the
important steps
in interpreting the
AP x-ray?

INDICATIONS FOR PORTABLE (AP) CHEST X-RAYS

AMSER emerg

The indications for portable chest x-rays are the same as for the PA and lateral chest x-rays. The decision to order a portable x-ray is based on the clinical condition of the patient. Portable chest x-rays are reserved for patients who are too ill to have routine PA and lateral examinations. These include critically-ill patients that cannot be moved, patients attached to life-support and monitoring devices, post-operative and post-trauma patients, and patients with severe cardiopulmonary symptoms.

In the intensive care unit (ICU) setting many patients require daily chest x-rays to monitor for changes in their clinical status. Unexpected findings in the ICU setting have been reported in 65% of the examinations – 25% of these leading to a change in clinical management (4,5,6).

Additionally, portable chest x-rays are performed immediately following endotracheal tube (ETT), nasogastric (NG) tube, central line, and chest tube placement, in order to monitor the positioning of these devices.

TECHNICAL CONSIDERATIONS AND THE AP EXAMINATION

The portable AP chest x-ray is performed at the bedside. The x-ray cassette is positioned behind the patient's back, and the x-ray camera is positioned in front of the patient. Ideally, the patient should be sitting upright at 90 degrees. However, in the emergency department (ED) and ICU, this is not usually possible, as many of these patients are intubated, paralyzed, post-operative, or post-trauma, and have very limited mobility. As such, the majority of portable x-rays are taken with the patient supine, or semi-erect.

Optimization of the portable chest x-ray can be achieved by making sure the patient's position is always ideal, and by using the best possible technical parameters.

What Are the Characteristics of a Good AP Examination?

The ideal portable chest x-ray is taken with the patient in full inspiration, sitting upright (Fig. 2a,b). As with the PA x-ray, the patient is positioned so that all of the lung fields are visible, there is no rotation, and the number of artifacts on the x-ray is minimized. Furthermore, like the PA and lateral x-rays, the AP examination should be sharp, and have optimized image exposure.

Figure 2. Technical characteristics of an AP x-ray. a, example of a technically good AP erect chest x-ray, b, example of a rotated AP erect chest x-ray.

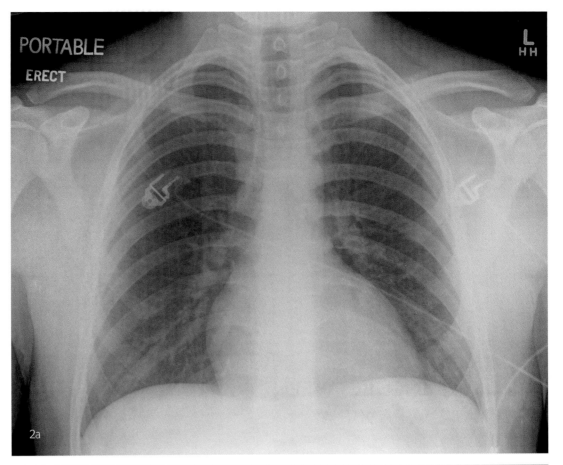

2a

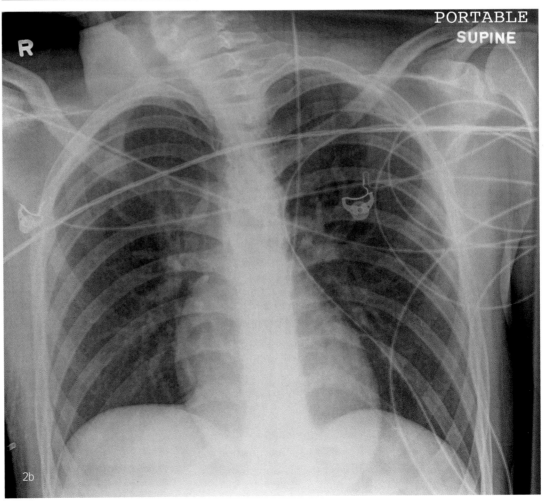

2b

THE DIFFERENCE BETWEEN AN AP AND A PA X-RAY

Quality

AMSER Obtaining a good quality AP chest x-ray is more difficult than obtaining a good PA x-ray – largely due to the patient's clinical status. Because these patients are critically ill, and many are on life support, there are more artifacts related to the presence of lines and tubes. Given the clinical condition of these patients, it is more difficult to ensure they are in the correct position – they are often rotated and not in midline. In addition, full inspiration may be difficult to obtain if the patient cannot follow instructions, is intubated, tachypneic, or cannot take a deep breath because of pain or cognitive issues.

Appearance of Thoracic Anatomy

AMSER The technique of the examination (PA versus AP) also causes some important differences in the appearance of normal anatomical structures in the thorax; for example, the altered appearance of the heart due to the magnification effect (**Ch. 2, Pg. 74**). Because the heart is closer to the x-ray source and farther from the x-ray detector during an AP examination, it will look larger on an AP x-ray (Fig. 3a,b). Furthermore, the cardiac magnification will be exaggerated by poor inspiration, and the supine position, that are common features of AP x-rays. This appearance can lead to overcalling congestive heart failure.

CHARACTERISTIC	CAUSE
Technical Considerations	
Rotation of patient	More difficult to position patient
Poor inspiration	Patient uncooperative, or unable to cooperate
More artifacts	Clinical status of patient (e.g., lines, tubes, etc.)
Overexposed or underexposed	Portable x-ray technology
Blurring	Slower exposure time
Anatomical Considerations	
Cardiac enlargement	Magnification effect
Widening of mediastinum	Magnification effect
Prominent upper lobe vessels	Supine position

Table 19.1
Specific Characteristics of an AP X-ray (Erect and Supine)

Figure 3. Difference between an AP and a PA chest x-ray. a, PA chest x-ray; arrows show the lateral edges of the heart, b, AP chest x-ray from the same patient; arrows show the lateral edges of the heart (the heart is magnified).

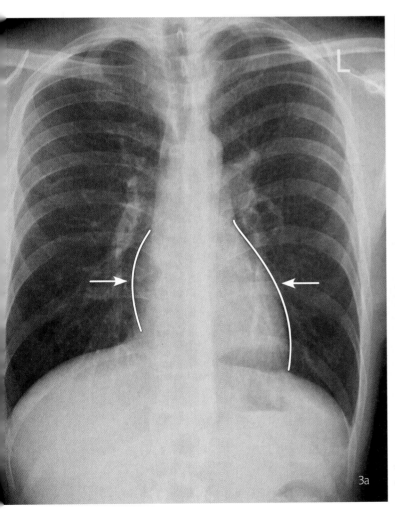

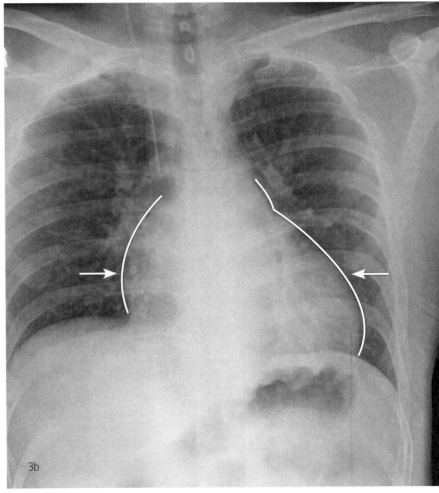

3a

3b

713

SPECIAL CONSIDERATIONS FOR THE INTERPRETATION OF THE AP X-RAY

The interpretative process for the AP chest x-ray is a modified version of the same six steps followed for the interpretation of PA and lateral examinations that are discussed in Chapter 16.

Acutely ill patients will usually require multiple chest x-rays during the course of the illness. Although each x-ray is very important, the initial chest x-ray examination in acutely ill patients is the principal examination for establishing or confirming the clinical diagnosis, and as such requires special attention (8).

After establishing the clinical diagnosis, follow-up x-rays are used to monitor for complications and for any change in the appearance of opacities.

When comparing with previous AP examinations make sure you understand the position that the patient was in when the examinations were taken. In order to accurately assess disease progression, or recovery, it is essential to compare sequential examinations with the patient in the same anatomical position (supine compared to supine, or erect compared to erect). It is very difficult to assess for change in fluid status when comparing a supine with an erect x-ray.

Supine Versus Erect X-rays (Fig. 4a,b)

1. Fluid will gravitate to the lowest part of the thorax, which in the supine position will be posterior and inferior. Air in the pleural space will rise to the anterior part of the thorax.

2. The supine position causes diverting of blood from the lung bases to the apices, with enlargement of the upper lobe vessels in the normal patient. The prominent vessels can mimic volume overload or failure. This finding disappears by positioning the patient erect.

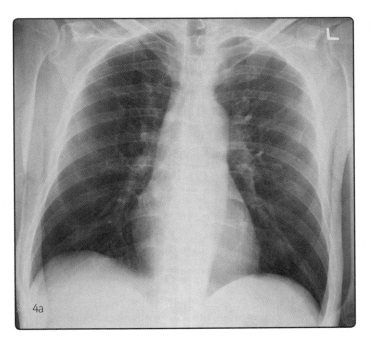

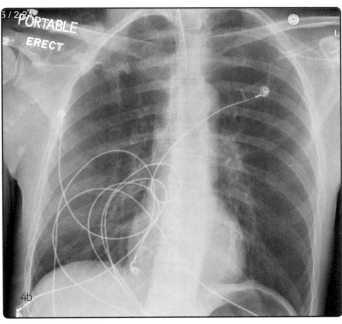

Figure 4. Supine versus erect chest x-rays. There are some important features of supine versus an erect AP chest x-ray. Fluid and air will distribute differently, and the upper lobe vessels will appear enlarged on the supine film. a, supine AP chest x-ray, b, erect AP chest x-ray.

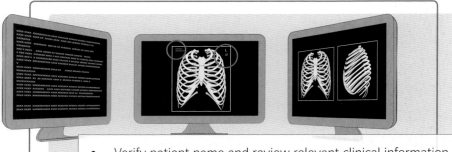

- Verify patient name and review relevant clinical information.
- Pay special attention to type of x-ray.
- Compare with previous radiological exams and reports.
- Review markers on x-ray.
- Make sure technically adequate.

1 **Preparatory phase**

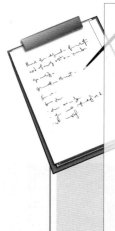

- Record information related to shape, size, borders, grayscale changes, position, distribution, secondary effects, etc.
- Describe information in context of acute setting.
- Are the opacities worsening or getting better?
- Is the volume worsening or getting better?
- Has there been a change in the position of the lines and tubes?

3 **Descriptive phase**

2 **Visual identification phase**

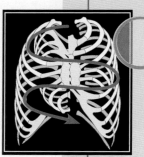

- Compare to normal.
- Scan x-ray using systematic approach.
- Make note of lines and tubes.
- Pay special attention to: cardiovascular status, parenchymal opacities, signs of barotrauma, effusions and rib fractures.

INTERPRETATION OF THE AP CHEST X-RAY

1. Preparatory Phase

The patient and examination identification is done on PACS; the same as for a PA x-ray. Because critically ill patients may have multiple chest x-ray examinations, sometimes on the same day, special care must be taken to understand the chronology of the examinations. Attention must be paid to how the examination was performed, the quality of the examination, and the patient positioning.

Was the patient supine, erect, or semi-erect? These positions will change the appearance (e.g., size) of the blood vessels, and alter the appearance of various pathologies (e.g., pleural fluid).

Is the x-ray technically adequate? The adequacy of the AP x-ray is assessed the same way as for a PA x-ray (**Ch. 1, Pg. 41**). You should assess the degree of inspiration, exposure, rotation, and positioning.

2. Visual Identification Phase

These patients are acutely ill therefore you need to look for changes in grayscale that can help diagnose acute abnormalities. Determine if the examination is normal or abnormal. If abnormal, determine if it is too white or too black. Comparison with previous x-rays is essential to identify subtle grayscale changes.

Similar to interpreting PA or lateral x-rays, use a systematic approach to scan the AP x-ray for abnormalities. Keep in mind that the systematic approach needs to be modified to accommodate for characteristics unique to the AP examination, and special attention should be paid to the following items.

- Location of lines, tubes and devices (**Ch. 20**).
- Cardiovascular status.
- Parenchymal opacities.
- Signs of barotraumas
- Effusions.
- Rib fractures.

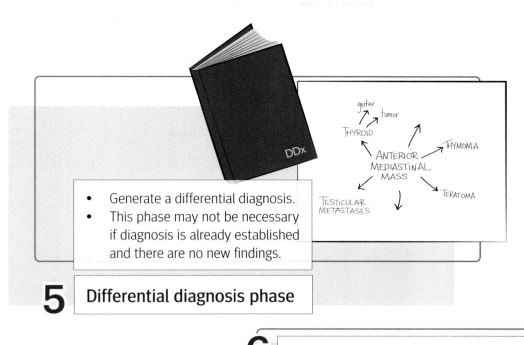

- Generate a differential diagnosis.
- This phase may not be necessary if diagnosis is already established and there are no new findings.

5 | **Differential diagnosis phase**

6 | **Communication (action) phase**

- Always review as soon as the x-rays are available on PACS.
- Communicate any unusual findings to the rest of the clinical team.

4 | **Summary phase**

- Generate summary statement(s) based on key findings.
- List all patterns and signs in order of clinical importance.
- Critically ill patients will often have multiple relevant findings!

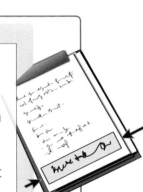

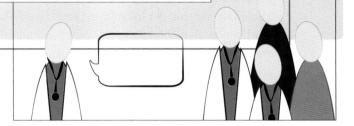

3. Descriptive Phase

The radiological findings must be described in the context of the acute setting, with special attention paid to line and tube position, cardiovascular status, possible barotrauma, and effusions. In many cases the clinical diagnosis has already been established, and the x-rays are used to determine any temporal change.

Are the opacities worsening or getting better?
Is the overall lung volume improving or worsening?
Has there been a change in position of the lines or tubes?

4. Summary Phase

Based on the radiological findings identify any patterns and signs, and list each. In these critically ill patients it would be very common to have several findings, all of which may be relevant. The findings should be listed in order of clinical importance.

5. Differential Diagnosis Phase

Formulate a differential diagnosis for each of the relevant findings. This phase is not necessary if the diagnosis has already been established and there are no new findings.

6. Communication Phase

Always review the images as soon as they are available for viewing on PACS. Communicate any unusual findings to the rest of the clinical team.

PROBLEMS SPECIFIC TO THE INTENSIVE CARE UNIT PATIENT

Lines, Tubes and Other Devices

As a priority, all medical lines, tubes and devices should be identified in patients in the ICU. Care must be taken to identify the correct location of each device separately. This can be challenging especially when multiple devices are present (Fig. 6a,b). A full review of proper device positioning is found in Chapter 20.

Watching the Hemodynamics of an ICU Patient

Typically, the hemodynamic status of an ICU patient is monitored using central venous catheters (CVCs) and Swan-Ganz catheters. Central venous pressure (CVP) is monitored by CVCs. Swan-Ganz catheters (pulmonary capillary wedge pressure monitors) are used to accurately assess the patient's volume status, and can help differentiate between cardiac and non-cardiac pulmonary edema (Table 19.2). A full discussion on the radiological features of heart failure is found in Chapter 10.

Although technically difficult, erect and supine AP examinations, when done properly, can also be used to follow the patient's hemodynamic status. The size of the upper lobe vessels and the size of the vascular pedicle can be measured on an AP x-ray, and closely monitored over time (Fig. 7a,b).

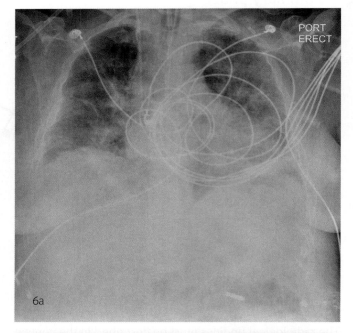

6a

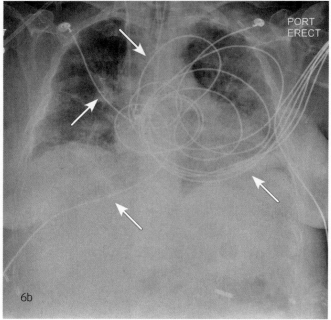

6b

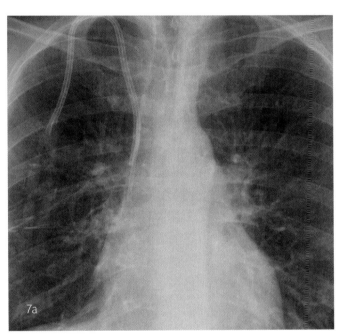

7a

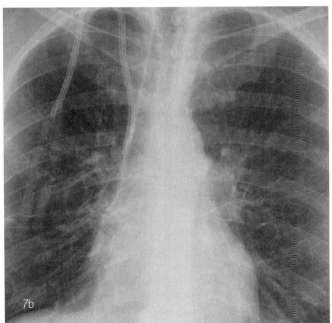

7b

	TYPE OF PULMONARY EDEMA	
	CARDIAC	NON-CARDIAC
Heart size	Increased	Normal
Vascular redistribution	Increased	Normal
Kerley B lines	Present	Absent
Peribronchial cuffing	Present	Absent
Vascular pedicle	Widened	Normal
Azygos vein	Enlarged	Normal
Alveolar edema	Present	Present
Pleural effusion	Common	Uncommon
Response to gravity	Yes	No

Table 19.2
Comparing Cardiac and Non-cardiac Pulmonary Edema

Figure 6. Lines and tubes on the AP chest x-ray.
Often AP chest x-rays will have numerous lines and tubes visible, which can be challenging to interpret. a, AP chest x-ray showing multiple tubes and lines, b, AP chest x-ray with the tubes and lines highlighted.

Figure 7. Hemodynamics on the AP chest x-ray.
AP chest x-rays can be used to monitor an ICU patient's hemodynamic status. a, AP chest x-ray with prominent upper lobe vessels due to vascular redistribution, b, AP chest x-ray from the same patient with normal upper lobe vessels, after the vascular redistribution has resolved.

Aspiration Pneumonitis

Acutely ill and post-operative patients are more prone to aspiration because of decreased consciousness, a decreased gag response, and because they may be intubated.

Chest x-ray features:

- Multi-focal airspace opacities that are gravity dependent (in the supine patient, and more commonly in the posterior segments of the upper lobes, or the apical segments of the lower lobes).
- Possible necrotizing pneumonia, and lung abscess.
- Possible atelectasis (if larger particles are aspirated).
- Possible ARDS (with aspiration of gastric contents).

Acute Respiratory Distress Syndrome (ARDS)

ARDS is a life-threatening lung condition that prevents enough oxygen from getting into the blood (8,9), due to a build up of fluid in the air sacs. ARDS needs to be differentiated from cardiac causes of pulmonary edema.

Chest x-ray features of ARDS (Fig. 8)

Present

- Diffuse airspace disease.
- More prominent in the periphery.
- Pleural effusions may occur.

Uncommon/Absent

- Kerley B lines.
- Peribronchial cuffing.
- Abnormal heart size.
- Vascular redistribution.

Temporal features of ARDS

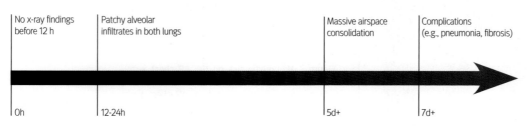

No x-ray findings before 12 h	Patchy alveolar infiltrates in both lungs		Massive airspace consolidation	Complications (e.g., pneumonia, fibrosis)
0h	12-24h		5d+	7d+

Figure 8. Aspiration pneumonitis. AP chest x-ray from a patient with aspiration pneumonitis. Note the example of aspiration in the right lung.

Figure 9. ARDS. AP chest x-ray from a patient with ARDS.

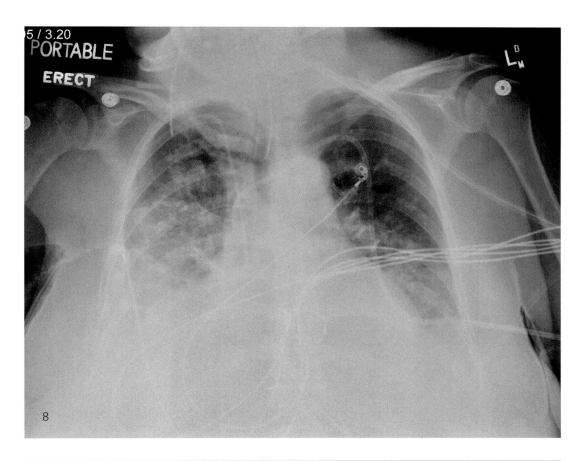

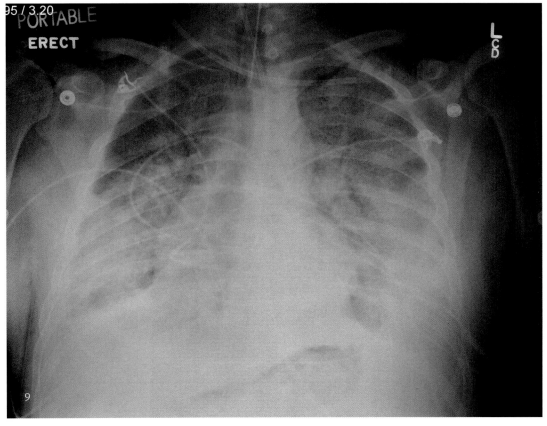

Suspect collapse if you see the following indirect signs.
- Elevation of a hemidiaphragm.
- Splaying or crowding of vessels.
- Triangular opacities.
- Hilar displacement.
- Mediastinal shift.

!

ATELECTASIS/COLLAPSE AND THE AP X-RAY

The presence of atelectasis in an ICU patient is important to recognize and treat. When evaluating the acutely ill ICU patient you will not have the luxury of a lateral x-ray, and therefore you will be limited to the single AP view for your diagnosis. The appearance of atelectasis on an AP x-ray is important to remember (Table 19.3)(Fig. 10a,b).

As we have learned the lateral x-ray is very valuable in determining fissure displacement. Without the lateral x-ray (as in the case of an ICU patient) we can suspect collapse, but in clinically problematic patients, confirmation will sometimes require cross sectional imaging (Fig. 10b).

LOBAR COLLAPSE	CHARACTERISTIC
RUL Collapse	• Minor fissure displaced superiorly. • Increased opacity in the right upper hemithorax medially. • Obscuration of the superior vena cava. • Apical opacity.
RML Collapse	• Obscuration of right heart border. • Increased opacity of the right lung base medially, adjacent to the heart.
RLL Collapse	• Triangular opacity of the right lung base medially, obscuring the medial aspect of right hemidiaphragm. • Right heart border normal.
LUL Collapse	• Opacity overlying the left hilum with a loss of the left side of the H-shape of the hilum. • Partial obscuration of the superior aspect of left heart border.
LLL Collapse	• Triangular opacity of the left lung base medially, obscuring the medial aspect of left hemidiaphragm. • Left heart border normal.

Table 19.3
Characteristics of Collapse on the AP X-ray

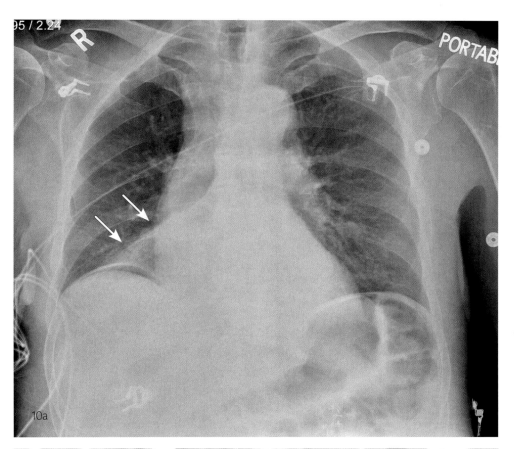

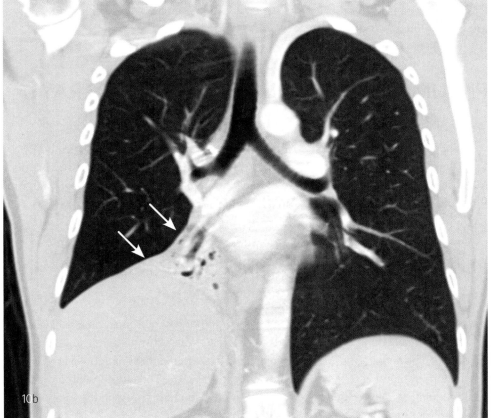

Figure 10. Atelectasis and the AP chest x-ray. a, AP chest x-ray from a patient with collapse of the right lower lobe (arrows), b, coronal CT scan from the same patient highlighting collapse of the right lower lobe (arrows).

PNEUMOTHORAX AND THE AP X-RAY

In the erect position, air in the pleural space will rise to the most superior part of the thorax, the apex. In the supine position air within the pleural space will rise to the most anterior part of the thorax, which is usually in the inferior aspect of the thorax. In this position the pneumothorax may be difficult to identify.

On the supine x-ray, the most reliable indicator of a pneumothorax is the deep sulcus sign (10,11) (Fig. 11)(Ch. 11, Pg., 430). Air accumulating in the pleural space anteriorly, inferiorly, and laterally will cause the otherwise sharp costophrenic angle to deepen, and this area will look too black – the deep sulcus sign.

PNEUMOMEDIASTINUM AND THE AP X-RAY

A pneumomediastinum on the AP x-ray will look exactly the same as on the PA x-ray. Air in the mediastinum will appear as black lines extending through the tissue planes within the mediastinum (Fig. 12). The air in the mediastinum will not be gravity dependant and will have the same radiological appearance on the erect, or the supine, AP chest x-ray.

PLEURAL EFFUSION AND THE AP X-RAY

Although more difficult to visualize, a pleural effusion can be seen on a supine x-ray, however, the fluid collection typically needs to be greater than 200 ml. On a supine x-ray, the pleural effusion can be detected as an increased opacity of the hemithorax, without a loss of the pulmonary vasculature or blunting of the costophrenic angles (Fig. 13). The effusion will be seen as a band of white running parallel to the lungs, vertically. If enough fluid is present, the lungs will be displaced medially from the ribs.

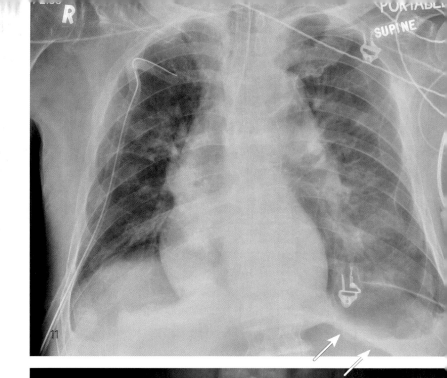

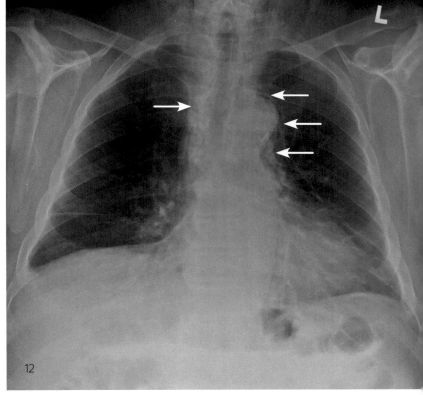

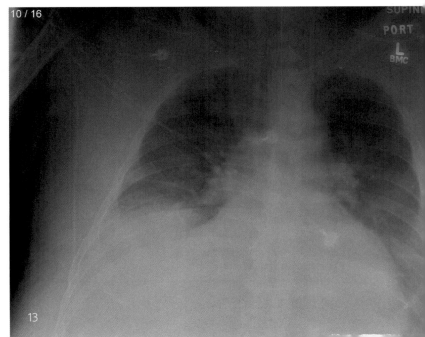

Figure 11. Pneumothorax and the AP chest x-ray. Supine AP chest x-ray from a patient with a treated pneumothorax. Notice the deep sulcus sign on the left (arrows).

Figure 12. Pneumomediastinum and the AP chest x-ray. AP chest x-ray from a patient with a pneumomediastinum (arrows).

Figure 13. Pleural effusion and the AP chest x-ray. Supine AP chest x-ray from a patient with bilateral pleural effusions; the pleural effusions can be seen as diffuse whiteness over the lower portions of the lungs.

725

AP X-ray Radiological Analysis Checklist

In order to make sure that the AP chest x-ray examination is of good quality, all parts of the checklist should indicate good quality.

PATIENT POSITIONING

1   Is the patient position correct?
     (rotation/centering)

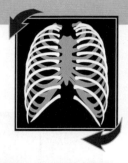
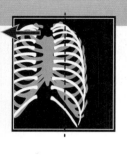

If **NO**, then describe.

Rotated right/left.
Shifted right/left.

QUALITY of INSPIRATION

2   Did the patient take a good
     inspiration?

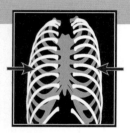

If **NO**, then describe.

Give number of posterior ribs visible.

EXPOSURE

3   Is the x-ray of adequate exposure?

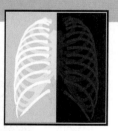

If **NO**, then describe.

Underexposed/overexposed.

LINES & TUBES

4   Are there lines and tubes present?

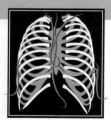

If **YES**, describe.

ETT/NG/CVC/SG/chest tubes/pacers.
Correct position/incorrect position.

BAROTRAUMA

5   Is there evidence of barotrauma?

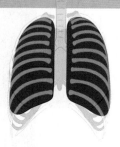

If **YES**, describe.

Pneumothorax.
Pneumomediastinum

CARDIOVASCULAR STATUS

6 Is there evidence of cardiac failure?

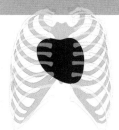

If **YES**, describe.

Vascular redistribution.
Edema.
Cardiomegaly.

LUNG PARENCHYMA

7 Is there evidence of airspace disease?

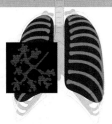

If **YES**, describe.

Right/left/bilateral.
Central/peripheral.
Better/worse.

PLEURAL EFFUSION

8 Is there evidence of a pleural effusion?

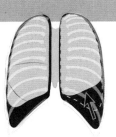

If **YES**, describe.

Right/left.
Give size.

RIB FRACTURES

9 Is there evidence of damage to the bony thorax?

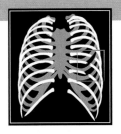

If **YES**, describe.

Right/left.
Give rib number.

COMPARE WITH PREVIOUS

10 Are there any changes compared to previous radiological examinations?

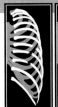

2013/05/13   2009/01/05

If **YES**, describe.

Improvement/progression.

If **NO**, state no change from previous.

14a

What are important steps in interpreting the AP x-ray?

CASE STUDY

You are working in the intensive care unit. Your non-ventilated patient on I.V. heparin developed acute shortness of breath and a drop in hemoglobin. You cannot hear any breath sounds on the right. You order a portable chest x-ray (Fig. 14a).

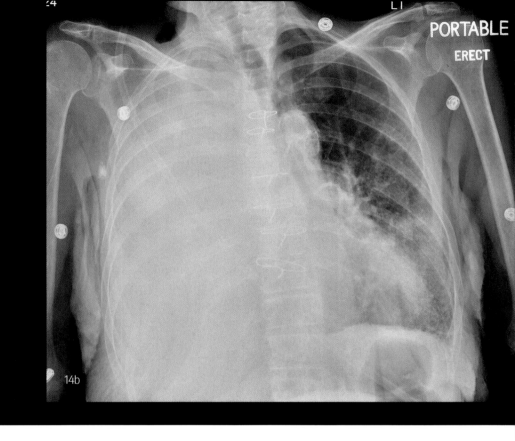

The examination shows complete whiteout of the right hemithorax. The mediastinal structures are shifted to the left consistent with mass effect on the mediastinum. The appearance is consistent with a massive right pleural effusion. The drop in hemoglobin suggests the pleural fluid is hemorrhagic.

Based on the findings, the diagnosis is acute right hemothorax.

DISCUSSION

References

1. Lewis, P.J., Shaffer, K., & Donovan, A. (Eds.). (2012). AMSER National Medical Student Curriculum in Radiology. http://aur.org/Secondary-Alliances.aspx?id=141.

2. Lewis, P.J., & Shaffer, K. (2005). Developing a national medical student curriculum in radiology. *Am. Coll. Radiol., 2*(1):8–11.

3. Amorosa, J.K., Bramwit, M.P., Mohammed, T.L., et al. (2011). Expert Panel on Thoracic Imaging. ACR Appropriateness Criteria® routine chest radiographs in ICU patients. [online publication]. Reston, VA: American College of Radiology (ACR).

4. Henschke, C.I., Pasternack, G.S., Schroeder, S., et al. (1983). Bedside chest radiography: diagnostic efficacy. *Radiology, 149*:23–26.

5. Bekemeyer, W.B., Crapo, R.O., Calhoon, S., et al. (1985). Efficacy of chest radiography in a respiratory intensive care unit: a prospective study. *Chest, 88*:691–696.

6. Graat, M.E., Choi, G., Wolthuis, E.K., et al. (2006). The clinical value of daily routine chest radiographs in a mixed medical-surgical intensive care unit is low. *Crit. Care, 10*(1):R11.

7. Adams, F.G. (1979). A simplified approach to the reporting of intensive therapy unit chest radiographs. *Clinical Radiology, 30*(2): 219–226.

8. Goldman, L., & Schafer, A.I. (Eds.). (2012). Cecil Medicine, 24th ed. Philadelphia, PA: Elsevier Health Sciences.

9. Khan, A.N., Al-Jahdali, H., Al-Ghanem, S., & Gouda, A. (2009). Reading chest radiographs in the critically ill (Part II): Radiography of lung pathologies common in the ICU patient. *Ann. Thorac. Med., 4*(3): 149–157.

10. Cummin, A.R.C., Smith, M.J., & Wilson, A.G. (1987). Pneumothorax in the supine patient. *Br. Med. J., 295*: 591–592.

11. Kong, A. (2003). The deep sulcus sign. *Radiology, 228*(2): 415–416.

CHAPTER 20
LINES & TUBES

importance

Many types of lines and tubes are used in the hospital setting for the care of patients; especially those who are critically ill. Chest x-rays are ordered to make sure that any tubes and lines used in patient care are in the right place. Simply identifying that a line or tube exists on a chest x-ray is not enough. Aberrant tube or line placement can lead to increased morbidity and mortality. For example, the placement of a nasogastric tube into the airways can lead to a pneumothorax. This chapter will help you localize lines and tubes with confidence, and hopefully minimize complications made by aberrant tube or line placement through accurate recognition.

objectives

Skills

You will identify

- an endotracheal tube, tracheostomy tube, nasogastric tube, chest tube, central venous line, and cardiac pacemaker, on the PA and lateral chest x-rays.

- the key radiological landmarks used for the assessment of line and tube placement.

- aberrant endotracheal and nasogastric tube placement on the PA and lateral chest x-rays.

associated resources

This chapter maps to the following AMSER curriculum content (1,2).

1) Iatrogenic pathology
    Malplaced endotracheal tube (e.g., too high, low, esophageal)
    Malplaced Dobhoff/nasogastric tubes (e.g., esophagus, trachea, bronchus)
    Malplaced central venous catheters (e.g., jugular, subclavian, right atrium)
    Other misplaced wires, catheters

2) Emergency radiology

3) Iatrogenic pneumothorax and pneumomediastinum

4) Correct position of chest tubes

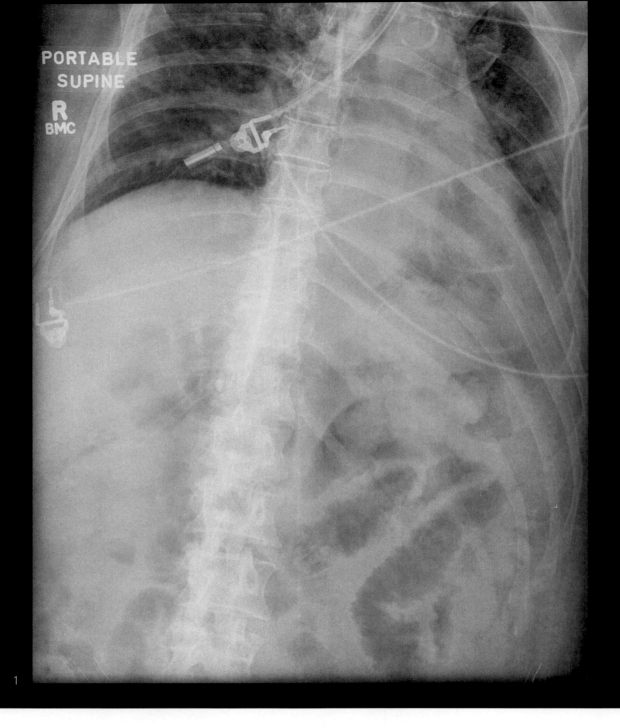

CASE STUDY

During your general medical rotation as an intern, you are asked to place a nasogastric tube into a patient that has suffered an ischemic stroke. You have some difficulty inserting the tube, and you are concerned about whether or not you placed it in the right position within the stomach. The patient has lost the ability to swallow, and does not have a gag reflex, so it is even more difficult for you to determine whether or not the tube is in the right place. You follow protocol and order an x-ray of the lower chest and upper abdomen (Fig. 1).

Can you determine if
the nasogastric tube
is in the right place?

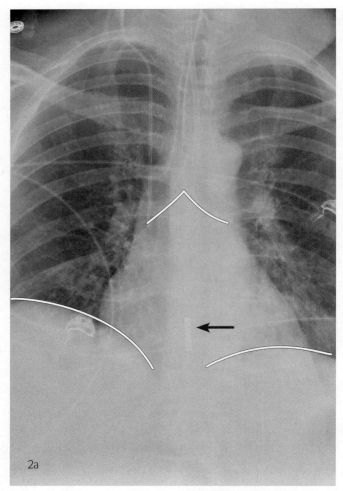

2a

LINES, TUBES & DEVICES

During the course of treating various thoracic and systemic diseases, lines and tubes are inserted into various thoracic structures for the purpose of:

- Maintaining physiological functions.
- Monitoring of physiological functions.
- Drug and nutrition delivery.
- Treatment.

Tubes and lines can be 'internal' (i.e., inserted into blood vessels, cardiac chambers, pleural spaces, the lungs, the esophagus, the spinal canal, and the airways).

Lines and tubes can also be seen on the surface of the thorax. These external lines and tubes need to be identified to avoid confusion with internal lines, because they can obscure relevant pathology, or may mimic disease.

Radiological landmarks are used to verify the position of all lines and tubes (Fig. 2a,b,c,d).

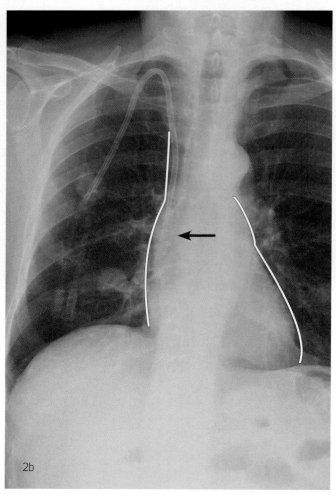

2b

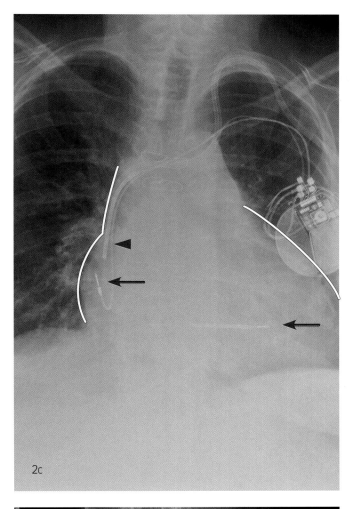

2c

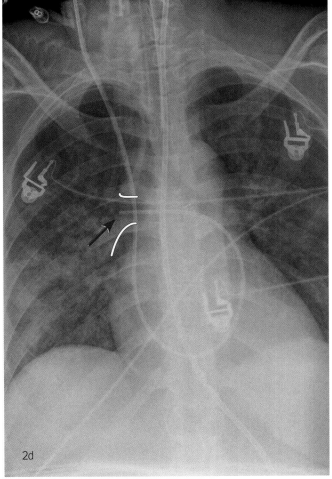

2d

Figure 2. Landmarks can be used to identify line and tube position. a, AP chest x-ray showing an NG tube (arrow) in relation to the carina and diaphragms, b, PA chest x-ray showing a CVC (arrow) in relation to the heart and SVC, c, PA chest x-ray showing an AV pacemaker (arrows) and a CVC (arrow head) in relation to the heart and SVC, d, AP chest x-ray showing a Swan-Ganz catheter (arrow) in relation to the right pulmonary artery (RPA).

THE AIRWAYS

Two types of tubes are inserted into the airways: the endotracheal tube (ETT), and the tracheostomy tube.

Understanding the Path of Airway Tube Insertion (Fig. 3)

Oral or nasal cavity (oral is shown)
Pharynx
Trachea

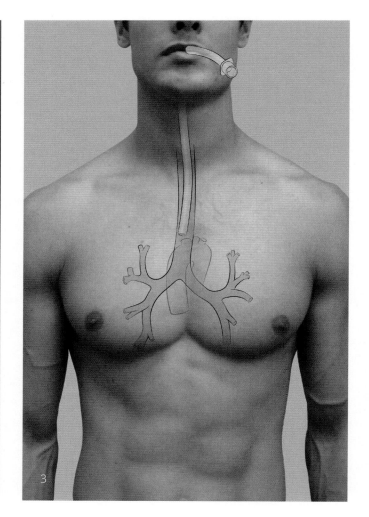

Figure 3. The path of airway tube insertion. Artistic rendition of the path of airway tube insertion via the oral route.

738

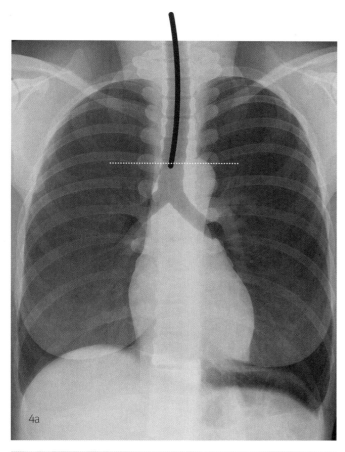

4a

Correct Airway Tube Positioning

The endotracheal tube (ETT)

The ideal position for the tip of the ETT is approximately 5 cm above the carina (Fig. 4a,b), whether the tube was inserted through an oral or nasal approach. To confirm the proper positioning of the tip of the ETT you need to first identify two structures. One is the carina (Ch. 7, Pg. 198), and the second is the tip of the ETT. Fortunately the identification of the ETT is facilitated by the presence of a longitudinal strip of radiopaque material that is embedded into the ETT during the manufacturing process.

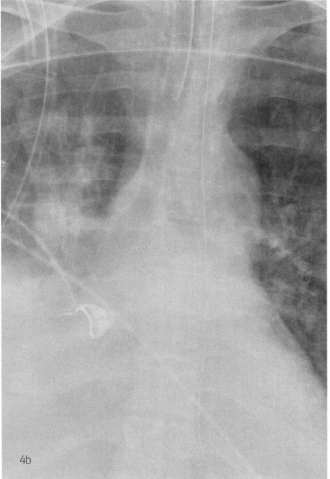

4b

Figure 4. Correct endotracheal (ETT) positioning. The ideal position of the ETT is 5 cm above the carina. a, illustration of ideal ETT tube position, b, AP chest x-ray with ETT tube correctly placed.

Neck position can be assessed by establishing the position of the mandible on the x-ray. In neutral position the mandible lies at the level of the fifth or sixth cervical vertebrae (C5-C6); in flexion it lies at the level of the first thoracic vertebrae (T1), and above the third or fourth cervical vertebrae (C3-C4) on extension. Unfortunately the mandible is frequently not visualized on the chest x-ray, and therefore cannot be used as a reliable landmark.

ai

Head and neck movement can partially displace the position of the ETT (3). Extension of the neck can cause withdrawal of the ETT up to 2 cm (range 0.2 to 5.2 cm), and potential vocal cord damage or extubation (Fig. 5a). Flexion of the neck can cause the ETT to advance up to 2 cm (range 0.2 to 3.1 cm), potentially into a bronchus (Fig. 5b). The ideal position of the tip of the ETT is therefore governed by the position of the head and neck.

The ideal position of the tip of the ETT with the neck in neutral position is 5 +/- 2 cm above the carina.

The ideal position of the tip of the ETT with the neck in flexed position is 3 +/- 2 cm above the carina.

The ideal position of the tip of the ETT with the neck in extended position is 7 +/- 2 cm above the carina.

Figure 5. Head and neck position influence the placement of the endotracheal tube (ETT). a, illustration of the change in ETT tube position when the head is extended, b, illustration of the change in ETT tube position when the head is flexed.

Figure 6. Correct tracheostomy tube positioning. The ideal position of the tracheostomy tube is 5 cm above the carina. a, illustration of the ideal tracheostomy tube position, b, AP chest x-ray with a correctly placed tracheostomy tube.

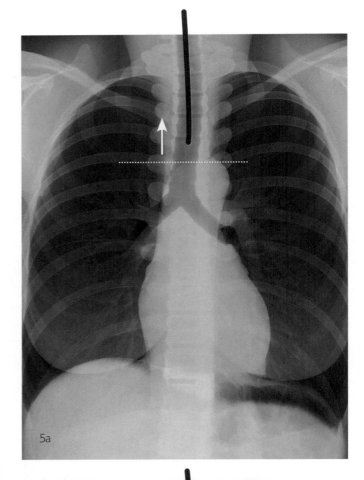

5a

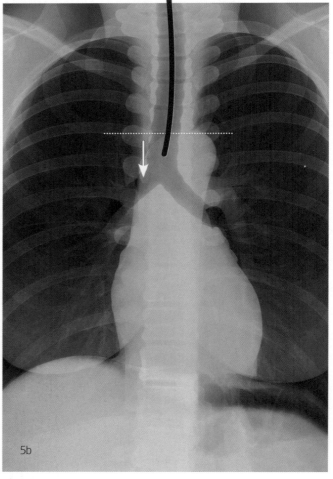

5b

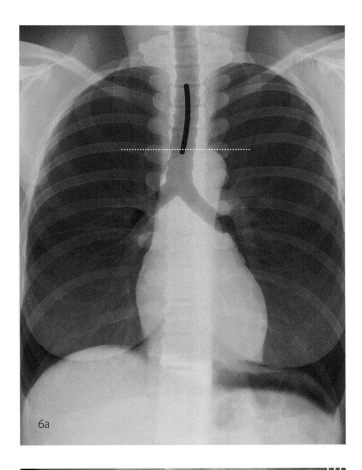

6a

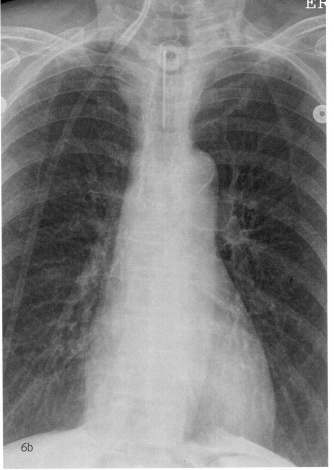

6b

The tracheostomy tube

A tracheostomy tube is inserted intraoperatively. An incision is made anteriorly in the upper trachea, and a curved tube with a cuff is inserted. Similar to the ETT, the tip of the tracheostomy tube should lie above the carina. Tracheostomy tubes are made of various materials. The visibility of the tube on x-rays will depend on the amount of radiopaque material present within the tube (Fig. 6a,b).

Airway tubes may be cuffed or uncuffed. The tubes may be preformed, and may be enforced. Endotracheal tubes may also be coaxial with endotracheal and endobronchial channels, and two separate openings allowing for the intubation of one lung selectively.

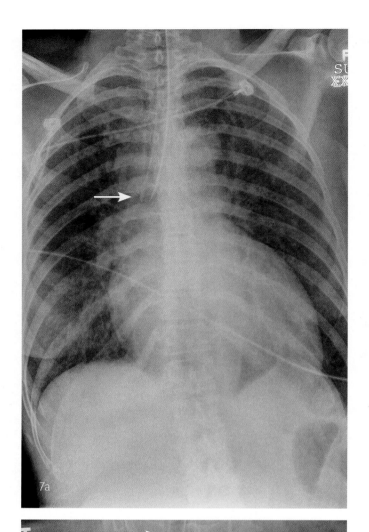

Abnormal Airway Tube Positioning

The ETT can be positioned too high or too low within the airways, or it may be positioned outside of the airways (4,5).

The ETT can lie too low at the level of the carina, or below the level of the carina within a main stem bronchus (Fig. 7a). This can lead to atelectasis or collapse of the non-ventilated lung.

The position of the vocal cords is at the fifth or sixth cervical vertebrae (C5-C6). Positioning of the inflated cuff of the ETT too high (Fig. 7b) can lead to damage of the larynx, especially the vocal cords. Tracheal necrosis or laryngeal nerve paralysis can also result.

Figure 7. Abnormal airway tube positioning. a, AP chest x-ray with the tip of ETT tube (arrow) within the right main stem bronchus, b, AP chest x-ray with the tip of the ETT tube too high (arrow), within the upper trachea.

THE UPPER GASTROINTESTINAL TRACT

Generally, upper gastrointestinal (GI) tubes are inserted into the esophagus and stomach to remove excess gas and fluid, or for the delivery of nutrition. Nasogastric (NG) tubes are used for suctioning and drainage, whereas Dobhoff tubes are used for feeding purposes.

Understanding the Path of NG and Dobhoff Tube Insertion (Fig. 8)

Nasal or oral cavity (nasal is shown)
Pharynx
Esophagus
Stomach
Duodenum

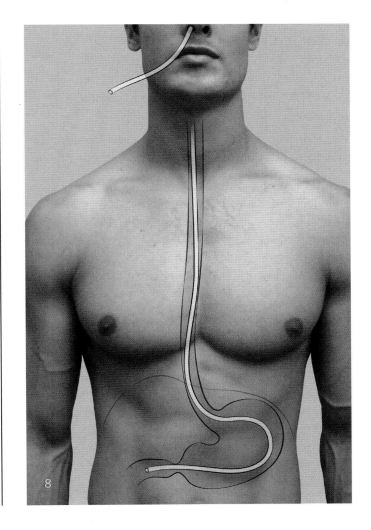

Figure 8. Path of the upper GI tubes. Artistic rendition of the path of the NG and Dobhoff tube insertion via the nasal route.

Correct Upper GI Tube Positioning

Nasogastric (NG) tubes

NG tubes are of various sizes, and most are easily identified radiologically because of the presence of a radiopaque longitudinal stripe. The tip of the NG tube should lie below the diaphragms, preferably in the region of the antrum of the stomach (Fig. 9a,b).

Dobhoff tubes

The Dobhoff tube is named after Dr. R. Dobbie and Dr. J Hoffmeister. The Dobhoff tube differs from the NG tube in that it comes equipped with a thin guide wire, and a weighted end. The guide wire is necessary to increase the rigidity of the tube and assists with initial tube placement. The tip of the tube is stiff, and is filled with metal and is easily identified on x-rays. The tip of the Dobhoff tube should be positioned in the region of the antrum of the stomach, or in the duodenum.

Abnormal Upper GI Tube Positioning

The main concern with abnormal NG or Dobhoff tube placement is the aberrant placement into the airways (6).

The NG or Dobhoff tube maybe placed in the trachea or a bronchus. If the aberrant positioning within the airways is not suspected and corrected, the tube can be advanced through the lung into the pleural space (Fig. 10a,b). Patients that are at high risk for tracheal or bronchial placement of NG tubes include the elderly, intubated and heavily sedated patients, patients with stroke, or comatose patients.

The NG or Dobhoff tube may also be positioned too high in the esophagus, within the thorax. Leaving the tube in this position puts the patient at a higher risk of aspiration. The tube may be coiled in the oropharynx, or within a hiatus hernia or an esophageal diverticulum. Intracranial placement of NG tubes through the cribiform plate has also been described (7). The tube can be coiled upon itself with formation of a knot, making the free removal of the tube difficult, if not impossible. Complications of tube insertion also include esophageal or gastric tears, or perforation (8).

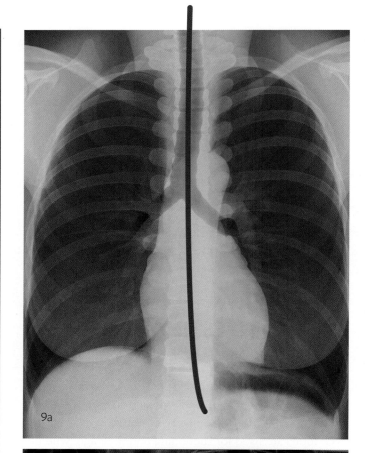

9a

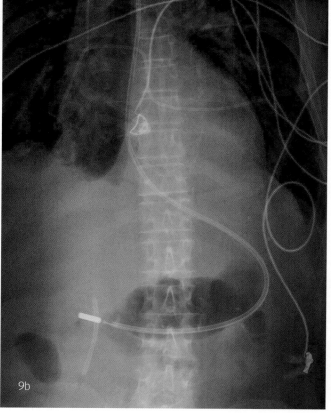

9b

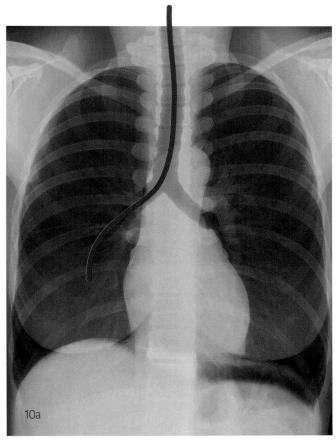

10a

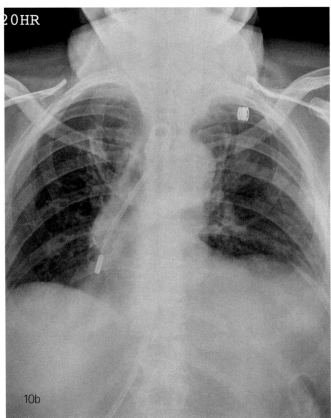

10b

Figure 9. Correct upper GI tube positioning. a, illustration of the ideal NG tube position, b, AP chest x-ray with a correctly placed NG tube.

Figure 10. Abnormal upper GI tube positioning. a, illustration of an incorrectly positioned Dobhoff tube, within the right lung, b, AP chest x-ray with an incorrectly placed Dobhoff tube, positioned within the right lung.

How to assess GI tube placement

Assessing the placement of an upper GI tube (NG or Dobhoff) is important to prevent lung injury and pneumothorax, due to aberrant line positioning.

STEP 1
Confirm that the patient is midline and not rotated (Ch. XX, Fig. XX).

STEP 2
Identify the carina (Fig. 11).

STEP 3
Identify the tube (Fig. 12).

STEP 4
If the tube extends in the midline of the thorax, and the tip lies below the diaphragm, the tube is in the stomach (Fig. 13).

STEP 5
If the tube is in the midline of the thorax, with the tip below the carina, the tube is in the esophagus (Fig. 14).

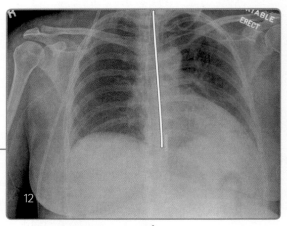

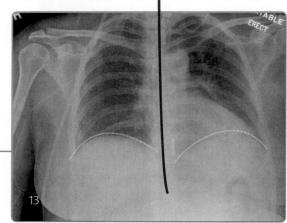

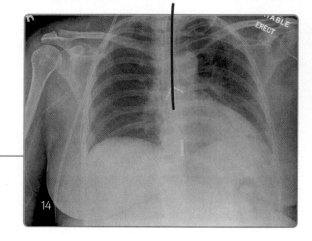

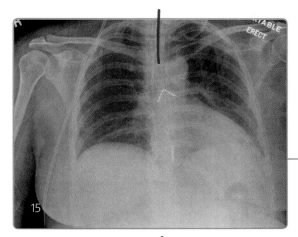

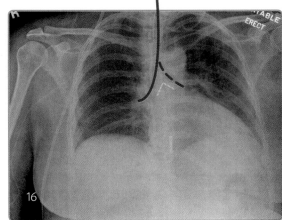

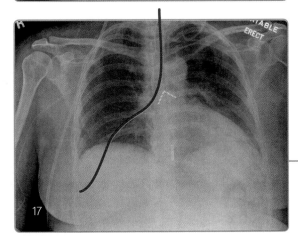

STEP 6

If the tube is in the midline of the thorax, with the tip above the carina, the tube is in the esophagus or the trachea (Fig. 15). *** ALERT ***

STEP 7

If the tube is in the midline of the thorax above the carina, but the tube deviates to the left or right below the carina, the tube is in a bronchus (Fig. 16). ***ALERT ***

STEP 8

If the tube is in the midline of the thorax above the carina, but the tube deviates to the left or right below the carina AND extends to the lateral chest wall, the tube has extended through the bronchial tree into the pleural space (Fig. 17). *** ALERT * Risk of Pneumothorax ***

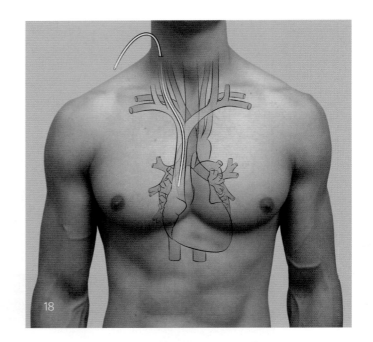

CARDIOVASCULAR

Central Venous Catheters

Central venous catheters (CVC) are inserted to monitor central venous pressure (CVP), to monitor pulmonary artery pressure, for transvenous cardiac pacing, or for the administration of fluids, nutrition and medications.

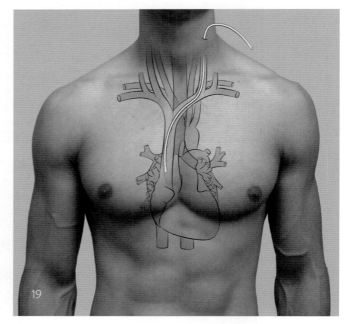

Understanding the path of CVC insertion

CVCs are inserted through the right or left internal or external jugular, subclavian, basilic or cephalic veins.

Right internal jugular vein (Fig. 18)

Right internal jugular vein
Right brachiocephalic vein
SVC

Left internal jugular vein (Fig. 19)

Left internal jugular vein
Left brachiocephalic vein
SVC

Right subclavian vein (Fig. 20)

Right subclavian vein
Right brachiocephalic vein
SVC

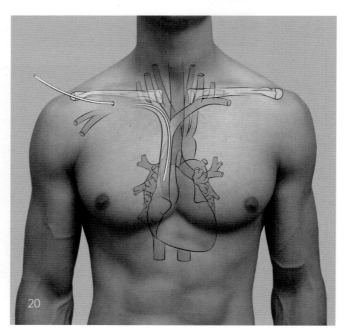

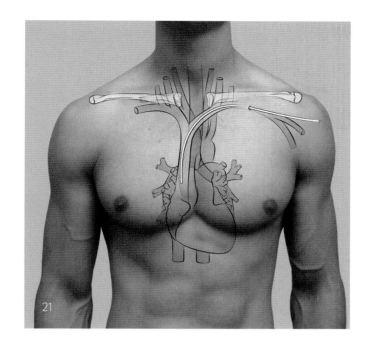

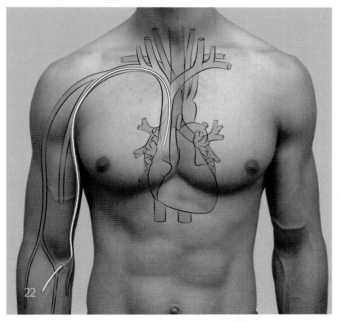

Left subclavian vein (Fig. 21)

Left subclavian vein
Left brachiocephalic vein
SVC

Right cephalic or basilic vein (Fig. 22)

Right basilic or cephalic vein (basilic shown)
Right axillary vein
Right subclavian vein
Right brachiocephalic vein
SVC

Left cephalic or basilic vein (Fig. 23)

Left basilic or cephalic vein (cephalic shown)
Left axillary vein
Left subclavian vein
Left brachiocephalic vein
SVC

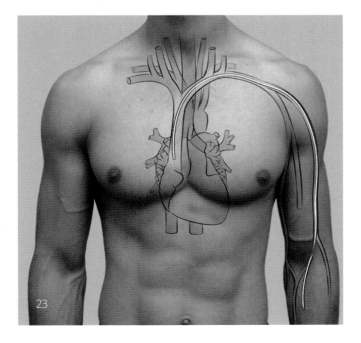

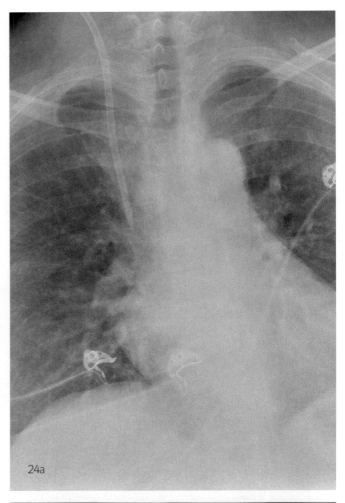

24a

> The pericardial reflection is the most superior border of the pericardium. If a blood vessel is perforated below the reflection, bleeding can occur into the pericardial sac, and can lead to cardiac tamponade.

Correct CVC positioning

The ideal position of the catheter tip is within the superior vena cava, with the tip pointing inferiorly (Fig. 24a). This position cannot always be achieved. The following provides guidance regarding the CVC position (9,10).

The great veins in the lower neck have been divided into three zones of significance for CVC placement (Fig. 24b).

Zone A – this zone lies at, and below the level of the carina, partially within the pericardial reflection. It contains the lower superior vena cava and upper right atrium.

Zone B – this zone lies at, and above the level of the carina, and it contains the upper superior vena cava and the junction of the left and right innominate veins.

Zone C – this zone lies on the left and contains the left innominate veins, proximal to the superior vena cava.

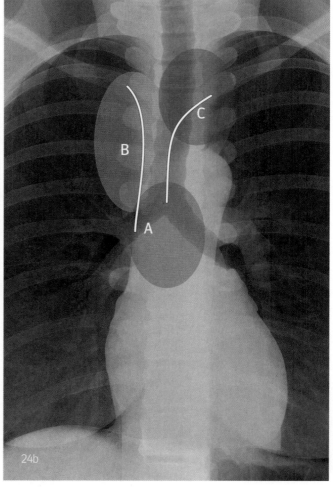

24b

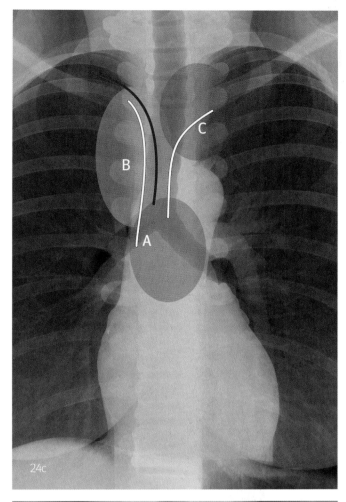

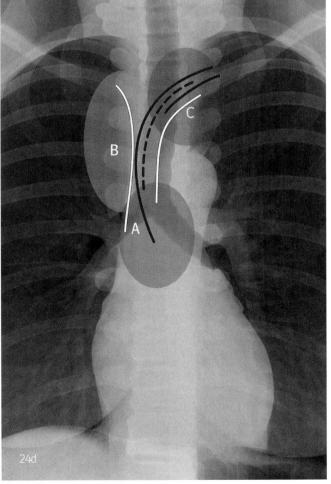

For a CVC inserted on the right side, the ideal position would be in Zone B, at, or just above the carina, with the catheter parallel to the long axis of the superior vena cava (Fig. 24c).

For a CVC inserted on the left, the ideal position is also in Zone B, at, or above the carina. Getting the catheter to lie parallel to the long axis of the superior vena cava can be more difficult to achieve from the left approach. If this position cannot be achieved then a compromise is to position the left CVC in Zone C within the left innominate vein, or in Zone A, at, or below the carina (Fig. 24d).

Figure 24. Correct central venous catheter (CVC) positioning. a, AP x-ray showing correct CVC positioning, b, illustration highlighting the anatomical landmarks used for CVC placement, c, illustration of the ideal right CVC catheter tip position, d, illustration of the ideal left CVC catheter tip position. Dotted line represents the most ideal position, solid lines represent acceptable alternates.

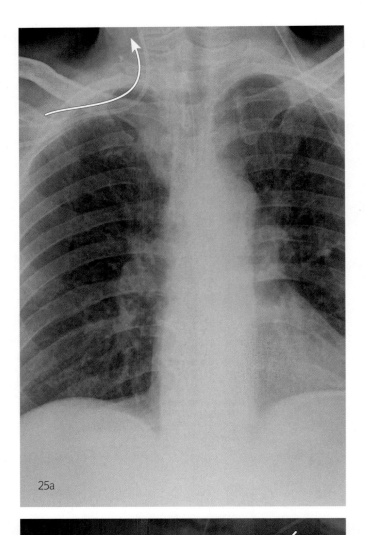

25a

Abnormal CVC positioning

AMSER The CVC can be positioned too far, or too short, relative to the ideal landmarks.

The CVC may be positioned in an aberrant vein.

Figure 25a shows a right subclavian CVC within the right internal jugular vein instead of the SVC. Figure 25b shows the aberrant placement of the left internal jugular CVC in the left subclavian vein.

Figure 25. Abnormal central venous catheter (CVC) positioning. a, AP chest x-ray with aberrant right subclavian CVC in the right internal jugular vein, b, AP chest x-ray with aberrant left internal jugular CVC in the left subclavian vein.

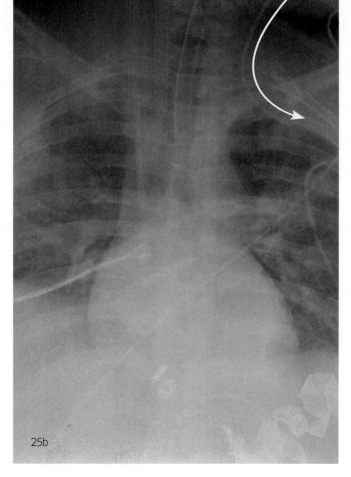

25b

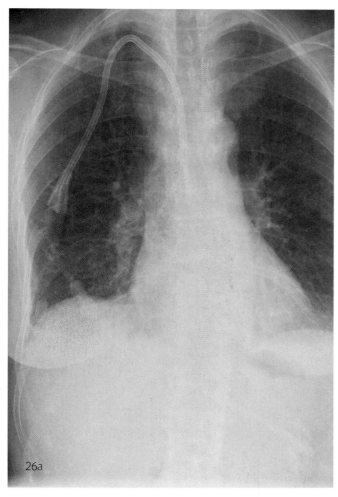

26a

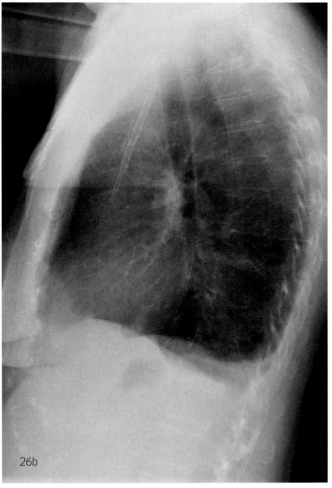

26b

Complications related to CVC placement include (11,12,13,14): **AMSER**

- Pneumothorax
- Pneumomediastinum
- Hydrothorax
- Hemothorax
- Hydromediastinum
- Cardiac tamponade
- Hematoma
- Arterial puncture
- Catheter positioned within an artery (Fig. 26a,b)
- Knot formed in catheter line
- Catheter line broken

Figure 26. Complications of abnormal CVC placement.
If a CVC is not placed correctly there are many potential complications. a, PA chest x-ray with a right CVC incorrectly positioned too medially within the mediastinum, b, lateral chest x-ray showing that the right CVC is aberrantly positioned within the aorta.

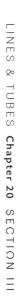

Swan-Ganz Catheter

Swan-Ganz catheters are used for monitoring pulmonary capillary wedge pressure.

Understanding the path of the Swan-Ganz catheter (venous and cardiac anatomy)(Fig. 27)

Example from the right internal jugular vein.

Right internal jugular vein
Right brachiocephalic vein
SVC
Right atrium
Right ventricle
Pulmonary outflow tract
Right or left pulmonary artery (right shown)

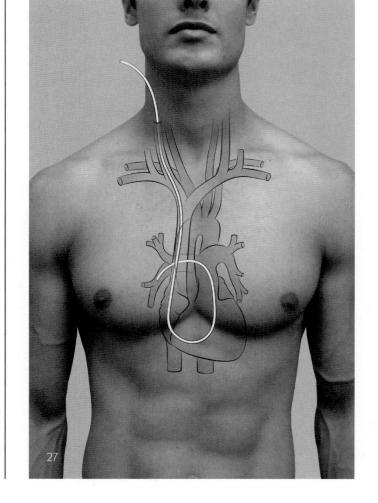

Figure 27. The path of a Swan-Ganz catheter. Artistic rendition of the path of the Swan-Ganz catheter.

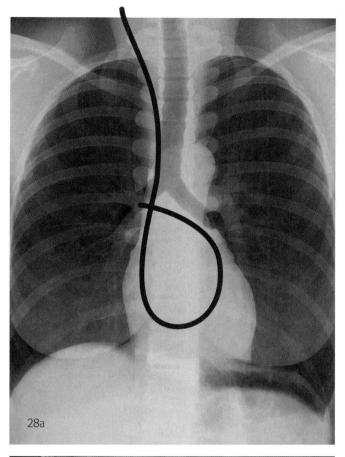

28a

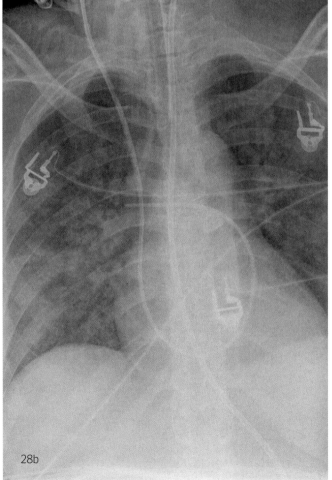

28b

Correct Swan-Ganz catheter positioning

The ideal position of the tip is proximal to the interlobar branch (Fig. 28a,b). The tip will advance with the flow of blood, when the catheter cuff is inflated.

Figure 28. Correct Swan-Ganz catheter positioning. a, illustration of the ideal Swan-Ganz catheter position, b, AP chest x-ray with a correctly positioned Swan-Ganz catheter.

Abnormal Swan-Ganz
catheter positioning (15,16)

The tip can be advanced too far distally (Fig. 29) – this can lead to pulmonary infarction because the blood supply is occluded.

The tip can be positioned in the heart or the coronary sinus.

The catheter can be coiled upon itself in the heart, with the potential creation of a knot in the catheter.

The tip can cause perforation of the heart or the pulmonary arteries (rare).

Aberrant positioning of the catheter tip will lead to erroneous wedge pressure readings.

Complications of Swan-Ganz catheter insertion are the same as those of CVC insertion (Pg. 753).

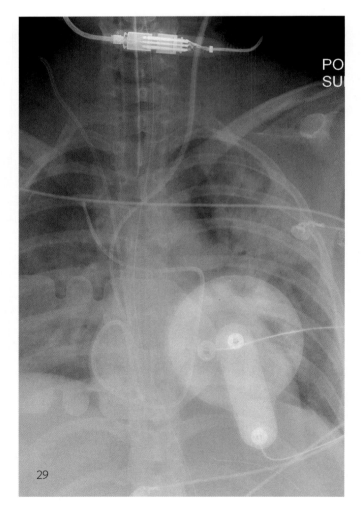

Figure 29. Abnormal Swan-Ganz catheter positioning.
AP chest x-ray with an abnormally positioned Swan-Ganz catheter tip; the tip is positioned too distally within the right pulmonary artery branches.

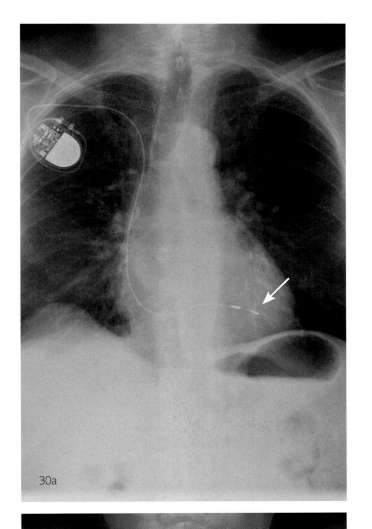

30a

Cardiac Pacing Devices

Cardiac pacing devices can be temporary or permanent, internal and external. There are two common types of cardiac pacemakers – the ventricular pacemaker and the atrio-ventricular sequential pacemaker.

The ideal position for a ventricular pacemaker is the apex of the right ventricle (Fig. 30a).

With the atrio-ventricular sequential pacemaker, the ventricular lead lies in the right ventricle and the atrial lead in the right atrium (Fig. 30b). Always carefully follow the leads to the battery pack to ensure continuity of the lead, because lead fractures can occur.

Figure 30. Correct cardiac pacing device positioning. a, PA chest x-ray with a correctly positioned ventricular pacer (arrow), b, PA chest x-ray with a correctly positioned atrio-ventricular (AV) sequential pacer (arrows).

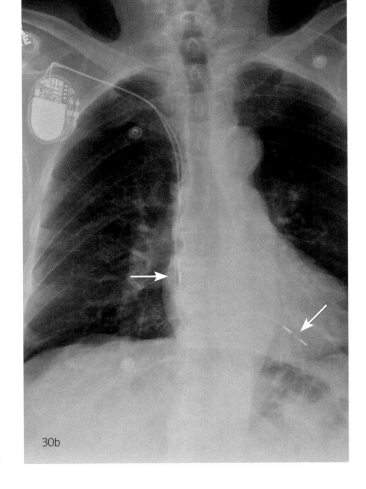

30b

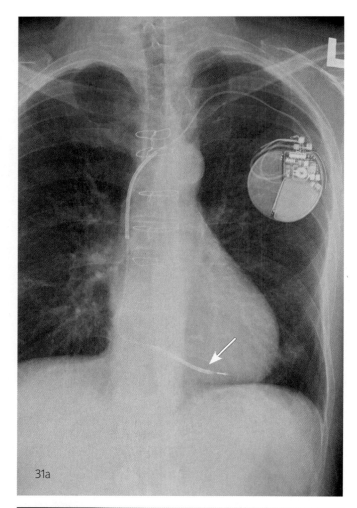

Implantable cardioverter defibrillators differ from regular pacemakers by larger battery packs, and the presence of wire insulation (Fig. 31a,b).

The position of the defibrillator leads is similar to regular pacemaker leads. The placement of the cardiac pacing device leads is usually performed under direct fluoroscopic control.

Figure 31. Implantable defibrillator. a, PA chest x-ray showing ideal defibrillator lead position (arrow), b, lateral chest x-ray from same patient showing ideal defibrillator lead position (arrow).

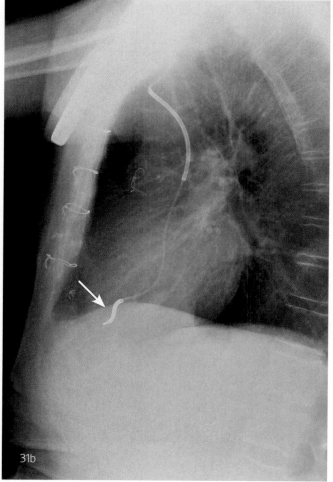

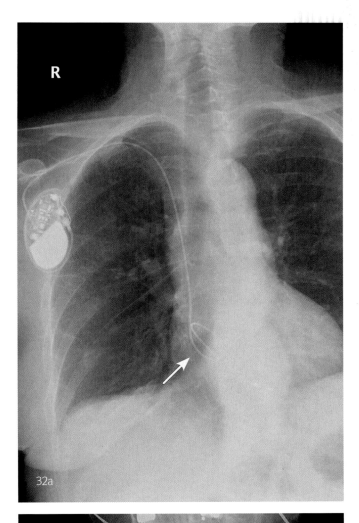

32a

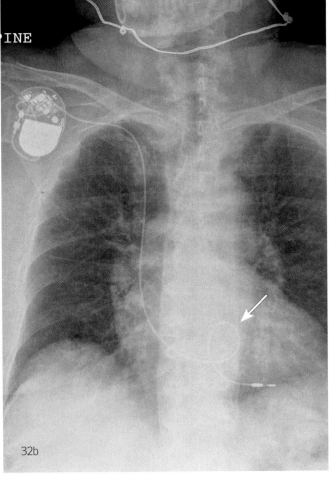

32b

Complications of pacemaker insertion are the same as those of CVC insertion (Pg. 753) but also include lead dislodgment and lead twisting (17,18). Lead twisting, or Twiddlers syndrome (19), is caused by the patient flipping the pacer battery pack on itself over and over again. This causes twisting and eventually shortening of the length of the pacer lead (Fig. 32a,b).

Figure 32. Complications of abnormal pacemaker positioning. a, PA chest x-ray showing a coil in a ventricular lead (arrow), b, PA chest x-ray highlighting coil in a ventricular lead (arrow).

THE PLEURAL SPACE

Chest Tubes

Chest tubes are inserted to treat a pneumothorax, to treat recurrent pleural effusions and emphysema, post lung surgery, and in patients with a high risk of pneumothorax during ventilation.

Chest tubes are placed in the pleural space through the skin and can be single or multiple, unilateral or bilateral. Depending upon the medical problem, the tip of the chest tube may be superior or inferior, medial or lateral. Usually for treatment of a pneumothorax, the tip is directed superiorly.

The visibility of chest tubes will depend on the presence of radiopaque markers (Fig. 33a).

The chest tubes have side holes, and when assessing chest tubes on x-rays, it is important to make sure that the side holes lie within the pleural space and not outside (Fig. 33b).

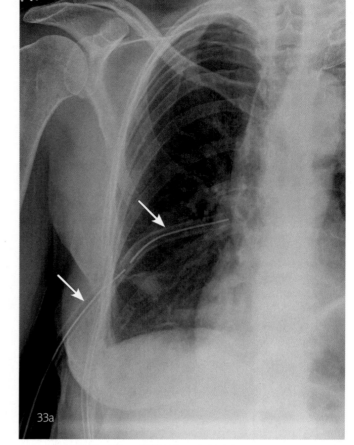

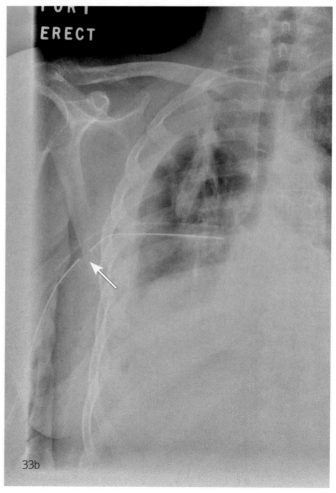

Figure 33. Chest tubes. a, PA chest x-ray with a chest tube; the chest tube is visualized because of a radiopaque linear stripe along the course of the tube (arrows), b, AP chest x-ray highlighting the side hole of a chest tube (arrow) visible within the subcutaneous tissues of the chest wall.

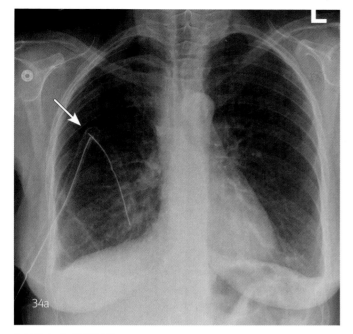

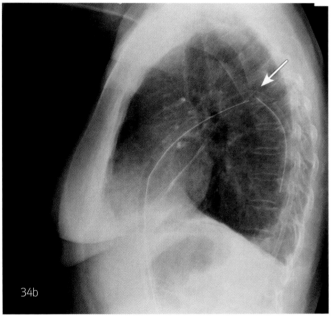

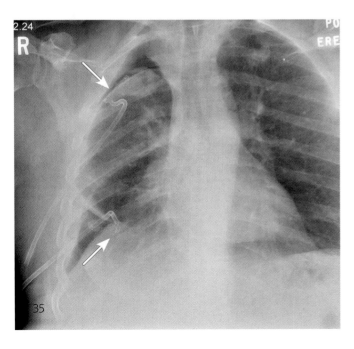

Abnormal Chest Tube Positioning (20)

Chest tubes can be positioned within the pleural space, but away from the pneumothorax or fluid, and therefore unable to treat the underlying condition. The side hole may be subcutaneous, leading to extensive surgical emphysema. They can be kinked (Fig. 34a,b). They can be erroneously positioned within the lungs, or pericardium.

Pleural Drains

On occasion, fluid collections in the pleural space are drained percutaneously with a pigtail catheter. This type of catheter can be identified by the characteristic pigtail coil at the catheter's end.

For treatment of chronic empyema, a sump drain can be used (in place of the original chest tube) (Fig. 35).

Figure 34. Abnormal chest tube positioning. a, PA chest x-ray highlighting a kink (arrow) along the course of the chest tube, b, lateral chest x-ray from the same patient highlighting the kink (arrow) along the course of the chest tube.

Figure 35. Pleural drains. AP chest x-ray highlighting two pigtail catheter drains (arrows) within the right pleural space.

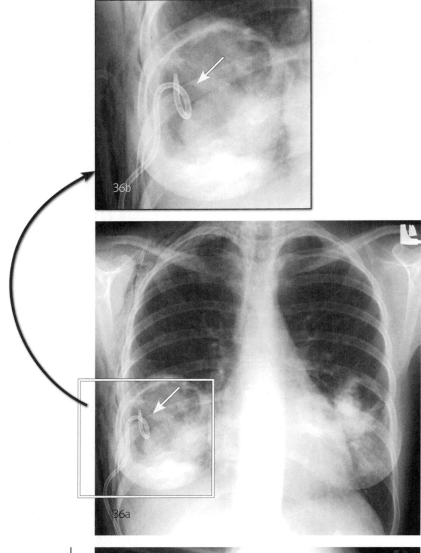

OTHER LINES & TUBES

Lung Drains

Lung drains are percutaneous catheters (Fig. 36a,b,c) that are used for the treatment of lung abscesses. They are introduced under radiological guidance, using either fluoroscopy or computed tomography (CT) imaging, so positioning is assessed during placement. A major complication of lung abscess drainage is a pneumothorax. Other complications include the shift of the drain to an incorrect position, or even falling out of the patient.

Figure 36. Lung drains. a, PA chest x-ray highlighting a pigtail catheter (arrow) within a right lung abscess, b, magnification of the same PA chest x-ray highlighting the pigtail catheter (arrow), c, lateral chest x-ray from the same patient highlighting a pigtail catheter (arrow) within a right lung abscess.

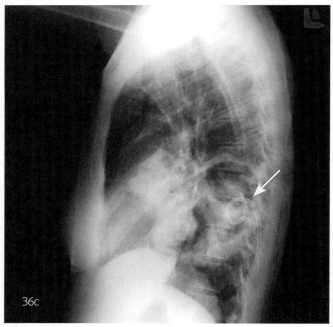

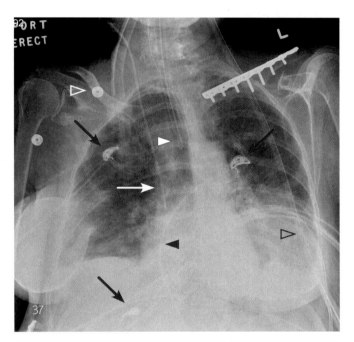

EXTERNAL LINES

In addition to the above mentioned internal monitoring devices, there are also external monitoring devices that are visible on the x-ray. Oxygen tubing can be visible as radiopaque tubing overlying the upper thorax. Cutaneous electrocardiography (EKG) leads can be identified by their metallic clips. Defibrillator pads are radiopaque, and rectangular in shape (Fig. 37).

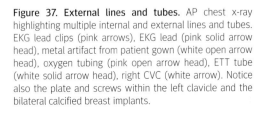

Figure 37. External lines and tubes. AP chest x-ray highlighting multiple internal and external lines and tubes. EKG lead clips (pink arrows), EKG lead (pink solid arrow head), metal artifact from patient gown (white open arrow head), oxygen tubing (pink open arrow head), ETT tube (white solid arrow head), right CVC (white arrow). Notice also the plate and screws within the left clavicle and the bilateral calcified breast implants.

DEVICE	IDEAL POSITION
ETT	Approximately 5 cm above the carina (depends on head position)
NG	Antrum of stomach/duodenum
CVC- right	Zone B – Just above carina
CVC- left	Zone B – Just above carina (Alternate Zone A or C)
Swan-Ganz	Proximal right or left pulmonary arteries
Cardiac pacemaker	Ventricle lead – apex of right ventricle Atrial lead – right atrium
Chest tube	All side holes in pleural space

Table 20.1
Summary of Ideal Device Positioning. ETT, endotracheal tube; NG, nasogastric tube; CVC, central venous catheter.

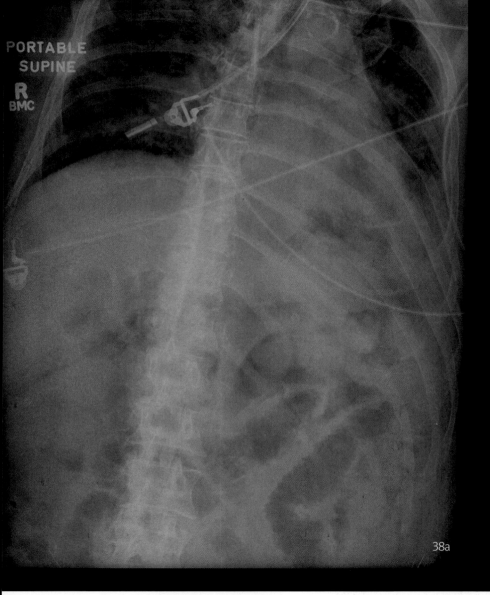

PORTABLE
SUPINE

R
BMC

38a

Can you determine if
the nasogastric tube
is in the right place?

CASE STUDY

During your general medical rotation as an intern, you are asked to place a nasogastric tube into a patient that has suffered an ischemic stroke. You have some difficulty inserting the tube, and you are concerned about whether or not you placed it in the right position within the stomach. The patient has lost the ability to swallow, and does not have a gag reflex, so it is even more difficult for you to determine whether or not the tube is in the right place. You follow protocol and order an x-ray of the lower chest and upper abdomen (Fig. 38a).

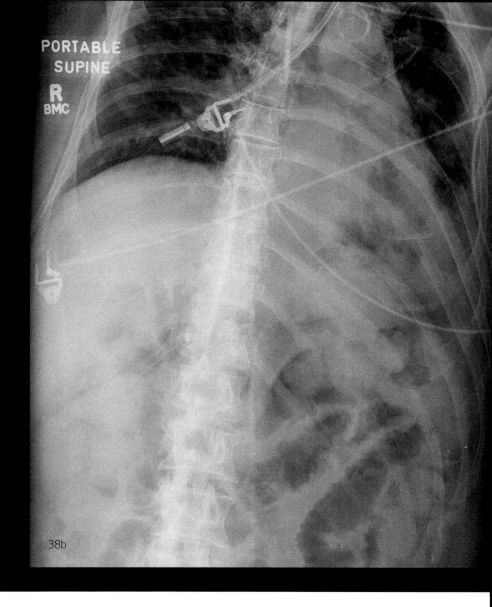

PORTABLE
SUPINE

R
BMC

38b

The main concern with nasogastric tube placement is the aberrant placement of the tube into the airways. It is always very important to check the placement of an NG tube by performing a chest x-ray. Figure 38b shows the incorrect placement of the NG tube. Notice how the NG tube has been pushed all the way into the right main stem bronchus. This can cause significant morbidity in a patient that has suffered a stroke.

Based on the chest x-ray there is aberrant placement of the Dobhoff tube into the right lung.

References

1. Lewis, P.J., Shaffer, K., & Donovan, A. (Eds.). (2012). AMSER National Medical Student Curriculum in Radiology. http://aur.org/Secondary-Alliances.aspx?id=141.

2. Lewis, P.J., & Shaffer, K. (2005). Developing a national medical student curriculum in radiology. *Am. Coll. Radiol., 2*(1):8–11.

3. Conrardy, P.A., Goodman, L.R., Lainge, F., & Singer, M.M. (1976). Alteration of endotracheal tube position. Flexion and extension of the neck. *Crit. Care Med., 4*(1):7–12.

4. Stauffer, J.L., Olson, D.E., & Petty, T.L. (1981). Complications and consequences of endotracheal intubation and tracheotomy: a prospective study of 150 critically ill adult patients. *Am. J. Med., 70*:65–76.

5. Goodman, L.R., Conrardy, P.A., Laing, F., et al. (1976). Radiographic evaluation of endotracheal tube position. *AJR Am. J. Roentgenol., 127*:433–434.

6. Dobranowski, J., Fitzgerald, J.M., Baxter, F., & Woods, D. (1992). Incorrect positioning of nasogastric feeding tubes and the development of pneumothorax. *Can. Assoc. Radiol. J., 43*(1):35–39.

7. Freij, R.M., & Mullett, S.T. (1997). Inadvertent intracranial insertion of a nasogastric tube in a non-trauma patient. *J. Accid. Emerg. Med., 14*(1): 45–47.

8. Pillai, J.B., Vegas, A., & Brister, S. (2005). Thoracic complications of nasogastric tube: review of safe practice. *Interact Cardiovasc. Thorac. Surg., 4*:429–433.

9. Stonelake, P.A., & Bodenham, A.R. (2006). The carina as a radiological landmark for central venous catheter tip position. *Br. J. Anaesth., 96*(3):335–340.

10. Fletcher, S.J., & Bodenham, A.R. (2000). Safe placement of central venous catheters: where should the tip of the catheter lie? *Br. J. Anaesth., 85*:188–191.

11. Tan, P.L., & Gibson, M. (2006). Central venous catheters role of radiology. *Clin, Radiol., 61*:13–32.

12. Amerasekera, S.S.H., & Jones, C.M. (2009). Imaging the complications. *Clin. Radiol., 64*:832–840.

13. Huyghens, L., Sennesael, J., Verbeelen, D., et al. (1985). Cardiothoracic complications of centrally inserted catheters. *Acute Care, 11*:53–56.

14. Gibson, R.N., Hennessy, O.F., Collier, N., et al. (1985). Major complications of central venous catheterization: a report of five cases and a brief review of the literature. *Clin. Radiol., 36*:205.

15. Coulter, T.D., & Wiedemann, H.P.S.O. (1999). Complications of hemodynamic monitoring. *Clin. Chest Med., 20*(2):249.

16. Slung, H.B., & Scher, K.S. (1984). Complications of the Swan-Ganz catheter. *World J. Surg., 8*:76–80.

17. Pfeiffer, D., Jung, W., Fehske, W., et al. (1994). Complications of pacemaker-defibrillator devices: diagnosis and management. *Am. Heart J., 127*(4 Pt 2):1073–1080.

18. Bailey, S.M., & Wilkoff, B.L. (2006). Complications of pacemakers and defibrillators in the elderly. *Am. J. Geriatr. Cardiol., 15*(2):102–107.

19. de Buitleir, M., & Canver, C.C. (1996) Twiddler's syndrome complicating a transvenous defibrillator lead system. *Chest, 109*:1391–1394.

20. Miller, K., & Sahn, S. (1987). Chest tubes. Indications, technique, management and complications. *Chest, 91*(2):258–264.

CHAPTER 21
The POST-OPERATIVE
& POST-RADIATION
CHEST X-RAY

importance

Surgery in the thorax can lead to significant changes in the anatomy and therefore, the appearance of the grayscale of the chest x-ray. The changes that can occur on a post-operative chest x-ray will depend on the type of thoracic surgery that was performed – surgery can be performed on virtually any part of the thorax. It is important to understand the changes that will occur following major thoracic surgery, and to correctly identify complications.

This chapter reviews both the acute and chronic x-ray changes, and complications, following thoracic surgery and radiation.

objectives

Skills:

You will identify:

- the key changes on PA and lateral chest x-rays of a post-operative and post-radiation patient;
- specific changes to the lungs, esophagus, chest wall, heart and aorta that are found on PA and lateral chest x-rays of a post-operative patient.

Knowledge:

You will review and understand:

- why radiological changes occur in a post-operative and post-radiation patient;
- the etiology behind the radiological changes of a post-operative and post-radiation patient.

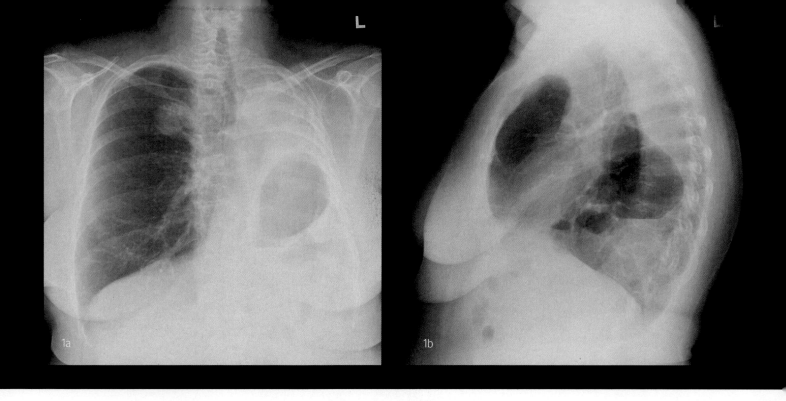

CASE STUDY

You are working as a resident in a thoracic surgery outpatient clinic. A 65-year-old female patient comes in for a follow-up appointment. The patient had undergone a left pneumonectomy for bronchogenic carcinoma three years earlier.

You are asked to interpret todays chest x-rays (Fig. 1a,b). You compare them to chest x-rays taken a year earlier (Fig 2a,b).

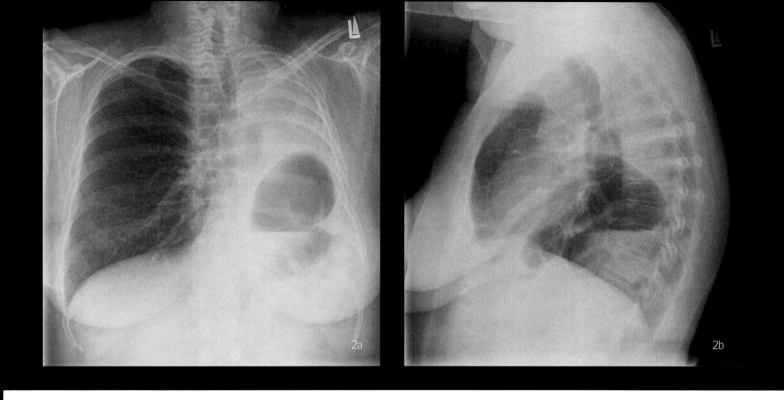

2a

2b

What are
your findings?

TRACHEA & BRONCHI

TRACHEOSTOMY (1)

Tracheostomy tube placement.

Early Post-Op Findings

Normal

- Tracheostomy tube visible in trachea

Abnormal observations/ complications

- Pneumothorax
- Pneumomediastinum
- Subcutaneous emphysema
- Bleeding and aspiration of blood

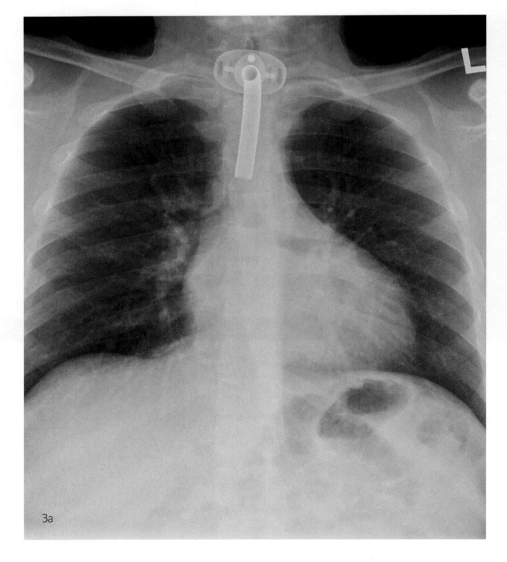

3a

Figure 3. Tracheostomy, late post-op. a, PA chest x-ray from a patient with a tracheostomy, b, lateral chest x-ray from the same patient.

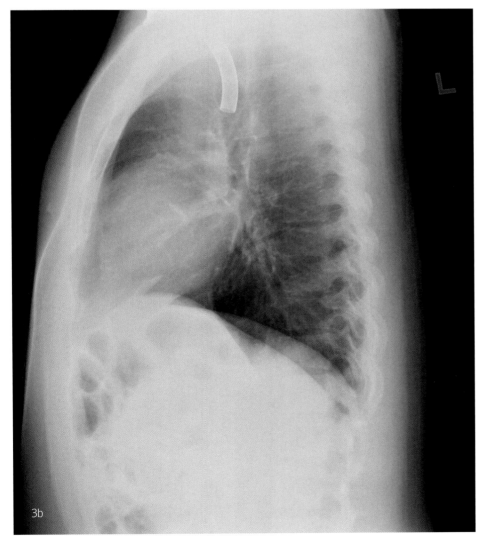

Late Post-Op Findings

Normal

- Tracheostomy tube visible in trachea

Abnormal observations/ complications

- Late complications are rare
- Tracheo-esophageal fistula

TRACHEA & BRONCHI

TRACHEAL/BRONCHIAL STENT PLACEMENT (2)

Tracheal/bronchial stent placement used to restore airway patency.

Early Post-Op Findings

Normal

- Tracheal/bronchial stent visible in trachea/bronchi

Abnormal observations/ complications

- Pneumothorax
- Pneumomediastinum
- Subcutaneous emphysema
- Bleeding and aspiration of blood
- Migration of stent

*** Complications are rare with bronchial stents***

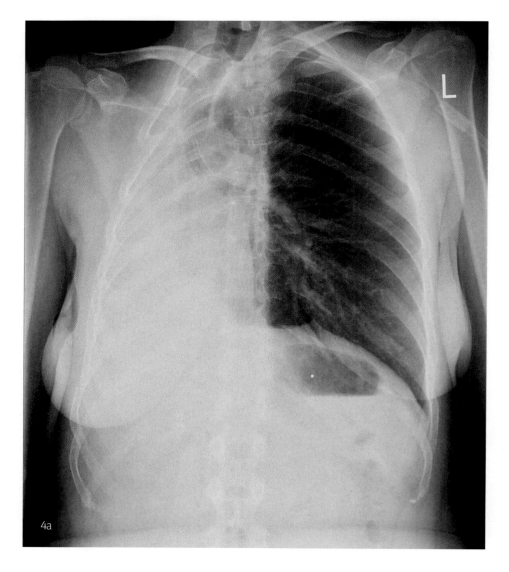

Figure 4. Endobronchial stent, early post-op.
a, PA chest x-ray from a patient with a recently placed endobronchial stent, b, lateral chest x-ray from the same patient.

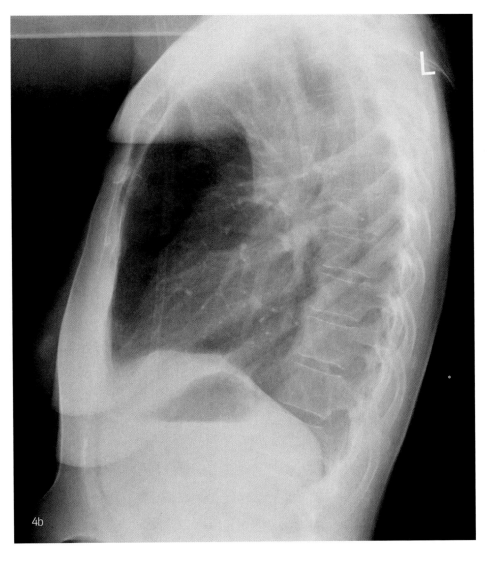

4b

Late Post-Op Findings

Normal

- Tracheal/bronchial stent
  visible in trachea /bronchi

Abnormal observations/
complications

- Tracheal/bronchial stent
  disruption/ unravelling
- Mucous plugging and
  atelectasis with bronchial
  stents

LUNGS

SEGMENTECTOMY (3,4)

Removal of lung segment.

Early Post-Op Findings

Normal

- Surgical sutures evident,
- Chest tube
- Atelectasis or bleeding may be present – should resolve quickly

Abnormal observations/ complications

- Bleeding
- Persistent air leak
- Pleural effusions
- Pneumothorax
- Infection of lungs (pneumonia)
- Infection of the pleural space (empyema)
- Postoperative atelectasis or collapse can occur as the result of retained secretions and edema at the anastomitic site.
- A bronchopleural fistula can occur (This is evident by persistent air within the pleural space.)

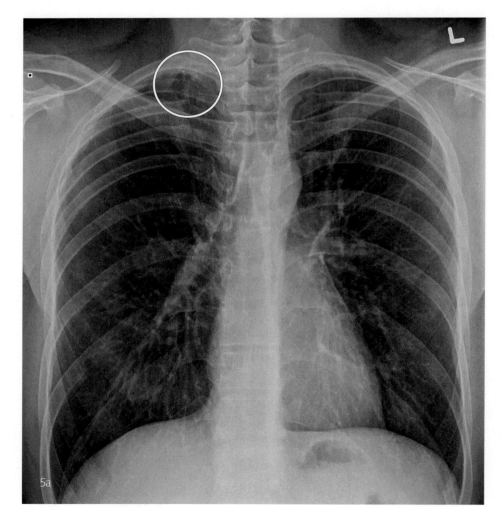

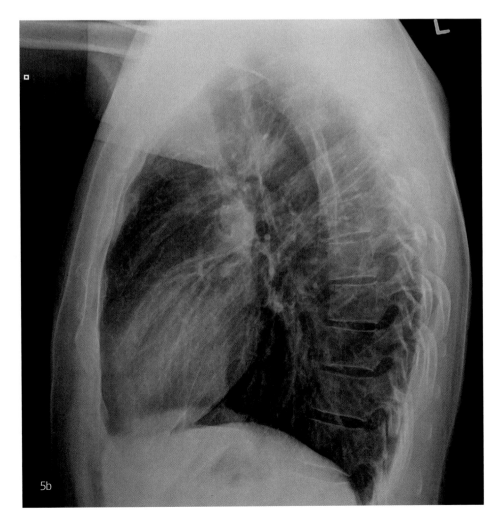

5b

Late Post-Op Findings

Normal

- Lung volumes normal
- No hilar distortion
- Line of fine metallic staples (use magnifying glass in PACS)

Abnormal observations/ complications

- Stricturing at the level of the anastomosis
- Possible esophgopleural fistula
- Tumor recurrence

Figure 5. Lung segmentectomy, late post-op. a, PA chest x-ray from a patient with a previous lung segmentectomy, b, lateral chest x-ray from the same patient.

LUNGS

LOBECTOMY (3,4)

Removal of lobe of lung.

Early Post-Op Findings

Normal

- Surgical sutures evident
- Chest tube
- Overall size of lung may be reduced causing elevation of diaphragm, and tracheal and mediastinal shift toward side of surgery
- Atelectasis or bleeding may be present (should resolve quickly)

Abnormal observations/ complications

- Bleeding
- Persistent air leak
- Pleural effusions
- Pneumothorax
- Infection of lungs (pneumonia)
- Infection of the pleural space (empyema)
- Postoperative atelectasis or collapse can occur as the result of retained secretions and edema at the anastomitic site.
- Bronchopleural fistula

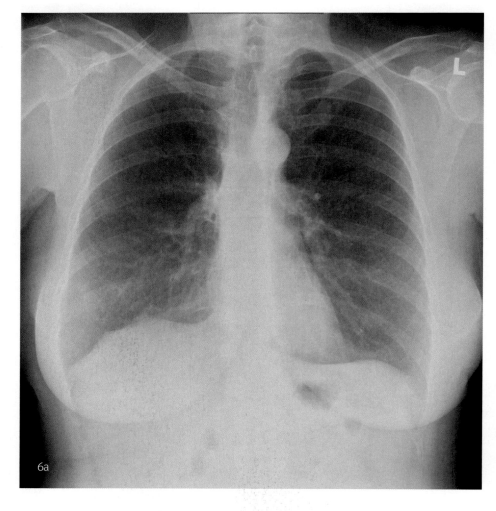

6a

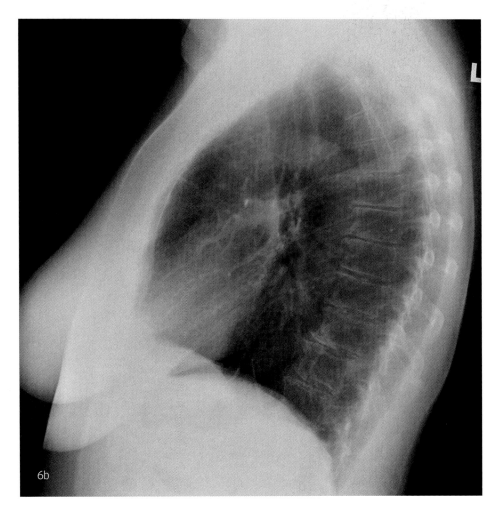

6b

Late Post-Op Findings

Normal

- Deformed rib
- Hilar distortion (might appear similar to chronic lobar collapse)
- Hilar position shifted: elevated/depressed
- Hilar size decreased
- Lung size decreased
- Mediastinal shift (toward surgery)
- Tracheal shift (toward surgery)
- If remaining lung is hyperinflated: lung volume, and mediastinal and tracheal position may be normal

Abnormal observations/ complications

- Bronchopleural fistula
- Empyema
- Tumor recurrence

Figure 6. Lobectomy, late post-op. a, PA chest x-ray from a patient with a previous right upper lobe lobectomy, b, lateral chest x-ray from the same patient.

LUNGS

PNEUMONECTOMY (4,5,6)

Removal of entire lung.

Early Post-Op Findings

Normal

- Air in pleural space
- Air/fluid level in pleural space (due to increase in serous fluid)
- Air Absorbed

Abnormal observations/ complications

- Bleeding
- Persistent air leak
- Pleural effusions
- Pneumothorax
- Infection of remaining lung (pneumonia)
- Infection of the pleural space (empyema)
- Postoperative atelectasis or collapse can occur in remaining lung.
- A bronchopleural fistula can occur.

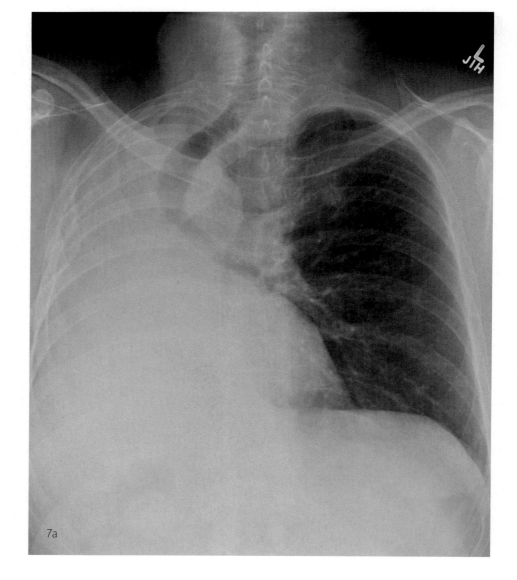

Figure 7. Pneumonectomy, late post-op. a, PA chest x-ray from a patient with a previous right pneumonectomy, b, lateral chest x-ray from the same patient.

7a

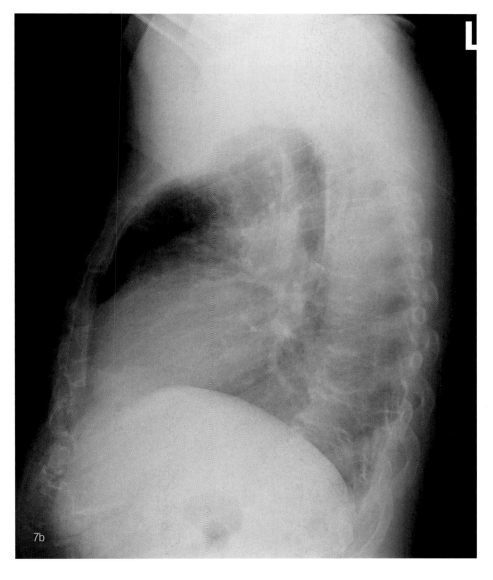

7b

Late Post-Op Findings

Normal

- Lack of one lung
- Fibrosis
- Pleural thickening
- Hyperinflation of remaining lung
- Minimal hyperinflation
- Fluid/fibrotic tissue on surgical side
- Remaining lung does not fill space of removed lung
- Minimal mediastinal and tracheal shift
- Maximal hyperinflation
- Fluid resorbed
- Remaining lung hyperinflates and fills void of removed lung
- Significant mediastinal and tracheal displacement

Abnormal observations/ complications

- Bronchopleural fistula
- Empyema
- Tumor recurrence

MEDIASTINUM - ESOPHAGUS

FUNDOPLICATION (7)

Repair of Hiatus Hernia by wrapping the gastric fundus around the lower esophagus. Currently performed laporoscopically (occasionally open surgery).

Early Post-Op Findings

Normal

- Expected to be normal
- Free air may be seen under the hemidiaphragms

Abnormal observations/ complications

- Atelectasis
- Free air under the hemidiaphragms.
- Surgical wrap may herniate above the diaphragms (complications will need to be assessed with upper endoscopy and computed tomography)

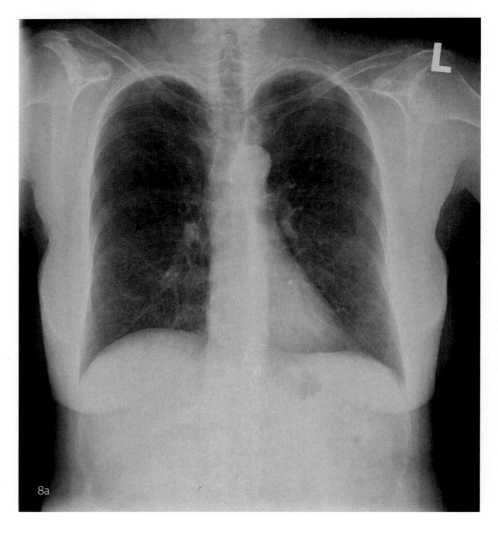

Figure 8. Fundoplication, late post-op a, PA chest x-ray from a patient with a previous fundoplication, b, lateral chest x-ray from the same patient.

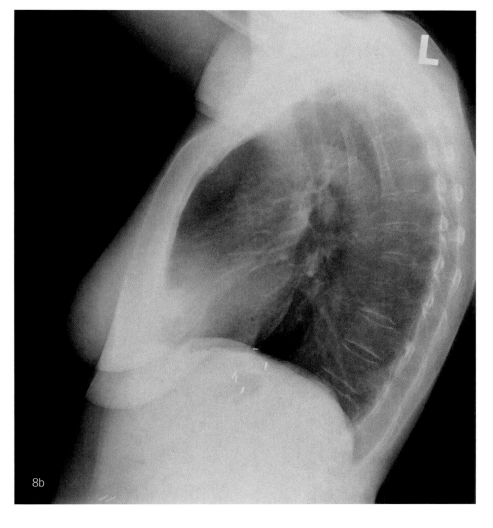

8b

Late Post-Op Findings

Normal

- Expected to be normal
- Surgical staples may be present

Abnormal observations/ complications

- Middle mediastinal opacity with an air-fluid level due to hernia recurrence
- Mediastinal air-fluid level visible due to accumulation of food (due to wrap being too tight)

TRANSHIATAL/TRANSTHORACIC ESOPHAGECTOMY (8,9,10)

Esophagus removed through cuts in neck and chest, and remnant stomach is anastomosed with the proximal esophagus.

Early Post-Op Findings

Normal

- Early changes relate to the surgery within the mediastinum with tubes and drains
- Stomach may be seen in the thorax

Abnormal observations/complications

- Atelectasis
- Free air under the hemidiaphragms
- Air present within the mediastinum (patients require chest tubes, mediastinal drains and nasogastric tubes)
- Breakdown of anastomoses
- Infections
- Bleeding
- Pleural effusion

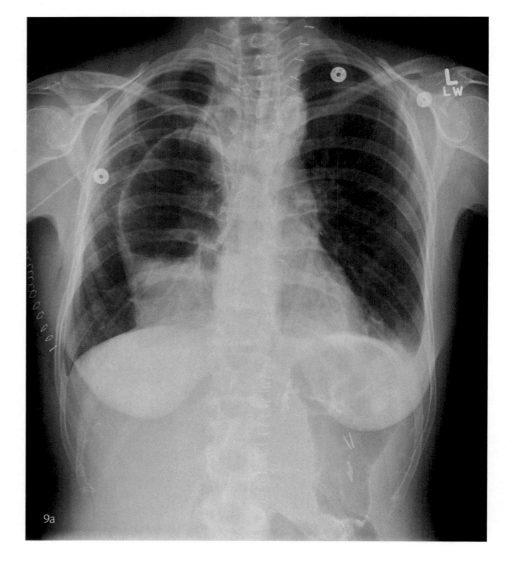

Figure 9. Esophagectomy, late post-op. a, PA chest x-ray from a patient with a previous esophagectomy, b, lateral chest x-ray from the same patient.

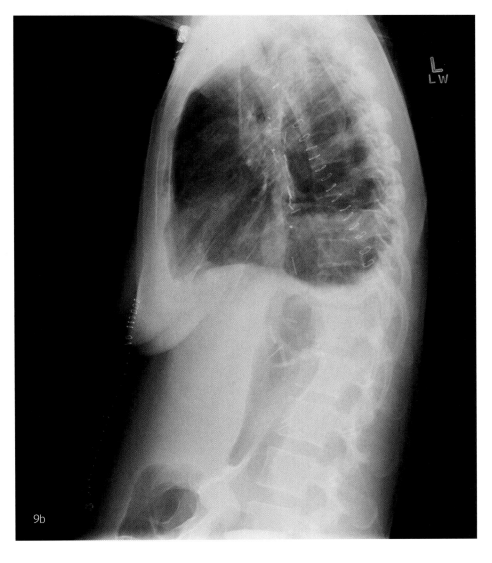

9b

Late Post-Op Findings

Normal

- Food and air within the esophagus

Abnormal observations/ complications

- Anastomotic strictures with air-fluid levels
- Tumor recurrence with air-fluid levels
- Chronic lung infections due to aspiration

MEDIASTINUM - ESOPHAGUS

ESOPHAGEAL STENT (8,9)

Esophageal stent placement to restore and maintain esophageal patency.

Early Post-Op Findings

Normal

- Esophageal stent visible in optimum position in the esophagus

Abnormal observations/ complications

- Esophageal Perforation
- Pneumomediastinum
- Pneumothorax
- Bleeding
- Migration of stent
- Incomplete expansion

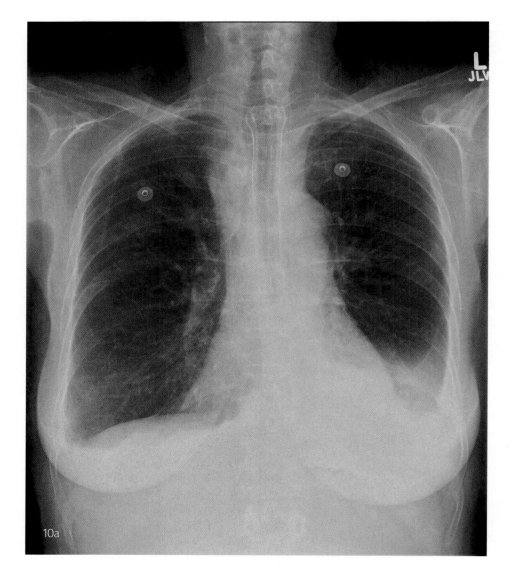

Figure 10. Esophageal stent, early post-op. a, PA chest x-ray from a patient with a recent esophageal stent placement, b, lateral chest x-ray from the same patient.

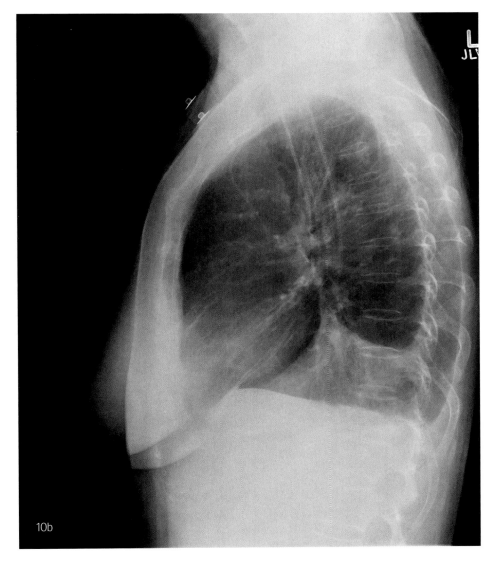

10b

Late Post-Op Findings

Normal

- Esophageal stent visible in optimum position in the esophagus

Abnormal observations/ complications

- Migration of stent
- Occlusion of stent
- Esophageal perforation
- Pneumomediastinum
- Pneumothorax
- Bleeding

MEDIASTINUM - SUPERIOR VENA CAVA

SUPERIOR VENA CAVA STENT (11)

SVC stent placement to restore and maintain venous patency.

Early Post-Op Findings

Normal

- SVC stent visible in optimum position in the superior vena cava

Abnormal observations/ complications

- SVC Perforation
- Bleeding
- Haemoptysis
- Pericardial tamponade
- Recurrent nerve palsy
- Cardiac failure
- Migration of stent

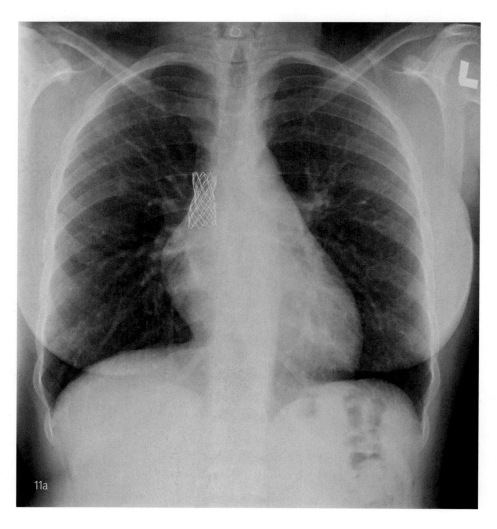

Figure 11. Superior vena cava (SVC) stent. a, PA chest x-ray from a patient with a recent SVC stent placement, b, lateral chest x-ray from the same patient.

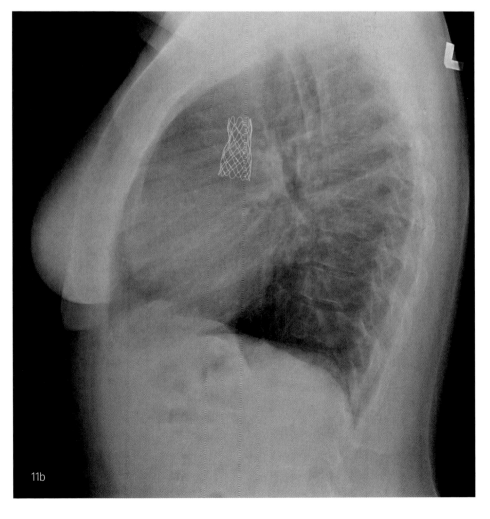

11b

Late Post-Op Findings

Normal

- SVC stent visible in optimum position in the superior vena cava

Abnormal observations/ complications

- Migration of stent
- Occlusion of stent
- SVC perforation
- Bleeding
- Haemoptysis
- Pericardial tamponade

MEDIASTINUM - THORACIC AORTA

ENDOVASCULAR ANEURYSM REPAIR (EVAR) (12)

Graft device placed into the aorta across the aneurysm to maintain the patency of the aorta.

Early Post-Op Findings

Normal

- Metal stent visible

Abnormal observations/ complications

- Infections
- Bleeding

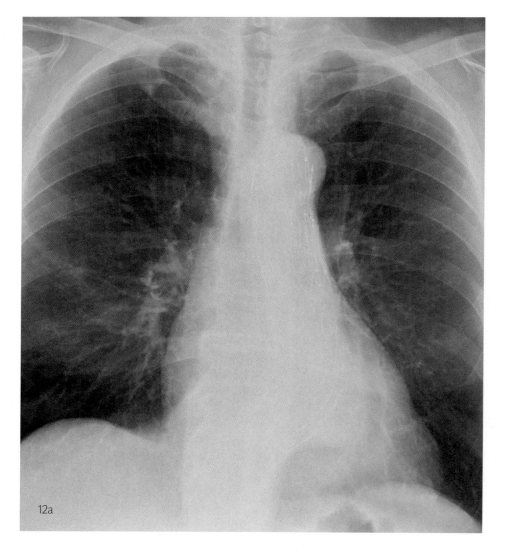

Figure 12. Endovascular aneurysm repair, late post-op. a, PA chest x-ray from a patient with a previous EVAR to restore patency of aorta, b, lateral chest x-ray from the same patient.

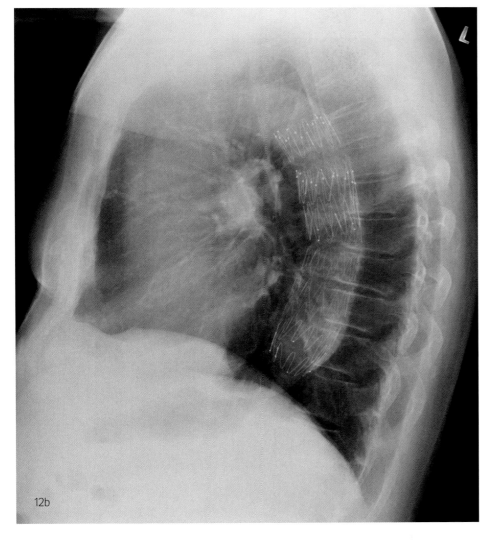

12b

Late Post-Op Findings

Normal

- Metal stent visible

Abnormal observations/ complications

- Graft Migration
- Graft failure and distortion

CARDIAC ZONE - HEART

CORONARY ARTERY BYPASS (CABG) (13)

Diseased coronary arteries are bypassed with an artery or vein harvested outside of the heart therefore restoring cardiac circulation.

Early Post-Op Findings

Normal Sternotomy wires

- Graft localizer wires

Abnormal observations/ complications

- Lines and tubes related to surgery

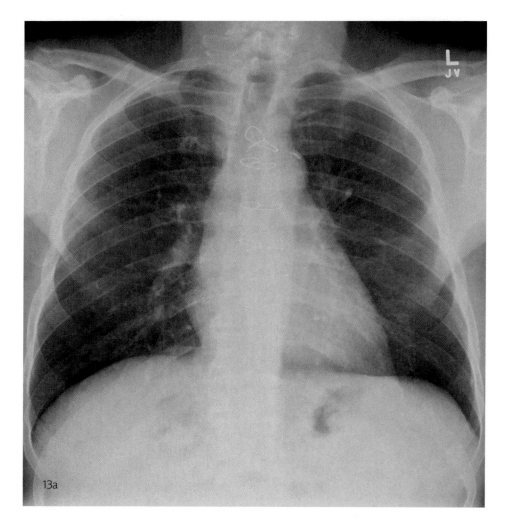

Figure 13. Coronary artery bypass (CABG), early post-op. a, PA chest x-ray from a patient with a recent CABG, b, lateral chest x-ray from the same patient.

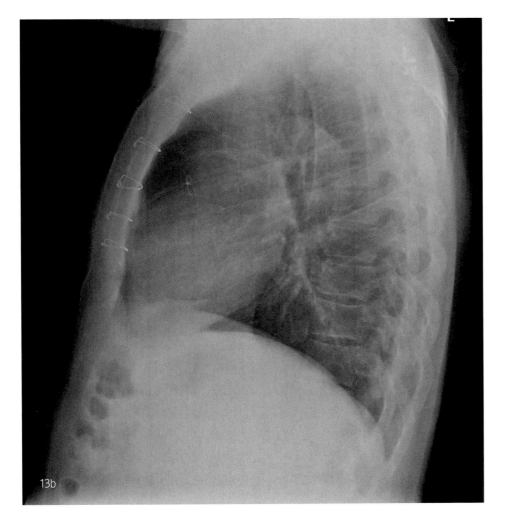

Late Post-Op Findings

Normal

- Sternotomy wires
- Graft localizer wires

Abnormal observations/ complications

- Infection
- Wire fracture
- Wound dehiscence

CARDIAC ZONE - HEART

VALVULAR REPLACEMENT

Replacement of faulty cardiac valves performed surgically through a thorocotomy.

Early Post-Op Findings

Normal

- Sternotomy wires
- Metal valves if present

Abnormal observations/ complications

- Lines and tubes related to surgery

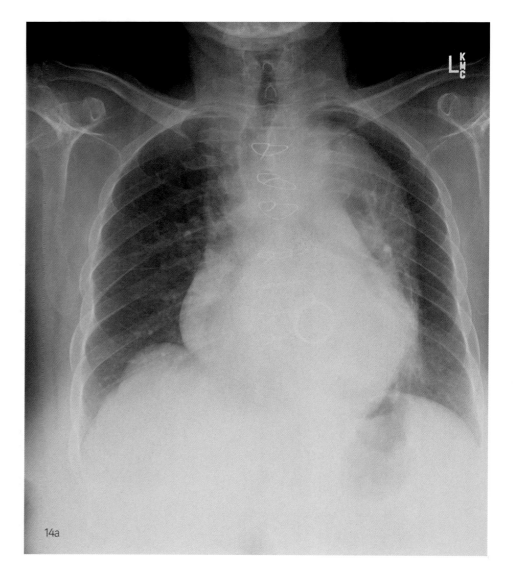

Figure 14. Valvular replacement, early post-op a, PA chest x-ray from a patient with a recent valvular replacement, b, lateral chest x-ray from the same patient.

14a

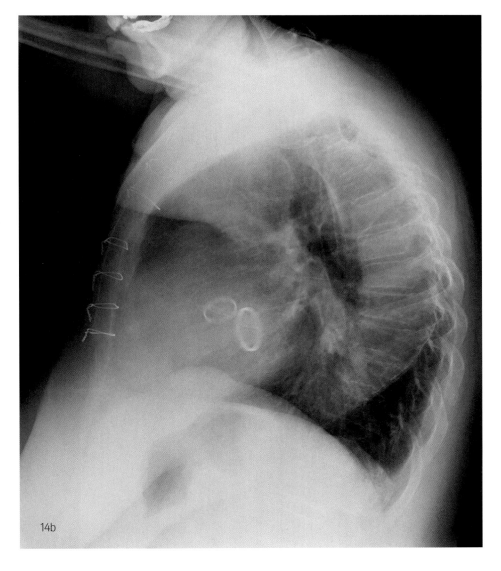

Late Post-Op Findings

Normal

- Sternotomy wires
- Metal valves if present

Abnormal observations/ complications

- Infection
- Wire fracture
- Wound dehiscence

14b

CHEST WALL - BONY THORAX

PECTUS EXCAVATUM DEFORMITY SURGERY (14)

Surgical correction of anterior skeletal chest wall deformity.

Early Post-Op Findings

Normal

- Metal support bar

Abnormal observations/ complications

- Post-op atelectasis

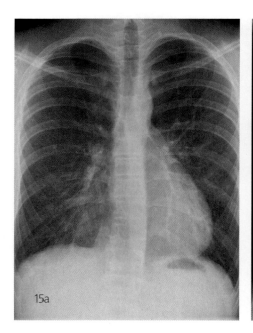
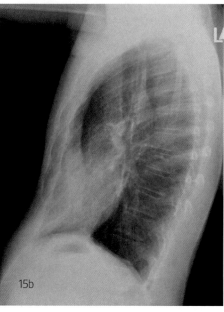

Figure 15. Pectus excavatum, pre-surgery. a, PA chest x-ray from a patient with pectus excavatum, prior to surgery, b, lateral chest x-ray from the same patient.

Late Post-Op Findings

Normal

- Metal support bar

Abnormal observations/ complications

- Metal support bar displacement
- Infection

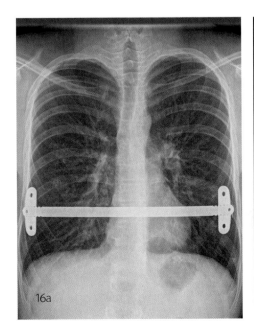

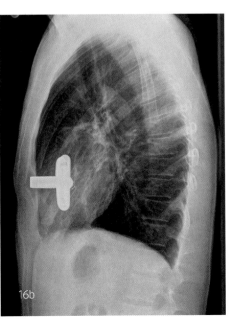

Figure 16. **Pectus excavatum deformity surgery, early post-op.** a, PA chest x-ray from a patient with recent pectus excavatum deformity surgery, b, lateral chest x-ray from the same patient.

CHEST WALL - RIBS

THORACOPLASTY

The surgical removal of ribs to repair thoracic deformities (e.g., scoliosis), or to cause the chest wall and underlying lung to collapse.

Of historical value: at one time tuberculosis was treated by causing collapse of infected lung lobes.

Early Post-Op Findings

Normal

- Multiple unilateral resected ribs

Abnormal observations/ complications

- Not applicable

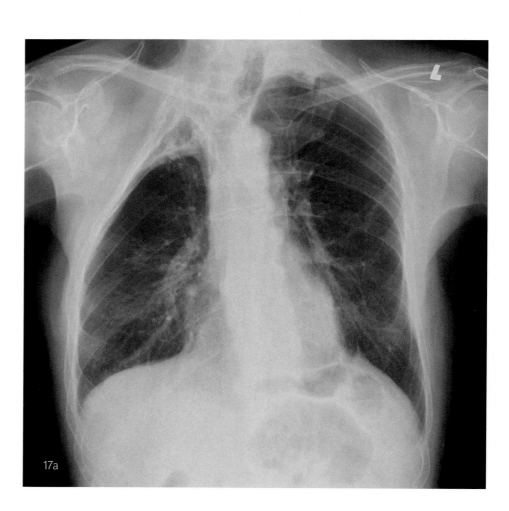

Figure 17. Thoracoplasty, late post-op. a, PA chest x-ray from a patient having undergone recent thoracoplasty, b, lateral chest x-ray from the same patient.

Late Post-Op Findings

Normal

- Multiple unilateral rib resections
- Deformed hemithorax

Abnormal observations/ complications

- Kyphoscoliosis

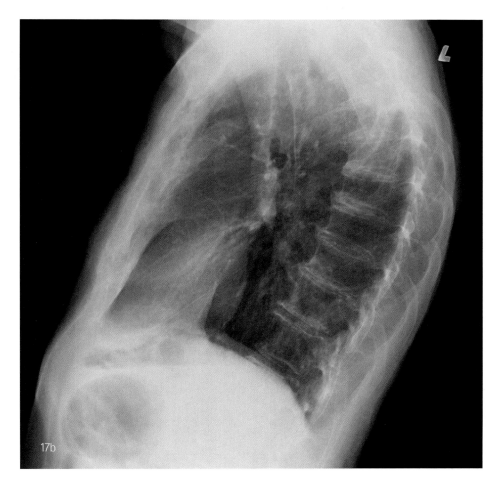

CHEST WALL - VERTEBRAE

HARRINGTON ROD PLACEMENT

For the treatment of scoliosis. Fusion of vertebrae in curved part of spine with the placement of a steel Harrington rod to allow vertebrae to heal.

Early Post-Op Findings

Normal

- Visible metal rods

Abnormal observations/ complications

- Infection

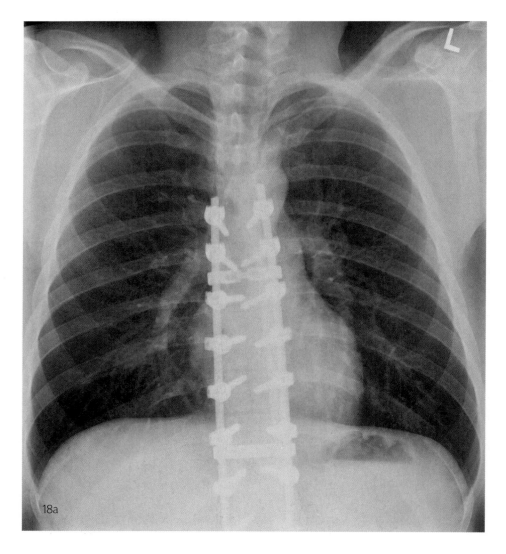

Figure 18. Harrington rods, late post-op. a, PA chest x-ray from a patient with Harrington rods, b, lateral chest x-ray from the same patient.

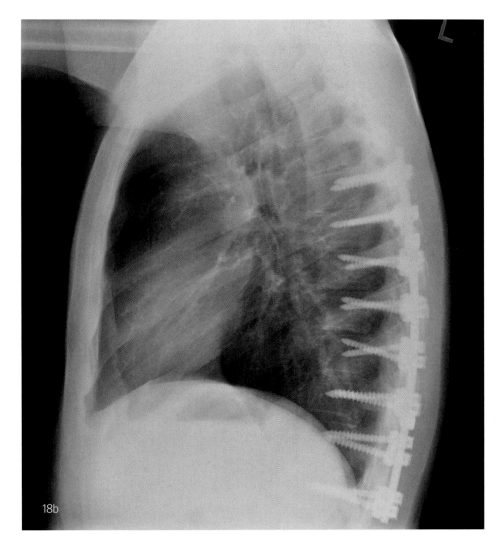

18b

Late Post-Op Findings

Normal

- Visible metal rods

Abnormal observations/ complications

- Broken rods
- Hooks or other metal pieces can migrate

CHEST WALL - VERTEBRAE

KYPHOPLASTY/VERTEBROPLASTY

Polymethylmethacrylate (PMMA) injected into vertebrae via a hollow needle to treat vertebral compression fracture (VCF) due to osteoporosis.

Early Post-Op Findings

Normal

• Cement within vertebral body

Abnormal observations/ complications

• Cement leakage

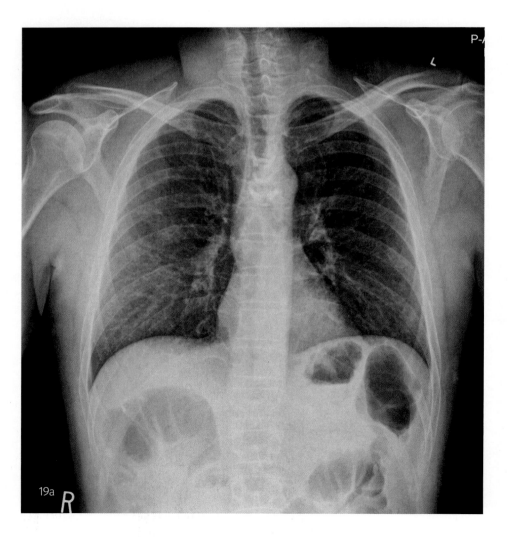

Figure 19. Vertebroplasty, late post-op. a, PA chest x-ray from a patient with recent vertebroplasty, b, lateral chest x-ray from the same patient.

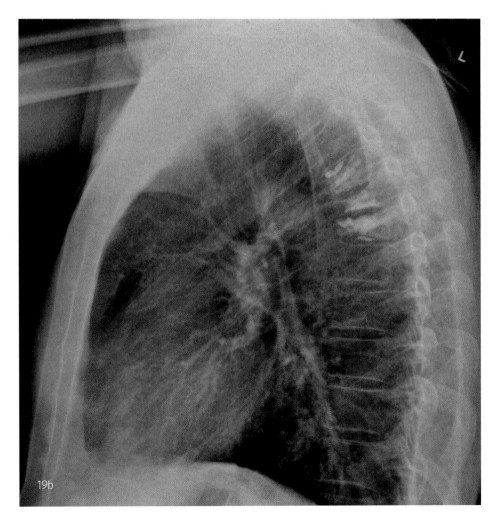

Late Post-Op Findings

Normal

- Cement within vertebral body

Abnormal observations/ complications

- Cement leakage
- Osteomyelitis
- Rib or transverse process fracture

CHEST WALL - STERNUM

STERNOTOMY

To gain access into thorax for various open thoracic surgeries.

Early Post-Op Findings

Normal

- Sternotomy wires

Abnormal observations/ complications

- Not applicable

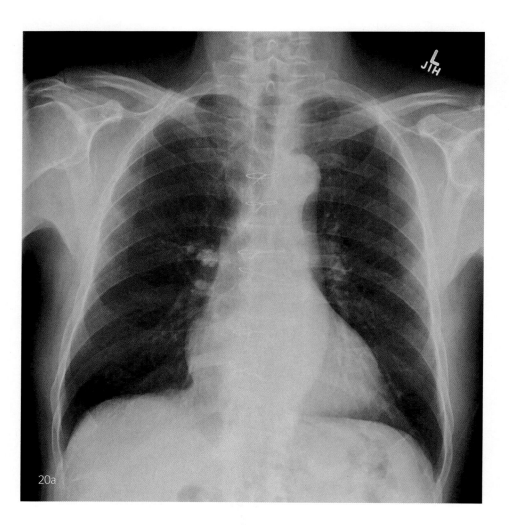

Figure 20. Sternotomy, late post-op. a, PA chest x-ray from a patient who underwent a recent sternotomy, b, lateral chest x-ray from the same patient.

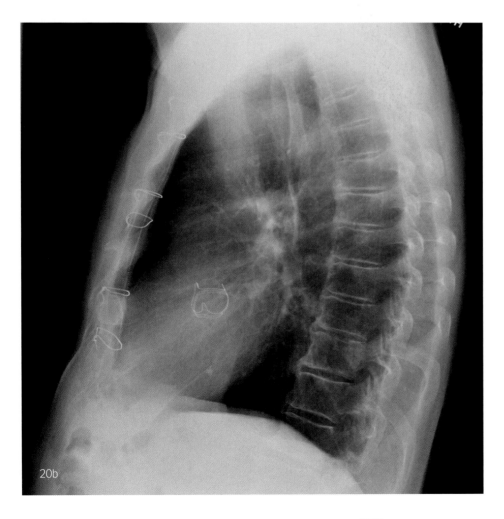

20b

Late Post-Op Findings

Normal

- Sternotomy wires

Abnormal observations/ complications

- Infection
- Wire fracture
- Wound dehiscence

CHEST WALL - BREASTS

MASTECTOMY

Removal of one, or both, breast(s).

Early Post-Op Findings

Normal

- Hyperlucent hemithorax on the side of the mastectomy
- Staples

Abnormal observations/ complications

- Hematoma
- Infection

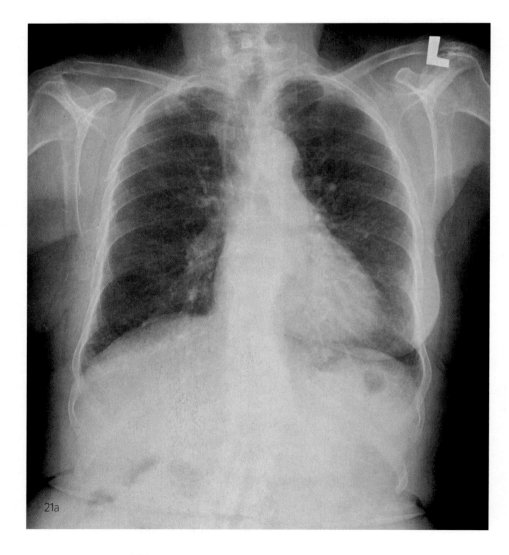

Figure 21. Unilateral mastectomy, late post-op. a, PA chest x-ray from a patient who had a previous right mastectomy, b, lateral chest x-ray from the same patient.

Normal

- Hyperlucent hemithorax on the side of the mastectomy

Abnormal observations/ complications

- Tumor recurrence

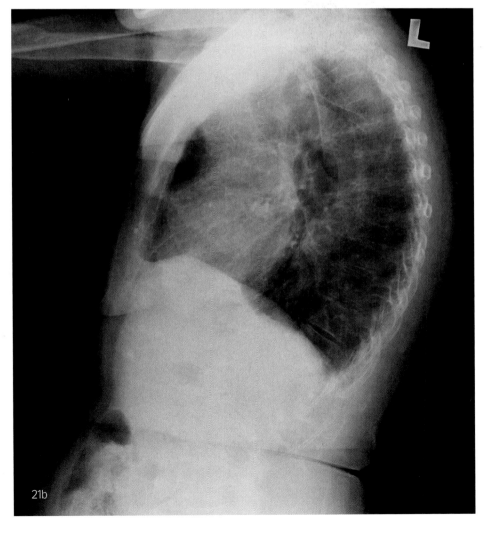

21b

CHEST WALL - BREASTS

BREAST IMPLANTATION

Silicone or saline breast implants to augment the size and shape of the breasts and for the correction of mastectomy related deformity.

Early Post-Op Findings

Normal

- Increased opacities (usually bilateral, but can be unilateral)

Abnormal observations/ complications

- Increased opacity from hematoma
- Gas in the soft tissues from infection (abscess) with gas forming organisms

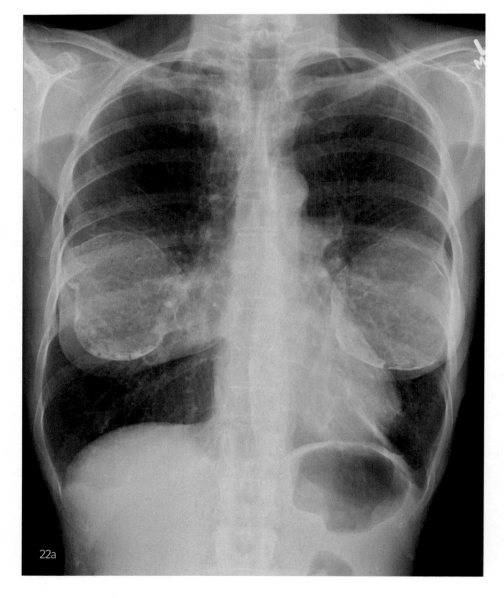

Figure 22. Bilateral breast implants, late post-op. a, PA chest x-ray from a patient who had previous bilateral breast implants, b, lateral chest x-ray from the same patient. Note calcification of breast implants.

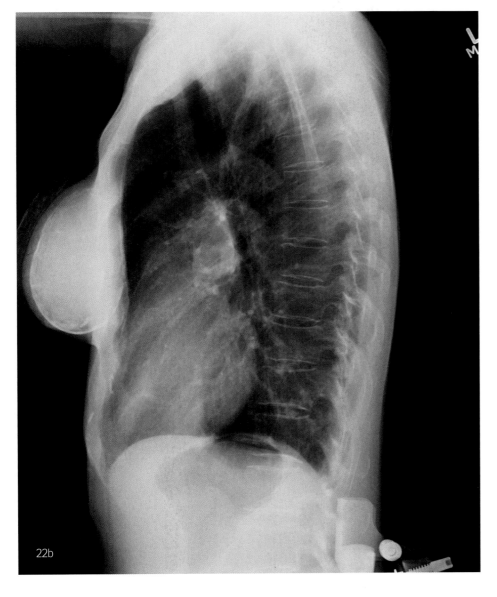

Late Post-Op Findings

Normal

- Increased opacities (usually bilateral, but can be unilateral)

Abnormal observations/ complications

- If implants calcify, there will be further increase in the opacities
- Implant migration
- Leakage of implant material

THE POST-RADIATION CHEST X-RAY

RADIOTHERAPY (15,16,17)

Radiation to treat chest wall or intrathoracic malignancies.
Risk of lung injury increases with radiation dose, and is frequently seen when the dose is greater than 40Gy.

Early Post-Op Findings

Normal

- No change

Abnormal observations/
complications

- Pneumonitis

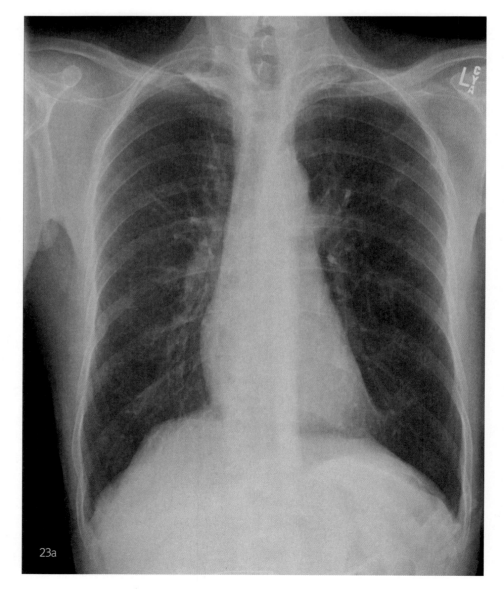

Figure 23. Post-radiation therapy, late. a, PA chest x-ray from a patient who had radiation therapy, b, lateral chest x-ray from the same patient. Note changes in lung apices.

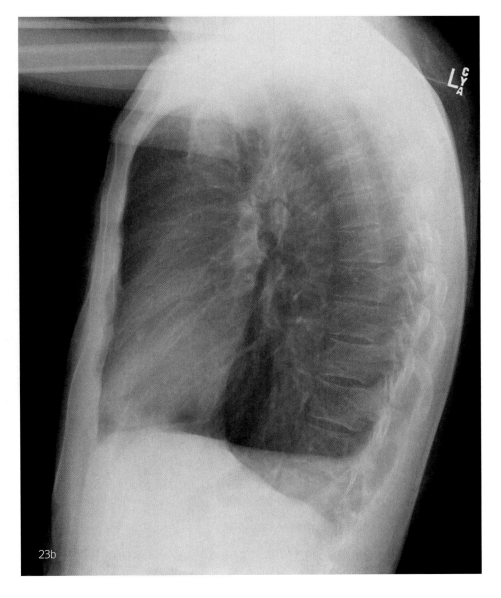

23b

Late Post-Op Findings

Normal

- No change

Abnormal observations/ complications

- Fibrosis corresponding to boundaries of radiation (edges are straight)
- Tumor recurrence

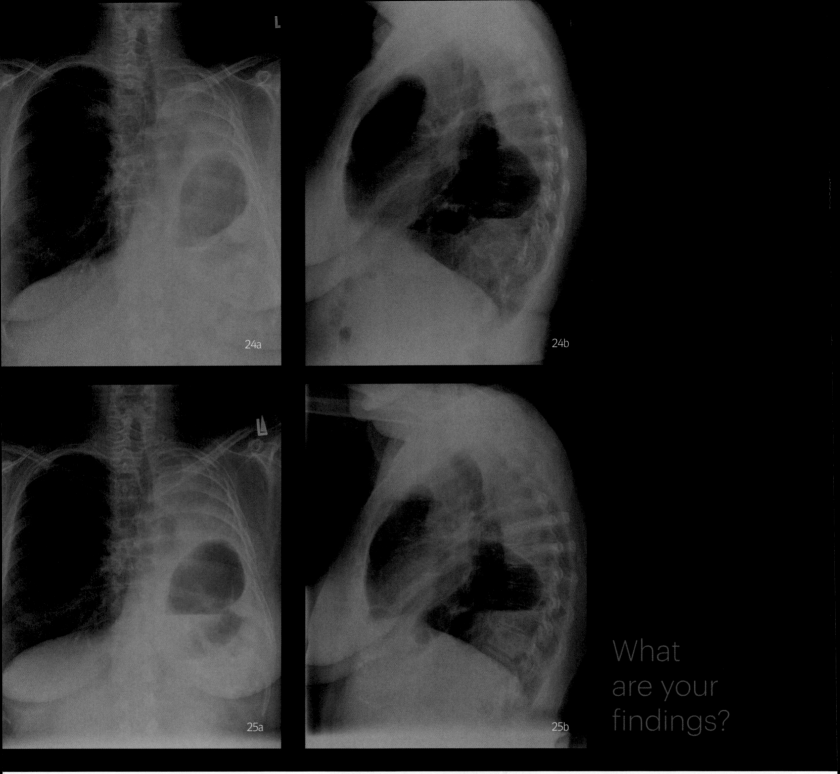

24a

24b

25a

25b

What
are your
findings?

You are working as a resident in a thoracic surgery outpatient clinic. A 65-year-old female patient comes in for a follow-up appointment. The patient had undergone a left pneumonectomy for bronchogenic carcinoma three years earlier.

You are asked to interpret today's chest x-rays (Fig. 24a,b). You compare them to chest x-rays taken a year earlier (Fig 25a,b).

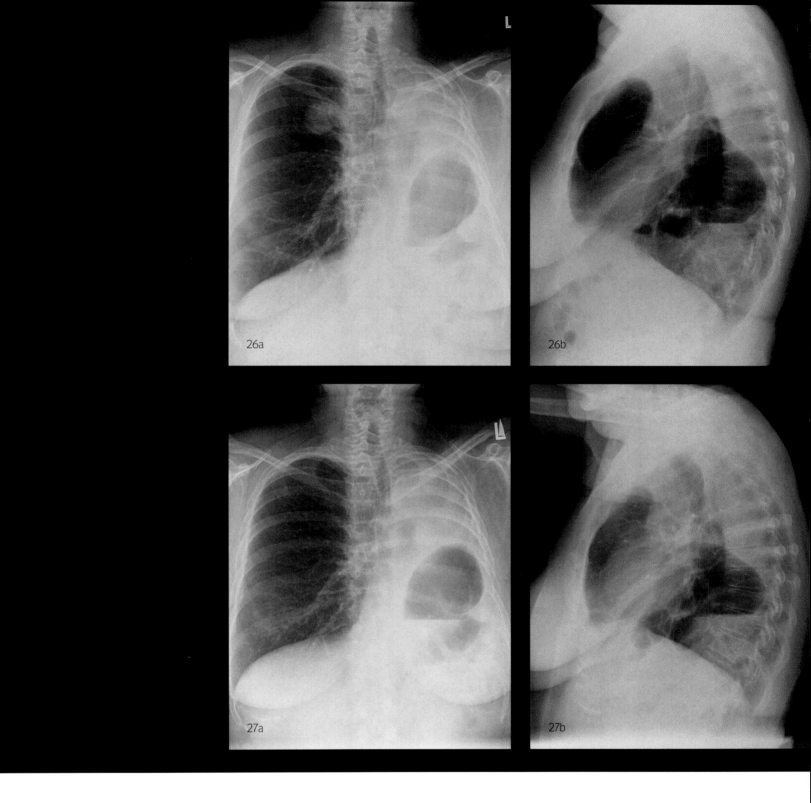

26a   26b

27a   27b

DISCUSSION

Since thoracic surgery can alter the way chest x-rays look, it is very important to differentiate between the post-operative changes and any new pathology. The post-operative changes essentially become the new "normal" for the patient. In this patient there is marked alteration of the grayscale of the x-ray (Fig 26a,b) related to the removal of the left lung, fibrosis within the left hemithorax and hyperinflation of the right lung. This appearance is the new postoperative normal appearance of the thorax. When you compare the current chest x-ray (Fig 27a,b) with the previous it becomes obvious that there is a new mass in the right apex. This may represent a metastatic deposit or a new primary bronchogenic carcinoma. Subsequently the patient successfully underwent a right upper lobe segmentectomy.

References

1. Orringer, M. (1980). Endotracheal intubation and tracheostomy. Indications, techniques, and complications. *Surg. Clin. North Am., 60*:1447–1464.

2. Burningham, A.R., Wax, M.K., et al. (2002). Metallic tracheal stents: complications associated with long-term use in the upper airway. *Ann. Otol. Rhinol. Laryngol., 111*(4):285–90.

3. Kim, E.A., Lee, K.S., Shim, Y.M., et al. (2002). Radiographic and CT findings in complications following pulmonary resection. *Radiographics, 22*(1):67–86.

4. Solaini, L., Prusciano, F., Bagioni, P., et al. (2008). Video-assisted thoracic surgery (VATS) of the lung: analysis of intraoperative and postoperative complications over 15 years and review of the literature. *Surg. Endosc., 22*(2):298–310.

5. Chae, E.J., Seo, J.B., Kim, S.Y., et al. (2006). Radiographic and CT findings of thoracic complications after pneumonectomy. *Radiographics, 26*(5):1449–68.

6. Valji, A.M., Maziak, D.E., Shamji, F.M., & Matzinger, F.R. (1998). Postpneumonectomy Ssndrome: Recognition and management. *Chest, 114*(6):1766–1769.

7. Goodman, R. (1980). Postoperative chest radiograph: I. Alterations after abdominal surgery. *AJR Am. J. Roentgenol., 134*(3):533–41.

8. Kim, T.J., Lee, K.H., Kim, Y.H., et al. (2007). Postoperative imaging of esophageal cancer: what chest radiologists need to know. *Radiographics, 27*(2):409-29.

9. Devenney-Cakir, B., Tkacz, J., Soto, J., & Gupta, A. (2011). Complications of esophageal surgery: role of imaging in diagnosis and treatments. *Curr. Probl. Diagn. Radiol., 40*(1):15–28.

10. Cassivi SD. (2004). Leaks, strictures, and necrosis: a review of anastomotic complications following esophagectomy. *Semin. Thorac. Cardiovasc. Surg., 16*(2):124–32.

11. Nguyen, N. P., Borok, T. L., Welsh, J., & Vinh-Hung, V. (2009). Safety and effectiveness of vascular endoprosthesis for malignant superior vena cava syndrome. *Thorax, 64*:2 174–178.

12. Maleux, G., Koolen, M., & Heye, S. (2009). Complications after endovascular aneurysm repair. *Semin. Intervent. Radiol., 26*(1): 3–9.

13. Peterson, L.R., McKenzie, C.R., Ludbrook, P.A., et al. (1999). Value of saphenous vein graft markers during subsequent diagnostic cardiac catheterization. *Ann. Thorac. Surg., 68*:2263–2266.

14. Robicsek, F., Watts, L.T., & Fokin, A.A. (2009). Surgical repair of pectus excavatum and carinatum. *Semin. Thorac. Cardiovasc. Surg., 21*(1):64–75.

15. Ikezoe, J., Takashima, S., Morimoto, S., et al. (1998). CT appearance of acute radiation-induced injury in the lung. *AJR Am. J. Roentgenol., 150*(4):765–70.

16. Loyer, E., Fuller, L., Libshitz, H.I., & Palmer, J.L. (2000). Radiographic appearance of the chest following therapy for Hodgkin disease. *Eur. J. Radiol., 35*(2):136–48.

17. Park, K.J., Chung, J.Y., Chun, M.S., & Suh, J.H. (2000). Radiation-induced lung disease and the impact of radiation methods on imaging features. *Radiographics, 20*(1):83–98.

CHAPTER 22
HOW TO READ
an X-RAY REPORT

importance

The radiology report is the final end product of the interpretive process produced by a radiologist. The report will provide a summary of the findings, and a differential diagnosis. Use this information to confirm your clinical suspicions, and to plan further patient care. PACS and voice-recognition dictation allow almost real-time reporting of x-ray findings by radiologists. The presence of a full radiology report is not only important for patient care, but also provides a valuable resource for students learning to interpret x-rays.

objectives

Skills

You will learn

- how to confidently uncover the key elements of a radiological report.

Knowledge

You will review and understand

- the basic structure of a radiological report.
- the process of interpreting a radiological report.

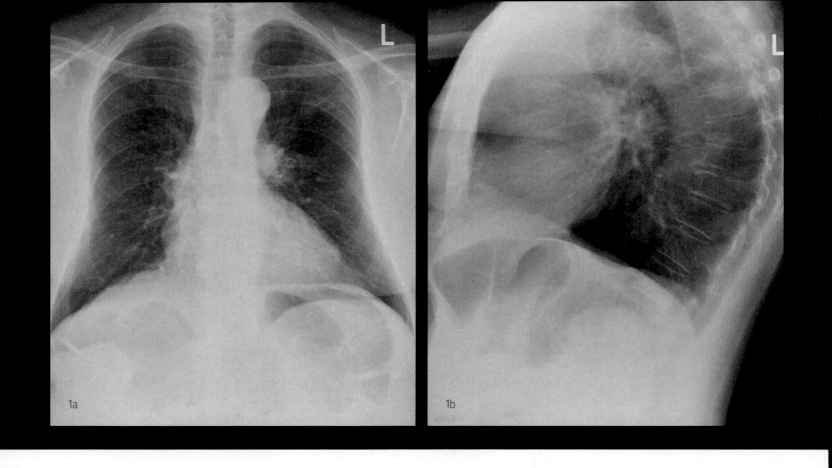

1a

1b

CASE STUDY

Earlier in the day you ordered a chest x-ray on your patient. You are concerned the patient may have lung cancer. On PACS you review the x-rays (Fig. 1a,b), and the radiologist's report (Fig. 1c).

**Hospital
Department of Radiology**

NAME: John Doe
DOB: May 15, 1947
PATIENT IDENTIFICATION NUMBER: 11111111
EXAM DATE: July 20, 2012

Chest 2 views PA and Lateral

Clinical indication: 65-year-old male smoker with a three month history of weight loss, hemoptysis and rib pain.
Comparison is made with previous study performed on October 7, 2006.
Good quality examination.

Findings:
2 cm ill defined nodule within the left upper lobe. There is no associated calcification or cavitation. The remaining lung fields are hyperinflated but otherwise clear.
There is mild enlargement and increased density of the right hilum.
Loss of the cortical outline of a 2.5 cm segment of the left 5th rib posteriorly. The remaining bone structures are normal.
There is no pleural effusion.
No other abnormalities.

Conclusion:
Findings suggest a primary lung cancer within the left upper lobe with evidence of spread to the right hilum, and to the left 5th rib.

Recommend urgent referral to lung cancer diagnostic assessment unit, and a staging CT scan of the thorax and upper abdomen.

How do you determine if the report is of good quality, and helps you with patient management?

STRUCTURE OF A RADIOLOGY REPORT

The radiology report is the communication tool between the radiologist and the referring physician. The report needs to contain accurate information, and needs to be presented in a format using language that is clear and understandable. The report needs to facilitate clinical decision making.

Report Content Items

In attempts to improve the quality of radiological reports, various organizations have produced guidelines that outline the essential components of a good quality report (1,2,3,4,5,6).

Based on these guidelines, the following list of report content items has been compiled, and grouped into four categories:

A. 1. Patient demographics
B. 2. Exam technique
    3. Relevant clinical information
    4. Comparison examinations
    5. Exam quality
C. 6. Findings
D. 7. Summary
    8. Diagnosis
    9. Differential diagnosis
    10. Recommendations

This list should look familiar. The items on this list form the foundation of the six phases of x-ray interpretation that were discussed in Chapters 5, 16 and 19.

Hospital
Department of Radiology

A. Patient demographics

NAME: John Doe
DOB: May 15, 1947
PATIENT IDENTIFICATION NUMBER: 11111111
EXAM DATE: July 20, 2012

Chest 2 views PA and Lateral

Clinical indication: 65-year-old male smoker with a three month history of weight loss, hemoptysis and rib pain.
Comparison is made with previous study performed on October 7, 2006.
Good quality examination.

Findings:
2 cm ill defined nodule within the left upper lobe. There is no associated calcification or cavitation. The remaining lung fields are hyperinflated but otherwise clear.
There is mild enlargement and increased density of the right hilum.
Loss of the cortical outline of a 2.5 cm segment of the left 5th rib posteriorly. The remaining bone structures are normal.
There is no pleural effusion.
No other abnormalities.

Conclusion:
Findings suggest a primary lung cancer within the left upper lobe with evidence of spread to the right hilum, and to the left 5th rib.

Recommend urgent referral to lung cancer diagnostic assessment unit, and a staging CT scan of the thorax and upper abdomen.

2a

Hospital
Department of Radiology

NAME: John Doe
DOB: May 15, 1947
PATIENT IDENTIFICATION NUMBER: 11111111

B. Exam technique, relevant clinical information, comparison examinations, exam quality

Chest 2 views PA and Lateral

Clinical indication: 65-year-old male smoker with a three month history of weight loss, hemoptysis and rib pain.
Comparison is made with previous study performed on October 7, 2006.
Good quality examination.

Findings:
2 cm ill defined nodule within the left upper lobe. There is no associated calcification or cavitation. The remaining lung fields are hyperinflated but otherwise clear.
There is mild enlargement and increased density of the right hilum.
Loss of the cortical outline of a 2.5 cm segment of the left 5th rib posteriorly. The remaining bone structures are normal.
There is no pleural effusion.
No other abnormalities.

Conclusion:
Findings suggest a primary lung cancer within the left upper lobe with evidence of spread to the right hilum, and to the left 5th rib.

Recommend urgent referral to lung cancer diagnostic assessment unit, and a staging CT scan of the thorax and upper abdomen.

2b

Hospital
Department of Radiology

NAME: John Doe
DOB: May 15, 1947
PATIENT IDENTIFICATION NUMBER: 11111111
EXAM DATE: July 20, 2012

Chest 2 views PA and Lateral

Clinical indication: 65-year-old male smoker with a three month history of weight loss, hemoptysis and rib pain.
Comparison is made with previous study performed on October 7, 2006.
Good quality examination.

C. Findings

Findings:
2 cm ill defined nodule within the left upper lobe. There is no associated calcification or cavitation. The remaining lung fields are hyperinflated but otherwise clear.
There is mild enlargement and increased density of the right hilum.
Loss of the cortical outline of a 2.5 cm segment of the left 5th rib posteriorly. The remaining bone structures are normal.
There is no pleural effusion.
No other abnormalities.

Conclusion:
Findings suggest a primary lung cancer within the left upper lobe with evidence of spread to the right hilum, and to the left 5th rib.

Recommend urgent referral to lung cancer diagnostic assessment unit, and a staging CT scan of the thorax and upper abdomen.

2c

The guidelines that apply to radiologists, apply to anyone performing a chest x-ray interpretation.

!

A differential diagnosis is not always necessary! (Ch. 5, Pg. 145 and Ch. 19, Pg. 717)

!

Hospital
Department of Radiology

NAME: John Doe
DOB: May 15, 1947
PATIENT IDENTIFICATION NUMBER: 11111111
EXAM DATE: July 20, 2012

Chest 2 views PA and Lateral

Clinical indication: 65-year-old male smoker with a three month history of weight loss, hemoptysis and rib pain.
Comparison is made with previous study performed on October 7, 2006.
Good quality examination.

Findings:
2 cm ill defined nodule within the left upper lobe. There is no associated calcification or cavitation. The remaining lung fields are hyperinflated but otherwise clear.
There is mild enlargement and increased density of the right hilum.
Loss of the cortical outline of a 2.5 cm segment of the left 5th rib posteriorly. The remaining bone structures are normal.
There is no pleural effusion.
No other abnormalities.

D. Summary, diagnosis, differential diagnosis, recommendations

Conclusion:
Findings suggest a primary lung cancer within the left upper lobe with evidence of spread to the right hilum, and to the left 5th rib.

Recommend urgent referral to lung cancer diagnostic assessment unit, and a staging CT scan of the thorax and upper abdomen.

2d

Common Problems with Radiological Reports

The prior section describes a well-formatted radiological report. Unfortunately, the quality of radiological reports varies. Elements of the report may be missing.

Issues related to the radiological reports can relate to:
• Lack of clarity.
• Missing components.

If this occurs, contact the radiologist directly to ask for clarification.

Figure 2. The radiology report. Example of a radiology report with various report content items highlighted. a, patient demographics, b, exam technique, relevant clinical information, comparison examinations, and quality, c, findings, d, summary, diagnosis, and recommendations.

STRUCTURED REPORTS

All radiologists wish to produce reports which accurately describe the findings, and provide information in a manner that facilitates effective clinical management of the patient. However, while radiologists will agree about what is important to include in a radiological report, a consensus about how the information should be presented has not yet been achieved. In fact, studies have shown considerable variability in the reporting styles of radiologists (7). This variability can lead to miscommunication of information, and suboptimal patient care.

Furthermore, the conventional narrative style radiological report is stored, and viewed, as free text (Fig. 3). In free text format, the details of the report are hidden within the report, and can only be found by reading the report in its entirety. In our report example, the fact that the heart size is normal can only be obtained by reading the full report, and deciphering this fact from the text. This makes extracting the necessary clinical information difficult and time consuming. In fact, referring physicians favor detailed reports that are in a tabulated format (8).

To decrease the variability and improve the quality of the radiology reports, structured reporting is being advocated (9,10). In a structured report, the details are presented in discrete fields in an organized format (Fig. 4). When creating the report, the radiologist is prompted to provide the necessary information to complete each of the discrete data fields. When all of the fields are completed a final report is generated. The referring physician reviewing structured reports knows that the information that is needed will be present in each report regardless of the reporting physician.

In the PACS environment the final report is stored in the radiology information system. To be stored structured reports are converted to free text. Therefore, structured reporting within the PACS workflow solves half of the problem – once the clinical report is stored, the information can no longer be accessed easily for future reference. Synoptic reporting aims to rectify this issue.

Synoptic reporting is the same as structured reporting, with the exception that the report is stored with the details remaining in discrete data fields. This allows retrieval of information by automated methods for future comparison, audit, and peer-review purposes.

Figure 3. Conventional radiology report. Example radiology report written in the conventional style.

Figure 4. Structured radiology report. Example radiology report in a structured format.

Hospital
Department of Radiology

NAME: John Doe
DOB: May 15, 1947
PATIENT IDENTIFICATION NUMBER: 11111111
EXAM DATE: July 20, 2012

Chest 2 views PA and Lateral

Clinical indication: 65-year-old male smoker with a three month history of weight loss, hemoptysis and rib pain.
Comparison is made with previous study performed on October 7, 2006.
Good quality examination.

Findings:
2 cm ill defined nodule within the left upper lobe. There is no associated calcification or cavitation. The remaining lung fields are hyperinflated but otherwise clear.
There is mild enlargement and increased density of the right hilum.
Loss of the cortical outline of a 2.5 cm segment of the left 5th rib posteriorly. The remaining bone structures are normal.
There is no pleural effusion.
No other abnormalities.

Conclusion:
Findings suggest a primary lung cancer within the left upper lobe with evidence of spread to the right hilum, and to the left 5th rib.

Recommend urgent referral to lung cancer diagnostic assessment unit, and a staging CT scan of the thorax and upper abdomen.

3

Hospital
Department of Radiology

Patient Name: John Doe
Date of birth: May 16, 1947
Patient Identifier: 11111111
Date of Examination: July 20, 2012
Type of Examination: Chest, 2 views
Comparison with: October 7, 2006

Indications: 65-year-old male smoker with a three month history of weight loss, hemoptysis and rib pain.

Exam quality: Adequate

Findings:
Heart Size: Normal
Lungs: 2 cm ill defined nodule in the left upper lobe. There is no associated calcification or cavitation. The remaining lung fields are hyperinflated but otherwise clear.
Hila: There is mild enlargement and increased density of the right hilum.
Mediastinum: There is a fullness of the right paratracheal region.
Pleura: Normal
Chest Wall: Loss of the cortical outline of a 2.5 cm segment of the left 5th rib posteriorly. The remaining bone structures are normal.

Summary :
Findings suggest a primary lung cancer within the left upper lobe with evidence of spread to the right hilum, and to the left 5th rib.

Differential Diagnosis : Cancer needs to be excluded.

Recommendations:
Recommend urgent referral to lung cancer diagnostic assessment unit, and a staging CT scan of the thorax and upper abdomen.

4

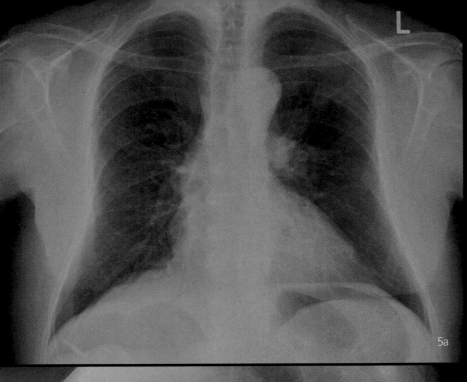

5a

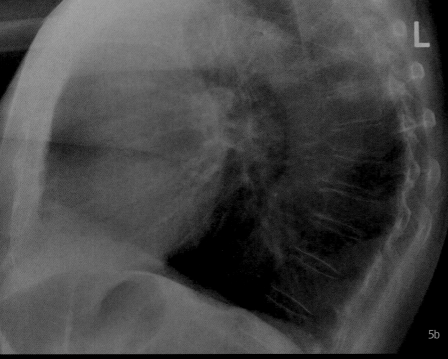

5b

How do you determine if the report is of good quality, and helps you with patient management?

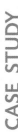
Earlier in the day you ordered a chest x-ray on your patient. You are concerned the patient may have lung cancer. On PACS you review the x-rays (Fig. 5a,b), and the radiologist's report (Fig. 5c).

Hospital
Department of Radiology

Patient demographics

NAME: John Doe
DOB: May 15, 1947
PATIENT IDENTIFICATION NUMBER: 11111111
EXAM DATE: July 20, 2012

Exam technique

Chest 2 views PA and Lateral

Relevant clinical information

Clinical indication: 65-year-old male smoker with a three month history of weight loss, hemoptysis and rib pain.

Comparison examinations

Comparison is made with previous study performed on October 7, 2006.

Exam quality

Good quality examination.

Findings

Findings:
2 cm ill defined nodule within the left upper lobe. There is no associated calcification or cavitation. The remaining lung fields are hyperinflated but otherwise clear.
There is mild enlargement and increased density of the right hilum.
Loss of the cortical outline of a 2.5 cm segment of the left 5th rib posteriorly. The remaining bone structures are normal.
There is no pleural effusion.
No other abnormalities.

Summary

Diagnosis

Conclusion:
Findings suggest a primary lung cancer within the left upper lobe with evidence of spread to the right hilum, and to the left 5th rib.

Recommendations

Recommend urgent referral to lung cancer diagnostic assessment unit, and a staging CT scan of the thorax and upper abdomen.

5c

DISCUSSION

Reviewing the radiological report (Fig. 5c), you have identified that the report contains all clinically important content necessary for directing clinical management. The report is therefore of good quality.

The radiological findings support your clinical concerns, and are suggestive of lung cancer. You refer the patient to the oncology service for confirmation of diagnosis, staging, and treatment.

References

1. Hall, F.M. (2000). Language of the radiology report: primer for residents and wayward radiologists. *AJR Am. J. Roentgenol., 175*(5):1239–1242.

2. Stolberg, H.O. (2002). Radiology reporting handbook. *Can. Assoc. Radiol. J., 53*(2):63–72.

3. Ridley, L.J. (2002). Guide to the radiology report. *Australas. Radiol., 46*(4):366–369.

4. Cascade, P.N., & Berlin, L. (1999). ACR standard for communication. *AJR Am. J. Roentgenol.,* 173:1439–1442.

5. Goergen, S.K. (2011). Radiology Written Report Guideline, Version 5. 2011: The Royal Australian and New Zealand College of Radiologists (RANZCR), Sydney, NSW, Australia.

6. Kahn, C.E. Jr., Langlotz, C.P., Burnside, E.S., et al. (2009). Toward best practices in radiology reporting. *Radiology, 252*(3):852–856 .

7. Naik, S.S. (2001). Radiology reports: Examining Radiologist and clinician preferences regarding style and content. *AJR Am. J. Roentgenol., 176*:591–598.

8. Grieve, F.M., Plumb, A.A., & Kahn, S.H. (2010) .Radiology reporting: a general practitioner's perspective. *Br. J. Radiol., 83*:17–22.

9. Langlotz, C.P. (2009). Structured Radiology Reporting: Are we there yet? *Radiology, 253*(1):23–25.

10. Dunnick, N.R., & Langlotz, C.P. (2008). The radiology report of the future: a summary of the 2007 Intersociety Conference. *J. Am. Coll. Radiol., 5*(5):626–629.

CHAPTER 23
APPROPRIATENESS & ORDERING of the CHEST X-RAY

importance

Appropriate ordering of a chest x-ray relates to patient safety and quality clinical care.

Throughout this book you have learned about the values and the limitations of chest x-rays. You can now apply that knowledge to clinical practice by ordering chest x-rays when there is evidence that they will benefit the patient. Lessons learned related to the appropriate ordering of chest x-rays can be used to understand appropriate ordering of other medical imaging examinations.

objectives

Skills

You will

- be able to quickly decide if you need to order a chest x-ray.

Knowledge

You will review and understand

- the definition of appropriateness.

- the indications for when it is appropriate to order chest x-rays and when it is not (contraindicated).

- what information you need to gather to judge whether or not it is appropriate to order a chest x-ray.

associated resources

This chapter maps to the following AMSER curriculum content (1,2).

1) Diagnostic situations/conditions that do NOT require imaging

Suspected rib fractures (unless complications – then PA/lateral chest x-ray (CXR), not rib films)

Pre-op CXR in asymptomatic individuals

2) Imaging algorithms (appropriateness criteria)

Appropriate imaging management algorithms for common diagnostic situations

Screening for metastases (CXR vs computed tomography (CT))

Staging for lung cancer (CXR vs CT vs positron emission tomography (PET))

Appropriate imaging for suspected pulmonary embolus

Appropriate imaging in trauma

Appropriate imaging for suspected aortic trauma

Appropriate imaging for suspected aortic dissection

Appropriate imaging for suspected small pneumothorax

Appropriate imaging for suspected foreign body aspiration

Appropriate imaging for solitary pulmonary nodule(s) seen on CXR

Appropriate imaging for pneumonia

Appropriate imaging for pneumomediastinum

Appropriate imaging for dyspnea in the non-immunocompromised patient

Appropriate imaging for dyspnea in the immunocompromised patient

Appropriate imaging for suspected interstitial lung disease

Appropriate imaging for total hemithorax opacification

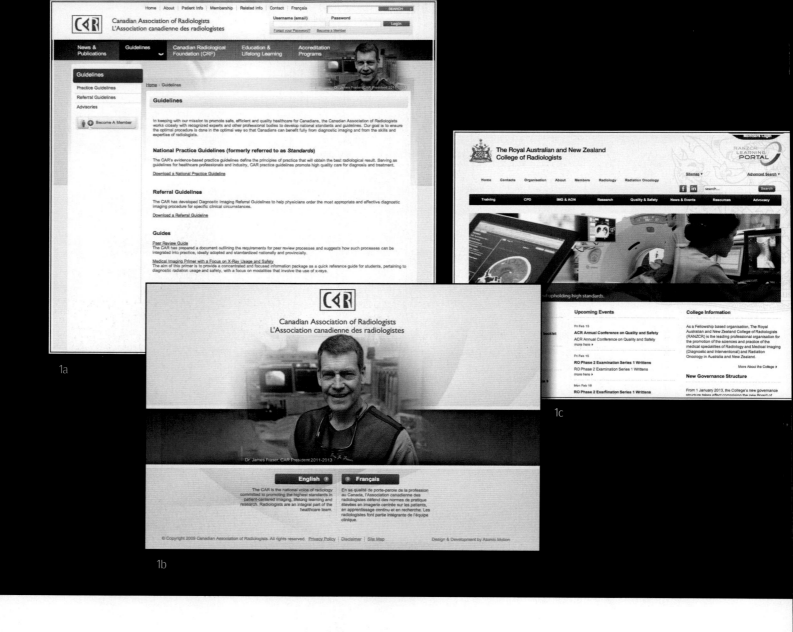

1a

1b

1c

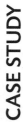
A patient is admitted into hospital with pneumonia. You are asked if the patient requires an order for daily chest x-rays.

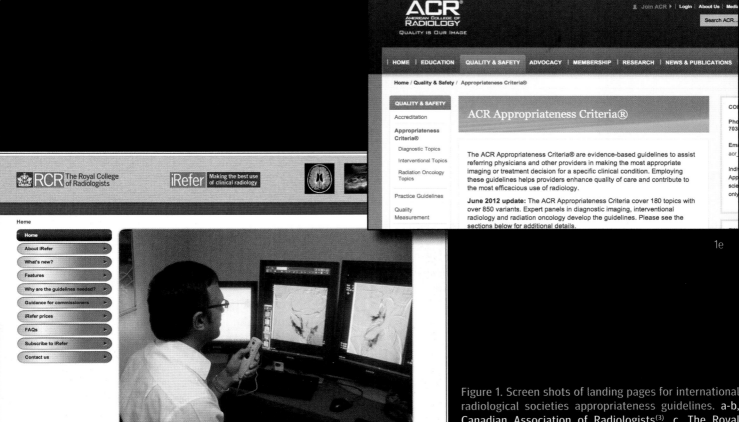

1d

1e

Figure 1. Screen shots of landing pages for international radiological societies appropriateness guidelines. **a-b,** Canadian Association of Radiologists[3], **c,** The Royal Australian and New Zealand College of Radiologists[4], **d,** The Royal College of Radiologists[5], **e,** American College of Radiology[6].

What is your response?

WHAT IS APPROPRIATENESS?

The indication to perform a medical procedure is appropriate when the expected health benefit (e.g., increased life expectancy, relief of pain, reduction in anxiety, improved functional capacity) exceeds the expected negative consequences (e.g., mortality, morbidity, anxiety of anticipating the procedure, pain produced by the procedure) by a sufficiently wide margin that the procedure is worth doing (7,8).

When is it Appropriate to Order a Chest X-ray?

Based on the above definition, the indication to perform a chest x-ray examination is appropriate when the expected health benefit (e.g., increased life expectancy, relief of pain, reduction of anxiety, improved functional capacity) exceeds the expected negative consequences (e.g., mortality, morbidity, radiation risk, anxiety of anticipation of the procedure, pain produced by the procedure) by a sufficiently wide margin that the procedure is worth doing (8).

Clinical Imaging Guidelines

Guidelines on the ordering of chest x-rays have been published and include:

1. The Canadian Guidelines (Canadian Association of Radiologists (CAR)).
2. The USA guidelines (American College of Radiologists (ACR)).
3. The Australian guidelines (The Royal Australian and New Zealand College of Radiologists (RANZCR)).
4. The UK guidelines (The Royal College of Radiologists (RCR)).

Figure 2. Clinical imaging guidelines. Screen shots of the landing pages of the, a, Canadian Association of Radiologists guidelines, b, American College of Radiologists guidelines, c, The Royal Australian and New Zealand College of Radiologist guidelines, d, The Royal College of Radiologists (UK).

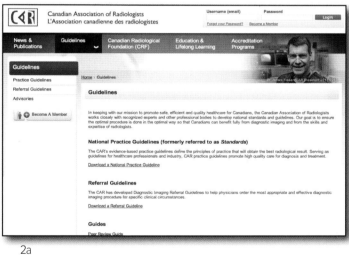

2a

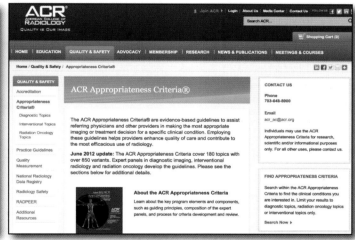

2b

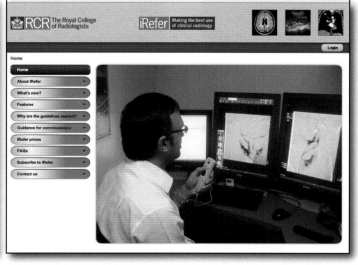

2c

2d

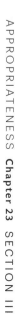

WHEN TO ORDER A CHEST X-RAY

Chest x-rays account for a significant number of x-ray examinations that are ordered. Judicious use of the chest x-ray is valuable in patient care. On the other hand, unnecessary use increases costs, increases radiation, may be in conflict with standards of patient care, and may trigger further unnecessary tests and procedures.

GENERAL	CARDIAC	RESPIRATORY
• Suspected tumor • Cancer staging • Tube and line positioning • Chest trauma	• Cardiomegaly or heart failure • Heart murmurs • Hypertension • Chest pain (acute) • Chest pain (sub-acute) • Suspected pericardial effusion • Suspected aortic dissection	• Infection (suspected pneumonia) • Chest trauma (suspected air leak, hemothorax or wide mediastinum) • Hemoptysis • Suspected pneumothorax • Asthma (if diagnosis not clear/severe attack/air leak suspected) • Shortness of breath (SOB) • Suspected pulmonary effusion

Table 23.1.
Common Indications for Chest X-rays (CXR)

> **!** The fact that an abnormality can be seen on a chest x-ray does not mean that a chest x-ray needs to be ordered.

WHEN CHEST X-RAYS ARE DEFINITELY NOT INDICATED!

In general, chest x-rays are NOT indicated if the results of the examination would make no difference to the patient's clinical outcome.

Chest x-rays are NOT routinely indicated preoperatively. In non-cardiopulmonary surgery, routine preoperative radiographs almost never contribute to better management and outcomes (9).

Chest x-rays are NOT routinely indicated on hospital admission, and should only be taken when they are clinically indicated (10).

Chest x-rays are NOT routinely indicated for the placement of NG tubes, unless there is suspicion the tube has been mal-positioned (11). (However, chest radiography is warranted for placement of central lines, chest tubes, pacemakers and endotracheal tubes.)

Chest x-rays are NOT routinely indicated for follow-up in cases of asthma, unless there are clinical suspicions of coexisting conditions during exacerbations (12). (CXR are essential to the initial diagnosis of asthma.)

Chest x-rays are NOT routinely indicated as follow-up in uncomplicated pneumonia cases progressing satisfactorily (13).

Chest x-rays are NOT routinely indicated (and are ineffective) for screening asymptomatic HIV-positive patients (14).

Chest x-rays are NOT routinely indicated as a screening tool (and there is strong evidence that it does not improve life expectancy) in patients with lung cancer (15).

APPROPRIATENESS Chapter 23 SECTION III

SPECIFIC APPROPRIATE IMAGING MANAGEMENT ALGORITHMS

CLINICAL SCENARIO	APPROPRIATE TEST	
	Step 1	Step 2
Screening for metastasis (16)	CXR	If CXR normal: consider CT in high risk patients (e.g., primary in bone & soft tissue sarcoma)
Staging of lung cancer (17)	CT (If superior sulcus tumor: MRI)	
Suspected pulmonary embolus – Low or intermediate pre-test probability, negative D-Dimer (18)	No further testing is needed	
Suspected pulmonary embolus – Low pre-test probability, positive D-Dimer (18)	CXR CTPA or V/Q scan	
Suspected pulmonary embolus – High pre-test probability, positive D-Dimer (18)	CXR CTPA or V/Q scan	
Suspected pulmonary embolus – Hemodynamically unstable (18)	Urgent CTA	
Suspected pulmonary embolus – Signs or symptoms of DVT (18)	Compression US of the lower extremities	
Blunt chest trauma / Aortic trauma (19)	CXR and CTA (Both should be done)	
Suspected aortic dissection (20)	CXR CTA	
Suspected small pneumothorax (21)	CXR: Inspiration and expiration	
Foreign body (21)	CXR	Depending on type of foreign body – may do repeat CXR as in case of small foreign body in esophagus Emergency bronchoscopy if in airways
Solitary pulmonary nodule seen on CXR (22)	Look for previous CXR	CT if greater than 4mm
Pneumonia (21)	CXR	Follow-up CXR if complications
Pneumomediastinum (23)	CXR	If high suspicion but CXR negative consider CT
Dyspnea in non-immunocompromised patient		
Cardiac origin suspected (24)	CXR	
Pulmonary origin suspected (suspected interstitial lung disease) (25)	CXR	Consider HRCT
Dyspnea in immunocompromised patient		
Cardiac origin suspected (24)	CXR	
Pulmonary origin suspected (suspected interstitial lung disease) (25)	CXR	Consider HRCT
Total hemithorax opacification seen on chest x-ray (21)	If mediastinal shift away from opacified hemithorax consider US to confirm pleural effusion If mediastinal shift toward opacified lung consider bronchoscopy and CT to exclude an endobronchial lesion	

Table 23.2

Specific Appropriate Imaging Management Algorithms. CT, computed tomography; CTA, computed tomography angiogram; CTPA, computed tomography pulmonary angiogram; CXR, chest x-ray; HRCT, high resolution computed tomography; MRI, magnetic resonance imaging; US, ultrasound; V/Q, ventilation/perfusion.

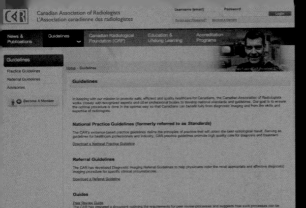

3a

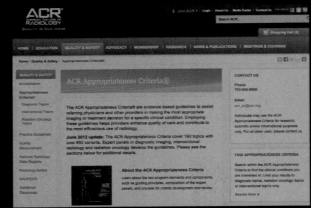

3b

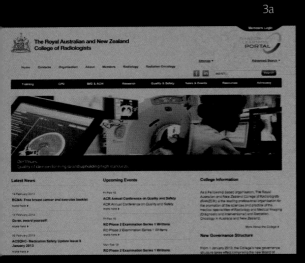

3c

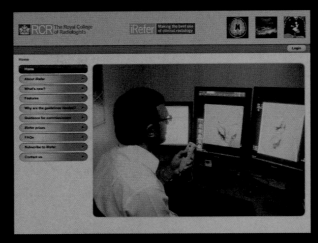

3d

What
is your
response?

CASE STUDY

A patient is admitted into hospital with pneumonia. You are asked if the patient requires an order for daily chest x-rays.

836

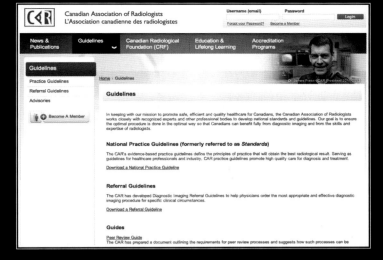

4a

Section F: Thoracic				
Clinical/Diagnostic Problem	Investigation	Recommendation (Grade)	Dose	Comment
F05. Hospital admission	CXR	Indicated only in specific circumstances [A]	☢	Routine CXR is not indicated. Admission CXR is indicated only in patients who have acute respiratory or cardiac disease and elderly patients with chronic cardiopulmonary disease with no recent CXR available.
F08. ICU patients	CXR	Indicated only in specific circumstances [A]	☢	Routine daily ICU CXR has been abandoned in most centers and replaced with on-demand CXRs even for mechanically ventilated patients.
F13. Pneumonia (For children see L43 – L45)	CXR	Indicated [C]	☢	Diagnostic Imaging should be guided by clinical findings. Initial imaging modality of choice when pneumonia is suspected. However, it should not be performed if pre-test probability is very high and a negative CXR would not preclude management.
	CT	Not initially indicated [C]	☢☢☢	Consider in cases of severe pneumonia, complicated pneumonia or possible atypical organisms. May help to diagnose pneumonia complicated with empyema and guide thoracentesis.
F14. Pneumonia: follow-up[1]	CXR	Not initially indicated [B]	☢	A CXR is only indicated in patients with signs and symptoms suggestive of a severe pneumonia. A CXR need not be repeated before hospital discharge in patients with satisfactory clinical recovery. A follow up CXR is recommended after at least six weeks for all patients who have persistent symptoms or physical signs or who are at higher risk of underlying malignancy (especially smokers and patients > 50 years), whether or not they are admitted to hospital.
	CT	Not initially indicated [B]	☢☢☢	CT is indicated only in cases with no radiological or clinical resolution within the expected time.

4b

DISCUSSION

A test should only be ordered if the benefit of the information obtained from the test outweighs any negative effects. In this case, unless there was a significant change in the patient's clinical condition, it would be inappropriate to order daily x-rays.

1. Lewis, P.J., Shaffer, K., & Donovan, A. (Eds.). (2012). AMSER National Medical Student Curriculum in Radiology. http://aur.org/Secondary-Alliances.aspx?id=141.

2. Lewis, P.J., & Shaffer, K. (2005). Developing a national medical student curriculum in radiology. *Am. Coll. Radiol., 2*(1):8–11.

3. Reprinted with permission of the Canadian Association of Radiologists (CAR). No other representation of this material is authorized without expressed, written permission from the Canadian Association of Radiologists (CAR). Refer to the CAR website at www.car.ca for the most current and complete version of the CAR guidelines.

4. Reprinted with permission of the American College of Radiology (ACR). No other representation of this material is authorized without expressed, written permission from the American College of Radiology (ACR). Refer to the ACR website at www.acr.org/ac for the most current and complete version of the ACR Appropriateness Criteria®.

5. Reprinted with permission of the Royal Australian and New Zealand College of Radiologists (RANZCR). No other representation of this material is authorized without expressed, written permission from the Royal Australian and New Zealand College of Radiologists (RANZCR). Refer to the RANZCR website at www.ranzcr.edu.au for the most current and complete version of the RANZCR policies and guidelines.

6. Reprinted with permission of the Royal College of Radiologists (RCR). No other representation of this material is authorized without expressed, written permission from the Royal College of Radiologists (RCR). Refer to the RCR website at www.irefer.org.uk for the most current and complete version of the RCR imaging referral guidelines

7. Buetow, S.A., Sibbald, B., Cantrill, J.A., & Halliwell, S. (1997). Appropriateness in health care: application to prescribing. *Soc. Sci. Med., 45*(2):261–271.

8. Sistrom, C.L. (2009). The appropriateness of imaging: a comprehensive conceptual framework. *Radiology, 251*(3):637-649.

9. Archer, C., Levy, A.R., & McGregor, M. (1993). Value of routine preoperative chest x-rays" A meta analysis. *Can. J. Anaesth., 40*:1022–1027.

10. Gupta, S.D., Gibbins, F.J., & Sen, I. (1985). Routine chest radiography in the elderly. *Age Aging, 14*:11–14.

11. Gray, P., Sullivan, G., Ostryzniuk, P, et al. (1992). value of postprocedural chest radiographs in the adult intensive care unit. *Crit. Care Med., 20*:1515–1518.

12. Brooks, L.J., Cloutier, M.M., & Afshani, E. (1982). Significance of roentgenographic abnormalities in children hospitalized for asthma. *Chest, 82*:315–318.

13. Jochelson, M.S., Altschuler, J., & Stomper, P.C. (1986). The yield of chest radiography in febrile and neutropenic patients. *Ann. Intern. Med. 105*:708–709.

14. Schneider, R.F., Hansen, N.I., Rosen, M.J., et al. (1996). Lack of usefulness of radiographic screening for pulmonary disease in asymptomatic HIV-infected adults. Pulmonary complications of HIV infection study group. *Arch. Int. Med., 156*:191–195.

15. Kubik, A., Pardon, D.M., Khlat, M., et al. (1990). Lack of benefit of semi-annual screening for cancer of the lung: Follow up report on the randomized control trial on a population of high-risk males in Czechoslovakia. *Int. J. Cancer, 45*:26–33.

16. Mohammed, T.H., Chowdhry, A., Reddy, G.P., et al., (2010). Expert Panel on Thoracic Imaging. ACR Appropriateness Criteria® screening for pulmonary metastases. [online publication]. Reston, VA: American College of Radiology (ACR).

17. National Collaborating Centre for Cancer (2011). Lung cancer. The diagnosis and treatment of lung cancer. 2005 (revised 2011). National Collaborating Centre for Cancer - National Government Agency [Non-U.S.], NGC:008662.

18. Moores, A. K. (2011). Current Approach to the Diagnosis of Acute Nonmassive Pulmonary Embolism. *Chest, 140*:509–518.

19. Demehri, S., Rybicki, F.J., Desjardins, B., et al. (2012). ACR Appropriateness Criteria® blunt chest trauma-suspected aortic injury. *Emerg. Radiol., 19*(4)287–292.

20. Paydar, S., Johari, H.G., Ghaffarpasand, F., et al. (2012). The role of routine chest radiography in initial evaluation of stable blunt trauma patients. *Am. J. Emerg. Med., 30*(1):1–4.

21. Canadian Association of Radiologists (CAR) (2005). Diagnostic Imaging Referral Guidelines. 2005: Canadian Association of Radiologists (CAR), Saint-Laurent, QC. pp.32–33,55–56,59.

22. MacMahon, H., Austin, J.H., Gamsu, G., et al. (2005) Guidelines for management of small pulmonary nodules detected on CT scans: a statement from the Fleischner Society. *Radiology, 237*(2):395–400.

23. Caceres, M., Ali, S.Z., Braud, R., et al. (2008). Spontaneous pneumomediastinum: a comparative study and review of the literature. *Ann. Thorac. Surg., 86*:962–966.

24. Abbara, S., Ghoshhajra, B., White, R.D., et al., (2010). Expert Panel on Cardiac Imaging. ACR Appropriateness Criteria® dyspnea -- suspected cardiac origin. [online publication]. Reston, VA: American College of Radiology (ACR).

25. Dyer, D.S., Khan, A.R., Mohammed, T.L., et al., (2009). Expert Panel on Thoracic Imaging. ACR Appropriateness Criteria® chronic dyspnea - suspected pulmonary origin. [online publication]. Reston, VA: American College of Radiology (ACR).

INDEX

Symbols

Bold items indicate a reference to a figure or table.

840

Bold items indicate a reference to a figure or table.

Bold items indicate a reference to a figure or table.

Bold items indicate a reference to a figure or table.

Bold items indicate a reference to a figure or table.

Bold items indicate a reference to a figure or table.

Bold items indicate a reference to a figure or table.

Bold items indicate a reference to a figure or table.

Bold items indicate a reference to a figure or table.

Bold items indicate a reference to a figure or table.

Bold items indicate a reference to a figure or table.

Bold items indicate a reference to a figure or table.

INDEX

Bold items indicate a reference to a figure or table.

Bold items indicate a reference to a figure or table.

Bold items indicate a reference to a figure or table.

Bold items indicate a reference to a figure or table.

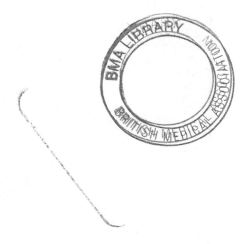

J2D Publishing Inc.